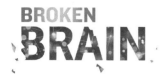

TABLE OF CONTENTS

Dr. Mark Hyman, Host

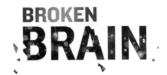

DISCLAIMER: The content of this book is based on research conducted by Hyman Digital, LLC, unless otherwise noted. The information is presented for educational purposes only and is not intended to diagnose or prescribe for any medical or psychological condition, nor to prevent, treat, mitigate or cure such conditions. The information contained herein is not intended to replace a one-on-one relationship with a doctor or qualified healthcare professional. Therefore, this information is not intended as medical advice, but rather a sharing of knowledge and information based on research and experience. Hyman Digital, LLC encourages you to make your own health care decisions based on your judgment and research in partnership with a qualified healthcare professional.

Please do not stop, adjust, or modify your dose of any prescribed medications without the direct supervision of your healthcare practitioner.

If you are at risk for suicide, homicide or other harm or injury, please call 911 or seek other help (such as a hospital emergency room or doctor's care) immediately. You are not alone and there is always hope. You can reach the National Suicide Prevention Lifeline anytime at (800) 273-8255.

These statements have not been evaluated by the Food and Drug Administration.
The information in this book is not intended to diagnose, treat, cure or prevent any disease.

BROKEN
BRAIN

EXPERT INTERVIEWS

BROKEN
BRAIN

DR. MARK HYMAN, HOST | Founder and Medical Director The UltraWellness Center

Dr. Mark Hyman:	You know, I first began to discover the mysteries of the brain when I personally got sick. I went from being very healthy, riding my bike 100 miles a day, being able to memorize 30 patients' charts and dictate them all flawlessly at the end of the day, to barely being able to walk up the stairs and not remembering where I was at the end of a sentence when I got there. It happened almost overnight and it happened, as I realized, because my whole system broke down from a number of insults I wasn't aware of. The main one was from being in China where I was exposed to huge amounts of pollution from coal burning, which releases mercury and lead and many other toxins.
[00:00:30]	
[00:01:00]	As it turned out, I ended up getting mercury poisoning, which essentially shut down all the systems in my body, my immune system, my gut, and my brain. It was pretty startling to be highly functional, highly capable of operating in the world, to being almost debilitated. I was really unable to function in any real way, and my brain wasn't working. I had trouble with remembering things. I had severe ADD and couldn't focus on anything. I had memory issues. It literally was like I had dementia, ADD, and depression all at once. Because no one had really figured out what it was, I sort of struggled from doctor, to doctor, to doctor.
[00:01:30]	
[00:02:00]	I went to see the psychiatrist who wanted to give me antidepressants. I saw the neurologist, who wanted to give me other drugs. It was just like a whole series of different doctors and a whole series of different drugs. I realized that I wasn't really depressed, I wasn't really demented, I wasn't really having ADD; that something was wrong and I needed to figure it out. That's when I discovered the world of Functional Medicine, which is essentially a model for getting to the root cause. In order for me to get better, I had to get to the root causes, which were, in my case, mercury and all the consequences of that. It turned out I had many other things I didn't realize. I had mold exposure, I had been exposed to Lyme disease and had Lyme disease. So, I would basically peel the onion of my story, and I was able to get to the bottom line of how to get better. It was really a powerful process for me to discover a whole new way of thinking about the brain.
[00:02:30]	I got all sorts of diagnoses, but no identification of the root cause. I was told I had chronic fatigue syndrome, which means nothing other than you're tired and feel lousy all the time. I was told I had depression. I was told I was stressed and was recommended to take anti-anxiety medication. I was given antidepressants, anti-anxiety medications, ADD medications. None of them really helped because I didn't deal with the root cause. I was very frustrated because they gave me all these labels, but they didn't actually tell me what was wrong with me. It was like I knew that something was real and it wasn't just depression or stress, because I was fine one minute and I wasn't the next.
[00:03:00]	
[00:03:30]	So, when physicians said that to me—when my doctors told me I was depressed or had ADD, or I needed medication, or I was anxious, it made me angry because I felt that I was given these labels but was given no roadmap to get better. I realize that, as physicians, we're trained to actually label people and often tell them it's psychological when it's very physical, because we don't know what to do and we don't know how to find the answer, and we don't know the questions to ask. So, we just assume, "Well, if you're having all these vague symptoms, it must be in your head." And I knew it wasn't, although it was affecting my head, it wasn't in my head.
[00:04:00]	I struggled for a number of years, going to doctor after doctor, specialist after specialist, to Columbia, to Harvard, to all the greatest minds in the country who I thought specialized in what I had and I got no answers. Then one day a nutritionist at Canyon Ranch invited me to a lecture by a Dr. Jeffrey Bland, who's a nutritional biochemist; studied with Linus Pauling. I listened to him speak and he painted an entire new view of medicine, an entirely new view of disease.

[00:04:30] I said to myself, "Either this guy is crazy or he's a genius. And if what he's saying is true, then I owe it to myself and my patients to learn about it." That's when I took a deep dive, first applying everything to myself, and incrementally I got better. I peeled the layers of what was wrong with me, using the roadmap of Functional Medicine, which doesn't really just look at symptoms, but looks at causes and understands the body as a whole dynamic integrated system where everything affects everything, and everything's connected. Because my brain was affected, the problem wasn't in my brain, the problem was in my body. And all the inflammation, the toxicity, and the gut dysfunction, it was then feeding back up to my brain. Once I understood that, I was able to apply the principles of Functional Medicine and get myself better.

[00:05:00] This was a really slow process because I didn't know what I know now, and if I knew what I know now I'd get better a lot faster. But essentially I had discovered I had mercury poisoning. It was by meeting a naturopath, who listened to my story and said, "Oh, you lived in China. You might want to check your mercury level." I had a level that was off the chart. If I see a patient with a level of 30, 40, 50, I think that's serious. Mine was 187. So, I was extremely toxic and I needed to figure out how to undo that. By getting the mercury out of my body, I slowly, slowly got better. There wasn't a moment where I just was

[00:05:30] better. It was a very slow process and I'm grateful that I was able to learn the things I did to actually help myself.

In Functional Medicine, we deal with root causes. I had to find all the causes. There's a principle that if you're standing on a tack, it takes a lot of aspirin to make it feel better. You've got to get rid of the tack, whether it's mercury or whatever it is. The second rule is, if you're standing on two tacks, taking one of them out is not going to make you 50% better. You have to find all of the tacks. So, it turns out I had

[00:06:00] many tacks and I had to deal with all of them. But I also knew from Functional Medicine that you have to create a healthy soil, that you have to create a foundation so your body can reset and heal. That foundation is really based on very simple principles, nutrition, exercise, stress management, sleep, and relationships and connections. All those really form the basis of creating a healthy human, and if you don't have those sorted, the rest of it may not work.

[00:06:30] Because my gut was so disrupted from the mercury, I went on an elimination diet. For months I ate turkey, broccoli, and brown rice, and that was it. I modified all sorts of things to try to get better. But it took a lot of time for those things to work. For some people, it's very quick if food is the issue. But my issue wasn't so much the food as it was the mercury. Then I learned how to do gentle exercise and yoga and meditation, and learned how to sleep at night in a regular rhythm, which I'd never done in my life. All those things really formed the foundation.

[00:07:00] And then I had to deal with the real issue, which was mercury. I did what we call chelation, which means to bind to metals. So, we bound up the metals with various medications and then supported my body's own detoxification system with things like glutathione, with a lot of cruciferous-rich vegetables, such as broccoli, collards, through various supplements like lipoic acid. All of which are designed to help boost my detox system and get rid of the mercury.

[00:07:30] You know, most of us have heard of mind-body medicine, which means the mind affects the body, that stress can impact almost any illness. We know that and that's well accepted. But what we don't know, or don't think about very often, is that the body can affect the mind. Everything from depression, anxiety, ADD, dementia, all these things can be affected by what's happening in your body and that's pretty much ignored by most psychiatry. This whole field of psychiatry was very descriptive, but it's not talking

[00:08:00] about causes. So basically, they think your body is disconnected from your head except from the stress response and that we shouldn't be looking for treatment for depression in your gut, or treatment for autism in your immune system, right?

So, we have a very different way of thinking in Functional Medicine, which is actually looking at how the body affects the brain. That is really a fundamental insight that I had. Once I started treating patients for their physical problems, their mental problems got better, their ADD went away, their autism improved,

[00:08:30] their depression went away, their anxiety went away, their panic attacks went away. I thought, "Wow! This is something that nobody's talking about: how our body affects our brain." The first thing to do when you have mental illness, when you have ADD, when you have depression, dementia, any of these things, is to start to treat the foundation. There may be psychological issues, there may be trauma and stress, but those things are much easier to deal with once you've built the foundation of health.

[00:09:00] Our approach to disease in general and to brain disorders is descriptive. So, we say, "Oh, you have memory loss, you failed these neurocognitive testing, you have these symptoms, you must have dementia." Or, "You can't focus, pay attention, you're distractible, and you have all these symptoms, that means you have ADD." Our entire diagnostic and statistical manual, which is what's used by psychiatry is descriptive. It's basically, "Here's this list of symptoms you have, here's what you have." But

[00:09:30] just because you know the name of the disease doesn't mean you know what's causing it. You could have 10 people with depression, or 10 people with autism, or 10 people with dementia and all of them have different reasons for those symptoms. I always say your brain has only so many ways of saying *ouch*, but there are a lot of things that can hurt it, and if we can identify those we can really help people. So, the fundamental problem with conventional medicine is that we describe disease by symptoms and not causes.

[00:10:00] We often think that our brain is separated from our bodies by something called the blood-brain barrier. We learn this in medical school, which means nothing gets above our neck. But nothing can be further from the truth. Everything we do, and think, and eat, and what we're exposed to, all affects our brain. Nutrition is probably the most important fundamental thing that's driving brain disorders, including sugar, which is a potent brain neurotoxin. It's addictive, in fact, it may be more addictive than cocaine. It's deliberately pushed into our society, where we're eating 152 pounds of sugar and 142 pounds of

[00:10:30] flour, which acts just like sugar in your body. That's been linked to everything from depression, to ADD, to even dementia, which is now called type 3 diabetes. So, we have to take this very seriously, so our high sugar, high starch diet is key.

The other problem with our diet is, we've been told for decades to eat a low-fat diet, which essentially is really bad for your brain, because your brain is made up of mostly fat. In fact, 60% of it is omega-3 fats. It's rich in cholesterol, it's rich in saturated fat. Without adequate fat, you have trouble with your brain.

[00:11:00] We also know that all the chemicals in our food, additives, preservatives, also potentially have negative brain effects, and they've studied this in children where they give kids colored water with additives and colorings, versus colored water from pomegranate. The kids who had the colored water from the additives all get ADD and hyperactive. So, we have really good evidence that these chemicals have a negative effect our brain.

[00:11:30] Our high-sugar, high-starch, low-fat diet, along with all the processing in our diet, is extremely harmful. In fact, we now know that omega-6 fats, refined omega-6 fats from processed oils, not naturally found in nuts and seeds and food, but processed oils, have been linked to depression, homicide, suicide, violence, and even poverty, in very well done studies by the NIH. I think we underestimate the impact of food on our mood. In fact, I got a letter from a prisoner, from a maximum-security prison, who was a murderer. He said he wanted to thank me for writing a book, which he was able to follow in prison that got rid of

[00:12:00] all the junk, all the sugar, and he said he realized he woke up like Rip Van Winkle from a bad dream, where his mood and his behavior and his attitude was driven by the processed food he ate. And now he felt like a new human.

[00:12:30] I think these are very powerful insights about how our nutrition affects our health. When I received this letter from the prisoner whose life was changed by eating real food in prison, which was probably hard to do, I realized two things: one—that I was happy for him and angry at our society for driving our industrial processed food system and our population. Our government creates policies that drive disease through supporting our processed food industry, through tax breaks, through subsidies, through lack of control of marketing to children, through poor recommendations from the government on what our diet should be, not based on science but based on industry interests; that our FDA regulates food based on

[00:13:00] lobby, not science. These are areas where our government is actually propagating poverty, violence, and more, by continuing this vicious cycle. Why do we spend $7 billion on food stamps for soda, when our government's also telling us to cut down on sugar? These hypocritical policies are actually driving a lot of what's wrong with our society.

[00:13:30] Another thing that drives brain dysfunction is gut dysfunction. We're now learning that your microbiome, this ecosystem of bugs in your gut, has been linked to depression, ADD, autism, even to Alzheimer's. We always thought the gut and the brain were kind of disconnected, maybe if you're stressed you get diarrhea. But the fact that your whole gut environment is driving changes in your brain, is a very new discovery. It has broad implications about what's wrong. Why do our guts get so messed up? Because we have a gut-busting culture. We eat processed food that's low in fiber, high in sugar, low in nutrients. We are exposed to inordinate amounts of antibiotics, even at birth. We're exposed to things like C-sections. One third of all births are C-sections, which don't allow you to develop [00:14:00] the healthy gut flora. We take gut-busting drugs like acid blockers and anti-inflammatories like ibuprofen. We take all sorts of other drugs like hormones, which all drive changes in our gut flora that end up affecting our brain.

[00:14:30] We've been exposed to 80,000 new chemicals in our environment, in food supply, in our house care products, in our facial and body care products, in our air and water and food, since the last century. These are having serious effects. We know from studies on infants, when they're born, looking at their umbilical cord blood, there are 287 known toxins. Over 200 of them are known neurotoxins, phthalates, PCBs, flame retardants, mercury, lead, and on and on, pesticides, DDT, PCBs; all of these have broad implications. We often study them one at a time, but we're seeing these as collective synergistic toxins, 287 in a newborn before they even took their first breath. We have to rethink our environment. We have to rethink what we're exposing ourselves to.

[00:15:00] For me, my broken brain was caused by mercury, and it is for many people. I've had patients with Parkinson's and dementia that we've reversed through using heavily focused detoxification approaches and getting rid of heavy metals and other toxins. These are really, really important insights about the role of environmental toxins, food toxins, our household products, our body care products, our water, our air. All of which can be remedied by very specific strategies to reduce your toxic load.

[00:15:30] Stress also has a negative impact on the brain. We know that physical stresses will cause emotional stress. We know that emotional stress will have physical effects. We know, for example, that if you're having an infection, or if you have heavy metals, or if your gut isn't working, or if you have infections with Lyme disease, this all affects your brain and can lead to all these broken brain issues. But we also know that stress itself, psychological stress, can have a serious impact on the body, but also on the [00:16:00] brain. We know that when you have high levels of sustained cortisol, which is the stress hormone, that shrinks the memory center in your brain, and you literally have an increased risk of dementia and cognitive issues, as you are more stressed. We know the opposite is true, that when you meditate or do yoga, these practices actually reform connections in the brain. We call that neuroplasticity. They help recreate new brain cells, we call that neurogenesis. We know that they increase stem cells, they decrease inflammation. So, learning how to regulate stress is really important.

[00:16:30] All of us are exposed to stress, and sadly most of us have far more stress than we ever did 1,000 years ago, with the advent of TV and Internet and all of our devices, and our constant workload, all these things are pretty abnormal. In fact, the average hunter gatherer tribe spent about 20 hours a week actually working trying to get food. The rest of the time they just hung out and chilled. We don't do that. We just go all day long and all night long sometimes. This creates really serious consequences for our health and our brain.

[00:17:00] I think less than 8% of Americans get their recommended daily exercise every day. And why is it important? Not only because it prevents heart disease, not only because it helps with weight, but because it has profound effects on the brain. We know that vigorous exercise three times a week is a

[00:17:30] better treatment for depression than most antidepressant drugs. We know that if you just take a walk every day, you dramatically reduce your risk of Alzheimer's and dementia. We know it's important for kids with ADD, we call that nature deficit disorder (they're not out playing and enjoying their bodies and stimulating their neural system in a positive way). They're overstimulated through video games and addictive behaviors. So, these are really profound effects of exercise across the board. In fact, one of the most powerful things it does is increase BDNF, that's called brain derived neurotrophic factor. It's like Miracle-Gro for your brain. What that does is it increases new brain cells, it increases the connection between brain cells. So, you can remake your brain at any age, and exercise is one of the most powerful tools to do that.

[00:18:00] We're seeing an epidemic of isolation and disconnectedness. But we know that being part of a group, that being connected, has profound effects on your health. Even if you're part of a bridge club or a bowling club, we know that those people live longer and are healthier. We know that from an extraordinary study in Roseto, Pennsylvania—where they looked at a group of immigrants from Italy who maintained their close-knit culture—they had a range of socioeconomic status within that group,

[00:18:30] but they all were together. They celebrated holidays together, they celebrated weddings and marriages and deaths, all as a community. But they actually started eating the horrible American diet. Even when they were eating the horrible American diet, they still had dramatically lower rates of heart disease and death than everybody else who lived in the communities around them. So, those social connections are powerful, and it's one of the ways that we maintain our health for so many reasons. In fact, altruistic behavior stimulates the brain in the same way as cocaine or heroin or sugar, so it's a much better way to get your high.

[00:19:00] We've seen a revolution in brain science in the last 20 years. We went from believing that the brain was fixed, that you had a certain number of brain cells at birth—if you damaged them that was your tough luck—to now understanding that even at the moment of death you are creating new brain cells and you are creating new connections, at any age. This revolutionized our view of what the brain is capable of. We know that these brain disorders are not fixed.

[00:19:30] This is one of the most powerful discoveries of the last 20 years, that we can actually modify what we thought were fixed brain disorders like depression, autism, and ADD, and even things like dementia and Parkinson's. The body and brain have the capacity to repair and heal when the insults are taken away and the right ingredients are put in the system. So, it's really a revolutionary time in brain science. Sadly, conventional medicine has just not caught up. At Cleveland Clinic, we are now doing a research program looking at how we can impact early dementia by using all these approaches and dealing with the root causes, infections, toxins, and diet. Then helping put in the right ingredients for health. It's a very

[00:20:00] powerful model, and we're seeing people actually start to reverse dementia and reverse common problems that we thought were not possible, like autism and ADD.

[00:20:30] We now know that sugar is a brain toxin. It's been linked to a whole host of brain disorders, from depression to anxiety. In fact, I remember a patient who came in with panic attacks. He was terrified he was having a heart attack and thought he was dying. I listened to his story and he said, he basically drank cokes all day long, and then he would stop and then his blood sugar would crash and he'd get a panic attack. So, the problem was the sugar was raising and lowering his blood sugar so much that it was an emergency. But we also know that it's been linked to what we call type 3 diabetes, which means that the brain becomes insulin resistant and that causes inflammation; it causes damage to your brain cells, and

[00:21:00] leads to dementia. We now know that sugar is a big cause of dementia.

[00:21:30] I first began to realize that dementia was not a fixed problem when I had a patient come in to me named Bud. Bud was about 70 years old. He ran a large corporation of his own family business. His wife said he was increasingly dysfunctional. He had to stop working, was highly depressed, and couldn't remember anything. He was told he had dementia and was on a slippery slope to death, and that he should get his affairs in order. I said, "Well, maybe there's something else going on." It was really the first case I'd seen where I said, "Let me just try some of the principles based on the theory of how the body actually works."

[00:22:00] We started looking for problems. First, he had pre-diabetes, which no one had diagnosed, and we know sugar and pre-diabetes are linked to dementia. If you're diabetic, you have four times the risk of getting dementia. We also found out he had high levels of mercury. He lived in Pittsburgh, which is a terrible place to live because they coat the streets with coal ash, they fertilize the fields with coal ash, and they have all the residue from the steel plants in the environment, which produced all this mercury. We also found out he had a number of genetic issues that affected his brain, leading to less likelihood of getting

[00:22:30] rid of mercury, a higher risk of B vitamin issues, we call them methylation problems. He also had problems with glutathione, which is detoxification hormones. He also had terrible gut issues, for 30 years his gut was not working properly and he had severe irritable bowel.

We addressed all these factors, not just one thing. We addressed his nutrition and his sugar in his diet. We made sure he had adequate levels of B vitamins. We made sure we got rid of the mercury in his body, by getting rid of his fillings and getting the mercury out of his system through chelation and IV

[00:23:00] therapy. We also gave him treatment for his gut and got his gut functioning again. All these things were dynamically interacting and we corrected all of them. It was like Rip Van Winkle—he came back to work, was functional, happy, and he had his memory back. He wasn't 100%, but he was really back into a normal functioning life and you wouldn't know anything if you talked to him.

[00:23:30] That case inspired me to really ask the questions of, "If that's true for one person, could it be true for more? And what else could we learn about this pathway that people go on towards dementia, without actually having to give them all these drugs?" What's really frightening is that we've spent billions of dollars, over 400 studies on dementia and really none of them have worked. A couple have had some slight benefit. But what I mean by benefit, is they delayed their going into a nursing home by three to six months, which is not really a benefit. So, we have to completely rethink our approach, and that's what's exciting about what we're doing at Cleveland Clinic, what people like Dale Bredesen are doing in

[00:24:00] reversing dementia. All these things are really key, and what we're doing here at the UltraWellness Center to reverse chronic disease, including dementia.

Most toxins are also neurotoxins. We pretty much ignored their effect, or if we haven't ignored it, we don't do anything about it. We know, for example, that there have been links between various environmental toxins and dementia. We also know very well that environmental toxins are linked to

[00:24:30] Parkinson's. In fact, conventional doctors all accept this because the data is so strong. We know that farmers have a much higher risk of dementia than the average person because they're exposed to pesticides. We know that people who work in tannery factories that tan leather are also exposed to toxic chemicals. We know that pesticides—all these things are driving brain dysfunction. So, we have to be very serious about identifying these toxins and helping people eliminate these toxins as a treatment, not just to say, "Oh well, you've been exposed to toxins, tough luck."

[00:25:00] I recall a patient who came in with early Parkinson's, who was 50 years old, which is very young to get Parkinson's. When I listened to her history and her story, she grew up in The Bronx and she had cockroaches and rats crawling all over her in bed every night, and she had a terrible pest phobia. So, when she moved to the suburbs in Long Island, she was obsessive about getting the exterminator to come every month inside and out, spraying her house and her garden. Then she was so terrified she also

[00:25:30] had a big vat of chlordane, which is actually a banned pesticide from decades ago, in her garage for decades. She was exposed to very high levels of these pesticides, and ended up having Parkinson's, and we were able to treat her by helping her body detoxify.

[00:26:00] When you actually deal with the root causes and then you optimize the body's function, with Parkinson's, people can have dramatic improvements in their wellbeing. I just talked to a patient today who has Parkinson's, and he was exposed at a very young age to all sorts of pesticides. When you were a kid, they used to have the pesticide trucks spraying the neighborhoods, and the kids would run through the pesticide fog. He had exposure, occupational exposures, and many, many other exposures, and he had Parkinson's. So, we found he had exposures to organophosphate pesticides in his urine, we found DDE, which has banned for decades from DDT, and still he had these in his system. We were able to actually treat him, and within a very short time using saunas and mitochondrial nutrients and things to help him detoxify, within a few days he said he was very much better.

[00:26:30]

[00:27:00]

What we see as aging in our culture is really abnormal aging. It's really preclinical disease or breakdown in the systems of the body. We see people decline as they get older. We see people have memory issues as they get older, but that's not normal aging. In fact, we now know that you can maintain a healthy cognitive status well into your 90s or 100s. I have a friend whose dad was 105, still sharp as a tack and lived by himself. So, the body is capable of that. The question is, why are some people able to do that and others not? It's because of the number of insults, and stresses, and toxins that we're all exposed to, poor diet, that affects our brain function dramatically.

[00:27:30]

At any age, we can reverse cognitive decline, we can improve our brain function. If you look at some of the work of Dale Bredesen, he's actually showing reversal of the brain size with testing that shows dementia. Literally, you can grow the memory part of your brain called the hippocampus, at any age, and even start to begin to change your brain trajectory by these interventions. We really have to think about our whole process of aging in a very different way, and understand that we have the capacity to regenerate, heal, and repair at any age.

[00:28:00]

It's interesting: as a doctor who treats both autism and Alzheimer's, they're very much the same. The brain is responding to a number of insults, and they're really the same disease at different age spectrums. So again, and we look at their diet, gut, exposure to toxins, their nutritional status, their immune system, and foods they're reactive to. And we optimize all those areas, and the patients often will get better. We don't treat autism, I don't treat Alzheimer's. I treat humans who have bodies that are out of balance. That strategy works to help reverse this brain dysfunction.

[00:28:30]

[00:29:00]

I've had many, many patients with autism. One of them comes to mind who was a little boy, two or three years old, who was quite dramatically affected. He had regressive autism. He had a number of insults, antibiotics, infections, vaccines, all these things affected his capacity to actually develop normally. His parents were told by the doctors, and by the way, his mother worked for a large pharma company, but they were told, "You need occupational therapy, you need behavioral therapy. Good luck. He'll probably end up in an institution, and we're sorry." That message unfortunately is something that parents get all the time, and it makes me angry, because I know there is so much we can do, because autism is not a brain disorder. It's a disorder that affects the brain. We now see dramatic amounts of inflammation in these children. We see exposure to toxins. We see all these gut dysfunctions in these kids, dysbiosis, we call it, imbalances in the gut flora. All these things drive brain dysfunction. So, by fixing those things, often the brain will recover.

[00:29:30]

I saw this one young boy came in, and he had terrible gut issues, he had stinky smelly stools, gas, diarrhea, horrible bowel movements. He had severe nutritional deficiencies, B vitamins, folate, B6, B12. He had mercury in his body. We were able to fix all these things one at a time, and he recovered. He went from not being able to speak to being fluent, from being in autistic class to being a normal kid in mainstream school. Now he's about 10-years-old and he's completely normal, completely lost his diagnosis. Happy, normal, well-adjusted kid. Not even on the spectrum at all.

[00:30:00]

Depression is just the name we give to people with a set of symptoms. You're hopeless, you're helpless, you're sad, you've no interest in life, sex, you don't want to eat. These are symptoms of depression. When the doctor sees you with those symptoms, they go, "I know what's wrong with you, you have depression." But depression isn't the cause of those symptoms, it's the name of those symptoms, which can have many, many causes.

[00:30:30] So, for example, it might be because you have a gluten sensitivity, or an autoimmune disease related to that called Hashimoto's that causes low thyroid function. Or maybe it's because you've been taking acid blockers for reflux because of your poor diet for decades, and you have B12 deficiency, which can cause depression. Or maybe because you live in the northeast you have vitamin D deficiency, and that can cause depression. Or maybe because you've take antibiotics that changes your gut flora—that can cause depression. Or maybe because you love sushi—too much mercury—that can cause depression. Or you hate fish and have omega-3 deficiencies—that can cause depression. Or maybe you eat a lot of sugar and have prediabetes—that can cause depression. I begin to look for all these things and more, and by treating those things, people often just recover.

[00:31:00]

[00:31:30] One of the things we've discovered in the last few decades is the importance of energy. I don't mean energy you feel, although it's related. I mean energy that your body produces from oxygen and from eating food. That gets burned in your cells in a little organ called the mitochondria. They're like tiny little energy factories or power plants. When those power plants start to become dysfunctional, which can happen from anything that causes inflammation—from toxins, from your gut, from nutritional deficiencies. When those little energy factories and power plants start to wind down, that's when disease occurs. What's striking is we've found this linked to autism, Alzheimer's, Parkinson's, to obviously things like diabetes, depression, these are all common pathways through which these diseases are affected.

[00:32:00] A leading autism researcher, Suzanne Goh, is studying mitochondrial therapy in autism, where she provides the nutrients to help the mitochondria to work better in a certain subset of kids with autism, and they recover. Things like CoQ10 and carnitine, lipoic acid, N-acetyl cysteine, ribose, these are just mitochondrial nutrients that we're often not having enough of, that can help reverse this. We see this in Parkinson's. We know Parkinson's is a mitochondrial disease that happens from insults like toxins, infections, inflammation, poor diet, and that when you support the mitochondria, you can help these patients feel better, function better, and stop their Parkinson's. We know that it's linked to Alzheimer's.

[00:32:30] All these conditions that we never really paid attention to, these mitochondrial dysfunction conditions, which are not particularly a disease, but they're actually a dysfunction that comes from all the insults in our life, they have been linked to all these horrible diseases that we now can do something about.

[00:33:00] Hormones are critical for your brain and they affect almost every function. We often ignore treating these problems because they may not be a true deficiency, they might just be an imbalance. As we age, we see a number of different hormones go out of whack. One: insulin goes up, and that causes pre-diabetes, which we know affects the brain. Also, we see cortisol go up as we age, which is the stress hormone. We see growth hormone go down, which helps our brains repair and grow. We see estrogen and testosterone, the sex hormones, decline, all of which are really critical in regulating our health. Melatonin for sleep.

[00:33:30] All these hormones are delicately balanced and when they're interrupted or dysfunctional, because of all these insults in our lives, lack of sleep, stress, poor diet, toxins, infections, gut dysfunction, etc., then we start to age fast and we start to break down. It's really important to optimize hormones. For example, thyroid, I had a patient who had Alzheimer's who just had a slightly dysfunctional thyroid. She wasn't full-blown hypothyroid, but when I gave her a little bit of thyroid hormone, it was like she had energy, she woke up, her memory got better. We see by tweaking these hormones as we age, particularly in things like dementia or dysfunction, we see really significant improvements.

[00:34:00]

One of the things we've been learning over the last few decades, in addition to the brain science of how we can increase our brain connections and build new brain cells, is that inflammation is a common denominator across a whole spectrum of diseases, pretty much all chronic disease, whether it's heart disease, cancer, diabetes, obesity, of course autoimmune and inflammatory diseases, but also brain disorders. We know that dementia, autism, and depression are all inflammation of the brain. In fact, they're recommending anti-inflammatory drugs to treat depression. That's the wrong idea, but it shows

[00:34:30] you the way the science is going.

[00:35:00] What causes inflammation? Well, guess what, it's the usual culprits, it's our diet. We have a very inflammatory diet, high in sugar and processed foods, low in the good fats that are anti-inflammatory like omega-3 fats. It's low in phytochemicals, which are plant compounds that are anti-inflammatory in our food, like vegetables and fruits, and spices like turmeric. All of these really promote inflammation in the body—sugar is probably the worst. Then of course, there are other insults. We have things like Lyme disease and tick infections, viruses. And we have gut dysfunction. Gut dysfunction is probably the other major driver of inflammation because when your gut is inflamed like most of our guts are, it creates inflammation, not just in your gut, but throughout your body and in your brain. Toxins also play a role in driving inflammation. Stress plays a role in driving inflammation. Lack of exercise is inflammatory, and

[00:35:30] exercise is anti-inflammatory. All these insults and factors are driving inflammation in the brain that leads to autism, Alzheimer's, depression, mood disorders, and more.

[00:36:00] Well, about 35 years ago the government told us we should be eating a low-fat diet. They had the food pyramid, which showed us to eat 6 to 11 servings of bread, rice, cereal, and pasta a day, which are low in fat. And then fats and oils only sparingly at the top of the food pyramid. What that's done is create a trillion-dollar food industry promoting low-fat salad dressing, low-fat cakes, low-fat cookies, low-fat processed food, and everybody's afraid of fat and is eating egg white omelets and avoiding fats. That's led to a huge problem because our brain is made up of mostly fat and requires fat to function. It's made up of omega-3 fats, saturated fat, cholesterol, all the things we thought were bad actually turn out to be very good for the brain and critical for its functioning.

[00:36:30] We also know that low-fat diets promote pre-diabetes, which also leads to brain injury. So, all of these factors are driving brain dysfunction, and the science has really flipped. The US Dietary Guidelines in 2015 said, for the first time in 35 years, that we should no longer worry about restricting fat in our diet, that we no longer have to worry about cholesterol. They still suggested reductions in saturated fat, but I think that data is going to be transformed in the next guidelines, because the evidence is so clear, and saturated fats are really not linked to heart disease or any serious illness.

[00:37:00] There are a number of fats that are mission critical for your brain function. The first are omega-3 fats. These are derived from fish, from wild fish, from algae, they're in some plant foods like walnuts and flax seeds, and they're very powerful for regulating inflammation. But they're also critical as they make up our cell membrane, and your cells are the interface where your body communicates with itself. So, in order for your cells to be working well, you have to have good healthy membranes. Omega-3 fats are critical.

[00:37:30] Also, saturated fats. In fact, a very specific kind of saturated fat called MCT oil, stands for medium-chain triglycerides, is derived from coconut oil, and it is very powerful as a fuel for brain cells and a fuel for your mitochondria. When you consume these fats, your brain is going to work better, you're going to be more focused, more clear, more energetic. And you will help prevent dementia, depression, autism, ADD, and a whole host of things, all of which are very effectively often helped by these healthy fats.

[00:38:00] In addition to eating these healthy fats—which come from grass-fed meats and grass-fed butter, from coconut oil, from avocados, from nuts and seeds—you also want to avoid the refined vegetable oils, which have been shown to be linked to depression, to violence, homicide, suicide, poverty. These are refined vegetable oils that we never consumed in human history. We've gone a 1,000-fold increase in our intake of refined soybean oil. That's 100,000% more of these refined oils than we had 100 years ago,

[00:38:30] and they're not really designed to be consumed in those massive quantities. As long as they're in your foods—eat the soybeans, eat the nuts, eat the seeds, but avoid the refined vegetable oils because they're bad for your brain.

[00:39:00] There are very few genes that will lead to a specific disorder. There have been 30-something genes identified that relate to obesity, and if you had all of them, your weight gain would only be 22 pounds, right? There are genes connected to Alzheimer's but they don't predestine you to Alzheimer's, they are risk genes. Now, there are some that are very strong, like the presenilin genes that are linked to early

Alzheimer's when you get it in your 50s. That's a different condition. There's later onset Alzheimer's, which is maybe something you might be predisposed to by certain genes like ApoE4. But they're not going to determine that you get it 100%.

[00:39:30] That's the good news, because we know now that you can't change your genes, but you can change your gene expression. You can change which genes are turned on or off, and how they affect health or disease. The way we do that, is what we call the exposome. The exposome is the sum total of things we're exposed to, primarily our diet, exercise, sleep, stress, environmental toxins, our gut flora, these are the things that are influencing our gene expression and turning them on or off, turning them up or down every single day, literally minute by minute. We have a tremendous capacity to change from being predetermined, which many of us think we are, to our being predestined to get something, to actually [00:40:00] being able to change that and not have to get those conditions.

We talk about trophic factors in the brain. What are the things that help it grow, develop, function, and connect? To be honest with you, the most important is food, and contained in the food are nutrients. Some of us have large variations in our needs. Some of us need a lot, some of us need a little. But there [00:40:30] are a few basic nutrients that are really critical for brain health, one of these is omega-3 fats. These are the fish fats that help form much of your brain structure and help it function properly, and help prevent Alzheimer's, ADD, autism, and even depression. Then there are other nutrients we need, the B vitamins, we call these methylating nutrients. B6, B12, and folate, are critical for the brain, and without them you end up with increased risk of dementia, increased risk of autism, ADD, and depression. So easy to get, the complex of B vitamins.

[00:41:00] Then we need vitamin D. Vitamin D is a critical brain nutrient, and has been linked to improvement in cognitive function and delay in many chronic brain disorders. So those are really critical. You add in a multivitamin and you pretty much have everything you need. If you're interested, you can add in probiotics, which help your gut flora, and lots of fiber, which also acts to fertilize the gut flora and help your gut function and, of course, your brain function. Those are foundational nutrients that I recommend everybody take who's worried about their brain.

[00:41:30] You know, we have Facebook, we have social networks, but there's never been a time in human history where we're more disconnected from one another in human contact. It's actually face to face, not Facebook. And that makes a huge difference in the functioning of our brain. We know, for example, that there's an emerging field called sociogenomics where your genes change when you're in a relationship with someone. If there's a hostile interaction, disease genes are turned on. When you're in a loving [00:42:00] happy interaction, health genes are turned on, immune system benefiting genes are turned on, inflammation is turned down. So, we know, in a very real way scientifically, how this works. When we have an epidemic of disconnection, it's creating more disease. When we have strategies for connecting, whether it's in faith-based groups, social groups, friends, parties, whatever it is that you can do to bring real connections with people, your health will dramatically improve.

[00:42:30] We learn through play; that's how we learn, that's how our brain develops. It's important at every age to encourage the development of play in your system, whether it's playing a game like bridge, or checkers, or chess. Whether it's learning to play tennis or learning to actually have other things that you enjoy, that challenge you, that you learn from, it's going to help your brain become more dense in terms of its connections, and also help bring about the development of new brain cells.

[00:43:00] The first thing you can do to optimize your brain function—a simple take-home—is change your diet. Get rid of the processed foods, get rid of the starch and sugar. Increase whole foods, plant-based foods, and increase healthy fats—omega-3 fats, avocados, nuts and seeds, healthy grass-fed animal protein, healthy grass-fed butter, coconut oil. All these things will help dramatically improve your brain function almost overnight. Then exercise is the other powerful thing. We know it benefits all sorts of brain [00:43:30] disorders, from preventing Alzheimer's, to depression, and of course, much more. Then lastly, I would say: sleep. Most of us underestimate the power of sleep. The reason it's important is that we've discovered a brand new system in the brain called the glymphatic system. It's not lymphatic. It's the brain's version of it, which is these glial cells, which detoxify your brain every night. If you don't clean out your brain every night and reset it, it will start to accumulate waste and end up causing damage to your brain. Getting adequate sleep is critical.

Adam Cobb:

[00:00:30]

Some of the biggest myths around exercise is that it's hard, is that it takes so much time. I always like to talk about that word—exercise—as in the myth, the fact that it could take 10 minutes. Exercise could be, rather than parking close at that first spot that you see and spending five minutes driving around the parking lot, actually, you just park a little bit further away where it is open. There are a lot of open spots at the grocery store and so, one: your car is not going to get hit. Then, two: you can walk a little bit extra in that moment, or if you're in a conference call and you know you have no time to get any exercise in, what would it look like to walk around the office, right? Or walk up and down the stairs? You just actually think of exercise as movement and if movement was the focus for exercise, then, what's possible?

[00:01:00]

[00:01:30]

Well, I'm not sure about most, but I feel like most people love movement, right? If movement's a thing, I mean, what did you love to do when you were a kid? What did you love to do? Did you love to dance? Did you love to get up and play? Then, you start thinking about exercise in the actual definition of play. Exercise involves the movement and involves the play. When you get to play, you think, "Oh, how could I play? How could I make play a part of my day?" I was telling everybody play like you're a puppy and it makes it simple.

Should everybody exercise vigorously? Well, vigorously could be ... that can be a different definition for everybody, but I think that everybody should be moving daily. Then, what would that look like? Would it look like waking up in the morning, every morning and starting your day off with a walk even around your block? As simple as that, walking your puppy or your dog; going for a walk.

[00:02:00]

[00:02:30]

For example, today I think I had a bit of brain fog and I saw a client and I still felt a little tired, a little funky. I grabbed my pup and I said, "Let's just ... let's go for a walk." He obviously said, "Okay." Then, as we went to the store talking to one person, all of a sudden, feeling really good and in probably a four-block walk but in that walk, you smile at some people, you're engaging a little bit and you're lighting up. It doesn't need to be long, right? But that idea of making it a priority and putting your priorities first is where movement really comes into place.

[00:03:00]

[00:03:30]

Exercise for our brains lights it up. As we talked about exercise sounding like movement, really lighting up the brain. We can be in a state of stuck and we can go from that state of stuck to feeling lit up just by movement, just by exercising. A simple 10-minute walk can start to fire those neurons and start to wake everything up and really turn the lights on. As far as issues with clients I've seen where they live a sedentary lifestyle and they're having a hard time feeling energized. People with that sedentary lifestyle typically are on a lot of depression meds, are typically more pessimists than optimists, and are typically more negative in general.

[00:04:00]

Not only that, but you just start to hear, you hear more excuses, you hear certain things on. I have a family member that was in line with that, and then all of a sudden, lost ... started moving, started exercising, lost 50 pounds and went from a pessimist to an optimist and recently just said, "What a beautiful day," at a family gathering. I was like, "A beautiful day?" "The sky is so blue." I thought, "What? I've never even heard you speak like that over the last 20 years," and now really lit up so there's something to that, right? There's something to, all of a sudden, getting fully lit up from the brain just by moving and being able to push.

[00:04:30]

I'll tell people that, yes, you can go on different medications. Yes, you might have to see somebody, but first start to move well. After that, I don't know. Maybe you'll eat well and I think you'll just have to think well and then, see how much of that other stuff, the medications, things that you actually need. Usually, it's very little. The absolute best exercise for the brain is the one that you do—real simple. The one that you do, the one that you commit to, that could be a walk, that could be me standing up from this chair right now and getting in 20 squats, or that could be just standing in place and firing off, doing some jumping jacks.

[00:05:00]

Some of the movements that I love that fire up the brain are really simple, especially if movement is hard or you have some injuries, is just taking a tennis ball and rolling your feet on the tennis ball and firing off. What that does is it starts to fire the fascia on the bottom of the feet and then, all of a sudden, these neurons start to fire, right? And so they create more blood flow in that. That would be one way, several ways, for ways to start to think of what are the best exercises. Again, the one that you do for the brain.

[00:05:30]

What I say to people that say they hate exercise is that, fine, you can hate exercise. Oftentimes, you're not going to fall immediately in love with exercise but you could fall in love with movement. Then, I put music on because what precedes movement at times could be music. For me, that's always the case. For my clients, always the case. It's really hard to listen to Michael Jackson and not move. I dare you to try it.

[00:06:00]

Easy exercises that people can do at home to really help that brain health but just to also ... Again, maybe while they're cooking, as simple as, just going for a walk, taking a call. I always think that's the easiest one because people often are cooking and on the phone and moments like that. Simply just walk around the couch. Keep it simple. I'm sitting down on the couch, up and down, right? The idea of doing a step up.

[00:06:30]

You might have a small stool at home and just stepping up on that stool and back down. Even as simple as isometric squeezing, so that could be something that people haven't thought of that they could do right now as they're watching this and just as simple. Just the idea of, you might be here and then opening up your chest and doing that 10 times and taking a deep breath and how good that feels. But also, you're squeezing your muscles, so you start to activate triceps, back of the shoulders, chest, core, everything like that.

[00:07:00]

Another one like that could be a pelvic tilt. You could simply lie down, take the first five minutes in the morning and the first five minutes at night. While you're speaking with a loved one, and you could actually, right now, just kind of tilt your hips a little bit, take your belly button, squeeze it close to your spine and you start to tilt. Oftentimes, I'll challenge my clients to always hold the pelvic tilt. I might karate chop them sometimes and make sure they're holding that tilt. Sometimes it doesn't work, ends up being pretty funny because I'll knock them up, but they get a little winded but then they go back to that tilt. You can easily lie down and do that.

[00:07:30]

Then, of course, stretching; I challenge everybody to stretch, not just forward and back, what they're used to, but stretch side to side. Give a little bit of lateral movement like a side lunge, movements like that. I'm always trying to stretch my calves. If there's a step, if I'm walking on a sidewalk and I see a little ledge, I'm just going to hang my heels off that sidewalk and create a little bit of stretch there, so stretch is also movement. Stretching is also exercise.

[00:08:00]

I tell everyone that oftentimes, they ask, "I just can't wake up. I cannot find time to exercise. I can't find time to move." They often want to know, "What can I do?" I tell them right off the bat, "What does your nighttime rhythm look like?" "Nighttime rhythm?" "Yeah, what does it look like before you go to bed? Do you turn ... For example, five tips, turning your phone off at a certain time, maybe having a limit, maybe saying, 'At 8pm, I'm going to put my phone on do-not-disturb or airplane mode,' and then also, setting your alarm but having that away from your bed." That's such a key thing. How many times do you roll over and hit the snooze button versus have to get out of bed and hit that and actually hit the alarm off? That's key, before you go to bed, making sure, one, you start to disconnect from your phone. Two: the phone's away from your bed when you go to bed when you set your alarm. What does it look like before you go to bed in a sense of flossing, mouthwash, brushing your teeth?

[00:08:30]

[00:09:00]

[00:09:30] What's that little rhythm like? Do you wash your face? Actually, having some type of rhythm, that you shower ... I always recommend some type of magnesium supplement because it simply calms the body down, right? Whatever that may be ... and then having a glass of water before you go to bed lightly and having one next to your bed, so those are a couple things as far as the PM rhythm.

[00:10:00] Then, next comes the AM rhythm, or that rhythm when you wake up in the morning. One: phone is away from the bed when the alarm goes off and that's not usually enough. Typically, you wake up in the morning, you shut your alarm off but hopefully, there's a song playing that stimulates your auditory, so, one: it wakes you up. Two: there's a song that might think of ... might motivate you, might make you think of something that's supposed to stir up some type of memory that puts the focus maybe on the desire of why you want to wake up in the morning and get moving.

[00:10:30] Maybe it's a family member and then, in that subject line on the phone, all these little things matter. In the subject line on your phone, maybe you have a quote or a saying that your mom or dad or somebody said to you that really spoke to you and motivated you. Those are a couple things, always having ... I personally, and I have my clients do this and it's really funny when I get the videos of them, but have a spray bottle next to your phone and when you shut your alarm off, you spray yourself in the face and you wake yourself up.

[00:11:00] I love having a tennis ball or a spiky ball there. I roll my feet in the morning. I recommend everybody do that right away in the morning and then having some type of glass of water right off the bat. Then another thing is always go right to the bathroom, brush your teeth. Because it's pretty hard to brush your teeth, do all those steps, and then try to get an extra 10 minutes of sleep that then goes to 30 minutes and you don't find time for movement. Those are the nighttime rhythm, the AM rhythm ... The PM rhythm and AM rhythm to get you going on your day.

[00:11:30] Momentum. You hear it a lot, people saying, "I just want momentum. I want to wake up in the morning." For me, I tell people that movement creates momentum. But even before that, movement creates freedom, so if you're waking up and you're in your body, you're moving, you start to feel that flexibility. You start to feel that freedom that movement creates in your body. Freedom has a feeling. That feeling that freedom creates goes right up into the mind and it starts to stimulate the biggest
[00:12:00] muscle of all—the muscle of your mind. Then, once that freedom's created—so that takes a daily practice—then that momentum starts to build. That movement now creates the momentum of your life. That momentum that's created, that momentum can kind of take you anywhere.

[00:12:30] If you imagine yourself on a surfboard and you're catching that wave, again, another example of exercise, but you're going on that surfboard and this wave's taking you a certain way and it's taking you ... because it's a good ride and it's taking you towards this reef, for example, well, you want to make sure that you steer that ride. Whatever ride momentum is taking you on, this is the same with exercising and movement, you want to make sure you're steering that. You want to make sure that you're directing it or you're designing it. Then, what would it look like to design your day, right? And making that priority first, which should be movement? Again, that challenge is always designing your
[00:13:00] day to create the most movement and the most momentum possible. It always starts with movement.

A key factor to being more present when we move is eliminating distractions. What would that look like, whether it's turning your phone on airplane mode, really focusing on you? It's a time to invest in you and your body feeling connected. Oftentimes, people will move and exercise and they're disassociated to the hand, to their own fingertips, and their own toes. They're not connected to their
[00:13:30] body. By the ability to turn things off, to focus on themselves for a minute and listen to their own breath; they can start to get present to their own body. If they can get present to their own body, they can get present to their own breath.

Then ... I don't know, maybe that breath and their body can become best friends. If they can do that, they can start to feel what's going on inside of them. They can start to know when it's time to move.

[00:14:00] They can start to know when it's time to eat—that thing that lights up. To be able to be fully present when we move, it takes that moment to step back and really have a breathing practice, I like to call it, really simple. It's hard to move your body on a daily basis unless you're familiar and friends with your breath. What that looks like could simply be stepping back, taking a deep breath in, holding your breath and then releasing it.

[00:14:30] A practice that a mentor shared with me and I share with all my clients is the four, two, six breathing pattern. That's simply breathe in for four. You're going to do it with me, right? Hold for two and then release for six. If you do that, it's four, two, six, that equals 12 seconds. If you do that five times, that's

[00:15:00] 60 seconds, so it takes basically five deep breaths of four, two, six to just get present, to get really in your body.

What do I eat for energy? I get that a lot. I think if there's one thing that ... We all know our superpowers. I think there's one superpower that I know they have, and that's being energized. Almost all the time, all my clients say they don't work with me to get a six-pack or anything like that. They work with me to never get tired again. What foods do I eat? I would say it has less to do with

[00:15:30] what I eat and has a lot more to do with when I'm eating. When do you wake up in the morning and how quickly are you eating? How much time from that meal to the next? How much time from that meal to the next and so on and so on and so on? So many people are skipping meals.

A simple, easy, one-step method to do this is after you eat in the morning. First, you wake up. You want to eat within the first 20 to 30 minutes when you wake up in the morning. Then, right after you finish, go to your phone. Click the timer. Set it for three hours if that's your choice and the program

[00:16:00] you're on. It is for me. I click the three-hour timer. Then, in three hours from that point, it goes off. I know around that time, I need to eat. Then, I set it again and I set it again right up until the full day. It's less about the what; more about the when.

Don't forget about the who. If you're eating with a certain group of people and you're getting certain results, then you can't think that you can eat with them and then have new results. Start to be mindful

[00:16:30] of the people that you're with and who you're eating with and then. And the how, like how are you eating? Are you slowing it down, right? Hashtag-putyourforkdown, right? Real simple. It's one of the most important things. It's probably one of the most vital things, because it starts to help you master your metabolism when you can just simply put your fork down and eat slower.

[00:17:00] How can we boost our mood? I think first and foremost, just getting associated to how you're currently feeling, having a way to do that. Number one: exercise to mood boosting is simply journal. It's to journal, to write down possibly one thing you're grateful for. I challenge people to write down the BID (beauty in the day) and what it looks like. I think the more beauty you can start to see throughout the day, the more you can uplift your mood. Number one: I would say journal. Number two: be able to get associated to that mood and understand you want to lift it up a little bit, creating

[00:17:30] some type of exercise. What works for you? What type of movement works for you? Can it be fast and quick because that works sometimes?

Say, you really want to be fired up that day. Well, maybe you want to go for a quick run, walk, run, walk, run, walk. Say you want to be a little bit calmer that day and a little more at ease. Well, maybe that exercise of the mind and that meditation component, that breathing component comes into place

[00:18:00] and maybe a nice long walk could then be that case for that calm kind of state. Foods also have a dramatic effect on mood. There are foods, and you can research what foods do that for you and your type, but realizing that foods can help you feel energized, certain food combining can slow you down, can make you feel sluggish.

It's not okay. Gone are the days where you eat a big meal and you go, "Oh, can't wait to have a big nap

[00:18:30] after this meal." Those days are gone. That was a thing of the past just like bodybuilding or just weightlifting, going to a gym and just throwing weights around; that has a place, but that's generally an old-school mentality now. Same thing with eating and just passing out. We know now that food is fuel and if food is fuel, then we eat for energy. How do we get energized from that? What does that look like? What foods do that for you?

[00:19:00] Are there certain grounding foods to help you ground? There are certain foods that kind of uplift a bit and there are other foods that make you feel really sharp. Getting associated to what those foods are for you. The best way to do it, because it can be different for everybody, the best way to do that is start to have your own clinical trial. How do you normally eat? Add one thing in. Add another thing in. Start to slowly add and subtract. Start to get associated to how those foods help you feel.

[00:19:30] Then, one of the best things in that is phytonutrients. I think that when people are feeling a bit sluggish, whether it's the metabolism that needs to pick up, whether it's that brain metabolism that needs to feel right because your brain could be bloated just like your body. If your brain feels bloated, then it needs to release. It releases by having greens, greens, and more greens. That's how people go green—go lean. It's really simple and you start to flush out those toxins.

[00:20:00]
It's a daily, starting your day with greens, having a shake with greens in it, making sure there's some association to one to two cups of green, whether that's kale, spinach, whatever that may be, with your meal in every meal. If you're eating three meals a day, great! Six meals a day, still making sure there's a green associated to that and especially for breakfast because I hear that all the time. Well, how can I have greens for breakfast? Well, there are many ways. Green drink is one of them, but adding
[00:20:30] something to your meal. It's a simple way but making sure that greens are in everything you do to create a better mood.

I would say the biggest stress relief technique, and we mentioned it, is that idea of writing because writing is releasing, so the more you can write, the more you can release; the more you can let go. Number one: writing and journaling, whatever that looks like for you. Having that practice of having a stress release, well, normally most people don't say at the end of the day or that next day, to say, "Oh,
[00:21:00] why did I read so much last night? Why did I write so much last night? Why did I drink so much tea last night and then stay up all night?"

People do say why they watched so much TV last night. TV can be an immediate stressor—too much TV. Obviously, documentaries, etc., things like that are fantastic but the idea of too much TV—you can
[00:21:30] start to go into monkey mind or this idea of ... You can know. You can start to pay attention to somebody and see them. If they watched too much TV, you know it. You know because it's just they're not really there. They're kind of there. It's a different take on things for real. With that, again, going back to that stress relief, that nighttime rhythm is one. Reading is another. Writing is another.

[00:22:00] A hobby. What is that? Is it coloring? Get a coloring book. That's really big nowadays, but having a coloring book and having association to colors and making sure that you're doing circles and shapes, having not only that, but whether it's painting, musical instrument, all these things are de-stressors. When it comes to movement and exercise, some of the things, I think, are real simple and that's just stretching at night, keeping it really, really simple. What's tight? It could be as simple as just stretching your neck and different movements like that. Standing and having one leg over like a pretzel stretch,
[00:22:30] one leg over the knee, the leg over the knee and just really stretching your lower back and just really stretching up nice and high, reaching the ceiling and doing that multiple times over and over again.

As far as brain optimization and what are the five things that you can do to have the most optimization of the brain and be firing every single day, feeling really energized? One: the association of movement
[00:23:00] and how movement can fit into your day every single day. I encourage most people, start with it in the morning because life can get crazy and you can always get some type of excuse but what does it look like in the morning? Number one: get moving in the morning, right? Number one.

[00:23:30] Two: start your day, in as far as optimizing the brain, with something in your belly. You better eat as soon as you wake up in the morning; so really, really, really important. Number three: journaling. Journaling is really a secret weapon. It really is. So many people don't make time for it but just the association of writing, I've heard once that writing is as therapeutic as a massage. Who wouldn't want to get a massage every single night before they go to bed? That's another way to do that.

[00:24:00] Simply having a conversation with a loved one, optimizing your brain and health—that's really important. And taking more time to sit back and breathe and having breathing being your most important exercise, but intentional breathing, going back to that four, two, six breathing and what that looks like for you. Making sure you're doing that, those five deep breaths of four, two, six, three times in a day. That could be you'd start your day with it, during lunch, before and after, have that there and then also before you go to bed and making sure of those things. Those are the five things I say that would optimize your brain.

[00:24:30]

ANAT BANIEL | Anat Baniel Method® NeuroMovement®

| Anat Baniel: | My work, which I call NeuroMovement, is embedded in the understanding of the brain's remarkable ability to change and to change for the better, because it can also change for the worse, but under very specific conditions. NeuroMovement is a very powerful way to communicate with the brain and |
| [00:00:30] | wake it up to start creating new connections that open the door to remarkable, new possibilities. |

It can be in the area of movement, flexibility, strength, and overcoming pain. It can be in the cognitive area—having more potent and more creative cognitive abilities—and also in the area of rehabilitation.

[00:01:00] If we think about adult stroke, for example, or vets that come back from the war, or a lot of work that we do with children with special needs; when we can access the brain and we do that through NeuroMovement, which we will talk more about, the trajectory of outcome, the possibilities that open up, have been and often times still are considered by more traditional approaches, as impossible.

[00:01:30] NeuroMovement, of course, utilizes movement but not as exercise. We can elaborate about that more and has what I call brain-friendly conditions for the brain to wake up and create new connections and positive brain change. I call those conditions the nine essentials, so that sort of wraps up concisely what NeuroMovement is. When we want to either solve a problem that we have—physical, emotional,

[00:02:00] or cognitive—or we just want to improve the level of our own performance. The question is always, what are we going to do? For example, if I want to be able to be more flexible, do certain movements with more flexibility, how am I going to go about getting more flexible, right?

[00:02:30] The usual way that we approach, or most people approach this problem or challenge, is what I call the mechanical approach. That means we look to stretch, to bend, or twist harder, to move the mechanical parts of our body, right? The arms, the muscles, the legs, the torso, in this example, with

[00:03:00] more force. That is because that's the model of the world that we first learn, from birth on. We learn that if we want to pick up something heavier, we need to use more force. If we want to push something, if we don't use enough force, it's not going to move. If we cry louder, maybe mother hears us faster.

The mechanical model is a very important and valid model, but then the brain doesn't work that way. If you hit real hard on the brain, all that happens is it's not going to work as well. The shift from thinking about ourselves mechanically and trying to problem-solve mechanically, to thinking about the

[00:03:30] brain as an information system, is a true paradigm shift. It's very counterintuitive and we can start talking about the essentials. Each one of those essentials, in many ways, contradicts what we believe. Or if we go automatically, we will do with the brain, which actually drives it in the negative direction rather than the positive direction.

[00:04:00] Everybody now that talks about brain and does research on brain or builds models of artificial intelligence or whatever you take, knows that the brain is an information system. The question is, what's the source of information for the brain? Normally, people would say stimulation and it's very true, but it's not the full answer. If we don't get stimulation from the eyes, or ears, or the sensation in our skin, or joints, or internal sensations coming from the body, or taste buds, we really don't have much to work with as new information.

[00:04:30] Stimulation alone is not enough. The real moment of creation of a unit of information is a perception of a difference. A difference between louder and softer, between harder and gentler, between red color and black color. If we don't perceive those, a difference, for instance, between colors, for

[00:05:00] whatever reason, we don't have colors. We hear the word colors, we know that people say they see something they call colors but we don't have it.

[00:05:30] When we talk later about the children, for example, children on the autism spectrum, they see, they hear. I mean, their eyes are intact, their ears are intact, but many of them—I believe, actually, all of them—have a challenge with perceiving. Their brain being able to what people call noise—signal-to-noise ratio. That means that the signal, the stimulation, is not clear enough for them to perceive relative to the background noise of the brain. What's very important to understand, that if we want to provide information to the brain and new information to work with, we need to make sure that the brain is actually perceiving differences. That's kind of like the baseline of my work, really.

[00:06:00]
[00:06:30] Another example that I think will be very clear to people is if you're in broad daylight and someone behind you turns on a flashlight, you're not going to notice it because there isn't enough added intensity to the light for your brain to notice that something happened behind you, right? Same thing with noise. You're in a room, in a restaurant where it's really noisy, or a party or something, and people talk, and people really sometimes almost yell and it's almost impossible to hear what they say. Because the signal that means the voice that comes from the person that talks to you is not sufficiently powerful to create enough distinction from literally the background noise. That is true for everything.

[00:07:00]
[00:07:30] The way the brain gets new information is when the brain itself perceives a distinction between a stimulation and the background so-called "noise of the brain." It's not like literal noise but it's the activity in the brain. When it notices that, it promotes the growth of new connections. You have to have that for new connections to happen. Otherwise, it just sort of does what it does; it doesn't do much new. The very first essential is movement with attention. Movement with attention is really the head essential, without which nothing will be there. Einstein said, "Nothing happens until something moves." My amazing teacher Dr. Feldenkrais said, "Movement is life. Without movement life is unthinkable."

[00:08:00]
[00:08:30] The brain, during waking hour, most of its activity is movement related. When we don't move, really nothing happens. Thinking is a form of movement and we can't see if the eyes don't do the subliminal movements. We don't know that movement is everywhere all the time. What I observed working with groups and working with individuals is that when people move, automatically they think about lunch, what they're going to have for lunch, or watching TV while they're doing something. When I teach there's no TV, but if people are just moving without paying attention to what they feel as they move.

[00:09:00] Once they get the instruction, whatever the instruction of the movement is, or when they just move spontaneously, that's done, right? They're going to do it. Then the attention to what you feel as you move, the sensations that occur: Does it feel light? Does it feel heavy? Does it hurt a little? Doesn't it? So on. Without attention to what we feel as we move, there are no detectable changes in the brain. There's a brilliant research that Dr. Michael Merzenich has done that shows that. When we feel, we pay attention to what we feel as we move. That's a whole other set of research studies, estimated 1.8 million new connections per second in the brain.

[00:09:30]
[00:10:00] You go from nothing happening to explosion. You're looking at billions of new connections if you look at 10, 15 minutes of process of that. Now, more and more people know that paying attention triggers brain activity and novelty in the brain. What I noticed, the most important and most potent attention to feel is to the self; what I feel as I do it. I've created programs, what I call NeuroMovement for Whole Brain and Body Fitness, that has four programs, six movement lessons each on different topics.

[00:10:30] One is the whole-body kind of focusing on different central areas of the body but in a dynamic way, not in a static way. That brings me to another concept that's called mapping. In order for me to be able to control my hand for instance, to do that, I couldn't do that intentionally when I was a month old; neither could you. It takes thousands of movements and variations of movements and permutations. You know how babies kind of watch their hands like that when they move and they're fascinated? They are paying attention. When we do that, connections start forming between the periphery to the brain, in the areas that are associated with the different parts of the body. We literally map ourselves

[00:11:00]   into our brains.

For instance, I've worked with quite a few babies and children that have what's called brachial plexus injury. That's an injury to the nerve that innervates the arm and the hand. If it's fully severed, then there's not much I can do with the arm. Very often, it's to the point where the arm cannot really move

[00:11:30]   but there are still some fibers that are intact. What happens is that the arm doesn't move. The child doesn't feel the arm and the brain doesn't know it has the arm, so it doesn't get mapped. Then gradually it gets a little mapped but it's very spastic because it can't get the complexity, the differentiation it needs.

[00:12:00]   I work with children like that and get their brain to gradually recognize, sometimes really fast. Actually, we have on YouTube a video of Devorah and she was eight weeks old. She never moved her left arm for long. They tried, they did therapy with her and so on, and in six minutes she started moving the arm. Once the brain recognizes the arm there—bang! The activity with an eight-week-old, the brain is just so... grows so fast, so yeah.

[00:12:30]   How do you apply movement with attention for adults? Norman, for five years, came and watched me work with the same children and I'm in his second book. He writes about my work with a girl who was never supposed to walk, or talk, or anything. Anyway, he talks about how I got her to talk. I didn't get her to talk, how she figured out talking. I know him well and the simplest way you can start the

[00:13:00]   process, you don't have to get my video tapes, you don't have to go anywhere, but you just start. As you move, you make your coffee or you brush your hair, and you start paying attention to what you feel.

What do I feel in my shoulder? What do I feel in the neck? What do I feel in my left foot? Gradually get more and more freedom to think of different ways to question and scan what you feel, you pay attention. You will do that; the movement will improve spontaneously. It just will improve because it

[00:13:30]   has never not worked for me and for the people I've trained. If you have a brain that is working, I've done it with the youngest who was five days old and the oldest was 98, so it works.

For more athletic, like if you go to the gym, let's say, and people lift weights, or do stretches, or something like that. If you just back off from the performance aspect of it for a moment, and one of my essentials is slow, I'll talk about it in a minute. You just slow down a little bit, so it gives you time.

[00:14:00]   That you're not just like jumping ahead of your ... Because attention, to pay attention and notice is slower than just doing, like running fast or something. You just say, "Okay, I'll do two, three, four movements and just pay attention to what I feel as I do them." Then you take a four-second stop, you just rest, and then you do the movement again, it will be better.

[00:14:30]   If you want to up your performance, you can just take any movement you're interested and engaged in, and start paying attention to what you feel. In the beginning, especially for people who are used to working hard and pushing hard, it feels like a waste of time. If you allow yourself and do this a few times, you will feel the jumps. It's really exponential; it's like quantum leaps. That's how you use it just

[00:15:00]   in your daily life. Hope couldn't basically do anything. She came to me, she was a little bit over a year old. I think she was about a year and a half, if I recall correctly. She didn't talk, she didn't roll, she didn't move.

[00:15:30]   I started working with her and, actually, I wasn't sure I could help her because she was just so inert. It seemed like nobody was home, but she started progressing. The parents were from Boston and they actually ... The father got a job in San Francisco and they moved to the West Coast so they could work with us more frequently. First of all, she woke up, she got some consciousness, some awareness. Before she could do much, she started feeling stuff; she started noticing stuff. That happens both with adults and the children that we work with. People just sort of wake up, they become like they're more there.

[00:16:00]   Then she gradually got more and more abilities, until she started walking independently. She was five years old when she actually walked independently. Initially clumsy, then it kept improving. Speech wasn't there. At that point she was put in a preschool. They wanted to teach her to talk. I asked the

[00:16:30]   parents actually to not put her with a traditional speech therapy because she had what one could call a very powerful aphasia. Anytime she tried to talk, she could yell or cry, so she could produce sound. When she tried to intentionally produce sound, she actually went the other way around. It's almost like the brain did it in reverse.

[00:17:00]   I was concerned that if she'd get therapy and people will tell her, "Say mama or say..." her name or whatever, that her brain would be trained to associate trying to speak with that reaction. Then that reaction gets grooved in very, very deeply and it goes with anxiety because she knows she's failing and all that stuff. I really wanted to avoid that. In school, they did this speech therapy. After about eight months, she was in school and she didn't see me during those eight months; she saw a local practitioner a little bit; they lived a little South of where I work.

[00:17:30]   I get an email and they say she has this wonderful therapist, everything else, but she can't talk. This therapist says that she has weak facial muscles. So, could I work on her facial muscles? I emailed the mother back and I said, "You know I don't work with muscles, I work with the brain." The mother emailed back, said, "Yes, I know. Could you do anything?" I said, "I will try." I didn't know how deep or engrained was her reaction, but I had written one condition that you give her six months to work with us. I said, "I'll start with two lessons." It was all I had that following week.

[00:18:00]   What I did with her that Dr. Norman Doidge describes in his book, is that I didn't let her talk. She came in and she expected that I'll work on the problem, right? I just talk, talk, talk, talk, talk, talk, talked about my daughter, talked about my daughter, talked about her experience in preschool and all that stuff. Then I'd ask her a question and didn't give her time to answer. In one of my questions she says, "Yeah." I'll just pretend that nothing happens and I keep talking, talking, talking, talking like that. I ask

[00:18:30]   with intonation a question and she goes, "Yeah."

It was only sitting. I was kind of creating and working with my hands, doing whatever I do with movement, and then I put her lying down. At that point, I started talking gibberish, so ... Like that. Like

[00:19:00]   I covered the whole time-span with my voice but it was gibberish. At a certain point, I got tired and I just got quiet. I hear from down ... She's lying on the table, I'm above her sitting, gibberish. I responded with gibberish, and she talked gibberish because it had enough freedom for her to be able to do. She couldn't do the precise stuff. That's why I did gibberish.

[00:19:30]   We did gibberish for a few months and what I started doing is, I started implementing words into the gibberish gradually. Her parents worried because they said, "Now she talks gibberish to everybody." I said, "Just tell them to take a deep breath and be okay." Now she talks. She doesn't talk with the fluency that I have, she's in a regular school, she's a good student, she has a life, she likes some kind of dancing, I don't remember. That's the story.

[00:20:00]   For me now the essentials are in my blood. I work with what is. The first thing I do, and I talk to people, and that is before you do anything, don't try to fix people. We cannot fix people. That's the

[00:20:30]   mechanical model. With a live being, the most powerful food for growth, change, and learning is connection. The essential, each and every one of them actually, is also a tool for powerful connection between two humans. In my world, in my imagination, I lend myself, I lend my brain, we become one brain. I know who I am, I know who they are, but I feel them, they feel me. I get informed by what I feel from them, which gives me a sense of possibilities of what they're ready to do next. That's like

[00:21:00]   really shifting approach.

Any therapy that looks to fix people, especially when we talk about psychology, and ability to move, and behaviors, might get some results but it's such a fraction of the potential of the person you're working with. Before even the essentials, from fixing to connecting. The essentials, so movement with

[00:21:30] attention. When I move and I pay attention to what I feel, guess who I'm connecting with? Myself, right? When I work with someone else and I pay attention as I move them to what I feel through them, that means I feel them, it gets them to pay attention to themselves.

[00:22:00] I have never had a child on the spectrum, no matter—autism spectrum—that didn't... Once I got to touch them and now they never resist touch, including the kids that are supposed to be really aversive to touch. I think it's so primal in our brain to be connected and to learn through touch and movement and feeling each other, that it's just an open highway. That's the first thing. Then, let's talk about the essentials.

[00:22:30] Slow. First, we can only do what we already know. The brain creates connections and then it creates myelination. That means it insulates the axons of the nerves, the nerve cells, to make the electrical current, very low voltage current that goes through those axons. Without that, the brain can't

[00:23:00] function. That's what happens in many of the neurological, the generative disease like Parkinson's and multiple sclerosis, and so on.

The more it is practiced, the more it's done, the more it gets insulated and the current can drive faster. When I want to move fast, my brain will always default into the most deeply grooved patterns that I

[00:23:30] have right now. If I want to improve, if I want to create something new, if I want a transformation, the way I am in the world, I have to slow down. If I want to facilitate for another human being to discover within themselves new possibilities, I need to facilitate for them to slow down. That's a very important essential, that people try to do things fast because they think, "If I do it fast, that means I'm doing it well."

[00:24:00] Really what it does, it makes that most people either cannot learn the thing or just get the very medial core level of performance. Another essential is subtlety. If you remember when I talked about the mechanical model versus the information model, in a mechanical model, if I want to do something that I can't do right now, I'm going to put more force into it. If you think about perception of

[00:24:30] differences, the way the physiology works and the perceptual system works, is again the more intense the stimulation; the more added stimulation I need to give it, to create a differential, to create a difference that I can perceive.

[00:25:00] For instance, if you just talk about movement and fitness: when people want to get more flexible, they think they should stretch the muscles. First of all, I would like all the world to know muscles are not supposed to stretch. They're supposed to contract and let go. You stretch a muscle, that means you're stretching a muscle that the brain is actively contracting. You're going against yourself, what the brain does. It creates tears in the muscle, it has to mend it, and then it gets tighter. If you want to create

[00:25:30] more mobility, you go on slow movements that are very gentle, you pay really close attention to what you do. The range of the movement will increase within seconds, guaranteed.

It's so counterintuitive to what we know, because in the mechanical world that's not the case. In an information world, and in a live information system like our brain, it's very much the case. Because the

[00:26:00] brain tells the muscles what to do. If a muscle is chronically short, the brain has to change. The muscle can't change itself, it's the muscle; reduction of force. Now, I want to talk about in the emotional level. You know how when somebody ... we try to convince them of something or we have an argument and we don't get what we need back, there's a tendency to raise our voice, to be more intense, to push

[00:26:30] harder, to try to make them get it. The more we do that, what happens? The less they get it, right?

It evokes in them a more powerful response. They get also defensive because it very often feels threatening, and they can't ... they don't understand what you're talking about. They just are not going

[00:27:00] to get it. It's true, and then it's true also cognitively. I work both with stroke patients and then my students that I train, I work on their thinking, becoming more potent. I want them to think better. Not what to think, but how to think, right? That they are more ... The thing with thinking is that when people have really strong beliefs, it's very powerful, very hard to see any other point of view or think a

---

novel thought. It's very hard to be creative.

[00:27:30]   Variations is nature's way of creating differences. When people analyze ... the Russians did that, they analyzed movement. Then, they put electrodes and they analyze which muscles participate in a person that's just walking forward. If you look at the person, the outcome is pretty much identical, right? They have their posture and they put one foot in front of the other and the muscles that get activated with each step change. A certain percentage changes. You never get the exact same thing again, it just keeps changing.

[00:28:00]   If you look at nature, if you look at genes, if you look at anything, you see that everything is built with variations. It's almost like saying like life and variations is the same thing. Again, when someone has a hard time understanding something or doing something, I don't tell them to try and do it. The one
[00:28:30]   thing I don't tell them is to do what they can't do. What I say is, "If you could, you would." If I'm asking you to do something you can't do, what are you going to learn if you can't do it? You're going to learn your limitations.

This is one of the big issues that Dr. Martha Herbert and I and my colleague Dr. Neil Sharp are looking at, working on a research proposal; to really transform how rehabilitation is done and we're focusing on adult strokes at this point. When somebody has a stroke, it's devastating. They've lost the... If it's
[00:29:00]   ischemic stroke, they're spastic, the arm is like that, they can't use the leg. It depends on the side of the brain, they can talk or they can't talk. People tell them, "Try to catch the spoon," right? The arm, they lost their neural connections ... they can't. It's like telling a three-week-old to catch a spoon.

[00:29:30]   You have a genius little being that's three weeks old but it's not going to catch a spoon, it's not going to say, "Mama," it's not going to go to Harvard—it's three weeks old. When somebody has a stroke, many of the functions that have been affected, the brain, they lost the connections, they lost the underlying neural networks. They cannot do it. When you ask them to do what they cannot do, you train them into their failure because the brain learns its experience. It doesn't learn what you want it to learn, it learns what it is experiencing and what it makes of it.

[00:30:00]   What I do, and my colleagues, people train with me. The very thing I do is not ask them to do what they lost. I start getting them to moving in ways that re-differentiate, recreate many of the connections that were lost, and hook up to the existing parts of the brain that were not harmed.
[00:30:30]   Again, with adults too, the results are remarkable. I have a center in San Rafael, I had a contractor that built my center, right? When he was 48, not long after he finished... Irish guy, ate a lot, smoked and drank, and had a stroke. Devastating stroke, two-sided, and on machines, breathing machine, and Propofol so he wouldn't move involuntarily with all the things that were in his veins.

[00:31:00]   I saw him once, so I just wanted to see whether I can connect to his brain. I didn't ask him to do anything and he was unconscious, but I had one of my graduates go twice a day, 15 minutes a day, and start moving him and getting to see where he responds. In 10 days, we started on the third day after
[00:31:30]   the stroke, which is perfect because the brain is a self-organizing system. No matter what happens, it's going to start organizing itself. When it has a stroke, it's all, like, way off; it's swollen, it's not going to do a job. I said to her, "Just get in there. Don't try to make him do anything."

He was laying down and every time she was there, since he was monitored, his oxygen absorption got better. It was very interesting. His need for the breathing machine reduced and he got calmer, so they
[00:32:00]   could do less and less of the Propofol. It was really remarkable because the brain got organized in a way that was on a higher quality. It was roughly two weeks, they took him off all the machines and within a few minutes he sat himself up. There were two people on either side but he wanted to go to the bathroom. He has his bed and the bathroom was just a few feet away. He got up and he walked to the bathroom.

[00:32:30]   The neurologist said, "One in a million." I said to the neurologist, "No, zero in a million. Because if you

[00:33:00] don't do what we did, you'll never see it again. If you do what you normally do, you won't see it." The variations is you work with where the person is at. Like another story, eight-year-old, a lovely boy, the autism pretty severe, couldn't learn to read and write. They tried to make him write the letters between two lines to contain it, right? Because they went everywhere. Then when that didn't work, they created a square. Now they contained it right and left and up and down. It didn't work.

[00:33:30] I did what I did with him, which will be too long to tell here. At a certain point I said to him to... I started by telling him, "Write a ... " I wrote the letter A, he recognized it. I said, "I want you to write it but I want you to write it really bad. Write a bad A." Now, to ask a child that writes badly to write a bad A is pretty easy. He's going to be successful. Success is important. He thought about it and then he just did a dot. I said to him, "This is so bad, maybe it's too bad because I know it's not a letter. It's a dot. Can you do a little bit of a letter but a bad one." You see what I'm doing there? I'm in the context of writing, right?

[00:34:00] Then, I did a bunch of variations and I wrote a bad one and he told me if it was bad or not. We went back and forth, all kinds of variations and different letters. Then he chose a letter and I drew a box and I could see him stop breathing. He held his breath; anxiety because he already knew that he was going to fail, right? I said to him, "Listen, you write whatever letter you choose, but on one condition: that

[00:34:30] part of the letter is going to be outside the square and part of the letter will be inside the square."

[00:35:00] You know how autistic kids don't look at you a lot of the time, or ever? It depends. His eyes just popped up, he looked at me straight and he said, "You're kidding me." I said, "No." He thought and he thought. What do you have to do when you have the instruction to write part of the letter out of the square? You have to know where inside the square is. I gave him an opportunity to distinguish between the inside and the outside. I said to the mother ... They flew, they were from out of town. They flew that afternoon back home. I said, "Don't ask him to write but he'll probably want to, and say nothing."

[00:35:30] She emailed us later when they got home. She said, "For an hour and a half on the airplane, he just wrote letters in between the two lines, perfectly. That's kind of what I call transformations and variations. Enthusiasm is another one of my favorite children, meaning essentials. I noticed working, that was a very specific client, that ... Again, another child, very severely impacted and the changes were there from the beginning but they were small, seemingly small, relative to her age. She started,

[00:36:00] she was a little over a year, and she could do nothing. She just cried, she couldn't roll, the eyes crossed. Bad, bad, bad, bad, bad, it was really serious. The doctor said to put her away in an institution, that she will never ... global brain damage, that was the diagnosis.

[00:36:30] For me, what people call small changes, are not small. Especially for the brain, it's a quantum system, it's an information system. It's either changing or not changing and it's either changing in a positive direction or negative direction. A small change is a judgment relative to our expectation. I worked with her and one of her parents was very attuned those small changes. Every time something little happened, I could see that the parent kind of, like, expanded, felt good, felt hopeful. The other parent was very devastated.

[00:37:00] It's very traumatizing for parents to have a child with special needs. Parents are a very neglected population in this equation and it's very important that we start doing more and more for the parents. Anyway, she, or I'd point out "a small change" and she'd get more depressed. The girl, her brain started feeling like wet cement. I wouldn't get that responsiveness and it's kind of like, oh, here we're going, and then in 10 minutes, all of a sudden something very new is there even though it's called small. It happened enough times that I made the correlation between which parent is bringing her.

[00:38:00] I requested that the parent that felt hopeful and well, be the one that brings her until she does well enough that the other parent can feel happy too. That's when I realized that we can either put water over the little flame or give it more oxygen and it grows more. What was fascinating for me is nobody

[00:38:30] said a word, but the child picked up without even seeing the parent. We pick up on people's feelings towards us. Whether we're aware of it or not, our brain knows on some level. She's fully functioning. Actually, Norman Doidge has her in his book too in the same chapter. That's enthusiasm.

[00:39:00]
[00:39:30] If we think about I talked before about perception of differences, enthusiasm is not a reaction. "Oh, I'm excited, I got the book I wanted or the gift." Whatever happened that I'm happy, but because of external conditions. It's a real emotional, mental, spiritual skill that we develop, that we choose to be enthusiastic about something that we could as easily be disappointed by. It's not fake; it's awareness, it's knowledge, it's enlightenment. The only reason I think I get the outcomes I get and the people I train are trying to do the same thing, is that those small changes, I go like, "Yeah, that brain is working really well." It doesn't matter how bad the picture looks, the brain is a good brain, so it's going to learn. That's enthusiasm.

[00:40:00] Flexible goals are so important and it's so important to people in our society. Goal setting is very valuable. Having a goal organizes our action, right? It sort of gives us directionality; it's very important. Again, the mistake that many, many of us do oftentimes in various areas of our life, is that we want to put the goal, getting the goal, upfront. If my goal now is to pick up a glass of water and I had a glass of water in front of me, I'll just pick up the glass of water. It's not a goal, it's an intention. I'm executing an intention.

[00:40:30]
[00:41:00] I talk about goals, to be able to do, be, feel, have, get, provide whatever area of my life, that I can't do right now. If I can't do it right now, I have no idea what it takes to get there. Even if somebody next to me got there a certain way, my way will have to be different. Even if it's a little bit different, but one is a little bit different and information system is different. I can have ideas from other people, I get variability, I get information, I get ... I have to find my path to myself, knowing and being able to execute that.

[00:41:30] I worked with a national runner and she was practicing to go to the Olympics. Her husband sort of semi-forced her to come to me, because she started getting injuries; one knee, and the same leg, ankle. She was really serious. I mean, she was dedicated, she was a serious girl. I looked at her body, and I saw that the muscles of her legs, especially the thighs are really big and thick, but her abdomen and torso, if you looked at profile, were like a little Japanese girl.

[00:42:00] Now, I know how the musculature needs proportionally to work. She needed to have a lot more work in her, more presentation, more mapping in the most powerful muscles in the body which are the muscles that are connected to the pelvis, right? She was using too much the periphery, so somewhere along the line she learned to do it that way. Now, she was good because she was a national runner, but she started getting injured. Her body couldn't sustain that because it was not well enough organized. It was organized enough for anybody who just runs a mile a week, but not somebody like her.

[00:42:30]
[00:43:00] What I did with her and I got her to agree ... My condition for her to work with me, talk about flexible goals, is that she is not going to run and practice the day after I give her a session. I said, "Otherwise, you'll just snap back to your old habits." She got an anxiety attack. I could see. I said to her, "If one day of not practicing, like really practicing, is going to fail you in getting into the Olympics, you may just give up now, right?" She had still a year to go, you know.

[00:43:30] The first time I worked with her I actually ... I didn't tell her I was doing it, but I was actually weakening her thighs and getting the center of the body much more represented in the brain. I get a call at 1pm and she says, "I did not run to train but I just ran without any ambition, and I got my best time ever." She got her best time ever three times through our process. That's flexible goals because she was trying to get there by more force doing what she was already doing, hoping to get it, and that's what her coach was doing. Then she changed the coach and I was very happy about that. Anyway, so that's flexible goals.

[00:44:00] I suggest to start cultivating enthusiasm, authentic enthusiasm away from where it's hard. Whether it's your child, can be autism or just a regular child that's maybe not doing that great, that moment in school, or your husband. You have a little, terrible wife or partner, or anything, it doesn't matter. Especially if you have a stronger attachment to it, don't try to practice enthusiasm there.

[00:44:30] Quite a few years ago I decided to practice enthusiasm. The first place I practiced it was in the supermarket. In the checkout line, the people in front of me, but especially the person that was punching in the products, the prices. Already it was easier for me because I could be grateful for them standing there and doing that job and then I would find something. Because if you look at a human being, it could be the belt, it could be buckle on the belt, it could be their smile, it could be the fact that they're there, it doesn't matter what. I would deeply, internally get really enthusiastic about it. Nobody had to know I'm doing it.

[00:45:00] Then I act it and I start expressing it. "I really love that buckle of your belt, it's really gorgeous." You have to say, and it's authentic. We can get to the point where I can choose to love you or choose not to love you. Because it's so much better to love you, I'm kind of unlikely to choose the other way, but sometimes, you know, for variations maybe I choose to hate somebody especially on the news or

[00:45:30] something. Anyways, so that's easy. Anyway, but even there, but you start practicing where it's easy, where it's neutral, where the risk is minimal, and you can do it internally. Then you start bringing it literally closer and closer to home.

By the way, one of the hardest places to do it for most people, ourselves ... Get enthusiastic about the gorgeous hair that you have, or enthusiastic of the fact that you have good shampoo for your hair, or

[00:46:00] you know ... It's more than appreciation, it's an active thing. Then what we train, and that's one of the chapters in my book because it's an essential in both books, is enthusiasm. Because we teach the parents to amplify, not to clap, not to say good boy or good girl; It has nothing to do with being good

[00:46:30] or bad. Internally, watch that child and say, "My goodness, if they can do this, they probably could do a lot more. They're brilliant if they can do that." Sometimes the brilliant activity is not what the parent wants the child to do.

I had one girl that was very, very affected...or even with my contractor. The doctor told me, the neurologist, they weren't sure he was going to stay alive. When I did some work with his feet, and soles of the feet; it doesn't matter because there's a lot of enervation between that and the brain, he responded. I went like, "We can do it, we can go for it. I just wanted to make sure it's not like a waste

[00:47:00] of time." He was still, like, not in good condition. The learning switch is ... Okay, so the brain puts order in this order and makes sense out of nonsense. That's the job of the brain. It does it through the ... It self-organizes, it creates patterns.

[00:47:30] It creates patterns within itself, and patterns of control of the body, and movements, thoughts, feelings, emotions, etc. The brain, I discovered either is in a learning mode or not in a learning mode, at any given moment. Very easy, if you're really tired, you're unlikely to be available to learn much. If you're really, really hungry, if you've had too much alcohol, probably higher math is not going to be what you're going to learn at that moment. If there's a lot of anxiety, right? If there's a lack of safety.

[00:48:00] There're certain conditions that are conducive for learning. Then, of course, we talk about nutrition, we talk about different things that are very important for the physiology of the brain to work well, but then the brain is either in a learning mode or not in a learning mode. All these essentials, what they do

[00:48:30] is they get the brain to operate itself on a higher level and a higher quality. It's not just like... The brain, again, that's not a mechanical system, it's an information system. It can upgrade its own quality of functioning and it can degrade its own quality of functioning.

The learning switch is when, either within yourself or when you interact with someone, you notice if there is responsiveness to what you provide. If there's responsiveness, that means the switch is on. By

[00:49:00] using the essentials, you tend to turn the switch on but you up the volume of the switch. What really happens with brains is that they learn to learn. We get better at learning, we get better, become potent, more and more potent learners. That's the most thrilling thing that I ... I know there are a lot of thrilling, wonderful things in life but actually this is one of the most thrilling things.

[00:49:30]

I discovered that when people become learners and more and more potent learners, the way I describe, a lot of the symptoms, even physiological things, improve. That means that when the brain itself works better, at a higher level, it impacts the vegetative nervous system. An example: digestion gets better, sleep gets better. Adults say, "Oh I did your whatever, your movement lesson and I sleep better at night." Children on the autism spectrum, they are very picky eaters, sometimes just one or two foods. Spontaneously, they start eating more foods.

[00:50:00]

[00:50:30]

I was just totally surprised and now, of course, this is the whole brain-gut connection, so it starts making more sense to me. I observed it, so the learning switch, and one of the ways to shut down the learning switch, is to ask somebody to do something over and over and over and over again. Thinking you're training them towards getting it. Lots of repetitions to move things into automaticity. We want the opposite of automaticity. When we understand that, we only engage a person if we can wake up that brain to go like, "What? What? What's going on? What am I to do here? Which connections am I going to grow? How can I make it better? How can I get what I want?"

[00:51:00]

Then, optimal amount of time for learning, like, that's really potent learning, 15 to 20 minutes. Done. Then, you can do something else or you can just walk ... I mean, you can learn something very different, but then after 40, 45 minutes, you have to give people a break or they don't really learn. We had our first teacher's conference, The Anat Baniel Method NeuroMovement Teachers' Conference. We had Michael Merzenich, we had Jill Bolte Taylor as keynote speakers; they both wanted to do that. Then Martha and I did a keynote and she did bottom-up and I did top-down things.

[00:51:30]

When you improve the physiology, it's fantastic. However, the brain still needs that kind of interaction to use the better physiology it has available for it, or the better nutrition, or whatnot. We're just starting to discover in research, an observation by different practitioners, that when the brain operates on a higher level, a lot of symptoms that look like they have nothing to do with learning or quality of brain organization improve in a variety of different areas because it's a generalized improvement of the whole system. Everything I'm saying, by the way, all those essentials, there are a lot of research findings that fully support all these finding.

[00:52:00]

[00:52:30]

Michael Merzenich wrote the foreword to my second book *Kids Beyond Limits*. He says that I defined, coming from a clinical place, what 20 years of research in neuroplasticity has done, more or less the same. We more or less define the same rules of what it takes to generate positive brain change. Imagination, there's wonderful research that shows that too, that when we imagine something vividly, when we think it and imagine it vividly, the brain changes as if we did it. That's why it's so important what we think. When people say you are what you think, to a great extent it's literally true in terms of the nervous system.

[00:53:00]

[00:53:30]

For instance, people who've had a real trauma to the brain, or again children on the autism spectrum, imagination is not something they generate. One of the ways I know that the kids on the spectrum or somebody who had brain damage is really improving, their imagination starts working. I use, especially with dancers, musicians, I get them to do stuff. Very often, I don't want them to go where there's already going to be pain because it will increase inflammation in the joints. That, of course, then reduces their ability to do things, increases pain. I have them imagine stuff, and then I have them do just like a tiny little movement or two, and then imagine.

[00:54:00]

It potentiates the brain; the brain gets really ... You can't imagine things if you're not using your brain in a really higher level. Dreams—something we all need to have. We all have to have a dream, something. It can be having a nice, vegetable garden, it can be changing how rehabilitation is done in the world. It doesn't matter the size of the dream, but I say that dreams pull us, direct us from the

[00:54:30]

future. If I have a dream, again it's sort of connected to flexible goals, I don't know if and how it will manifest, but it gives a context in which all my experiences can start getting a direction.

[00:55:00] When I work with people, I really care that they have a dream. I don't care what their dream is, but it's important they have a dream. Healthy people have a dream, it doesn't matter what age they are. Awareness is the final one, because I see awareness as the youngest function of the brain, the slowest.

[00:55:30] There's thinking and then there's awareness, and extremely potent and central for our ability to learn and to be well for health. For me, awareness is an action. First of all, most people talk about consciousness and awareness as if it's interchangeable.

For me, consciousness is kind of like general consciousness that I believe all vertebrate animals at least have, to some degree. Like a dog knows if you're going to take a trip and you take out your suitcase, the dog gets really mopey. Because they connect that with, "My beloved human is going to be gone for a while." They know where their food normally is. That's consciousness, awareness. I'm very

[00:56:00] specific about it, that I know that I know. I know that I've just moved my hand up and I move my hand down.

From my observation, infants, young children, are very aware. They're not verbal about it, but they notice and you see their eye movements and they make connections. It's also how their cognition

[00:56:30] develops. Awareness is the... At least the degree of awareness that we have, is a unique human quality. I believe that, to a great extent, that's what makes us human. When people act, and they have no idea what they're doing, and they have no idea how they are impacting other people, and they have no idea to look to become aware, and their tunnel vision, and they don't perceive around themselves, they can function, they can live, but they're more like lower vertebrate.

[00:57:00] When we become aware, it's ... First of all, awareness is, in my experience, the glue of learning. When I work with people—let's say a musician—I have them play their instrument before we start working, and then I have them feel the changes, become aware of the changes, and then take the instrument again—let's say a violin player—and play again. It's really easy with a musician because they hear the

[00:57:30] music and they hear the difference. They feel the difference in their body, and they hear the difference.

I work with some, the really top classical musicians in the world, and when their music quality goes up, oh my God, does that wake them up, right? It glues, because then that guides them. They don't know what they did with this shoulder, that shoulder, it doesn't matter. The brain recognizes it, integrates it, glues it in really fast. Awareness is a real shortcut to gazillions of repetitions. Repetition is important to

[00:58:00] automate something, when you have it—the quality—you want it, but it really fast-forwards learning remarkably.

You become aware of it, you notice it. Whatever the brain does with that, and it's much more yours, much more available, you also perceive the difference when you're not that way, or not doing it that way. You'll be like, "Okay, that feels different. How did it feel when I did it the way I liked it?" The brain

[00:58:30] can take you back there. I have Facebook and the Internet and all that stuff, we have a lot of ... Mostly children, not so many adults ... we have one amazing Tessa, who had a stroke at 28, and she came to us after she graduated. A month after she graduated her rehab, and left side, so she was aphasic. She

[00:59:00] had a very hard time saying words at all, and her vocabulary was way, way down, and she couldn't really speak, communicate.

Paralyzed on the right side. I didn't even know it at the time, she had no sensation except for pain. The arm paralyzed. Beautiful girl, she was cheerleader for the Colts, she was an athlete and... devastating.

[00:59:30] She wasn't discovered for 36 hours, so the swelling in the brain had a lot of time to do more damage. After the very first session she had ringing in her ears. I didn't know because nobody told me. She didn't tell me or her father who brought her, and the ringing was gone.

[01:00:00]   After the second lesson, she could feel her face for the first time, and a session is like 30 minutes. She was with a brace on the leg, and she got rid of the brace after two days. It was easier to feel the ... She started feeling the floor with her foot. There's a video, six-minute video on YouTube, Facebook, where she talks. Her fiancé is in the film industry, so he made a film, six, seven minutes, where she talks about her process and it's just remarkable. It's just remarkable.

[01:00:30]   People can get the professional help but they can also use the essentials right away. I started saying that we get letters. I mean not letters, but emails, we get Facebook messages where parents say, "We watched those videos, we read your book, we tried this, and now my child can do this." I have a letter from an 83-year-old woman. She wrote a letter, old-fashioned. She actually mailed us a letter that she had a stroke. She started doing our work daily, from videos. We never met her, and she's back to
[01:01:00]   driving, back to everything. Her neurologist says, you know, they can't explain it.

ANN HATHAWAY, MD | AnnHathawayMD.com

Dr. Ann Hathaway: I found that I had certain health problems. I had a lot of GI (gastrointestinal) issues. My kids had certain medical issues, not serious ones, but certain medical issues. My friends had issues. My sisters had issues, and none of these issues were being solved by regular medicine.

[00:00:30]   I started on a search to find better answers. I started looking at organizations, especially organizations of physicians that looked at things more deeply, more carefully, more profoundly, to look for underlying causes. I went to quite a few organizations and learned from them; the American Academy of Environmental Medicine, the American College for Advancement of Medicine (A4M), several others.

[00:01:00]   There's an organization in the San Francisco Bay Area where I live, Orthomolecular Health Medicine.

[00:01:30]   Eventually, I found The Institute for Functional Medicine (IFM). Actually, a friend of mine, another health practitioner, dragged me to a lecture, an all-day Saturday lecture on detoxification given by Dr. Jeffrey Bland. This was about 1996. I went to the lecture. I sat there, I imagine, with my jaw hanging open for the entire day. I was hooked. I only understood maybe 25% of what he was saying, but I knew that it was different, and that it was important, and that that was the kind of medicine that I wanted to take a look at and practice.

[00:02:00]   I had a lot of gastrointestinal issues my entire life. Starting as a pre-med student, as a medical student, I went to probably eight or nine different gastroenterologists over a long period of time. When I finally

[00:02:30]   ... By the way, I got absolutely zero help from them. And one of the important things about what they didn't talk about—what they never mentioned—was that diet could have anything to do with gastrointestinal health.

[00:03:00]   When I got to study environmental medicine, Functional Medicine, what I found was that—wow!—diet is super important in what your gastrointestinal health is like and what your total health is like. At around age 40, when I was getting into Functional Medicine, I stopped all dairy. Guess what? Within 10 days, my gastrointestinal tract was 90%, 95% better. A few years later, I stopped gluten, and I recovered the rest. I still have a sensitive stomach. I have to watch my gut. I'm one of those people

[00:03:30]   that has ongoing gut issues, but it's not like it was the entire rest of my life, prior to changing my diet. I take a probiotic, I take digestive enzymes. All these things make a huge difference, but Functional Medicine, compared to a mainstream gastroenterologist ... it's like night and day, the difference in terms of my quality of life, and I think the quality of life for my patients.

[00:04:00]   When you feel better physically, your brain works better, but also, of course, my microbiome was much, much healthier. Back in those days, there wasn't that much talk about the microbiome, but I'm sure ... When you have a symptomatic gastrointestinal tract, you have an unhealthy microbiome. As we know, as we've been learning a lot this weekend, having a healthy microbiome has a huge impact on the brain. What you eat has a huge impact on the brain. If you are eating foods that are

[00:04:30]   inflammatory in your gastrointestinal tract, that affects a multiplicity of things in your gastrointestinal tract.

[00:05:00]   We now know that two-thirds of our immune system is embedded in our gastrointestinal tract. When you have an inflamed, irritated GI tract, that lymphatic system, that immune system, is inflamed also, sending all kinds of cytokine messages, inflammatory messages, to the entire rest of your body, including to your brain. Guess what your brain has? Your brain has an immune system, the microglia, the astroglia, and those cells respond to cytokines. Guess what they do? When they get a message

[00:05:30]   from the gut, "We're under attack. We have a lot of invasion going on of something. We don't know what, but we have a lot of invasion going on in the immune system that's embedded in the gut." Then the brain's immune system also gets overactive, starts producing cytokines. Inflammatory cytokines in the brain can interfere with mood, with cognition, with everything that's going on in the brain.

[00:06:00] The role of estrogen, especially estradiol, in the postmenopausal female brain, is a topic that is very near and dear to my heart. I feel very, very passionate about this topic, because estradiol is extremely protective of the postmenopausal female brain. On top of that, this is a very poorly understood factor.

[00:06:30] Many, many doctors do not know this, do not understand the science behind this, and the general public certainly is not aware of how protective estradiol is to the postmenopausal female brain.

[00:07:00] Estimates are that estrogen provided to postmenopausal women, starting at the time of menopause, and continuing on, who knows how long, but possibly on into their 60s, 70s, and 80s, could reduce Alzheimer's disease by as much as 40% or 50%. It's really, really a big factor, and yet, it is not known to the general public, to women who are postmenopausal. They don't see this information. In general, their physicians are unaware of it.

[00:07:30] To the contrary, what they do think is that giving postmenopausal estrogen increases breast cancer risk. The combination of not knowing that it's protective of the brain and thinking that it increases the risk of breast cancer creates a really sad situation, because the reality is, we don't really have enough information about estrogen and breast cancer to know the answer for sure. There's not enough

[00:08:00] research. But the research we do have, the real double-blind, placebo-controlled trials, which are the only trials that are very reliable, with estrogen alone, without the synthetic progestins, which are definitely problematic and increase breast cancer risk, but with estrogens alone, there's only two

[00:08:30] double-blind, placebo-controlled studies. Neither of them show an increase in breast cancer risk.

[00:09:00] We have this situation that's very frustrating to me. It's one of these things where you feel like you're in a topsy-turvy world, where the reality that should be is the opposite. For the last 20 years, I've been reading all the literature on estradiol, estradiol and brain health, estradiol and breast health, estradiol and bone health, estradiol and mood ... all of that literature. There is quite a significant amount of

[00:09:30] literature. But a lot of that literature is basic science, in other words, animal studies.

When you get to clinical studies, human studies, a lot of those studies are studies where they're using an estrogen and a synthetic medroxyprogesterone. Once you throw in that medroxyprogesterone,

[00:10:00] guess what you get? Medroxyprogesterone is terrible for the brain, it's terrible for the breast, and it's terrible for the bone. Yet, in lots and lots of observational studies, meta studies, and review articles, they'll lump all the different research, estrogen alone, estrogen with medroxyprogesterone together.

[00:10:30] Now we have, starting around the time that the Women's Health Initiative (WHI) study came out, we have much more, what we refer to as oral micronized progesterone, available to combine with the estrogen. Because it is true that when you give estradiol to a postmenopausal woman, if she has a uterus, and most of them do still have their uterus, although not all of them, you need to give a progesterone, because estradiol grows the uterine lining, and progesterone will reverse that growth. If

[00:11:00] you grow the uterine lining without reversing it, you will potentially increase the risk of endometrial or uterine lining cancer. We do need to have a progesterone available in most cases.

What we don't have, we don't have enough research with real progesterone, oral micronized progesterone. There's only one short study, four-year study, in early menopausal women. It's called

[00:11:30] the KEEPS study, with bioidentical estrogen, estradiol, and oral micronized progesterone, real progesterone. In that study, there was no increase in breast cancer. But we need much, much more to be able to convincingly tell women, and convince their physicians, as well, that this is safe.

[00:12:00] But I will tell you the following and it's important in benefit-risk balancing: if you have a 60-year-old woman, her risk, lifetime going forward, of developing breast cancer is 9.3%. If you take a 65-year-old woman and you want to say what is her lifetime risk going forward, of developing Alzheimer's disease,

[00:12:30] it's 17.2%, almost twice as much. Yet what unbalance is going on in our society? Everyone's afraid of breast cancer, and no one understands that estrogen will protect their brain. There are many, many ways that estradiol is protective in the brain. That is a really important point. I go through that research in great detail when I'm teaching physicians.

[00:13:00] Estradiol receptors, an estrogen molecule needs to bind to something, either on the surface of the cell, or it binds to something inside the cell. There's cell surface, or membrane receptors, and there's intracellular estradiol receptors. These receptors are in very high density in the brain, in the parts of

[00:13:30] the brain that deteriorate with Alzheimer's disease, the hippocampus, the amygdala, the pituitary gland, the hypothalamus, the frontal cortex, the posterior cingulate cortex. All these areas have a very high density of estradiol. These receptors, estrogen acts in those parts of the brain, for example, the hippocampus. In the hippocampus, when the estrogen acts there, it maintains the density of the neurons, the actual nerve cells there are in higher numbers and packed together more tightly. In

[00:14:00] addition, the number of connections between cells, the synapses, are increased with estradiol present.

[00:14:30] The actual dendrites, the little stems that grow out of the neurons that connect to the synapses and connect to other cells, the dendrites are increased. The way estradiol increases the dendrites is by increasing a very, very important brain trophic molecule called BDNF, or brain-derived neurotrophic

[00:15:00] factor. At this conference here, the Neuroplasticity and Neuroprotection Conference, there is a mention of brain-derived neurotrophic factor in every single lecture that occurs. It's extremely important in the brain.

In addition, we have estradiol receptors in our mitochondria, in our mitochondria throughout our body. But in those parts of the brain that I mentioned, the mitochondria, which are our energy-making machinery, every cell in our body, the mitochondria function to make more energy when estradiol is present. The estradiol produces less reactive oxygen species, or so-called free radicals, less molecules

[00:15:30] that damage the cell, when estrogen is present. The membrane potential of the mitochondria is higher, which is better, because there's less leakage of cytochrome c outside of the mitochondria, when estradiol is present, and that means that the mitochondria is better at making energy.

[00:16:00] Also, intracellularly, there are estrogen receptors. When the estrogen binds to these particular intracellular enzymes, they increase the production of antioxidants. For example, if someone has a

[00:16:30] stroke, when estrogen is present, they will have less damage from that stroke. After the stroke, or in any other kind of cognitive damage, say you have a head trauma with estrogen present, you will have better neuronal repair.

There are many, many ways that estrogen is very protective, but I have to talk again about my nemesis, the medroxyprogesterone molecule. In the United States and most of Europe, starting in the

[00:17:00] late 50s, early 60s, that was the first time they started to give hormone replacement to menopausal women. For whatever various reasons, what they decided to give them was Premarin, which is conjugated equine estrogens. It's a mixture of estrogens from pregnant mares' urine. That, and then when they gave that, they realized, we have to give a progesterone as well. Instead of giving regular

[00:17:30] progesterone, for various reasons, they decided to use medroxyprogesterone, a synthetic molecule that has progesterone-like activities and, in particular, it protects the uterine lining.

[00:18:00] Unfortunately though, although it does protect the uterine lining, it has a number of other very deleterious effects. Almost every benefit of estrogen is wiped out when you add medroxyprogesterone to the mix. Medroxyprogesterone, remember I talked about the up-regulation of mitochondrial function, if you give medroxyprogesterone—boom!—it negates that up-regulation of the mitochondrial function.

There was a very important study done, a collaboration between Stanford, UCLA, and several other

[00:18:30] medical centers, looking at women who had been on postmenopausal hormone replacement for at least 10 years, for an average of 10 years. They did a study where they did these very elaborate PET

[00:19:00] scans, called FDG PET scans, on their brains. Then they took half of them off their hormones and they left half of them on. Two years later, they repeated the PET scans.

[00:19:30] What they found was that if the women were on estradiol, transdermal estradiol alone, or conjugated equine estrogens, the Premarin, alone, they had some protection of their brain. Their brain was very similar to two years earlier, in terms of how active it was, and the size of certain areas of the brain, particularly the areas that tend to deteriorate in Alzheimer's disease. Whereas the women who had gone off the hormones and were measured two years later, they had a lot of areas of deterioration in their brain, hippocampus, amygdala, frontal gyrus, posterior cingulate gyrus, etc.

[00:20:00] However, the women on the hormones, conjugated equine estrogen, or transdermal estradiol, who were also on medroxyprogesterone, you can probably guess what happened to them. They did not have significant protection. That medroxyprogesterone negated the benefits of those estrogens.

[00:20:30] I just saw a patient last week who came to me for a consult, for advice. She decided that she wanted to go back to her own physician to get her hormones because she thought that that would be better covered by her insurance, which is totally fine. Her doctor did indeed write her a prescription for a transdermal estradiol patch, very nice, that's great. But she also wrote her a prescription for medroxyprogesterone, 5mg, which, first of all, is a higher dose than is usually given. But that was a

[00:21:00] gynecologist. I'm just astounded with the amount of medical literature that exists, that explains in great detail, how deleterious medroxyprogesterone is, that it's used. I will say, for the most part, it is not used. For the most part, most gynecologists, most people who prescribe bioidentical hormones, are using transdermal estradiol and oral micronized progesterone, or some other form of bioidentical

[00:21:30] progesterone. But there still are people prescribing this, sadly. There's absolutely no reason to be prescribing it.

[00:22:00] When you go through the menopausal transition, your estradiol level drops about 90% over, for some women, over a one-month period. For some women, it's more gradual and takes a year. But that drop in estrogen begins the process of neurodegeneration, those areas that deteriorate in Alzheimer's disease. The process of developing Alzheimer's disease is a slow, gradual process. Even though your

[00:22:30] estradiol drops precipitously at age 50, or 52, whenever your ovaries cease production, you still, for the most part, don't see dramatic cognitive impairment in any immediate sense. But the process, the process of deterioration, the loss of the estradiol, begins a process, an atrophic process, a slow, gradual deterioration. Whereas if estradiol is present, you get neuroprotection, and you get trophic

[00:23:00] support. Those cells remain dense, and plump, and intact, and their connections remain intact. But without it, it gradually begins to deteriorate.

Every once in awhile, I do see a woman who has an absolute dramatic cognitive decline at the time of menopause. Usually, it'll be someone who's very high functioning, a CEO. She runs a huge operation.

[00:23:30] She has to constantly prioritize and delegate and she's constantly working with a lot of complexity. All of a sudden, she feels like a deer in the headlights. She can't organize her thoughts. She can't be, "Okay, your team, do this. Your team do that. Your team, do this. Your team, do that. You guys have a week. You guys have a month. You guys ..." She can't do it. It's completely gone. She's like, "I can't

[00:24:00] even think." We get her estradiol level up from two, to maybe 40, maybe 50, and she will generally be amazed to find that she's completely back. She can do everything she used to do.

[00:24:30] Estradiol levels, before menopause, for most women, run somewhere between 100 and 450. We find we don't need to take women back to that level of estradiol. Usually 40 or 50, for many women, even 30, works quite well to give them back their neuroprotection and their cognitive abilities.

[00:25:00] Most of the speakers at this event here have mentioned that two-thirds of those who have Alzheimer's disease are women. You might be surprised to know that most men at age 70, 75, or 80, have more estrogen than women in their brains because guess what happens with their testosterone? Yes, their testosterone goes down, but they have an enzyme called aromatase that turns some of their testosterone into estrogen. Especially in their brain, they have aromatase enzyme. Men at age 70, 75, or 80, will have more estradiol, and they also have more estradiol receptors in their brain than women do. That's one of the reasons women are more estradiol-dependent than men for cognitive function.

[00:25:30] But men also have more estrogen, more estradiol present, than women do when they're older.

[00:26:00] I have been working for the last year and half or so, with something called the Bredesen Protocol for reversal of cognitive decline. That's a very intensive program where we work with people with mild, usually with mild, cognitive decline, but we also will work with people with moderately advanced Alzheimer's disease. It is a very multi-factorial project to reverse someone's cognitive decline.

[00:26:30] But the very first thing on the list, the very first thing that we address, is diet. We want people to have a low insulin and a low blood sugar, and a low hemoglobin A1c. All of those things help reverse cognitive decline. Alzheimer's has been called pre-diabetes of the brain. Certainly, if you have diabetes, you're at increased risk for Alzheimer's disease. When your blood sugar is high, it pumps your insulin high, and insulin is inflammatory. Inflammation is a major factor in cognitive impairment and Alzheimer's disease.

[00:27:00]

[00:27:30] Also, high blood sugar causes something called glycation, where the proteins throughout your body, including in your brain, are having a sugar molecule added to them. That addition of a sugar molecule to a protein is damaging. That's actual damage to that particular molecule in your brain. If you picture a loaf of bread baking, when the top of the bread turns that darker brown color, that's glycation. That's actually the part of the bread is very hard, and that's damage. That's glycation. The more that happens in our brain, the more prone we are to neurodegeneration and Alzheimer's disease.

[00:28:00]

[00:28:30] In the Bredeson Protocol, we work with ... I will say, a little bit more about diet, because we actually move people from a regular standard diet, or even a good diet, whatever diet they're on, to a ketogenic diet. We want people to be, at least part of the day, in ketosis. What that means is that your body is burning a lot of fat. We move people from maybe, possibly a good diet or a terrible diet, to a diet that's high in low carb vegetables, no grains in general, or very, very low grains, no sugar, low fruit, high in certain kinds of fats, the beneficial fats.

[00:29:00] What are the beneficial fats? Obviously olive oil, avocado oil, avocados, high-quality nuts and seeds, even high-quality animal protein in moderate amounts. Chicken, fish, lamb, etc., are an important part of the diet, eggs. In most people, we're really increasing the fat content in their diet.

[00:29:30] We often add something called medium chain triglycerides, one to two tablespoons a day, to their diet, because medium chain triglycerides help them get into and stay in ketosis. Medium chain triglycerides are absorbed really easily from the gastrointestinal tract into our bodies. Also, our mitochondria, which can either burn a molecule of sugar or a molecule of fat, will suck up these medium chain triglycerides easily and burn them very efficiently for fuel. A Paleo, high-vegetable, high-fat, ketogenic diet is where we go with diet.

[00:30:00]

[00:30:30] Treatment of cognitive impairment, I will have to say, it is not for the faint of heart. This is for people who are willing to make a very intensive commitment, who are highly motivated, and are willing to do things that are, for most people, somewhat pretty difficult to do. Making this kind of dietary change is, for many people, quite difficult. You're giving up desserts. You're giving up most of your fruit. You're giving up grains. You're giving up alcohol, because alcohol is fundamentally, essentially, in the end, it's metabolized as a sugar. There are a lot of pretty dramatic changes that people have to make to really do this protocol. If you're not going to really do the protocol full on, we recommend that people don't do it. You either have to be all in, or it's not going to work.

[00:31:00]

[00:31:30] Exercise: people have to exercise every day. We will accept six days a week, but we tell them every day. And it's vigorous. They have to do either interval training or some kind of vigorous exercise. We also highly recommend that they do strength core training so that you don't get injured doing your intensive kind of workout.

[00:32:00] By the way, these are things that if people take them on early, I think they're very preventative of cognitive impairment. It's good to know early on if you're APoe4 carrier and are at increased risk. I test every single patient who comes through my door for APoe4.

[00:32:30] Exercise, stress—we have a very intensive stress reduction program for every person. They can do Tai Chi. They can do yoga. We use HeartMath a lot, which is a guided meditation program where you actually can look at the app, which follows your breathing and your heart rate and takes you to a physiological lower state of excitation. You want to go from a stimulated state to a relaxed state and HeartMath teaches you how to do that very incrementally. We like that a lot for stress reduction.

[00:33:00] Sleep is very important. People need to get eight hours sleep. If they're not getting good sleep, we need to work very hard to change that. We make sure everyone who comes through our program does not have sleep apnea. Many, many people who are overweight, of course, have sleep apnea, but the sleep apnea that often gets missed is people who are the skinny sleep apnea people. Central sleep

[00:33:30] apnea, or just a configuration of their mouth and the back of their throat, where they have an upper airway spasm, and unbeknownst to them, are having episodes of low oxygen throughout the night. Those people tend to be tired throughout the day, even though they think they're getting plenty of sleep.

[00:34:00] Those are the four important lifestyle premises: diet, exercise, stress, and sleep. Then after that, we go into the biomarkers. There's a huge battery of blood testing, urine testing, that we do on folks who are coming through this protocol, lots of inflammatory markers that we look at, infectious markers that we look at. Are they carrying one of the Herpes viruses? Are they carrying Lyme disease? Are they carrying the Lyme co-infections? Do they suffer from mold biotoxin illness? All those things need to be looked at, and if they have those, they need to be treated.

[00:34:30] Are they methylating well? If they have a high homocysteine, we need to correct that. Their B12 needs to be corrected. Their thyroid needs to be optimized. We don't look at the numbers and say, "Okay, are they in the so-called normal range on the lab tests?" No, we have a particular optimal range that we're looking for. Is their vitamin D optimal? Are all their B vitamins in an optimal state? Are all their minerals in an optimal state? Do they have heavy metal toxicity? Do they have a high mercury, a high

[00:35:00] lead, a high cadmium? If they do, we need to treat that. We need to get rid of it, because any of those things can be a cause. Yeah, there's a lot that goes into the program.

[00:35:30] As far as food goes, it's important to have a lot of detox foods in your diet. What are detox foods? The cruciferous vegetables are very important detox foods. In fact, all vegetables are important in one way or another in detox. We like for two-thirds of what someone ... as far as volume, when you look at your plate, we want two-thirds of what you put into your body to be a vegetable. We want a variety of

[00:36:00] colors. We want a variety of types of vegetables. We want non-GMO. We want organic as much as possible, because pesticides and insecticides are potential toxins.

[00:36:30] We are trying to remove toxins, to the degree we can, from all of our patients' bodies. We use R-Lipoic acid, and glutathione, and N-acetyl cysteine as part of our program to remove toxins. If someone is, we think, is particularly toxic, we might use intravenous glutathione or intravenous lipoic acid, intravenous phospholipids, which are membrane support molecules, all of that.

[00:37:00] Those are some of the foods and some of the methods we use to detox. We, of course, advise people to avoid things like trans fats, avoid GMO if at all possible. You want to get as much organic when you're getting your olive oil. If at all possible, you want to get cold press; first coldpress organic olive oil. The higher quality food you eat, the better off you are. Lots of my patients who are not cognitively impaired also take these supplements. There are lots of people who are toxic in various ways, who are not cognitively impaired.

[00:37:30]	Certainly, anybody can take glutathione; it's available orally now, Liposomal glutathione is available. R-Lipoic acid is very available and N-Acetylcysteine. Occasionally, there's a person who runs a high cysteine and it's a little disadvantageous for them to take N-Acetylcysteine if they already run a high cysteine, but it's not especially dangerous.
[00:38:00]	
[00:38:30]	A lot of times in my patients, I'm looking at full-on nutritional evaluation that's going to look at some of those things I mentioned before: every vitamin level, every mineral level, their organic acids, their amino acids, their fatty acids. It's going to look at their omega-3 level, their omega-3 to omega-6 level, their oxidants, their actual blood glutathione level, their lipid peroxides, which is the measure of damaged fats that are coming out in their urine. We use this test and many other tests to decide what are the optimal supplements for this particular individual going to be.
[00:39:00]	If I were going to be advising everyone about preventing cognitive decline, or to put it a better way, to optimize your own cognitive function for as long as possible, I would say that it's very important to eat well, to lower your stress.
[00:39:30]	What are all the things that lower stress? Make sure that you have a good support system in your life. Have a good social life, get out in the world and do things that you enjoy, and do stress reduction techniques whenever you need to. If you're in a terrible situation at your job, get out of it, if at all possible. These are obvious things. Make sure that you're getting good sleep. If you're not getting good sleep, get some help to make sure that you are getting good sleep.
[00:40:00]	Exercise every day. Find something that you enjoy—dancing, running through the woods, whatever it is. Make sure that you have a habit, a well built-in habit of doing it every day. The more you do exercise, the more endorphins you get from it.
[00:40:30]	Have a good Functional Medicine doctor that can take care of you and advise you on which biomarkers are most important to be aware of in you, and which ones need to be adjusted with changes in your diet, and changes in your supplement regimen. Make sure your gastrointestinal tract is working for you. If you have GI symptoms, get a full-on, comprehensive GI evaluation and make sure you get it corrected.

ANNIE HOPPER | Founder – The Dynamic Neural Retraining System

Annie Hopper: [00:00:30]	The limbic system is basically an area of the midbrain and it is responsible for our security. It's filtering billions of bits of sensory information and emotional information coming in at any point in time and it's actually categorizing that information into two very succinct categories, either "threat" or "no threat." The limbic system is primarily involved with our survival, so survival of an individual and survival of our species.
[00:01:00]	There are various forms of trauma that can affect neural circuits within the limbic system. That trauma could be viral, chemical, psychological trauma, emotional trauma, mold exposure, or various bacteria can actually affect the circuits in the limbic system as well. There are various forms of stressors that can actually impair neural circuits in the limbic system that cause the brain to disorganize and start to encode information that wouldn't necessarily be threatening, as threatening in the brain.
[00:01:30]	I guess you could probably sense if you have some kind of limbic system impairment if you have sensory distortions. Say, for instance, you have sensitivity to certain smells, in particular, chemical smells. A lot of people would say they're really sensitive to perfume or they get headaches or they start to get different kinds of symptoms as a result of exposure to various chemicals in their environment.
[00:02:00]	It could be perfumes or colognes or it might be typical cleaning products or laundry products that people might be using, and they can find themselves getting sensitive to those products for sure. That's one way you can tell that you might have limbic system impairment. Other things like anxiety, depression, the inability to get over illness, like just this chronic state of hyperreactivity or chronic state of almost like an anxiety, but the person isn't aware that they're actually feeling anxious at all.
[00:02:30]	It would mostly be symptom-based that you would come to that conclusion. However, you could have some kind of brain scan that would probably show hot sections in the brain, over-firing of threat and protective mechanisms within the brain that would show that that area of the brain is firing too rapidly and too much.
	In 2004, I lived in Kelowna, British Columbia, Canada, and at the time I was a core belief counselor, so I really looked at working with people on belief systems that might hold them back from love, joy, or success in their life. I looked at a lot of patterns that might be running in their life, like emotional patterns, psychological patterns or behavioral patterns that might be contributing to belief systems that would stop them from moving forward in life.
[00:03:00]	I also wrote a newspaper column at the time called *Emotional Rescue* where I would teach people how to become the internal observer, how they could actually take a bird's-eye view of patterns that they might be writing in their life. Now, I was also featured on a local talk radio as a guest host in emotional wellness.
[00:03:30]	At the time, I moved into an office building where my office actually was right next door to the janitor's supply room. I actually had an adjoining wall with the janitor's supply room, where they had all the cleaning chemicals for the building. Slowly, over a course of five months, I started to get just more sensitive and more sick. I went to a lot of well-meaning practitioners, both in the medical field and alternative practitioners, and I was diagnosed with toxic overload.

[00:04:00]	I started to do whatever I could to detoxify and clean my system, yet unfortunately, even though I did every protocol that was recommended, I continued to get more sick. In the beginning, I just became sensitive to perfumes and colognes and things like that. Then it escalated to cleaning products and then it escalated to chronic pain, then it escalated to depression.
[00:04:30]	Then, at one point, I couldn't actually walk down my street anymore because if someone was doing their laundry and I was walking outside and walking by someone's laundry fumes, I might go into seizures. It became really difficult to navigate my life because I couldn't actually go anywhere anymore.
[00:05:00]	At one point it actually escalated to being sensitive to electromagnetic fields and you could imagine electromagnetic fields are around us all the time. They're in wireless, they're in all your electronic appliances. When that happened, I actually had to leave my home and that is at the point where I became what I like to call houseless, not homeless.
[00:05:30]	I became houseless in a sense that I didn't have anywhere to live anymore because my sensitivities were just through the roof and my central nervous system was picking up on minute amounts of stimuli as if it was life-threatening. I started to camp and lived on a broken-down houseboat and did whatever I could to survive. That's what it looked like.
[00:06:00]	Illness is a really good motivator and I recognize that of all the well-meaning physicians and people that I went to for answers, that no one actually had an answer for me. So, I started to research the brain because intuitively I knew that I had some form of brain injury. I started to research the limbic system because it seemed like the most natural place to look because I knew that my sense of smell was altered.
[00:06:30]	I could smell chemicals from a mile away and not only smell them, but my actual sense of smell had changed. Things that used to smell good now smelled like some kind of toxin. It was bitter and acrid and I felt like I was being poisoned by everyday things in my environment. I began to wonder what part of the brain was responsible for my sense of smell.
[00:07:00]	Then I looked at a lot of research that had already been done on the brain and a lot of overlapping conditions like chronic fatigue, fibromyalgia, anxiety, and post-traumatic stress disorder, and recognized that the common denominator was over-firing of these threat mechanisms and fear centers in the brain that were the common denominator in all of these illnesses. I went to work at really understanding what the limbic system did and how I could influence it.
[00:07:30]	Self-directed neuroplasticity basically means that through your own will, through your own thoughts, through your emotions, through your behaviors, you can actually act back on the brain to change brain structure and function, which is really quite remarkable. We were taught for 400 years that the brain was hardwired and that we couldn't change it and now we know that the brain is actually changing all the time. Self-directed neuroplasticity basically means that there are ways in which you can change brain structure and function if you know the right tools and how to do that.
[00:08:00]	In my own recovery from limbic system impairment, I used a lot of resources. Not only information that I was finding out about the brain, about the limbic system, how to influence the limbic system, and looking at all the brain research that I was doing, also my own experience in being that curious observer and looking for patterns within myself, because I recognized that I was no longer the Annie that I used to be.

[00:08:30] I was a happy-go-lucky, really bubbly, extroverted person, who had become this closed-down, scared person who was struggling for survival on a moment-to-moment basis. I was really looking at how could I influence different circuits in the limbic system and I was reading a lot of different books about neuroplasticity and about the brain-body connection and how emotions can actually change the brain-body connection that really started to influence how I would work with myself.

[00:09:00] Looking at the work of Candace Pert, who wrote the book *Molecules of Emotion*, the work of Dr. Bruce Lipton, who writes about epigenetics or working above the level of the genes, the work of Dr. Jeffrey Schwartz, who wrote a book called *Brain Lock*. It was interesting in Norman Doidge's book, *The Brain That Changes Itself*, when I was reading his book he interviewed a lot of leading neuroplasticians at that time.

[00:09:30] I incorporated principles that they were using in their own practice, like Dr. Pascual-Leone was talking about the power of thought and how thought alone changes the brain, and Dr. Edward Taub, who was working with stroke patients and how you could use a restraint kind of technique to get people to start using different pathways of the brain.

[00:10:00] I think most importantly it was Dr. Jeffrey Schwartz's work, when I was reading Doidge's *The Brain That Changes Itself* and his work with patients who have OCD. He was talking about how there was a part of the brain called the caudate nucleus that wasn't working functionally in people with OCD, and that's why it leaves them with this feeling of contamination. They just can't move from one thought to the next.

[00:10:30] Although I didn't have OCD, I did think, "What if the threat mechanisms in my brain are just not working functionally and that's what's causing this heightened sensory awareness," and also this state of ... I was in a chronic state of fight-or-flight and I couldn't get out of it. I was wondering if it was just that threat and survival mechanism that was at play. Really, using myself as the experiment, changing my thought patterns, changing my emotional patterns, and changing my behaviors, I was able to actually rewire those circuits in the brain.

The first thing that happened, that I knew it was working, was that my sense of smell started to normalize for very small moments in time. Things that were actually making me go into convulsions weren't making me go into convulsions anymore. Things that used to have a putrid kind of smell were actually smelling normal again.

[00:11:00] That happened for small moments at a time and I knew, without a shadow of a doubt, that it was a brain-related illness. That there was a mechanism in my brain that had gone rogue, and through self-directed neuroplasticity, I was able to regulate that system again and basically shut off a chronic stress response.

[00:11:30] Nutrition came into play in terms of—I went to see an environmental doctor at one point and I was on a lot of detoxification treatments, I cut out gluten, I was eating a really, really clean diet—extremely clean, clean as a whistle—and I got worse; It didn't actually work. Although nutrition is a big aspect of health in general, certainly changing my diet wasn't actually advantageous when it came to limbic system impairment.

[00:12:00] There's a very specific sequence of events that have to happen in order to change your limbic system. One is to recognize the impairment to begin with. What does limbic system impairment look like? What does it sound like? What does it smell like? How is your physical body actually expressing when you have limbic system impairment? What are your thought patterns? What are your emotional patterns? What are your behaviors?

[00:12:30]   First, recognizing what those patterns are and how they're affected with limbic system impairment and then recognizing when you're in that specific pattern. When you recognize and you have awareness of that specific pattern running, whether it's in your thoughts, your emotions, in your body, or in your behaviors, you can actually stop in that moment and redirect your brain pattern.

[00:13:00]   The redirect is about redirecting to a heightened emotional state, a different thinking pattern, and different behaviors in that moment in time. It's a very specific, step-by-step process, so if I just said, "Change your thoughts," I think it would be simplifying a very complex issue. The program that I've developed is not super complicated. However, it takes a lot of dedication and a lot of focus and
[00:13:30]   repetition, in order to create those new neural pathways.

In fact, we ask people to practice for at least an hour for six months. A lot of people have been diagnosed with ... That they have something impaired with their methylation genes and so sometimes people say, "Well, I don't think that this program will work for me because I have the dreaded gene." Regardless of whether you have that gene or you don't, it actually does not make a difference in terms
[00:14:00]   of rewiring your limbic system. You can still rewire your limbic system regardless of genetics.

I didn't actually know that I had fibromyalgia for a long time; I would just go to work and come home in the evenings and I'd be in chronic pain, but the pain would shift from one location to the next. I would often ask my husband James, "Do you think you could massage my shoulders or massage my neck?" He asked me at one point, he said, "Is there ever a moment when you're not in pain?"

[00:14:30]   I had to stop and think about that for a second, and the answer was no; I was in pain all of the time. It was impossible to sleep. It was impossible to find a comfortable sleeping position. If I slept on one side then my shoulder would hurt or my hips would hurt. So, I'd turn over, but no matter how many times I flipped during the night, I could never find a comfortable position because I was just in chronic pain.

[00:15:00]   Anyone who's suffering from some form of chronic illness, where they think there might be a stress response, or a maladapted stress response that's involved with that illness, would be a good candidate to take this program. That means people with chronic fatigue syndrome, fibromyalgia, chemical sensitivities, chronic Lyme disease, anxiety, depression, chronic pain, food sensitivities, the list is just endless.

[00:15:30]   In the beginning, we created the program for people that have chemical sensitivities, chronic fatigue or fibromyalgia. We've recognized that, through reports from people that have been taking the program, that it works for much more than that. In fact, even people with something called postural orthostatic tachycardia syndrome are recovering with the program as well and that's an autonomic nervous system dysfunction disorder.

[00:16:00]   It works for a lot of people, and we're getting reports of people reclaiming their life. I think in terms of who's a good candidate for the program, you have to be dedicated. You have to put in the work. It's not easy. However, the work is well worth it; you can basically get your life back.

What I would say to enhance brain function in terms of looking at just even thought patterns in itself, and your emotional set point, the brain has a natural negativity bias, meaning that we're more likely
[00:16:30]   to see what's not going right in the world than what is going right. I think that that can become a habit, and especially with the media is really focused nowadays on what's not going well.

I think as a general rule of thumb, noticing the goodness in life is a really good habit to get into; to really train your brain to look for what's going well. Other than that, certainly increasing our emotional
[00:17:00]   state, too. Instead of getting anxious or worried about small things, really put it into perspective. Is it worth it for me to get upset about this, and what are my choices? Become empowered in your life, and make those moment-to-moment choices that will provide you with happiness in life.

[00:17:30] I think that a maladapted stress response and limbic system impairment is really common. In fact, we know in Canada in 2014, according to a Canada health statistics survey, they estimated that 1.4 million people in Canada are suffering from chronic fatigue, fibromyalgia, or chemical sensitivities. If those numbers are the same in the US, that's close to 13 million people.

[00:18:00] We're obviously doing something really wrong. Something's happening that we're in this mode of life where we're exposed to so many things all of the time that are causing limbic system impairment and a maladapted stress response. The one thing that I would like to talk about with people is simple things like, let's look at your home environment. Let's clean up your home. Start using natural organic products, stop using things like perfume and things that have parfum in it.

[00:18:30] Parfum, which is an ingredient in a lot of products, has about 200 chemicals in it. The thing about the chemical industry is that it's not regulated. We get away with just marketing this stuff and nobody actually recognizes what's in it or how harmful it is. Even if studies have been done, they haven't really been done in unison. By the time the average woman leaves a house, they've probably applied, oh, I don't know, at least 27 different chemicals to their body, just in personal hygiene products.

[00:19:00] We really want to be consciously aware of what we're putting on our body, what we're putting in our body, and also what we have in our home. So, how we're cleaning our home, how we're furnishing our home. A lot of people will end up getting sick. A lot of times what we find with people that end up with limbic system impairment is that they've had the perfect storm of stressors.

[00:19:30] They've had maybe some kind of emotional stress, like a divorce or separation, and they move into a new home where they've got all these new products, right? They've got new furniture, new carpets, new paint, and everything's off-gassing, so we have all of these volatile organic compounds that we're absolutely immersing ourselves in. Most homes are really airtight, so we don't have any ventilation happening in that space anymore.

[00:20:00] Maybe they've gone through something that's been upsetting like a divorce or a separation. They move into someplace new that's had a lot of renovation, so they have new products, and perhaps they've had a virus or bacteria. That can be it; that's the perfect storm for limbic system impairment. Then the brain goes into this distorted chronic stress response, and people just can't get out. No matter how hard they try, they can't get out.

[00:20:30] Unfortunately, we see a lot of people that have gone through the medical system and still don't have answers. People that have spent $100,000, $200,000, sometimes up to $1 million, and they're still struggling. Even though they're really motivated to get well, they just haven't been able to find the answer.

I think it's really important, when we're talking about viruses, bacteria or chemical injury, that we recognize that there's an overload happening in the body. It's really important to address that virus. It's really important to address the bacteria. It's really important to address the toxic overload.

[00:21:00] At the end of the day, if the person is still sick and they're still suffering with that state of unwellness, then there's something else happening. The brain has been affected too. It's really important that we also address brain function, and specifically, what's happening in the limbic system, because the threat mechanisms in the brain are now firing really rapidly and really quickly because of that initial

[00:21:30] trauma. It's really important that we also look at how can we correct the brain so that the brain and body can go from that state of survival into a state of growth and repair where healing can actually take place.

[00:22:00] In terms of detoxification programs, I was on some IV detoxification protocols. I was taking a lot of nutritional supplements. I had a very strict diet as well. I did a lot of detoxification protocols. In fact, for most people, you would think that detoxification would be a good thing, right? We want to make sure that we detoxify our body.

[00:22:30] With someone with limbic system impairment, you actually have to be really careful. Because the exit pathways aren't really working functionally, you can imagine if you're in a chronic stress response and you're running away from a tiger, because you feel like you're being threatened. You're running away from a tiger. You could imagine that it's not important to go to the bathroom in that moment; what's important is to run for your life.

[00:23:00] Someone with limbic system impairment, it affects their communication, the way that the cells in your body are communicating to each other. It affects your detoxification systems as well. Because it affects the detoxification pathways, it's really important that we bring the limbic system back online so that the detoxification pathways are functioning normally. For someone else who might respond really well to a detoxification treatment, someone with limbic system impairment might not actually respond in the same way, because that threat mechanism is stuck on.

[00:23:30] When I was seeing an environmental doctor, who was very well-meaning, I was put on a lot of detoxification products, which actually made me worse. I developed electromagnetic sensitivity after that. I phoned this particular doctor and I said, "Hey, I don't know what's going on, but now I can detect even wireless in my house and I can't live in my house anymore." He didn't have a response. He didn't have an answer. His answer was just to continue what I was doing.

[00:24:00]
[00:24:30] I couldn't continue what I was doing, because at that point I was houseless. The only thing that mattered was my survival and that's a really hard place to be. I think that the suffering that people go through is unimaginable. There is a whole segment of society that people don't know about. They live out in the desert because they have no place to live anymore. They don't have jobs. Their family has abandoned them. A lot of them commit suicide because it's just hard to live like that.

The illness runs in a spectrum, right? Unfortunately, we see a lot of people who are on the severe end of that spectrum. What I would like to see, and that's why I'm speaking at this conference, is for people to be diagnosed early on so they don't have to go through years of suffering, through years of debilitating illness.

[00:25:00] There's an answer. It's here, it's available to everyone, and there's a way that we can stop suffering. I can't say it loud enough or shout it from the rooftops loud enough to say there is an answer. I'm in the very blessed position to be able to witness what other people would call medical miracles every day. It's not a miracle, it's the brain.

[00:25:30] When you understand the brain, you understand the limbic system, you understand how it's been impaired, and how you can go in and change those neural circuits and move the body from a state of survival into a state of growth and repair, that's when the miracles start to happen, because the body starts doing what it's naturally meant to do, which is to rejoice in life, to be able to handle these day-to-day stressors that are coming at us at any given time.

ARSALAN DARMAL, MD | Amen Clinics

Dr. Arsalan Darmal: I'm an adult, child, and adolescent psychiatrist by training. I've done my residency at the Albert Einstein College of Medicine in New York. Then I also completed a child fellowship at Albert Einstein

[00:00:30] College of Medicine. After graduation, I accepted a position as a professor of psychiatry at John Burns Medical School. I was there for about 12 years and, at that time, I came across Dr. Amen's work and joined the Amen clinic. Most of the knowledge and experience of working in a holistic area was at the

[00:01:00] Amen Clinic. I was very fascinated by his approach, so learned a lot from him. I started using natural supplements myself and learned from my patients and noticed the response. As I continued to use, especially in younger children, I was impressed by minimal side effects or actually no side effects. I got a very good response; the parents were happy, the kids were tolerating it well. That is how I came

[00:01:30] across kids with ADHD. They have a difficult time reading social cues, and so boundaries are a big challenge for them and expression of empathy becomes a big challenge for them.

[00:02:00] Oftentimes, friendship becomes a big problem because they cannot express empathy or show empathy. They may have empathy, some, but some don't even have empathy, so lack of empathy causes a lot of problems. Impulsivity becomes a major issue especially in the younger group. In

[00:02:30] adolescent time, impulsivity is a major issue and because of impulsivity they get into a lot of legal problems. These kids are usually labeled as class clowns and because of that the classmates or friends will avoid contact as much as possible and so they become isolated. In order to get the attention, they will get into more antisocial types of behaviors.

[00:03:00] Because of impulsivity, they're almost always in trouble, and trouble in school causes problems at home. Parents are usually called in and so it affects the child and parents' relationships. Even, at times, it can cause some problems among the parents because the parenting style becomes an issue.

[00:03:30] Sometimes both parents will be compatible with their parenting style and sometimes they may not be. It creates a challenge in their parenting strategies.

Eventually what happens is these kids are moved from one school to the other, from one academic setting to the other, and so that in its own turn affects their friendship. Eventually, they graduate with

[00:04:00] a lot of difficulties, but usually, turn into more antisocial issues. About one third of these kids, the ones that don't do well academically, start cutting classes and get into substance abuse. Substance abuse is a major issue for about 30% to 40% of these kids, and then with that, with impulsivity, substance abuse and a lot of legal problems, eventually they develop a lot of mood disorders, anxiety, and

[00:04:30] depression become their main issues.

There's about 20% to 40% of these kids, they can outgrow ADHD, and those are the ones who are more academically successful and do well in school. Then about one third of these kids continue to

[00:05:00] have ADHD as an adult. As an adult, again, impulsivity and lack of attention, motivation, and drive, become the main issue for them as an adult.

The DSM diagnostic criteria classifies ADHD as inattentive type, the impulsive and hyperactive type,

[00:05:30] and then a combined type. We classify ADHD much differently; our classification is based on what we see clinically, but also the SPECT finding. Also, we have classical type of ADD, inattentive ADD, overfocused ADD, temporal ADD, limbic type ADD, and anxious type ADD.

[00:06:00] Depending on the different classifications, the symptom presentations are different. Usually kids with inattentive type, they are on the low side of the spectrum. They manage to do okay, they don't get involved that much in legal problems, and impulsivity is not the major issue. The ones that have a combined type where impulsivity, hyperactivity, and inattention are combined, those are the ones that are on the severe side of the spectrum.

[00:06:30]	One would be a very comprehensive way, and that means that before coming into the clinic, they get screened. Sometimes they do a consultation with a physician, they complete a symptom checklist where there's about 84 questions that the child answers, and then the parents on their own, both parents answer those questionnaires. Then sometimes we ask for teachers to complete the forms.
[00:07:00] [00:07:30]	Then there's a thorough history: the patient sits with a historian, and the historian runs a very thorough history. At times, in the majority of the cases, especially for the first-time evaluations, we ask for a SPECT (single photon emission computed tomography) scan. The SPECT scan is to look at the activity in the brain and to determine comorbid conditions. Oftentimes in history, either the parents or the patients may miss a certain type of comorbidities. The scan will alert us to possible comorbidities.
[00:08:00] [00:08:30]	Then there are other tests that are done, what's called Beck Depression Inventory, the child behavioral checklist. We complete a child depression inventory, we also do anxiety scales, and Conners' Continuous Performance Test, another test called WebNeuro, we complete those tests. Then, all of the information comes to the physician. The physician will review all of the information before seeing the patient, and then the patient is seen with the family or, at times, without, just individually.
[00:09:00]	It gives us quite a bit of time to spend with the patient. The luxury of the style is that we have a lot of information before seeing the patient and you're well informed about the patient's weaknesses. That's why it allows you to inquire more about the areas of deficits and get a very thorough history. Because you've also had the ability to look at all the different areas including a SPECT scan, which is at times very helpful. It gives you a lot more confidence in your diagnosis.
[00:09:30] [00:10:00]	Then the treatment plan that you develop is also a very comprehensive treatment plan. The treatment plan includes dietary interventions, which are very, very important in our clinic. It also includes physical exercise, which we also believe that's very important, especially in kids and adolescents, where their brain is growing, and the exercise makes a significant impact on the shaping of the brain.
[00:10:30] [00:11:00] [00:11:30]	Also, recommendations about Cognitive Behavior Therapy, psychotherapy, natural supplements. In cases where we have ADD, we do ADHD coaching. We also recommend 12-step programs for our substance abuse cases. In cases of traumatic brain injury, we consider hyperbaric oxygen treatment. We also consider natural supplements, that's the first step of treatment is that almost always we try to consider natural supplements. In cases that are more severe and refractory to treatment, we almost always get those type of cases where patients have not responded, and at the endpoint they come into the clinic, and so at that time we're a little bit more aggressive in our treatment. We consider medication, and in cases of depression or anxiety, we consider Transcranial Magnetic Stimulation. We also consider neurofeedback, especially for anxiety and ADHD; almost always we consider neurofeedback. Then in more severe cases we have more aggressive interventions.
[00:12:00]	SPECT is a nuclear medicine technology. It's a functional brain imaging in that it determines the activity in the brain. What it does—it tests the blood flow in the brain and based on the blood flow in the brain, we consider metabolic activity. The theory is that those areas of the brain that are working well, those areas demand more oxygen and nutrients, so the blood flow is higher to those areas. Those areas that are lazy, damaged, inflamed, or not working well—those areas do not demand that much oxygen and nutrient, so the blood flow is lower.
[00:12:30] [00:13:00]	What we do is we give you an isotope; the isotope is the radioactive isotope called Ceretec and it flows with the blood, goes to the brain, and then gets absorbed by the brain cells, gets fixed in the mitochondria and under the camera it lights up. Those areas of the brain that are working too much will absorb most of the isotope, those areas that are lazy or damaged will not absorb the isotope. Those areas that don't absorb the isotope, it looks like a hole or a dark area, and so based on the different activity patterns throughout our practice, we have learned to apply that into the diagnostic criteria for the patients.

[00:13:30]

[00:14:00]

In the majority of cases, we see a decreased perfusion in the prefrontal cortex area of the brain. The prefrontal cortex is right above the eye socket, it's the front part of the brain, which is the executive functioning of the brain, in a normal setting. You should have normal activity; we don't see any kind of a deactivation in that area. In cases of traumatic brain injury, or in cases of ADHD ... in 70% of the cases, we see a deactivation in the prefrontal cortex area. That deactivation by itself means that the executive function area of the brain is not working well. This is the area that we call the braking mechanism of the brain, where it tells you not to do this and allows you to do certain activities.

[00:14:30]

[00:15:00]

That braking mechanism is impaired, meaning that the individual will be impulsive, hyperactive, and will have very limited control of his or her behavior. That's the prefrontal cortex, and when we see a decreased activity in the prefrontal cortex, the treatment approach will be more towards stimulating the prefrontal cortex area. At times, we see that the brain already is overstimulated, especially when we see cases where the limbic system, including the basal ganglia (the limbic system and basal ganglia are basically the alarm center of the brain), when it's overactive it indicates mostly anxiety. The limbic system, when it's overactive, indicates more mood disorder.

[00:15:30]

When we see that type of activity, we pay more attention to the mood component or the anxiety component and target our treatment more first towards that type of treatment where you treat the anxiety and the mood first and then consider other areas. That has been used for 25, 30 years. The case studies in the 90s, there were a lot of case studies—Lu et al., Zeng et al., Dr. Amen has a lot of studies. There's another guy, Putt et al., he has done a lot of his work on traumatic brain injury.

[00:16:00]

[00:16:30]

I'm especially very fascinated with the traumatic brain injury and application of SPECT in mild to moderate traumatic brain injuries. In mild to moderate traumatic brain injury, you cannot determine the extent of the damage by doing an MRI or a regular scan like a CAT scan. Those are structural brain imaging, and in structural brain imaging you cannot see the impairment. In order to see the impairment in mild to moderate traumatic brain injury, the only study that can help is a functional brain imaging.

[00:17:00]

[00:17:30]

[00:18:00]

There are three different functional brain imaging: the PET scan, the functional MRI, and then there's the SPECT scan. Functional MRI is very, very expensive, it's very limited in its usage, and it's new. PET scan is also very expensive and a lot more radioactive. The only reasonable study one could do in a mild to moderate traumatic brain injury is the SPECT scan. Most of my clinical work, in the area of ADHD and the traumatic brain injury where we did a study on the NFL players, was five or six years ago, and these were NFL players that had significant traumatic brain injuries. They came in, we did a SPECT scan, we developed a protocol of treatment, we treated them, and then we did a re-SPECT on them and there was a significant improvement from baseline to posttreatment.

[00:18:30]

I was very impressed by that study, and then my own patients where I've used a lot of SPECTs imaging with the treatment response and/or lack of response for that matter. In my experience, there are several effects. One is that I see a lot in a psychiatric practice is the aggression. Almost always, we see that the individual becomes more aggressive—testosterone by itself or growth hormone by itself can make you more prone to aggression.

[00:19:00]

[00:19:30]

Aggression is one thing that we see; mood instability, because of the aggression, we commonly see it. There are some cases that physically they could get a little bit more hyperactive, physically they develop some sort of hypertrophy or swelling of the muscles. Their physical appearance changes, and that has implications on their behavior.

[00:20:00]

[00:20:30]

Sexual behavior gets impacted; gets overstimulated sexually. We also see certain other changes such as development of acne, some changes in their overall ability to focus, concentrate, and even sleep pattern could change. Those are the initial effects. Then there are long term effects after several years of using it. It becomes even more problematic, and at this point the individual has to have the steroid hormones in order just to feel normal, just to feel a normal level of energy. Initially they get energized quite a bit, and then later on when their own reproductive organs are not able to produce these hormones, they become more and more dependent on the steroid hormone. If they stop, they develop even more mood instability and depression, almost always. But if they continue to use, the complications are there.

[00:21:00] In sports, they become more aggressive in the early stages. Later on, they develop some sort of muscle weaknesses. The initial muscle strength that they develop, later on, after years of using it, is not there. There is an inheritance component in anxiety; depending on what type of anxiety we talk about. I
[00:21:30] believe that the general anxiety disorder and social phobia has a stronger genetic component in it, but other types of anxiety, for example posttraumatic stress disorder, which does have a genetic component to it, but you almost always need the environmental factor to unmask the underlying condition.

[00:22:00] In general, I believe that there is 60% to 70% genetic predisposition, and another 30% to 40%, we have to have the environmental factor that will contribute to it. PTSD almost always have to have a traumatic life experience where you feel like your life is in danger. Panic disorder, you don't see it
[00:22:30] before age 11 and 12, but then it gets more unmasked after age 11 and 12. We feel that the genetic predisposition is there but the environmental factors also play a role.

In general, I believe almost all psychiatric history has a strong genetic component to it. If the parenting
[00:23:00] style is different and the parents are aware, the parenting style is different and try to minimize exposure to anxiety-provoking situations, the more you minimize the risk factor, the less the likelihood that they will develop as a disorder. All of us have anxiety, and actually anxiety is a good thing. Anxiety
[00:23:30] protects us against danger and threats, so a person who has no anxiety is actually very problematic. We all have an alarm system in our brain, the question is that whether this anxiety becomes too excessive and out of control; that is where the problem is, that is when it turns into a disorder.

[00:24:00] The environmental factors including diet, personal development, exercise, substance abuse, relationship, friendship, social life, and parenting style, they all have an impact on the anxiety and
[00:24:30] development of the anxiety. Yes, if you implement more protective factors, then the anxiety or depression for that matter will not emerge. Depending on the age of the child, you would want to, first of all, avoid exposure to certain movies or video clips, or video games that increase the level of anxiety. So, horror movies you would want to avoid it as much as possible. In fact, I tell my patients,
[00:25:00] no, no, for kids who are 13, 14 years old. I tell them no horror movies.

Some of these kids, as they become 11, 12, 13, 14, they talk more about horror movies and so they're more inclined towards watching the horror movies. There's an excitement there, there is that adrenalin rush there, so then that will lead to insomnia and nightmares. That is, once the sleep is disrupted, a lot of things will show.

[00:25:30] Then to avoid very harsh parenting strategies that can put the child at danger of a stress axis activation. The stress axis gets activated, the child feels more threatened. Generally, these kids already
[00:26:00] feel more threatened when they start going to school. They're very threatened in their interpersonal relationships and home is the safest place for them. Then when they come home and they feel that home is also not a safe environment, the likelihood of developing anxiety disorder is very, very high. Almost always be supportive and practice certain strategies like meditation, self-relaxation, deep
[00:26:30] breathing, yoga. In some families, yoga works quite a bit for children and adolescents.

Regular exercise regimen almost always increases the serotonin level in the brain. As your serotonin
[00:27:00] levels are high, you feel less anxious. Even diet, avoiding caffeine or stimulants and increasing healthy fats, or even food that can increase your serotonin level or tryptophan level that will lead to high level of serotonin can by itself reduce the anxiety. Just avoiding gluten in a lot of families, by itself, helps
[00:27:30] prevention of the anxiety. Self-calming behaviors, deep breathing, relaxation, thought blocking. Thought blocking is the practice where the parents learn to teach the child or themselves how to block

certain negative thoughts that are too excessive and out of control.

[00:28:00] One of my biggest challenges in my practice is how to convince a child to avoid sugar and food colors. Also, they get exposed to a lot of toxic red dye, food colors … all the snacks, they almost always have food colors. Sugar is a big challenge. I almost always recommend an elimination diet for the parents and spend quite a bit of time in teaching them how to eliminate the food and then reintroduce, and

[00:28:30] then develop insight, child's insight into how that particular food is affecting. It's a big challenge, it's very difficult to control the diet of a 10, 11, 12-year-old child, because if they don't get it at home they can get it from outside and so it becomes a real big challenge. Once the child develops some insight that know this is causing this problem for me, then they will avoid it.

[00:29:00] Elimination diet is that we believe, and I think there are so many studies that have established as a diet, all what we eat, what we put in, we express that—we show that—especially when it comes to

[00:29:30] behavior and especially during our phase of development. A child or adolescent, the brain is growing really fast, and so the more nutritious your food, the less toxic your food, the better the brain will develop. What we try to eliminate a lot is sugar, gluten, and in some cases, dairy. There are times that kids may be allergic to peanuts or certain other nuts, where we kind of go with that.

[00:30:00] Sometimes the parents know themselves, but it's hard for them to implement the diet. We kind of use some different strategies and I have felt more successful when the child agrees with you. Most of the

[00:30:30] work is to educate the child and to educate the parents. So, an example: elimination of gluten. I tell kids and the parents to not take gluten for two weeks. So, you'd want to avoid anything that has gluten, going to a gluten-free diet for two weeks. Then after two weeks for lunch, take gluten containing food, pasta, or whatever it may be. Then in an hour or two, observe your behavior. Most

[00:31:00] kids would say that, "I feel sluggish and tired," or they'll say, "I feel awful," and then you're successful. Some kids will not even notice that, even if they notice, they probably minimize it. It's almost always depends on the intensity of the presentation. The intensity, the severity of the symptoms—that's a very important determinant.

[00:31:30] The second factor is the age factor. Because younger than 12 years old, the black box warning for using antidepressant is high, so you try to avoid as much as possible for kids who are younger than 12. Kids who are older than 12 and more aggressive, kids who are young adults, like 16, 17 years old,

[00:32:00] they're closer to adult life, then I'm even more aggressive. It's almost always it's their support network that they have that also is very helpful. If I see a child that doesn't have that good of a support network, the parents are not around, or the child has more of a high risk to commit suicide or to hurt themselves or someone else, that's when I go more aggressive and consider medications.

[00:32:30] Generally, I'll say here in about 75%, 80% of the cases, we consider the holistic approach. We usually try to use a supplement that increases your serotonin and norepinephrine level—there are certain

[00:33:00] supplements that can help. It all depends on the intensity of the risk factors, the risk factors for suicide, those are the things that really helps in our determination.

Sometimes we get cases that have not had any response and so we're very aggressive in our

[00:33:30] treatment. I think a child born today gets overstimulated from the beginning compared to a child born 50 years ago. So, that overstimulation by itself can cause some effect on the overall brain development.

[00:34:00] I see children one-year or younger-than-one-year-old sitting in front of the TV and watching cartoons, and so I think all of those have an impact, so clearly there's overstimulation. On the other hand, there is so much exposure to things that are very exciting and children will be more inclined towards that.

[00:34:30] An example would be access to video games. Children will sit down for hours and hours and hours and will play video games. Not only the video game, the type of video game they play will have an impact on their social, emotional, and moral development of the brain. As you're practicing that video game, you're basically activating one part of your brain. There are particular circuits that get activated or

[00:35:00] overactivated at the cost of lack of development in other areas of the brain. The other circuits in the brain that need to be developed, for example, reading would activate certain circuits, writing will activate certain circuits, social interaction will activate certain circuits. Those circuits from a developmental point of view are not activated, and so they don't develop that well.

[00:35:30] I believe the brain circuits are like muscles: the more you use those circuits, the stronger those circuits get. That's what I feel that a lack of balance and lack of exposure to different types of activities in life will eventually lead to development of certain disorders: ADHD, anxiety, or depression. The more

[00:36:00] you're educated, the more you understand what depression is, what anxiety is, what ADHD is, the better it is. The more information you have from school about the child, or from a daycare about the child, and listening to them and basically accepting their point of view, because they see the child in a

[00:36:30] different setting, they see the child with other children, so that input is very, very important, always listen to them.

One point that I always tell the parents is: the more you know your kid's friends, the better you know your child. Almost always try to know who they hang out with, who they're socializing with. The more

[00:37:00] you know your children's social setting, who they hang out with, where they go, that's very important. Educate yourself about diet, how diet could affect a child, how obesity could affect a child, in their emotional development, in their moral development, in their interpersonal development, on their self-

[00:37:30] image, all of those factors. They're things that could easily be controlled in the beginning. Obesity is, in my opinion, something that a lot of kids today struggle with, and they continue to struggle as an adult, because the eating habits don't change.

[00:38:00] All of these habit formations start from early childhood. I guess more attention to what they eat, their physical appearance, and their overall well-being is there. Sleep is another factor. A lot of adolescents struggle with falling asleep and have no energy during the day. A kid comes here is falling asleep right in front of me. When you continue to investigate, the kid pretends to be going to sleep, wakes up

[00:38:30] around 12:00, 1:00 in the morning, continues to play their video games until 4:00, 5:00 in the morning. And then they go, and they're tired for the rest of the day. Kids could be sneaking, so the more attention you pay the more you get to know them, the better. Then, bonding is a very important

[00:39:00] factor. You have to bond with your kid. If you don't have bonding, it'd be very difficult to control your child. It's a very important part.

Compatibility with your partner's parenting style is important. Try to avoid conflicts amongst each other in front of the kids, like arguing or fighting. The more you avoid that, the better it is. We have

[00:39:30] this elephant brain theory where kids who are obese, in their cognitive abilities, they suffer a lot more.

Generally, kids who are more obese are also more anxious. They're in class, they're more afraid of

[00:40:00] being teased by their peers or in school. So, they almost always have a school phobia. They try to not be exposed. Because of that, they develop a lot of challenges with focusing, attention, concentration, and memory. Anxiety also affects them. Even when they sleep, the sleep pattern, the normal breathing pattern is affected by weight.

[00:40:30] If you are overweight, your sleep architecture changes, and if you're not in a deep sleep for too long, that clearly affects you from a developmental point of view, especially when kids hit 12, 13, 14, that's when the body image becomes a very, very serious issue. The kids are already overweight. From my personal experiences, some kids will start restricting their diet or practice other types of eating

[00:41:00] disorders such as purging and eliminate certain food, use laxatives and then develop eating disorders, and that can make things even more complicated.

[00:41:30] Exercise is almost always our number one intervention. We believe that 45 minutes to an hour of cardio or aerobic exercise is as effective as taking Zoloft or Prozac for a child. That is very, very important.

CHRIS KRESSER | Founder, Kresser Institute

Dr. Mark Hyman: [00:00:30] [00:01:00]	So, Chris, welcome. You've been studying the human body for a long time, and you go deep into subjects that most people just skim over. The brain is something you really focused on as something we need to care for in specific ways to enhance its function, to reverse disease and prevent future disease. The ways you do it are pretty diverse and unique. The things that nobody talks about like being in nature, our rhythms of our biology, and using substances that are available to us through food or different kinds of dieting. I want to sort of dive into some of these specifics. We have access to our brain through the external world, through our diet, through all kinds of inputs that most people don't realize they have the power to change. Yet a lot of the things you're talking about are simple things that people can do without seeing a doctor, without having a lot of tests done, that make an enormous difference. Let's start in with diet because it's something that people have easy access to, and it's a doorway to the brain that most people don't access. So, tell us about how you use diet—things like ketogenic diets, fasting, other foods—to actually enhance brain function.
Chris Kresser: [00:01:30] [00:02:00] [00:02:30]	Great. Thanks again for having me. It's always a pleasure to talk to you. I mean, at the fundamental level, the brain is so important because it's the mediator of our entire experience of the world. Everything that we experience, every thought we have, every feeling, every sensation that we have is mediated by the brain. If the brain is not healthy, you know, nothing will work well. I always start with the basics. The basics are really easy to overlook. It's easy to focus on supplements and all the sort of hacks and advanced tricks that you can do to support your brain, but that's all pretty worthless if you're not doing the basics. So, diet is often the starting place, as you pointed out. First of all, just a really nutrient-dense diet is, I think, the most important thing. The brain needs a variety of nutrients to function properly, and these include B12, B6, folate, DHA, choline, zinc, and copper. All of these play a really vital role in the brain. Studies show that a significant number of Americans and people in the industrialized world, and in the developing world, are deficient in these nutrients. We have a diet that's dense in calories, and rich in calories, but really poor in nutrients.
Dr. Mark Hyman:	Yeah.
Chris Kresser:	So that's, I think, the first thing.
Dr. Mark Hyman:	Yeah, I think that people don't realize. People have a very high-calorie and nutrient-poor diet, so it's calorie-dense, nutrient-poor. The question is what is a nutrient-dense diet?
Chris Kresser: [00:03:00]	Yes, that's a great question because there's a lot of misconceptions out there. I think people, when they think of nutrient density, the first thing they think of is vegetables, perhaps. Certainly, vegetables are very nutrient-dense, particularly in phytochemicals and things like that. But when you consider essential nutrients like the vitamins and minerals that I just mentioned, as well as fatty acids, most people might be surprised to learn that animal products tend to be more nutrient-dense even than vegetables in that case. Particularly organ meats and shellfish.
Dr. Mark Hyman:	Liver.
Chris Kresser: [00:03:30]	Liver. You know, you always hear me talking about liver. But, any organ meat, and shellfish as well, are super, super nutrient-dense. So just like a three-ounce serving of oysters, for example, one time per week, will meet your entire dietary need for copper and zinc for that week. If you're talking about bang for your buck, organ meats and shellfish are super nutrient-dense.

Dr. Mark Hyman:	Most people think that those meats are protein only.
Chris Kresser:	Right.
Dr. Mark Hyman: [00:04:00]	But they're actually very rich in minerals, and vitamins, and antioxidants.
Chris Kresser:	They think they're protein, or they think they're just big blobs of saturated fat that should be avoided, because of all the fat phobia that we've had for so many years. Unfortunately, that's transitioning, I think, at this point.
Dr. Mark Hyman:	Thanks to you.
Chris Kresser:	And you, and many other people. But these foods are really nutrient-dense and should be a part of a healthy diet, and of course includes vegetables, fruits, whole fruits, nuts, seeds, and a wide variety of plants. So that's number one.
[00:04:30]	But beyond that, and beyond what I hope are the obvious steps like removing processed and refined foods, and sugar, and minimizing stuff that comes in a bag or a box, which really comprises the majority of what many Americans are eating these days ...
Dr. Mark Hyman:	And it's not just because they make you fat, it's because they're neurotoxins.
Chris Kresser: [00:05:00]	They're neurotoxins and they're totally depleted in nutrients. Again, they're high in calories. You know, we're well fed, but we're starving for nutrients. That's another way to put it. The more empty calories that we eat that don't have nutrients in them, the worse our brain is going to function. So that's the basic level.
[00:05:30]	But then there are some tweaks or hacks that we can do with diet that can potentially prevent and reverse neurodegenerative conditions. So, someone that's already starting to suffer from neurodegeneration like early onset dementia, Parkinson's—things like that—and even for healthy people, these can increase brain function. One of them is a ketogenic diet.
Dr. Mark Hyman:	What is that?
Chris Kresser: [00:06:00]	Ketones are produced when we restrict the intake of carbohydrates, and to a lesser degree, protein. These ketones substitute for glucose as a fuel source for the brain. And the brain ... There's quite a bit of evidence that suggests that the brain actually prefers ketones to glucose as a fuel source. That's especially true when people have conditions that inhibit the brain's ability to use glucose. This has been referred to as Type 3 Diabetes, where the brain's use of glucose is impaired, and then ketones can substitute for that glucose and make the brain function better.
[00:06:30]	We have a lot of studies now that show that the ketogenic diet improves mitochondrial function in the brain. It increases GABA signaling, which is a major neural transmitter. It increases the expression of something called glutamate synthase, which mops up extra glutamate, which is an excitatory neurotransmitter that can cause harm if there's too much of it in the brain. These ketones have, in some cases, a pretty miraculous effect in conditions like epilepsy or, again, Parkinson's, dementia, and Alzheimer's.
	When healthy people do a ketogenic diet, what they often report is increased feelings of mental clarity, focus and attention, and just feeling a sense of alertness that they haven't felt in years, or maybe have never felt in their entire life.
Dr. Mark Hyman: [00:07:00]	Yeah, that's so true. I'm a physician seeing patients and I've used this therapeutically in patients with dementia who came out of fog and were able to converse, remember things. I've done it with autism, kids who are violent and very disruptive. It dramatically changed their behavior. And in Parkinson's ... you just see the power of food as a drug.

Chris Kresser: [00:07:30]	Yes.
Dr. Mark Hyman:	So, most people think of food as just energy I'm eating to get energy. But they don't realize, by understanding the nuances of how to use diet as a drug, that you can either help, treat, prevent, or even reverse many common problems. Everything from depression to anxiety to autism to ADD, Alzheimer's to Parkinson's. And, you know, we don't use it. I mean, it's being used clinically in epilepsy, you mentioned. It's being researched in Alzheimer's. Even in brain cancer. It's seen to reverse brain cancer.
Chris Kresser: [00:08:00]	Mm-hmm.
Dr. Mark Hyman:	Yes. A very powerful tool. So, tell us about this concept of fasting because it's kind of a unique thing that most people would never want to do, which is, "Why would I not want to eat," you know?
Chris Kresser:	Right. Here we've been talking about the importance of nutrients, and food, and inputs. Now we're talking about not having any inputs at all. It seems counterintuitive but ...
Dr. Mark Hyman:	I'd just get hangry.
Chris Kresser: [00:08:30] [00:09:00]	Right. Well, you do at first, especially if you're not used to fasting. But actually, over time, when you become accustomed to fasting, that initial period of discomfort gets shorter and more manageable. But the reason fasting works ... There are several reasons that it works for brain function. One is that it's the fastest way of getting into ketosis. So not only ... When you're fasting, you're not only restricting fat and protein, you're restricting carbohydrate, and that's what starts ketone generation. Second thing is it upregulates a process called autophagy, which is like a cellular cleanup and repair process.
Dr. Mark Hyman:	Like the garbage truck.
Chris Kresser:	The garbage truck of the cells. The interesting thing is, if you think about it from an evolutionary perspective, human beings often had periods of food scarcity where they were fasting. You know, probably involuntary—not something they were choosing to do—but we evolved in that environment and so our bodies come to expect these periods of food scarcity and even depend on them, perhaps, for these important cellular repair and clean up processes.
Dr. Mark Hyman: [00:09:30]	Mm-hmm.
Chris Kresser: [00:10:00]	Third thing that fasting does is it upregulates stem cell generation. It actually can create completely new cells. If you're suffering from any kind of neurodegenerative condition, this is absolutely crucial. The reality is, after about age 40, all of us are suffering from neurodegeneration. The question is just to what degree. So, if we do things like fasting and ketogenic diet ... It doesn't have to be all the time. I'm not, you know ... Obviously you can't fast all the time. You're not going to make it very long if you do. But cyclical periods of fasting and ketosis. So, for example ...
Dr. Mark Hyman:	Do you mean completely no food?
Chris Kresser: [00:10:30]	There are different ways to do it. I don't generally recommend pure water fasts because they can cause cramps and electrolyte imbalance, and they're often really difficult for people to do. But a bone broth fast can be a really good option because the broth contains a lot of minerals—phosphorus and magnesium—things that can help prevent the cramping and the discomfort. Another popular option these days is called a fat fast. You eat maybe 400 calories per day of pure fat in the form of medium-

chain triglyceride, or MCT, or even exogenous ketones that you can buy now over the counter and supplement with, or perhaps just some coconut oil in your coffee.

Dr. Mark Hyman: Like Bulletproof Coffee, yeah.

Chris Kresser:
[00:11:00]
You know, like a Bulletproof Coffee type of thing. This can help to take the edge off the hunger a little bit, but it also speeds up ketone generation because you've got more fat coming in, and this fat makes it easier to get into ketosis, so it can help you get through that uncomfortable period more easily.

Dr. Mark Hyman: So, it's a fat fast that makes you skinny.

Chris Kresser: Absolutely. And it totally amplifies your brain power at the same time.

Dr. Mark Hyman:
[00:11:30]
So, you know, there are different ways of fasting and we're going to talk about the concept, but let's get a little more granular about different ways of fasting. Most people probably hearing this are going, "I'm not going to stop eating." Do you do it for an hour, for a day, for a week?

Chris Kresser:

[00:12:00]

[00:12:30]
There are so many different ways of fasting, but I'll cover the ones that are most popular and I think are most effective. One is called intermittent fasting. There has been a lot of research and media attention on this lately. Intermittent fasting can take many forms. It can be an alternative day fast, so you eat one day, you don't eat the next day. But the form that seems to be most doable for most people is compressed food intake. It means you only eat food in an eight-hour period during each day. So, you eat between 12 p.m., let's say, and 8 p.m. That means you're doing a 16-hour fast from 8 p.m. until 12 p.m. the next day. You're doing an intermittent fast each day. You're skipping breakfast, essentially, not eating until noon. But during that morning period, you could, if you wanted to, have some coffee, for example, or tea with some fat in it just to help with the ketone generation and to help take the edge off the hunger. So that's one way.

Dr. Mark Hyman: So, no more Häagen-Dazs before bed?

Chris Kresser:

[00:13:00]

[00:13:30]
No more Häagen-Dazs before bed and no bagel with cream cheese when you wake up. Then there are more extended fasts. These can last anywhere from one day to seven or even 14 days. You know, three-day fasts have become more popular. I see more and more people trying these. In some ways it can be more difficult though, because the hardest day when you're fasting is the second day, typically. That's when you really start to be hangry, as you suggested. You know, the hunger gets intense, and especially if you're not used to it, it can be really challenging. But by the third day, most people report feeling an elevated mood, heightened clarity, focus, attention. They start to actually really enjoy it. So, if you end on the third day, you're kind of like continually getting past the hardest part of the fast and less of the benefit and the enjoyment from it.

If people are going to do seven-day fasts, it's generally better to do it under the supervision of a physician because there are ... Especially if they have kind of a low body mass index, because there are some issues.

Dr. Mark Hyman: Maybe you're skinny, like you and I.

Chris Kresser:
[00:14:00]
Yes, exactly. There's something called refeeding syndrome that can happen once you start to eat again. It involves an electrolyte imbalance and it's pretty rare, but it can happen in people who are really skinny, who do an extended fast. If you're overweight, there's less of a concern and it can really help with weight loss, of course, too. You generally lose about half a pound of fat a day when you're fasting. So that's another benefit of fasting is the metabolic reset. If we now are understanding brain conditions to be ...

Dr. Mark Hyman: For diabetes.

Chris Kresser: [00:14:30]	Not just for diabetes, for your brain, because now we understand that a lot of brain conditions, neurodegeneration is caused by metabolic problems. If you're hitting the reset button on metabolism, that's going to have big benefits for the brain.
Dr. Mark Hyman:	Great. Let's talk about something else you share that's not too common in a medical prescription, which is being in nature.
Chris Kresser:	Yes.
Dr. Mark Hyman:	Why is that important, and how does it affect our brain?
Chris Kresser: [00:15:00]	Well, again, if you think about it from an evolutionary perspective, humanoids have been around for about two million years. That's 66,000 generations.
Dr. Mark Hyman:	Way before there were skyscrapers.
Chris Kresser: [00:15:30]	Way before iPhones and skyscrapers and, you know, working inside. We spent most of our time outside and we lived in nature, a natural environment with the natural rhythm of night and dark, and slept outside. Really you could say nature is hardwired into our DNA. Fast forward to today, when the majority of people spend the majority of their time indoors, completely disconnected from the natural environment. What studies are showing now, is that spending time in nature downregulates or dials down the prefrontal cortex, which is like the command center of the brain. So, it basically allows us to step away from that command and control kind of mentality, it relaxes that prefrontal cortex, and allows the brain to rest. That's probably the easiest way to think about it.
[00:16:00]	There's actually even a term now that's been coined called nature-deficit disorder. It's rampant, especially in kids. It's thought to be a risk factor for ADHD and autism spectrum disorders, and all kinds of other brain and neurodegenerative conditions in both kids and adults. I think it's really important and often overlooked.
Dr. Mark Hyman:	It's great, you were mentioning your kid goes to a forest school.
Chris Kresser:	She goes to a forest school.
Dr. Mark Hyman:	Where you go in the forest and you just play and have fun?
Chris Kresser: [00:16:30]	That's right, yes. Which is what kids at that age should be doing. She's almost six.
Dr. Mark Hyman:	I mean, it had a huge impact on me when I was a kid. I went on canoe trips, I was riding horses outside, I was camping, I was being in nature a lot of the time, and it really, I think, imprinted on me, that as a therapy.
Chris Kresser:	Absolutely.
Dr. Mark Hyman:	And, for me, it's kind of my go-to therapy.
Chris Kresser: [00:17:00]	They're now doing that with kids who have ADHD, depression, anxiety, and other behavioral problems. They're sending them essentially on camping trips where they don't take any technology. They're not allowed to play video games, they disconnect from their phone. The first few days are really hard for the kids, but then all of the kids almost unanimously report feeling a sense of calm and well-being that they haven't felt possibly ever in their life. They want to go back and they want to keep doing it, so it's really powerful.

Expert Interviews – Chris Kresser

© 2017 Hyman Digital. All Rights Reserved.

Dr. Mark Hyman: [00:17:30]	So, there's something else that you sort of talked about, which is sort of related to this, which is this concept of circadian rhythm and how that plays a role on our brain, in our hormones, in our neurotransmitters, which is basically how we live in rhythm or out of rhythm. Can you talk about that and the brain?
Chris Kresser: [00:18:00]	Yes. This is really fascinating because it goes way back, way before humans, actually all the way back to the first single-celled organism that evolved on this planet. We're talking about billions of years here. Every organism that ever came to be on this planet evolved in the 24-hour light and dark cycle that we have on planet Earth. So, every cell of every organism is entrained to that 24/7 light dark cycle. We now know that, in humans, that light-dark cycle affects every aspect of our physiology, from our endocrine system, our hormones, to our brain function, to our metabolism, everything.
Dr. Mark Hyman:	Sleep.
Chris Kresser:	Sleep. Of course, sleep.
Dr. Mark Hyman:	Most importantly.
Chris Kresser: [00:18:30] [00:19:00] [00:19:30]	Most importantly, sleep. So, what happens, you know, essentially our bodies are hardwired to expect a period of light followed by a period of darkness. When we wake up in the morning, our bodies start producing cortisol, which is a kind of like a get-up-and-go hormone. And then when night falls it starts producing melatonin, which helps us to fall asleep and stay asleep. So, the problem is now, you know, in the last 150 years, we've developed artificial light, which is awesome. It allows us to be more productive and, you know, entertainment and art and all kinds of things are possible with artificial light that weren't before. But the downside of that is now we can sit in our bed at 11pm staring at our iPad, which is emitting blue light, the same spectrum of light that the sun emits, and that basically tells your body it's time to wake up, time to get the cortisol production going. And then the melatonin drops totally messing with your circadian rhythm, and then that can have downstream effects like increasing the risk of obesity and metabolic disease, increasing the risk of depression and anxiety, seasonal affective disorder. We know even that flight personnel and people who do shift work are at much higher risk for cancer.
Dr. Mark Hyman:	And heart disease.
Chris Kresser:	And heart disease.
Dr. Mark Hyman:	Diabetes.
Chris Kresser:	So, it just affects our immune system, our cardiovascular system, everything. So, getting closer to that natural rhythm of light and dark is really important. It doesn't mean we all have to live in a tent in the back yard ...
Dr. Mark Hyman:	Can we put a mattress in it?
Chris Kresser: [00:20:00] [00:20:30]	You could do that if you want. I mean, actually it would be really good for you. But we can do things like, for example, if we have to use a computer at night, there are now glasses that you can buy that filter out the blue light that comes from those screens, or even if you're watching TV. So, if you came to my house at night, you'd see my wife and I wearing these funny glasses with kind of an orange tint that filters that light out. You can take steps to try not to use electronic media within an hour or an hour and a half of bedtime, because that has that effect that I just described. And then get some bright light exposure during the day. So, if you work in an office or in an indoor environment, make sure to go outside for a walk at lunchtime, or in the morning take a walk, with no sunglasses. Make sure you let that light hit your retina and stimulate that cortisol production.

Dr. Mark Hyman:	It's basically like candle therapy. When the sun goes down, switch to candles, get off your screens.
Chris Kresser:	Absolutely.
Dr. Mark Hyman:	And if you can, wear those funny glasses.
Chris Kresser:	Yeah. Turn the lights down, get some mood lighting, and yeah.
Dr. Mark Hyman:	Yes.
Chris Kresser: [00:21:00]	And then, you know, it's pretty widely recognized now, which is why even computer operating systems now, like, the latest update for Mac (High Sierra), their latest operating system has something called night shift. A lot of people might not even know that this is on their computer, but when you turn night shift on, what happens is when the sun goes down, the type of light that's emitted from the screen changes. It becomes warmer, which is meant to mimic more of a kind of light that you would be exposed to at night, not during the day time.
Dr. Mark Hyman: [00:21:30]	Yes.
Chris Kresser:	So, this is really well-established research. It's gone so far that computer makers are now incorporating this into the operating systems.
Dr. Mark Hyman:	And now we have these LED lights and fluorescent lights that we're exposed to all the time and have a huge impact. Cleveland Clinic—we created a clinic that is meeting environmental standards and also health standards.
Chris Kresser:	Right.
Dr. Mark Hyman:	So, we actually changed the lighting.
Chris Kresser:	It doesn't look like a hospital when you go in there.
Dr. Mark Hyman: [00:22:00]	No. We changed the air fluctuation, we changed the materials that are in there to actually optimize well-being. We know we can actually access the brain through all these external inputs: light, sound, music, touch, taste, and environment. All those things are really powerful doorways ...
Chris Kresser:	So important.
Dr. Mark Hyman:	... that we can access the brain, that we don't even utilize as brain therapy.
Chris Kresser:	Absolutely.
Dr. Mark Hyman: [00:22:30]	So, this is really pretty exciting research. Let's talk about ways of ... Besides the obvious, which, you know, we've talked about diet. Exercise we didn't chat about, but it's a powerful tool. Meditation. I want to get into some of the hacks you talk about, some of the doorways ... Given all the stresses of our life, given the deficiencies in certain activities or nutrients, how do we use substances that are available to us through diet or through supplements to actually optimize brain function?
Chris Kresser: [00:23:00]	Right. So, this has been an area of pretty intense study and also experimentation within the biohacker community. There's a new class of nutraceuticals, you know, supplements, herbs, and nutrients that provide a kind of therapeutic effect called nootropics. These are things that have been shown to improve cognitive function or have some effect on some aspect of brain health like mood. I mean, it's a huge topic. There are so many potential things we could talk about, but I'm just going to mention a few of them that I've found to be the most helpful with my patients and with my own experimentation.

[00:23:30] So, one is choline. Now choline is a very important substance found ... You know, that we need in our brain. It's sometimes referred to as a B vitamin. It has important effects in the brain, but it's importantly a precursor to acetylcholine.

Dr. Mark Hyman: Which is a neurotransmitter.

Chris Kresser: So, acetylcholine is a neurotransmitter that is really heavily involved in attention and concentration and focus.

Dr. Mark Hyman: And by the way, it's what goes down in Alzheimer's.

Chris Kresser: [00:24:00] Absolutely. It goes down in Alzheimer's and you see ... It's involved with memory and cognition in general. We want to keep our acetylcholine levels high, and taking choline as a supplement is one way to do that. Of course, choline is also in liver, egg yolks, and many other foods, but if all of that's not working and you need an additional boost, choline can be really helpful. There are many different kinds of choline and ways to supplement with it. For the brain, I think the most effective form is Alpha-
[00:24:30] GPC, which is a form of choline that's been shown to very easily enter the brain and have a bigger impact on acetylcholine levels. So that's number one.

Number two is there's a whole class of acetams like Piracetam, which is similar to an amino acid called pyroglutamate. What it does is it increases the activity between neurons. Neurons are always sending messages back and forth, and if you increase that activity, you sort of enhance the cognitive function of the brain. Piracetam does that. It's generally better, I've found. One side effect of Piracetam that can happen is headaches, mild headaches. Those are generally mitigated or alleviated if you take the Alpha-GPC or choline with the Piracetam.

[00:25:00]

[00:25:30] Another one is Noopept, which is a peptide that inhibits glutamate synthesis. It basically increases the availability of glutamate in the brain. So, glutamate is an excitatory neurotransmitter. It's one of those Goldilocks things. You don't want too much of it, but you don't want too little of it either.

Dr. Mark Hyman: One of the main drugs for Alzheimer's blocks the effects of glutamine, because it overexcites the brain creating inflammation and brain damage.

Chris Kresser: [00:26:00] Yes. Overexciting the brain. So, I think you need to be ... I should have mentioned this in the beginning, but all of these things are, you know, they have different effects on different people. I encourage people, if they're going to do these things, it's probably best to do them under supervision if they can. But if they are going to try them, to take it slowly. You know, start with a really low dose. Try only one thing at a time. A lot of people will stack nootropics. They'll take three or four of them together that all
[00:26:30] have slightly different but complementary effects to try to get the best effect, and that's not a bad thing if you are already familiar with the individual effects of each of them. That's the caveat I should have mentioned from the beginning.

Dr. Mark Hyman: To start slow and build.

Chris Kresser: Start slow and use one thing at a time until you figure out how it affects you, and then you can add other things in.

Dr. Mark Hyman: Are these medications or supplements?

Chris Kresser: These are supplements that are available over the counter. And then, you know, plain old caffeine, actually, and coffee, they're both ... They're not technically nootropics because they're stimulants, but they have nootropic effects. Caffeine, for example ... I mean, it has many effects, but one of the big ones is it increases dopamine production. Dopamine is another important neurotransmitter in the
[00:27:00] brain, and that one regulates what we call executive function. Attention and focus, and even motivation, are strongly influenced by dopamine. So those are four that fall into that nootropic

category that can be helpful.

Dr. Mark Hyman: Let's just talk about the caffeine and the coffee for a minute. You know, there's evidence that it
[00:27:30] depletes adenosine, which is the energy in the cells, that it depletes over time and adrenaline. So, you get this spike in these stimulatory hormones or neurotransmitters and then you crash, which is actually my experience, you know? When I went to medical school, I started drinking coffee. I would notice every afternoon about three of four, I would just want to fall asleep. I connected it to the coffee. How do you explain that where you're kind of artificially boosting these things and then you crash?

[00:28:00]

Chris Kresser: So, we can speak in general terms and then individual terms. I think that's always important when we're discussing any of these topics. If you look at the research on caffeine, overall, it's very positive, I think. There are some areas, like you mentioned, that raised potential for concern, but when you look at the research on a kind of net basis, you see positive outcomes with mild to moderate caffeine or
[00:28:30] coffee consumption. Because it's not just the caffeine, it's also the antioxidants and the other compounds in the plant.

Dr. Mark Hyman: Yeah. I mean, coffee, sadly, is the number one source of antioxidants in the American diet.

Chris Kresser: Right. For most people, yeah. So, I think coffee on the whole can have a positive effect, but that's if it can be tolerated by the individual person. We now know that there are a lot of genetic polymorphism and factors that influence how we metabolize caffeine. One person might be what we call a slow
[00:29:00] metabolizer. These are the people, like me, and perhaps like you, that if I have coffee after 12pm, my sleep is tanked for that night. I'm not going to sleep at all. And yet, there are also fast metabolizers. These are people like my dad who can drink a cup of coffee after dinner and go to sleep and not have a problem. So, there's a wide variation in how people respond to caffeine, and I think you have to ... You don't necessarily need to know your gene status, you just ... You figure out, you know, kind of on your own.

Dr. Mark Hyman: Yeah, sure.
[00:29:30]

Chris Kresser: If you drink coffee and you're like this, and you can't sleep, and you're crashing in the afternoon, it's probably not going to work for you.

Dr. Mark Hyman: Yes.

Chris Kresser: And that's the same for any of the other nootropics that I mentioned, you know? Some people take Piracetam and feel really jittery and amped up, and it doesn't work for them, whereas they do better with choline, and for other people it's the opposite.

Dr. Mark Hyman: I always say the best doctor is your own body.

Chris Kresser: That's right.

Dr. Mark Hyman: ... Because it's going to tell you what works and what doesn't work if you listen to it.

Chris Kresser: It's got the final word.

Dr. Mark Hyman: Yeah.
[00:30:00]

Chris Kresser: You can have all the best theories, but if your body doesn't respond then it doesn't matter.

Dr. Mark Hyman:

[00:30:30]

So, you know, in my own practice I've noticed that when I treat people's digestive system, their brain gets better, whether it's autism, Alzheimer's, Parkinson's, or MS. Particularly we're now learning that depression and mood disorders, which we often thought were emotional, are maybe physical, and that the key doorway might be the gut. Depression we're learning may be an inflammatory disorder. Like the brain might be inflamed from various factors. So, talk to us about the gut and these mood disorders, and how we can think about what we can do.

Chris Kresser:

[00:31:00]

[00:31:30]

It's really interesting because I feel like a lot of what we're doing in modern medicine is rediscovering things that we have known for a long time. 2,000 years ago, Hippocrates said, "All disease begins in the gut," right? All the way back then, he knew something about that. And then even in the US, in the 1930s, there were a couple of researchers, physicians, at Duke University - Stokes and Pillsbury, who wrote a seminal paper explaining the gut, brain, skin axis, and the connection between disruption of the gut microbiome. There wasn't the term microbiome at that point, but they were talking about Lactobacillus, you know, low levels of Lactobacillus and Bifidobacteria, and conditions like depression or anxiety, and also skin stuff, which we won't go into. This was in the 1930s.

Dr. Mark Hyman:

Like almost 90 years ago.

Chris Kresser:

[00:32:00]

Almost 90 years ago, and then we lost that thread for, you know, many, many decades. But in the last 10 or 20 years, the gut-brain access has been a really hot topic in the research literature, and even now in popular media. I think a lot of people have heard that there's a connection between the microbes that inhabit our gut and our brain, that things like intestinal permeability or leaky gut, when the gut barrier breaks down, that can cause problems with our brain, and it may be connected to conditions like autism spectrum disorder and ADHD.

[00:32:30]

And then as you mentioned, the most current theory on what causes depression is known as the inflammatory cytokine model of depression. That's a fancy way of saying that when our gut becomes inflamed, it produces chemicals that travel through the bloodstream, cross our blood brain barrier, and suppress the activity in the frontal cortex. And that produces all of the telltale signs and symptoms of depression.

Dr. Mark Hyman:

They should be taking Advil for a depression?

Chris Kresser:

[00:33:00]

Absolutely not. That's actually going to make the gut worse over the long term. We know that Advil can cause ulcers and a whole bunch of other problems in the gut. But what we should be doing is tending to our diet. You know, diet is a crucial factor for gut health. If we eat a lot of heavily processed and refined foods, that causes a pro inflammatory microbiota, which means it feeds pathogenic bacteria and bad bugs. It allows them to proliferate and then they produce compounds that can be toxic to the brain.

Dr. Mark Hyman:

[00:33:30]

[00:34:00]

I'm going to stop you there for a minute. There's fascinating research on the different types of molecules that get produced by bacteria. In our diet we have high levels of probiotic acid, which is toxic to the brain, and it's been linked to autism and many other conditions. Most people are not aware that any bran products they eat, or flour products, have high levels of probiotic acid because it's a preservative. It's put in there. So, when you eat at a fast food restaurant, eat processed bread ... I mean, if you make bread yourself, that is different, but it's a very common ingredient. We're ... huge levels. And the good products that come from healthy bacteria called butyrate actually heal the brain. We're not even aware of what we're doing to our brains by the food we eat and it's so connected. And yet, you know, just cutting out all processed foods and cutting out all fast foods and refined grains, can have a huge impact.

Chris Kresser: [00:34:30] [00:35:00]	Mm-hmm. And then eating prebiotic foods. You know, these are foods that can be fermented by our beneficial bacteria, like Bifidobacteria that produce the butyrate that you mentioned is really important. There's been a big decline in the consumption of these foods that can be fermented, fermentable carbohydrates. These would be things like onions and garlic, Jerusalem artichokes, some starchy plants, some nuts and seeds. They're all whole foods. They're all foods with fibers that can be fermented by our gut bacteria. These fibers are really important because we can't digest them. We don't extract any nutrients from them, but the gut bacteria living ... You know, the hundred trillion bacteria or microorganisms living in our gut can. So, every bite of food that we put in our mouth, we need to think of how it nourishes us and how it nourishes our bacterial community, because feeding both of those systems is equally important.
Dr. Mark Hyman:	Historically, we eat a lot of fermented foods because that's how we preserve things.
Chris Kresser:	Absolutely.
Dr. Mark Hyman:	Sauerkraut, kimchi, and these foods that are ways of preserving foods that otherwise would go bad.
Chris Kresser:	That's right. And if you look at hunter-gatherers, they consume on average—in many cases—over 100 different plant species. You know, for Americans, it's like six or seven.
Dr. Mark Hyman:	Yeah.
Chris Kresser: [00:35:30]	Tomatoes and lettuce on burgers, you know, maybe carrots and a few others, and that's it. So, when you have that lack of diversity of fiber and plant foods, your gut bacteria isn't going to work as well.
Dr. Mark Hyman:	Historically, you know, the original data on this was from Dr. Dennis Burke who went to Africa and found that the average hunter-gatherer's stool weight was two pounds, and the average stool weight of the industrialized group that was living in the cities was like four ounces. You know, we eat about eight grams of fiber on average—maybe 15 if you're good—in America, and, you know, we need over 100 grams of fiber, which is a lot.
Chris Kresser: [00:36:00]	They're eating over 100, and most of the dry weighted stool is bacteria. That's exactly what explains why their stool weighs more, because it's full of these beneficial bacteria.

So, then there are other conditions. We know that infections like H. pylori, parasites ... There have been some peer-reviewed published studies connecting fungal overgrowth in the gut, which used to be looked at as a sort of ... |
Dr. Mark Hyman:	Wacky.
Chris Kresser: [00:36:30]	... quacky, wacky condition, but there was a study associating it with inflammatory bowel disease. I recently saw a study connecting it with worse outcomes and alcoholic liver disease. They're starting to come out and say, "Okay, everyone does have yeast and a digestive tract, that's normal. But what happens when the bacteria that protect against the proliferation of that yeast become depleted?" Or if you have an infection or you're eating foods that that yeast thrives on, then this yeast becomes ...
Dr. Mark Hyman:	Sugar.
Chris Kresser: [00:37:00]	Yeah, exactly. And that's how wine is made, you know? We know this. So, if you have an overgrowth of yeast in the digestive tract, that's when things can become problematic. Yeast produces aldehydes and other chemicals that can literally make us feel like we're drunk.
Dr. Mark Hyman:	Yes.

Dr. Mark Hyman:	There are actually cases and reports of people who had high blood alcohol levels from eating too much sugar and flour that led to the fermentation of starches in their gut that really produced alcohol, and they absorbed it, and they got arrested for drunk driving.
Chris Kresser: [00:37:30]	Right. Right. And I know you see this in your practice, but I see a lot of kids with yeast overgrowth, because kids these days are eating a lot of sugar and processed and refined food, they're not eating whole nutrient-dense foods. Guess what, these kids have behavior problems, they have mood issues, they are not able to even attend school in many cases because of this. When we treat the gut and we deal with the fungal overgrowth and the dysbiosis ...
Dr. Mark Hyman:	They get better.
Chris Kresser:	... you can see remarkable changes.
Dr. Mark Hyman:	Yes.
Chris Kresser: [00:38:00]	You can see kids going from being almost non-verbal to speaking. You know, physical contact becomes a possibility where it wasn't before. You get kids ...
Dr. Mark Hyman:	They look in your eyes.
Chris Kresser:	They look in your eyes. You get kids getting off of these Ritalin and other stimulants, and being able to actually participate in their lives. I mean, it's amazing.
Dr. Mark Hyman:	It is amazing, yeah.
Chris Kresser:	And it's all just with the gut, you know, diet and focusing on the gut.
Dr. Mark Hyman:	Chris, you're a practicing clinician and you treat patients.
Chris Kresser:	Yes.
Dr. Mark Hyman: [00:38:30]	You're not just making up all these theories, but you're connecting what you see in the clinic with the research, and then you implement therapies that aren't typical. I'd love you to share maybe a few case stories, patients who you've approached this way, through a different doorway into the brain, and what kind of outcomes you've seen.
Chris Kresser: [00:39:00]	Yeah. So, a couple of years ago I had an 86-year-old woman who was ... She had a diagnosis of dementia and early onset Alzheimer's. Her family members brought her in. She was living with her daughter and her daughter's husband. They had kind of reached the end of their rope, you know? They went through what most patients with Alzheimer's go through. They'd have a really expensive battery of tests and then the doctor says, "I'm sorry, there's nothing we can do. Here's a drug. And by the way, that drug has not been proven to even slow the progression of Alzheimer's, much less reverse it. And good luck," you know? I mean, that's essentially the play.
Dr. Mark Hyman:	Get your affairs in order.
Chris Kresser: [00:39:30] [00:40:00]	Yeah, get your affairs in order and seek out some help for the family members, and that's it. These people weren't, you know, didn't want to accept that, understandably. So, they were seeking out other approaches, and they came to see me. First thing I did was I put her on a ketogenic diet, which is what I often do in patients with neurodegenerative disorders. She, you know, until that time, was eating a pretty standard American diet. A lot of flour and bread. She loved cookies and cakes and things like that. So, it was difficult for her to make that transition, but her family, since she was living with her family, they made that easier. And within ... I got a call from her daughter a couple of weeks later saying, "I don't even recognize ... This is like my mom used to be. I haven't seen this person in 10

years." Her memory was better, she could actually ... You know, her short-term memory improved. She was able to function in a way that she hadn't been able to. She was able to take care of herself. And this was just by doing a ketogenic diet.

[00:40:30] And then we started to add in some additional cognitive supports. Some of the things that we talked about earlier—as well as some herbs like ginkgo, bacopa, and ashwagandha, that increase glutathione levels in the brain and are neuroprotective and actually can reverse amyloid—you know, can actually get rid of some amyloid formation. Then she started to improve further. She was already fairly far
[00:41:00] along the progression; she didn't recover completely, but she's still doing well years later. She's still doing that program and she hasn't progressed any further.

Dr. Mark Hyman: Which is unheard of.

Chris Kresser: Unheard of. Completely unheard of. The second case that comes to mind is a child with pretty severe behavioral disorders. He would basically have, you know ... It was really, really hard for his parents.
[00:41:30] Like even something like his shoes not being tied correctly would send him like into a complete fit, spasm, you know, tantrum on the floor, beating the floor, you know, which was really problematic if they ever tried to go anywhere. He wouldn't use the bathroom anywhere outside of the house, so that really limited ... He couldn't go to school for that reason, or they had to go pick him up at school and
[00:42:00] bring him home during the day. He was very sensitive to any kind of contact. This is now referred to as sensory processing disorder. So certain types of clothing on his skin, or even physical contact, would send him into a tail spin.

I did a whole work-up, mostly focusing on the gut, and found that he had significant fungal overgrowth. He had a condition called SIBO, which is an overgrowth of bacteria in the small intestine where it shouldn't be. He had disrupted gut microbiome. He had a lot of food intolerances. He was gluten intolerant. He was still eating gluten, but he was also intolerant of dairy and eggs and other food proteins. So, we cleaned up his diet. We treated him with herbs and supplements for the fungal
[00:42:30] overgrowth. We used prebiotics and probiotics to support beneficial protective bacteria, and within a month and a half of that, he was already coming off of the psychoactive drugs that he was taking. The psychiatrist called and said, "What did you do to this kid? I don't even recognize him." They got a call
[00:43:00] from the teacher at school saying, "Where is this kid? Have you sent his twin brother?" because they'd never seen him operate in this way, and be able to get along with his peers, and actually go use the bathroom at school, and start to be able to function like a normal kid.

This was just with some pretty simple dietary changes and some supplements and botanicals that you can buy over the counter, and probiotics and prebiotics to support gut health. So, again, this kid would have been on a lifetime of medications. He was already in the situation that a lot of people are in, where they take one medication and that causes side effects, so then they need to take another
[00:43:30] medication to deal with the side effects of that drug. He was already starting that treadmill. Most kids, unfortunately, in that situation, are facing a lifetime of that, just escalating more and more and more. It's so sad, but it's ... Like the most rewarding part of my work is being able to help a kid in that way.

Dr. Mark Hyman: Yes, I see this all the time. You know, what's striking is that we often think of these things as
[00:44:00] behavioral disorders, but they're biological disorders that are caused by various insults irritating the brain and inflaming the brain.

Chris Kresser: Yes.

Dr. Mark Hyman: When you take away all the stuff that's bothering them and you put in some food stuff, it's dramatic. It can happen very quickly, like in days or weeks.

Chris Kresser: Absolutely.

Dr. Mark Hyman: [00:44:30]	You know, I do recall a number of my patients who had the same story. One little girl was a beautiful little girl, but was like nine years old and was violent. She would attack her sister, she would get kicked out of class 10 times a day. She was on the bus home from school, they'd have to stop the bus. She would cut her family out of pictures that she was in. It was just really powerful. She didn't have any gut symptoms, and I found that she had terrible overgrowth of yeast, terrible bacterial overgrowth like you mentioned. I treated her gut, and it was like the same story. It was, "Where is that kid?" You know?
Chris Kresser:	Yeah. Yeah.
Dr. Mark Hyman: [00:45:00]	She was sweet, and loving, and kind, not disrupting school anymore, riding the bus home. And how many of these kids are sort of struggling like this that really, we can impact through these doorways to the brain?
Chris Kresser:	I think you raised a great point that all parents should be aware of, which is when the problems in the gut don't always cause obvious gut symptoms. That's tricky because when a parent sees the behavioral problems, or the doctor for that matter, they don't think about the gut automatically. They don't think this could be a gut issue. So that's the message that we need to get out there.
Dr. Mark Hyman:	They just think it's some troubled kid or some fat kid, or ...
Chris Kresser: [00:45:30]	Exactly. I mean, consider the effect on the kid. The kid will spend their whole life thinking there's something wrong with them, they're bad, they don't fit in, you know, and there's some fundamental defect, which is just horrible for the child's development and self-esteem. But when they understand that there was actually something physiologically that's contributing to this and causing this, it doesn't just improve their symptoms, it totally shifts their awareness, their self-awareness, their self-concept, and can really dramatically change the outcome of their life for that reason.
Dr. Mark Hyman: [00:46:00] [00:46:30]	So, what you're talking about Chris is, you know, reversing conditions that are irreversible—Alzheimer's, ADHD, autism, depression—that people suffer with throughout their life. And this is relatively simple: changing your diet, changing your lifestyle, a few supplements, fixing some problems that occur that are common like the gut. And, you know, we are looking at an epidemic of brain disorders in this country and around the world, and it's something we actually know what to do, but is sadly void in conventional therapy.
Chris Kresser:	Yeah. We've been searching for the magic bullet, you know? A single drug that's going to treat each of these conditions, and that's just not the way it works. They're all multifactorial, which means they have a number of different causes, and all of those causes need to be addressed instead of just trying to slap a band aid on the problem-
Dr. Mark Hyman:	That's right.
Chris Kresser:	... which clearly isn't working but has been our approach in this country to chronic disease for the last several decades.
Dr. Mark Hyman:	Yeah.
Chris Kresser: [00:47:00]	You know, with one in two people now having chronic disease, and one in four having multiple chronic diseases—and that is just expected to increase over time—we're in big trouble if we don't make a shift in our paradigm and how we approach chronic disease.
Dr. Mark Hyman:	No, it's so true. So true. You know, we just kind of missed the boat on this.

Chris Kresser: [00:47:30]	Yeah. Well, you know, our medical system evolved at a time where the top three causes of death were all acute infectious diseases like typhoid and pneumonia. It was like you have one disease; you want to see one doctor, you got one treatment, and you were either better or you died. Those were pretty much the outcomes. But, today, you know, people have multiple diseases. They see multiple doctors, usually a different doctor for every different part of the body. Those doctors are not communicating with one another—not seeing it holistically—and you end up with this sort of patchwork approach that is not only ineffective; it's actually harmful.
Dr. Mark Hyman: [00:48:00]	Yeah. We talk about evidence-based medicine, which means you've had to have something studied: a single agent against a single disease. It's randomized control trials. The truth is, and when we practice medicine, we're not practicing evidence-based medicine, because we might have five drugs for five different diseases, all in the same patient, that's never been studied.
Chris Kresser:	And most of those drugs are being used off-label in many cases in ways for indications that they were never actually studied for.
Dr. Mark Hyman:	Or approved for.
Chris Kresser:	Abilify, for example. Number-one selling drug right now used for depression and behavioral issues. It wasn't actually approved as an antidepressant.
Dr. Mark Hyman: [00:48:30]	No. It's true. And, you know, some of these practices of pharmaceutical companies to push these drugs for off-label indications has been found to be criminal, and they've been actually fined billions of dollars. But if they do, they don't care, because they're making more billions.
Chris Kresser:	Drop in the bucket.
Dr. Mark Hyman:	You know, they may be fined a billion, but they made 10 billion, so who cares?
Chris Kresser:	It's only the oil industry that makes more than the big pharma, so they've got deep pockets.
Dr. Mark Hyman: [00:49:00]	Just one last thought, you know, sort of reminded me what you're saying: that Functional Medicine has a saying—based on the thinking of Dr. Sidney Baker—which is called The Tack Rules. If you're standing on a tack, it takes a lot of aspirin to make it feel better. Get rid of the tack.
Chris Kresser:	Yeah. Yes, absolutely.
Dr. Mark Hyman:	And so, you're talking about like bacterial overgrowth or yeast in these kids, you can give them psychotic drugs, or anti-depressive drugs, or all these medications, stimulant drugs, but they're not going to work unless you get rid of the cause. The other issue is there are many causes. If you're standing on two tacks, taking one of them out doesn't make you 50% better.
Chris Kresser:	No.
Dr. Mark Hyman:	You've got to find and remove everything.
Chris Kresser: [00:49:30]	Yeah. Another analogy that's similar is like if you're in a boat and it's got a lot of leaks, you can bail water out and that might help slow the sinking; but ultimately you have to plug all of the leaks, not just one, for you to be able to stop bailing water.
Dr. Mark Hyman:	That's so great.
Chris Kresser:	It's really important and I think we see some positive signs, things are shifting and moving in direction, thanks largely to work from people like you at the Cleveland Clinic and all of the pioneers in the

[00:50:00]   Functional Medicine community. But I'm just, you know, hoping it moves quickly so we can prevent unnecessary suffering, especially in kids.

Dr. Mark Hyman: That's really the take-home here, is that there are millions of people suffering unnecessarily and that we can end that suffering.

Chris Kresser: Yes.

Dr. Mark Hyman: So, thank you, Chris, for your work.

Chris Kresser: Always a pleasure.

Dr. Mark Hyman: Thanks for joining us.

DALE BREDESEN, MD | UCLA and Buck Institute

Dr. Dale Bredesen:

[00:00:30]

[00:01:00]

I did not come through a Functional Medicine background. I became interested in the brain when I was a college student and read a book called *Machinery of the Brain* by Dean Wooldridge, and I got very excited about the brain and how it worked and began to be interested in the neuroscience of the brain. How does it actually work, what actually goes wrong? I went to medical school and trained in neurology; and in neurology there are a lot of diseases that we can't do much about, in particular the neurodegenerative diseases. Alzheimer's, Parkinson's, Lewy body, frontotemporal dementia, PSP, on and on—where we have not been successful—and you could argue that it's the area of greatest biomedical failure; for the successes that we've had in HIV and the successes that we've had in cancer, we've not had successes in neurodegeneration. I went back to the lab then after clinical training so that we could understand what are the mechanisms that actually drive these diseases? Why do you get neurodegeneration?

[00:01:30]

[00:02:00]

And over the years, with the collection of information, we began to see a pattern for what Alzheimer's disease actually is. Why you have specific molecules involved, why they actually feed into a specific set of path ways, and we realized that Alzheimer's disease is really about a critical balance that has many, many different inputs to it dozens and dozens of inputs; not from what we can see thousands and thousands, but many, many inputs that we had to address. So, what happened was, when we started to look at what are actually the things and we tell the patients to imagine 36 holes in a roof; you can cover one hole, it doesn't really help you that much. We want to be able to address all of the different holes and when we started doing that we realized it actually fits in very nicely with what Functional Medicine has been doing in terms of approaches to many different things.

From brain disease to hypertension, to type 2 diabetes, to autoimmune problems. We realized that what we were seeing from the test tube actually fit in very nicely with a Functional Medicine approach, so that's how I became interested in Functional Medicine.

[00:02:30]

[00:03:00]

What has happened is that we are practicing medicine that is a century out of date, basically. While things have moved forward in Silicon Valley and things have move forward with iPhones—and look at what you can do today that you couldn't do even 10 or 15 years ago—medicine is still being practiced in an old fashioned way, where we look for a specific diagnosis. We ask, "What, what is it?" Is it measles, is it a broken bone, is it rheumatic fever, what is it? And then for each thing, what it is, we get the right prescription, we give them the right thing to do it. That's not the way physiology works. What we need to do then is to ask in 21st century medicine, instead of to ask what it is to ask why it is. What are all the contributors and so we need to close what I call the complexity gap. For example, you have a computer that can fly a plane, you have to match the program with what is required for the plane, with the complexity of what it takes.

[00:03:30]

[00:04:00]

In medicine, we have a tremendous gap, we have human organisms that are incredibly complex; they have complex chronic illnesses like neurodegeneration, and what do we ask? Serum sodium, serum potassium—a few things like this—it doesn't come close to addressing it. Therefore, what do we come away with? The idea that these diseases that are complex chronic illnesses are ineluctable; you can't stop them, you can't see them coming, there's nothing you can do—but that is wrong. If you use larger data sets, if you look further at what is actually driving the problem—we can see this from the laboratory research—here are the things that actually drive the problem. Then you can see that in fact there are specific contributors and it's virtually never one; it's a combination of contributors that add up to an overall change that leads to a complex chronic illness, like one we would call Alzheimer's disease.

[00:04:30] What's accurate to say is reversal of cognitive decline in pre-Alzheimer's and Alzheimer's disease. What we've reversed is the cognitive decline. You can't say that you reversed the Alzheimer's, because there's no pathology yet to say that it's gone. What we can say is that the cognitive decline—which continues down—has now changed and now reversed and now people have improved, and we see this, this is now several hundred people. We reported the first 19 in two different reports, but this is now in several hundred people.

[00:05:00] We recommend though that everybody—just as everyone should get a colonoscopy when they turn 50—everyone should get a cognoscopy when they turn 45 or over. If you're 55, 60, whatever, check out where you stand. You can do this with genetic testing, blood testing, functional testing; and if you're already symptomatic, then including imaging in that. But if you're not, you don't necessarily need to include the imaging, but you should know where you stand; and definitely, if you have one
[00:05:30] copy of APoe4, you have an increased risk for Alzheimer's disease over someone who has zero copies; and if you have two copies, of course that's increased further and it's very likely that you will develop it during your lifetime.

The reality is, Alzheimer's disease should be a rare illness, because if everyone simply checked ahead of time and got on the appropriate program, we would not see such a high incidence of Alzheimer's disease. So, we do recommend that anyone—especially people who know that they're APoe4 positive
[00:06:00] or have a family history of Alzheimer's disease—get a cognoscopy, get checked out, and get on an appropriate program that will minimize your risk for developing full-blown Alzheimer's disease.

We've all heard a lot about the gut microbiome and its importance in various diseases, but it is true that the rhino sinus microbiome is also critically important. In fact, the neuropathologists have been
[00:06:30] telling us for many years that whatever causes this pathology of Alzheimer's disease looks—if you look at the neuropathology of it—looks as if it has come from the nose. It is the rhinencephalon, the nose brain that is typically affected in this illness, and as they've said over the years, we just don't know what that agent or agents are. The reality is that if you look at what happened with neurosyphilis and in some ways, Alzheimer's disease is the neurosyphilis of the 21st century. If you look at what happened in neurosyphilis, you had a single organism, treponema pallidum, which set up a chronic
[00:07:00] inflammation in the brain for years and years that could lead to dementia and frequently did. With Alzheimer's it's different. What we see as Alzheimer's, the amyloid, the tao, the changes that we see in pathology are the result of a protective response and that's a 180 degrees from what people have claimed.

[00:07:30] This is a protective response to three fundamental different insults and one of them is infection, chronic infection or inflammation, and so when you look at the brains of Alzheimer's patients, what has been reported? Organisms from the mouth, like P. gingivalis organisms from the lip, like herpes simplex virus one and then various fungi and molds that are actually living in your sinus. So, in fact
[00:08:00] your rhino sinus microbiome is going to turn out very important and some of the work, for example, I'm looking at bio films—looking at so called MARCoNS that actually secrete specific factors—that reduce the trophic support to your brain and enhance cognitive decline; this supports the idea that, ultimately, you wanna have an optimal rhinosinal microbiome. Not terrible surprising, from what
[00:08:30] we're seeing with the gut, the oral microbiome, the skin microbiome—these microbiomes are turning out to be critical for complex chronic illnesses like Alzheimer's disease.

The amyloid again is a protective response and there is some nice work coming, for example, from Robert Moyer and Rudy Tanzi and Harvard, showing that it's an antimicrobial peptide. We've also seen previously that when you have trophic withdrawal, you change the balance of the molecule that is the precursor for amyloid. So, amyloid comes from a parent molecule called amyloid precursor protein,
[00:09:00] which functions as a molecular switch, so that it actually can go in a trophic direction—which supports neuroid formation elongation—and inhibits program cell death. It can be cleaved in an alternative way that pushes it in an anti-trophic, in a downsizing direction, so you're going back and forth with the
[00:09:30] switch. When you're young, then you are balancing these beautifully; but as you begin to get older,

you can be too much on the wrong side of this, which produces the amyloid. So yes, the things that push that in the direction that is ultimately going to give you what we Alzheimer's disease.

[00:10:00]

Although we recognize subtypes of these, but what we call Alzheimer's disease can be inflammation, chronic infection, can be trophic withdrawal or can be exposure to toxins. For example, amyloid is a very good binder of various metals like iron or like copper—things like that—so all of these things can push you in the direction that we associate with Alzheimer's disease and hence the amyloid is literally a protective response under these conditions.

[00:10:30]

[00:11:00]

Toxins contribute in many different ways. As you know there are many, many different mechanisms for toxins to contribute to many human diseases, and we're exposed to toxins at an unprecedented level, unfortunately. One of the things that's critical, though, and especially the biotoxins, things like mycotoxins, is that ... And these are a little different than the metallotoxins, for example; so different mechanisms, but in the biotoxins, one of the mechanisms is that these activate your innate immune system. You essentially take two steps when you're exposed to a pathogen. You've got step one, which is a general activation—it's a little bit like if you had a bomb, a terrorist who had bombed some area. The first thing that would happen is that you would go into a general alert level and people would stay home, people wouldn't go out—you'd have this general alert. The second step would be much more specific.

[00:11:30]

[00:12:00]

You would have some film potentially that had been caught of the person. Now you would know, which person to respond to; so in the immune system, the first part is called the innate immune system, and the second part—the more specific part—is called the adaptive immune system. These toxins trigger the innate immune system. For people who respond better, they ultimately have an adaptive response. They get rid of the toxin, you don't have more exposure, things are good. But with continued exposure or with a poor response where the innate system responds but the adaptive system does not respond—and Dr. Ritchie Shoemaker and his group have done a lot of nice work in this area—then you get this chronic activation of the innate immune system and guess what one of the things is for that innate immune system? Amyloid beta. You've now got this chronic activation, which is producing the very stuff that is collecting in the brains of the Alzheimer's patients. It turns out that amyloid is also a very good binder of metals.

[00:12:30]

Especially divalent metals, things like mercury and copper, and things that can be in a divalent state, like iron for example—and actually the epidemiology work suggests that there may be—turn out to be some other metals as well, that will turn out to be important. For example, if you look at the RNA— that is going to lead to the amyloid precursor—that RNA actually has a region that binds to iron. You interact and you actually increase the production of the APP, of the amyloid precursor in the presence of iron.

[00:13:00]

[00:13:30]

We actually identify, there are six different subtypes, but they all are related to those three major processes. What happens is, you have this balance and you've got many different things that are on the side what we would call synaptoblastic; just like if you look at osteoblastic—someone who has osteoporosis—has too much osteoclastic activity for the amount of osteoblastic activity. They've gone in the wrong direction. Same story with Alzheimer's. There is a whole set of signals that are synaptoblastic that are forming synapses, and they're supported by things like nutrients. There's a whole set of signals that are synaptoblastic that are literally pulling back and downsizing, and the things that are signaling on a synaptoblastic side fall into three general groups. They are inflammatory things, whether inflammatory due to pathogens, chronic pathogens like borrelia and molds and chronic viruses and chronic bacteria, things like that. Or sterile inflammation, such as people eating trans fats and too much sugar and things like that.

[00:14:00]

Advanced glycation end products, and similar, that's what we would call type one. Then, there is a type 2. If you suddenly withdraw trophic support, nerve growth factor, BDNF, estradiol, progesterone, pregnenolone, testosterone, 3T3, thyroid, B12, Vitamin D—all these things are critical support factors. If you withdraw them, especially suddenly, then you will move to the wrong side of that balance and,

[00:14:30]

[00:15:00]

in fact, enhance your likelihood of developing amyloid, so we call that type 2. There is a type 1.5, which has some of both and that's what we call glycol toxic; so people who have chronically high insulin and glucose, people headed for prediabetes and type two diabetes—but this happens before you actually get to type 2 diabetes—you're already at increased risk. They have both the inflammatory part, because of things like the advanced glycation end products; and they have the atrophic part, because they have insulin resistance.

[00:15:30]

Insulin is no longer functioning as a trophic factor in the way it did before. They have a little bit of type 1, a little bit of type 2—so we call that type 1.5. Then there's a separate group and they present very differently: the so-called type 3. These are people who've been exposed to things like biotoxins, like mycotoxins or metallotoxins. And these people often have—instead of an amnestic presentation where they will come in with difficulty storing new information—they often have cortical presentations: so problems with calculation, problems with visual perception, problems with word findings, problems with organizing. These are the things that they often present with. It is a different presentation; they're often younger people.

[00:16:00]

[00:16:30]

Very different story and these people virtually all end up turning out to have an exposure to these various toxins. So, we call that type 3 and it has to be treated differently actually; and then there's a type 4, which is a vascular contribution; and type 5, which is traumatic contribution. But they largely go by these same three major mechanisms. The most important thing initially is to get in early, and to find out how far along you are, and then as you say the subtypes. We want to know … People frequently have more than one; so you might find someone who's 70% type 1 and 30% type 2, that sort of thing. So yes, they have that personalized approach to addressing type 1 and type 2. There are a lot of things that we can all do to give ourselves Alzheimer's.

[00:17:00]

[00:17:30]

Most of us don't want to do that, but if you look through all the things that you can do to give yourself Alzheimer's disease … In fact, a lot of us are doing most of these already, and one of them is to eat a very high-carbohydrate diet. A pro-inflammatory diet, a diet that gives you insulin resistance. You drive up your insulin levels and you develop a change … And there's some beautiful work from professor Ed Goetzl at UCSF showing that if you actually look at neural exosomes—so these are tiny fragments of cells that you can find in the blood that are derived from neurons—you can actually see this change, where you see that the signaling molecule IRS1, which normally should have high tyrosine phosphorylation low serine/threonine phosphorylation. The tyrosine is the on switch, the serine/threonine is the off switch; because of chronically high glucose and insulin levels, it has switched. You now have high on the off button and low on the on button, so you're not getting the same signaling that you had before. You are literally changing your brain chemistry by this chronically high consumption of a high-carbohydrate diet.

[00:18:00]

[00:18:30]

[00:19:00]

The reality is, we did not evolve as human beings to have a high-simple-carbohydrate diet but we are awash in simple carbohydrates now. There may be a number of links between leaky gut and Alzheimer's but an obvious one is that with leaky gut, you produce a state of chronic inflammation, and inflammation unquestionably is pro-Alzheimer's. For example, just the activation of NF-κB, one of the inflammatory mediators—some of the genes that this affects turn out to be the very ones that cleave the amyloid precursor protein to produce the amyloid. So, you are putting yourself in a pro-Alzheimer's state if you have chronic inflammation, and leaky gut is a great way to produce chronic inflammation. In addition, of course, you end up with fragments of bacteria that actually end up in the brain. You can see them sticking literally at the side of the amyloid plaques. Leaky gut is something we all want to avoid, if we're trying to avoid cognitive decline. You have to remember that the amyloid precursor protein actually is an integrating receptor.

[00:19:30]

It is sampling many, many different things. Trophic factor support, like nerve growth factor and brain-derived neurotrophic factor. Sampling things like estradiol level, testosterone level, pregnenolone level, and nutrient levels, things like Vitamin D. So, in fact, the reality is, as you start to add, you have more of these things. You are increasing your risk. It's not typically one thing. Now, having said that,

[00:20:00]

there are certain things that in our world situation, people are particularly poor. So, for example, there are one billion people on earth who are zinc-deficient. That is a relatively common contributor. And by the way, zinc is important in appropriate use of insulin, so in fact it will increase your likelihood of having the very poor state of insulin usage that is associated with cognitive decline. Vitamin D, another very common ... Many, many people are deficient in Vitamin D. Magnesium, another one ... Very, very deficient. And for people who are taking proton pump inhibitors, they're at increased risk for having still lower zinc and still lower magnesium and low B12. B12 is another one that's been recognized for many years as being important in cognitive decline.

[00:20:30]

[00:21:00]

It's many, many different nutrients, and again with our poor soils that we now have, our depleted soils, the processed foods that we are eating, we're all contributing to our own cognitive decline. So yes, you want to do the best you can with food and that includes things like prebiotics and probiotics; but yes, it's also helpful to know and so rather than saying, "Well, we suggest you eat this or do that," check the biochemistry, see where you stand, and you can actually see when you do need supplementation and when you can do it with food, then great. Of course, food is the best way to do it. The things that you want to start with are diet, exercise, sleep, and stress reduction. Those are the big four, but if those aren't enough, then of course you want to add additional things like specific supplements, herbs, and brain training—another critical one.

[00:21:30]

[00:22:00]

Social interaction, on and on, meditation. As a scientist who spent many years in a lab, I'm in shock to see ... I never thought I would be telling people you should be doing things like meditation and relaxing your stress, because I always thought we'd be developing a very targeted monotherapeutic pill that's going to help you. This is not a monotherapeutic disease. The monotherapeutics can be helpful, but in the background of the whole program. As a researcher, we're typically not running a clinic; we're typically training many practitioners who run clinics. Right now, seven different countries and all over the US, who then will look and interact with us and look at specific markers. So yes, you want to know again, how far the person is along? What are the drivers of the process? Their biochemistry and their genetics, and then their functional status, and then you want to go from there to look at what is an optimal program.

[00:22:30]

We developed an algorithm and software that will evaluate how much of each subtype a person has, and then from there develop an initial program. Of course, the final decisions are up to the patient and the physician, but this at least gives you some background to understand what is driving the process.

[00:23:00]

[00:23:30]

The whole idea of recode, which is reversing cognitive decline, is to obtain larger data sets in order to determine specific subtypes, and give us an optimal plan for how to reverse cognitive decline. It's worked very well so far in the first few hundred people, and so the first steps are to determine your subtype, to determine your status, and then to look at the beginnings. Optimal diet, optimal exercise, optimal sleep, optimal stress reduction—those turn out to be very helpful for many, many people. Then beyond that, what else can you do to optimize your biochemistry? Brain training and specific brain training, that focuses on the underlying pathophysiology. Very helpful, and then beyond that, specific supplements can be very helpful. Right place at the right time ... Things that, for example, increase brain-derived neurotrophic factor, which increases to a small extent with exercise, of course—very important—but also can be increased still further with specific supplements. Then specific herbs that have been used for thousands of years.

[00:24:00]

When these are used as monotherapies, they're not as helpful, so there been many studies that looked at one monotherapy or another monotherapy and said, "Oh yeah, we don't see much of an effect of this." Yes, you need to have it as an overall concept. If you were to ask somebody, "What's the instrument that makes the orchestra?" Well, there's not one instrument; they're all playing together, and this is a network. This is a network function and a network dysfunction, so you need to hit all of the different linchpins in the network in order to make this function; and that includes bio identical hormone replacement, where indicated. It includes specific addressing of specific pathogens; so if you have a chronic Lyme infection that hasn't been recognized, it should be treated.

[00:24:30] If you have other tick-born blood infections, babesia, bartonella—these things are important—they're critical to treat, and if you're going to get your optimal cognition, you need to address those things, you need to optimize your immune system function. You may need intranasal VIP, you need the Shoemaker protocol for CIRS-related markers, which are markers specifically for mycotoxin and other

[00:25:00] inflammagen exposures. Until you address the things that are actually causing your cognitive decline, you're not going to get the optimal outcome. One of the most exciting things is to see people get better, because I was taught that these people don't get better, and I thought that I would die still studying transgenic mice and cells and culture and things like that. To see people changing their lives has been very exciting and ... For example, we had one person who got much, much better and still at

[00:25:30] three and a half years doing very, very well.

He had had PET scan-proven APoe4 positive repeated neuro psych evaluation Alzheimer's disease, and has done extremely well, and one of the things he said is, "I've allowed myself to talk to my grandchildren about the future once again."

[00:26:00] He had given up on talking about the future because he knew that the future didn't include him, and so he's gone back to doing that. Another person said that her husband ... The nuance in his guitar playing has come back, which was really exciting to hear. Another person was going to commit suicide before first being evaluated and treated, and has done very, very well and, of course, did not commit suicide, actually said to her family member after, "Did you know that I had Alzheimer's disease?" And the family member said, "Well, of course, I did; it was obvious from your symptoms, but I didn't want

[00:26:30] to say anything to you about it." Another person said that it has allowed her to enjoy life again, and to get out and do the things that she always enjoyed doing. Another one said that she went back to playing golf, and she was able to remember what everyone was doing and her own strokes on the course and everything, and so now a little harder for people to cheat, because she actually is seeing who's doing what on the golf course.

[00:27:00] Just to see the changes, we had another young woman, who said, "My mother is back. My mother is back interacting with the family again." These sorts of things are really exciting to hear. There's no question, the epidemiology shows that women are at greater risk than men. It's not 100% clear yet why that is. One of the guesses is that women have a more rapid decline in hormonal support. Men

[00:27:30] have a slower decline as they go through andropause; it's a slower decline and we know that sudden declines are one of the things that change the APP signaling. There are other possibilities, we don't know all of them yet, but there is no question that about 65% or so of the Alzheimer patients are indeed women; and in fact, today, your chance of developing Alzheimer's disease during your lifetime if you are a woman is greater than your chance of developing breast cancer. So, of course, Maria

[00:28:00] Shriver has done a wonderful job of pointing out that this is really a woman-centric illness.

Yes, men do get it; they do represent about a third of the patients. By the way, about 60% of the caregivers are women, and so there's an undue burden on women of Alzheimer's disease. We've always recognized, as with other complex chronic illnesses, that the earlier you intervene the better. The best, of course, is pre-symptomatic; and if not then during SCI (subjective cognitive impairment)

[00:28:30] which may last for a decade; and if not then, during mild cognitive impairment, MCI; and if not then, during early Alzheimer's. But recently we have seen people, even late in stages. And first and recently with a MoCA score of one, who has indeed shown definitive improvement. We don't know where the cutoff is, but what we do know is the earlier you are, the better overall you're going to do; so the people who are later on can get improvement, but they may not get improvement all the way back to

[00:29:00] normal. We're still trying to understand what can we do to help the people who are further along to actually improve them dramatically.

My advice to anyone who is starting to experience cognitive decline is, do not wait. We've taken the other approach in the past saying, "Well, it's probably not Alzheimer's." We keep saying that until, "Oh, it is Alzheimer's and there's nothing we can do about it." What I recommend is, everybody come in as early as possible. If there's no problem, great, get on prevention. Make sure that you never have

[00:29:30]   a problem. By the way, the current program makes you healthier. The side effect is some weight loss, some better insulin sensitivity, and some better energy ... That's not such a bad side effect. Get in as early as possible and get evaluated. We have the ability now to evaluate and to reverse cognitive decline that we haven't had in the past.

[00:30:00]   What we need ... Of course, we need many more people to come through. We need clinical studies; so, what we've had so far are patients coming through who we see get better, but we need a standard clinical trial. Here is the problem with that. Standard clinical trials change one variable. This all started with a clinical trial that was proposed—the first comprehensive clinical trial proposed—for mild cognitive impairment, pre-Alzheimer's back in 2011, and it was rejected by the institutional review

[00:30:30]   boards because it was too complicated, and because the feeling was the people wouldn't do the things that we'd asked them to do. And as the IRB said to us, "You guys obviously don't understand how to do a clinical trial, because you're changing more than one variable." We said, "Obviously you guys don't understand Alzheimer's disease, because it's not a one-variable disease." For the future, what we need

[00:31:00]   to do is develop a way in which we can have a programmatic approach and have that approved for a clinical trial. A fundamental change has to occur in the way that we do these trials.

BROKEN BRAIN

DANIEL AMEN, MD | Amen Clinics

Dr. Daniel Amen:

[00:00:30]

The biggest myth about brain health is you can't change it. When I was in medical school, we were taught that you were born with all the brain cells you'd ever have, and if you lose them, you're out of luck. We now know that was completely false, that your brain actually makes new cells every day, and your behavior is either growing them or hurting them. Your behavior has a big impact on how healthy or unhealthy your brain is.

[00:01:00]

ADD or attention deficit disorder, also called ADHD, attention deficit hyperactivity disorder—they're just different names for the same thing. And, in fact, it's probably 10% of the population. So, most people who have it actually don't know that they have it. Short attention span, distractibility, restlessness, disorganization for things like time and space, so their rooms tend to be a mess. They tend to be late and have impulse control issues. ADD, in our research and many others, lowers activity in the front part of the brain. The front part of the brain is the brain's brake. It stops you from saying every stupid thought you have.

[00:01:30]

[00:02:00]

When it's low, people with ADD get themselves into trouble because they say things that might hurt someone else's feelings. They do things without thinking it all the way through. Now, all of us do that at some point in life; we didn't sleep, we had a bad day. But people who have ADD—it's just been part of their life for most of their life. People who have ADD—really anybody who's struggling with their mind—should seek help when their symptoms are really beginning to interfere with their life.

[00:02:30]

They're interfering with reaching their potential at school, at work, in relationships, or with their health. The thing I love about what we do here at Amen Clinics is we actually look at people's brains and, yes, you can change them. That's the coolest thing, but when you optimize someone's brain, their schoolwork is better, their work is better, their relationships are better, and people begin to head toward their potential, which really makes them happy.

[00:03:00]

[00:03:30]

When I first started looking at the brain in 1991, I thought ADD was one thing. There was already published research then that ADD was low activity in the frontal lobes. But the more ADD people I saw, the more I realized it wasn't one thing in the brain. Initially, I made four subtypes based on the imaging work, and then it was five, and then it was six, and, recently, we added a seventh type. The important thing about that is if you give everybody Ritalin, two types get better, five of them get worse, which is why Ritalin has a bad reputation. For the right type, it's amazing. For the wrong type, it's a nightmare.

[00:04:00]

Blood flow is just such an important issue. Blood is essential to life. It brings nutrients to cells and it takes away toxins so without adequate blood flow, you're in trouble. The imaging study we do here at Amen Clinics is called SPECT (Single Photon Emission Computed Tomography), and it's a study of blood flow. It looks at blood flow to the brain, and the number one brain imaging predictor of Alzheimer's disease is low blood flow. When you don't get adequate blood flow, brain cells start to suffer, many of them start to die, and it can cause lots of problems.

[00:04:30]

[00:05:00]

I often talk about brain envy. If you want to get your brain really healthy, it's simple: just three things. Brain envy: you got to care about it, avoid bad, anything that hurts it; do good, engage in regular brain healthy habits. Then, as I started to think about blood flow, I'm like, "It's the same thing." Really, it's blood flow envy—well, love your blood vessels and take care of them because if they're struggling, your brain is going to struggle. Blood flow envy, avoid anything that hurts them. Caffeine constricts blood flow. Nicotine constricts blood flow. Having high blood pressure, low blood flow, because it's harder to get through. Heart disease, I mean, your heart is this magnificent pump so keeping your heart healthy, exercise, boost it.

[00:05:30]

What are the horrifying statistics about blood flow? 40% of 40-year-olds have erectile dysfunction—that's blood flow. Do you know what that means? If you have blood flow problems anywhere, it might likely mean it's everywhere: 40% of 40-year-olds have brain dysfunction, 70% of 70-year-olds have erectile dysfunction, which means 70% of them will also have brain dysfunction. If you have erectile

[00:06:00]

dysfunction you want to be serious about reversing that. So how do you do that? Love the supplements ginkgo and vinpocetine. The prettiest brains I've ever seen take ginkgo. Exercise, incredibly healthy ... And beets, they have a compound in them, nitric oxide, that helps increase blood flow.

[00:06:30]

Food is medicine or it's poison, and having worked with Dr. Hyman on *The Daniel Plan*, it's the number one thing to get right if you want your brain and body ... because we're eating constantly. I'm a huge fan of smart calories, but it's not just any calories, right? You can go on an 800-calorie Twinkie diet and you

[00:07:00]

will lose weight, but you'll also increase your risk for inflammation, heart disease, dementia, depression, and cancer.

Let's just get this clear: I think calories matter but you need to make them high-quality calories. Water is absolutely critical: 78% of our body is water, 80% of our brain is water, so being properly hydrated is

[00:07:30]

critical, and then clean protein is essential. I actually think you should have protein in every meal because it helps to balance your blood sugar, but you want it clean. That means things like hormone-free, antibiotic-free, free-range, grass-fed. Healthy fat—I'm a huge fan of fat—60% of the solid weight of your brain is fat. If someone calls you a fat head, say, "Thank you."

[00:08:00]

Carbohydrates are really important; they're essential to life, but I want to eat smart carbs. These are carbs that are loaded with nutrients and fiber but low glycemic carbs, which means carbs that don't raise your blood sugar. High blood sugar levels are a terrible predictor of premature aging and

[00:08:30]

Alzheimer's disease. Think colorful carbs—berries, red bell peppers, orange bell peppers, carrots—and kill the sugar before the sugar kills you. What I like to do, what we like to do here at Amen Clinics is actually put people on an elimination diet because there are just so many people who are sensitive to

[00:09:00]

dairy, to wheat, to corn, to soy. I have one guy, he had multiple suicide attempts and was very sad and those are often the patients we see here at Amen Clinics: people who failed other people.

He went on an elimination diet and immediately felt better. It was like, "Wow! I was like taking all these meds, they didn't help," and then we added one thing back at a time to see if there was something he was sensitive to. Twenty minutes after we added back corn, he had his first suicidal thought. I was like,

[00:09:30]

"Whoa!" He broke up with corn. You want to know what you're sensitive to.

I wrote a book called *The Brain Warrior's Way* with my wife and we argue in the book the real weapons of mass destruction are highly processed, pesticide-sprayed, high-glycemic, low-fiber food-like substances stored in plasticized containers that are destroying the health of America, with two-thirds of Americans overweight and nearly 40% obese. The food and fake food we serve people is a huge cause of

[00:10:00]

this national epidemic. I published two studies that showed as your weight goes up, the actual physical size and function of your brain goes down. It's the biggest brain dying in the history of the United States, and it's not okay because my babies, my grandbabies, will never be able to afford the tsunami of illness coming our way.

[00:10:30]

Food is one of the most important interventions, but whenever we think of people here at Amen Clinics, we always think of people in four circles. We look at their biology so that's where diet comes in. It's also where the scans come in and it's also where, if you had a head injury, that comes in there. We look at their psychology, how they think. We look at their social circle, who do you hang with because people

[00:11:00]

are contagious—you become like the people you spend time with; and there's this spiritual circle, which is why you're on the planet. What is your deepest sense of meaning and purpose?

Whenever we intervene with someone, we have biological interventions: food, exercise, nutrients. Psychological interventions: learn to not believe every stupid thing you think. Thoughts lie. They lie a lot. There are social interventions: who do you hang out with, let's assess that. There are spiritual

[00:11:30]	interventions: why do you care? When we use those four circles, people get better.
[00:12:00] [00:12:30]	I had a really hard day at work. I saw four suicidal people; it's a lot for a psychiatrist. Two couples who hated each other, and two teenagers who ran away from home. I went home feeling worn out and I came home to an ant infestation in my house. There were thousands of them. I remember as I'm getting the ant spray and cleaning up all the ants, I began to think my patients are infested with ants: Automatic Negative Thoughts. I have to bring ant spray to work the next day. I did put it on the coffee table and I started talking to people about we need to kill the ants, and they liked that. I got rid of the ant spray because it's toxic, and I found an ant puppet and an anteater puppet, and I started playing with the kids I see. I'm also a child psychiatrist, but also the adults, and ultimately, it's come down to this exercise.
[00:13:00] [00:13:30]	Whenever you feel sad or you feel mad or nervous or out of control, I want you to write down what you're thinking; just write it down and then, you ask yourself, is it true? Can I absolutely know that it's true? How does the thought make me feel? Who would I be without it? We turn it around to the opposite and researchers show that this one simple technique—learning how to not believe every stupid thing you think—is as effective as antidepressant medication. That it helps people lose weight, it improves their work productivity and improves their relationships.
[00:14:00] [00:14:30]	I see this LPGA golfer who I love; she's awesome and when I saw her first, she's very depressed and would spend hours a day crying. She's just the most disciplined person except when it came to her mind. No one had ever taught her and she's like 40 years old. No one had ever taught her to not believe every stupid thing you think, and when she started journaling and questioning and correcting the negative thoughts that were going through her head, she's not been depressed for over a year. I mean, yes, I could have given her four antidepressants and then all the side effects that go with that, but I have this little thought in my head, first do no harm. What's the least toxic thing I can do is to teach you to discipline your mind and that's really helpful.
[00:15:00]	Here at Amen Clinics, we see little kids and old people and everybody in between. I think what we're famous for is brain imaging. We do a study called brain SPECT imaging that looks at blood flow and activity, and helps us to guide treatment. We do another imaging study called quantitative EEG that looks at the electrical activity in the brain. Once you have the map, it's like, well, how do you change it? We'll use medicine if it's appropriate, but we also love natural treatments, hyperbaric oxygen. It's one of the mainstays of our treatment for people who have low activity in their brain.
[00:15:30] [00:16:00]	We see another one called Transcranial Magnetic Stimulation using powerful magnets to stimulate or calm certain areas of the brain depending on what we see on the scans. We also do neurofeedback which helps change the electrical activity patterns. We do hypnosis. We do psychotherapy and family therapy. We have a new treatment we're really excited about called ketamine infusion, using a dissociative drug that has actually been found to rescue many people who are in suicidal states. I mean, really helpful for a resistant depression and other things.
[00:16:30] [00:17:00]	We also have integrative medicine services. A long time ago, I realized you really can't divorce your brain from your body, so if your thyroid is not right, your brain is not going to be right. If you have a toxic load, your brain is not going to be right so we offer integrative medicine services, too. We have another very cool treatment called microcurrent treatment. It's called the Equiscope. It helps with pain and you give low volt microcurrent electricity into joints or into areas of pain, and it helps you feel better. One of my friends, Mark Victor Hansen, who's the co-creator of the *Chicken Soup for the Soul* series, he said, "Daniel, you have to learn about this." I'm like, "People do this to me all the time." It's like, "Leave me alone." He's like, "No, you have to hear about this."
[00:17:30]	My knees were hurting, I played football in high school and in college intramural football. I tore my ACL and I've always struggled with knee pain. I had it operated on and it was acting up again and I'm like, "Okay. I need to get surgery, get a knee replacement, something. I'm tired of being in pain." I met the guy who promotes Equiscope, and for 90 minutes, he worked on my knee and I had no pain and I could

[00:18:00] run. And I'm like running up and down the stairs, the hallway, and I'm like, "No," because I don't think of myself as a placebo responder. Maybe I am, but after that, the next day, I went on a plane to Italy and I got an Airbnb apartment. I'm like thinking I'm not going to stay in a fancy hotel, I want to be in their

[00:18:30] community, 72 steps up. I'm like, by the end of this trip, my knees are going to be trashed and I'm going to be on serious drugs, I'm going to be strung out, I'm sure.

No pain and I must have walked 10 miles every day, and three times up and down those stairs. I'm like, "Okay, I'm paying attention." We also use the microcurrent therapy here. If somebody is interested,

[00:19:00] when it comes to brain imaging, we're better than anyone in the world. We've done 130,000 scans on people from 111 countries. I mean, literally, people come from all over the world to see us. Yes, you can get a SPECT scan in Ohio or in Massachusetts, but no one with our experience.

Hyperbaric oxygen—there are people doing that all over the country, all over the world. Neurofeedback,

[00:19:30] there are many great people. The thing that makes us special is we do scan-guided treatment. Almost everyone who's got a brain issue or a mental health issue, no one's looking at their brain, and I've been doing this a long time—that's crazy, right? I know, I'm a psychiatrist, I'm not supposed to call things crazy. That is just freaking crazy. You've heard it said, a picture's worth a thousand words, but a map is worth a thousand pictures.

[00:20:00] A map tells you where you are and it gives you direction on how to get to where you want to go. Without a map, you're lost. Virtually 100% of people if they're homicidal, if they're suicidal, if they're losing their memory, if they're depressed, if they're failing in their marriage or at school, no one is

[00:20:30] looking at their brain. They're looking at the symptoms and then they're diagnosing and treating them based on symptom clusters and that's just stupid. There is no other specialty in medicine, not one, that treats people without biological data, not one.

[00:21:00] We made it our goal to try to change how psychiatric medicine is practiced by adding imaging. That's the first thing and the natural way is to heal the brain because as soon as I started looking in people's brains, they were taking Xanax or they're on opiates. The brain looks terrible and I'm like, well, what are the natural things we can do which is what always connected me with Dr. Hyman.

[00:21:30] A long time ago, I realized that nobody wants to see a psychiatrist. No one wants to be labeled as defective or crazy or abnormal, but everybody wants a better brain. What if mental health was really brain health and we just believe that. I mean, it's so clear to us when your brain works right, you work right, and when your brain is troubled for whatever reason, you have trouble in your life. If we can

[00:22:00] actually see it as an organ that we can evaluate and optimize, who wouldn't do that? Rather than so many of the people that initially come here and their parents are like, "Well, I can't get them here," because they say they're not crazy. It's like tell them, "Crazy or not, that's not the issue. The issue is we want them to have a better brain because with a better brain, their life is better."

[00:22:30] If you have someone in your life that's depressed—and depression is one of the most treatable illnesses on the planet—the important thing is to give them information and give them hope. I have a 14-minute TED Talk. It's got almost four million views, called *The Most Important Lesson from 83,000 Scans*, so I did it three years ago. It just inspires people, it gives them hope, it gives them an alternative to where they

[00:23:00] are. Stop telling them not to feel bad because they feel bad. Stop telling them to count their blessings because they've probably done that.

You have to know why they're depressed. Like ADD has many different types, so does depression. Some brains work way too hard, some brains don't work hard enough. You have to know what you're dealing with so you can properly target treatment. We know that if you have depression, in girls, females, it

[00:23:30] doubles their risk of Alzheimer's disease, so the chronic stress hormones associated with depression, with the negativity, with the sadness, the tearfulness, can actually damage some of the circuits in your brain. If you're a guy and you have depression, you have four times the risk of Alzheimer's disease.

[00:24:00]

[00:24:30]

Some people actually think it's a precursor to dementia. The quality of your thoughts really matter. We did a study here on appreciation so I scanned the psychologist who was writing a book called *The Power of Appreciation*, and she focused on what she loved about her life and her brain looked awesome and I'm like, "Well, you have to do the opposite so that we can compare." I had her think about what she was afraid of, what was negative in her life, and it completely deactivated her frontal lobes, so the judgment center of her brain, completely deactivated her temporal lobe, which is where Alzheimer's disease starts, and it dropped out her cerebellum, which is the processor in the brain.

[00:25:00]

[00:25:30]

Moment by moment, thoughts matter and if you tend to be depressed, you tend to have way more negative thoughts than people who aren't. Growing up, I got beaten up virtually every day of my life until I was about six. I had an older brother who has ADHD. He wouldn't be still at all and he decided it was fun to pick on me so I was an anxious kid. Now, at six, he decided I'm a better playmate than I am a punching bag and we've been great friends ever since, and every chance I got to beat him in tennis, I do badly. But when I was a little kid, I used to bite nails and pick my skin and I used to be masterful at predicting the worst possible things that would happen.

[00:26:00]

[00:26:30]

Doing what I do, it really helps me not to believe every stupid thought I have. I'm masterful at using hypnosis for my patients; anytime I put myself in a trance or one of my patients in a trance, I go with them. Learning mindfulness and meditation, cognitive therapy has all been incredibly helpful to me. I do the things I tell my patients to do: hypnosis and meditation, not believing in every stupid thing I think, and it has helped me tremendously because, I mean, another time of my life I went through great anxieties when I started doing imaging and I just thought it was cool. My problem is I had a national platform when I thought it was cool.

[00:27:00]

[00:27:30]

I had written my first nationally published book in 1991 when I started doing scans. When I started doing them, I started writing about them and then a group of my colleagues go, "No. You shouldn't be doing that. Psychiatrists don't do that. You're a charlatan. You're a snake oil salesman," and I got freaked out because I didn't go to medical school for people to be disrespectful to me or to bully me. I mean, I really felt bullied and I had a flaw then that I have subsequently lost, which is I used to want people to like me. Now, I had a lot of people who hated me and my patients always loved me but it was hard for me. I stopped talking about what I did.

[00:28:00]

In 1995, I had a personal experience where my nephew had attacked a little girl on the baseball field for no reason, out of the blue. And when I scanned him, I found he had a cyst the size of a golf ball causing his behavior to be deranged. I mean, there's just no better way to say that. I mean, he was like Columbine ready to happen and when they took the cyst out, his behavior went back to normal. For me, I took that as a sign, lose the anxiety and fight for what you know was right, which is if you don't look, you don't know. Sometimes to lose anxiety, you actually need almost a conversion-like experience of, "Okay, why are you doing what you do?"

[00:28:30]

[00:29:00]

I wrote a book once called *Unleash the Power of the Female Brain*, and I did it because I have five sisters and three daughters, and the female brain is just wildly different than the male brain. I'm not even sure we're the same species, it's that different. There's this study from Canada showing that females have 52% less serotonin than men and that's the neurotransmitter that helps you feel happy, that helps you feel positive, relaxed, and birth control pills drop it further. We know women have twice the amount of depression as males, three times the amount of anxiety disorders as males.

[00:29:30]

[00:30:00]

[00:30:30]

There are ways to increase serotonin; one of them is truly toxic, and a couple of them are more helpful. The most common way people increase serotonin in their brain that helps them be happier, less anxious, and less worried is they get a sugar burst. Anything that increases an insulin response in your body pushes tryptophan, the amino acid building block for serotonin, into your brain and makes you happy. Cookies, cake, candy, frappuccinos made with a lot of sugar, pasta, potatoes, rice—those things that are high glycemic, you just feel happier. A woman once told me she'd rather get Alzheimer's disease than give up sugar. I'm like, "Did you date the bad boys in high school?" I mean, it's clearly, it's a bad relationship, right?

[00:31:00] If you kill the sugars, many people will go, "Well, what am I going to do?" Well, exercise raises serotonin in the brain, 5-HTP, one of my favorite supplements, and the spice saffron, the most expensive spice in the world, is not that expensive as a supplement. We actually make something called serotonin mood support with 5-HTP and saffron. If you can exercise and then during those times when you're getting anxious or sad, saffron and 5-HTP, it can help you in such a positive way.

[00:31:30] Brain fog is really interesting and what I've seen is there are 35-year-olds that go, "I'm foggy and my memory is no good. That's normal, right, because I'm 35." I'm like, "No, you have bad habits." Someone who's 45 goes, "I have brain fog and my memory is no good, but that's normal because I'm 45." I'm like, "No. You don't love your brain enough." "I'm 70, that's normal," I'm like, "No. It's not normal." I mean, come on, but it's usually the sign that there's trouble.

[00:32:00] No matter your age, if you have brain fog and it's not because you drank too much the night before or you didn't sleep, but it's becoming more a part of who you are, it's time to get assessed and treated. I have a new book, I'm so excited about, called *Memory Rescue*. It's the best reference book I've ever
[00:32:30] done. It has 1,600 scientific references and it's based on this simple idea that I have. If you want to prevent Alzheimer's disease, if you want to keep your memory strong, if you want to rescue it from going to the dark place, you have to prevent all the risk factors that we know destroy your brain and we know what they are. I mean, there's a lot of science behind this and I put the 11 major risk factors into a mnemonic called Bright Minds.

[00:33:00] If you can remember these 11 things, it will rescue your memory. It will also rescue you from an addiction, from depression, from anxiety. Bright Minds: "B" is for blood flow. Low blood flow is the number one predictor of Alzheimer's disease. If you have things like hypertension, heart disease, erectile
[00:33:30] dysfunction, you're not exercising—that's a predictor of trouble. Exercise, and ginkgo and vinpocetine—two supplements I like a lot—and eating things like beets, can be really helpful.

[00:34:00] Know your risk and do something simple to help it. "R" is retirement and aging. When you stop learning, your brain starts dying. New learning needs to be part of your life. "I" is inflammation, a major cause of depression and dementia. We measure everybody's C-reactive protein here. We also measure their omega-3 index, and omega-3 fatty acids are amazing as anti-inflammatory intervention. The spice turmeric, because it has the curcumins that have been shown to have powerful anti-inflammatory properties.

[00:34:30] The "G" is genetics—if you have it in your family, you need to be concerned. It is not a death sentence, it's a wakeup call. Curcumins actually have been found in combination with vitamin D to decrease the plaques thought to be responsible for Alzheimer's disease. If you have it in your family, you want to learn to like curry. I didn't like it. Now, I like it. It's an acquired taste, at least for me. "H" is head trauma,
[00:35:00] a major cause, and our society's so stupid. I mean, so stupid that we cheer at boxing matches. Mixed martial arts is legal—it shouldn't be legal. There's money in it; we know the connection between playing football and long-term brain damage.

[00:35:30] The American Soccer Association just came out and said, "If you're under 11, you cannot hit soccer balls with your head." Because they realized it's associated with long-term brain damage. You don't like 12-year-olds, 13-year-olds, 14-year-olds ... Their brain is not finished developing until you're 25 so it's like, seriously? Are we engaged in high-risk behaviors? We need to have more love, more respect for the brain, so protect it—that's the big strategy for H. Hyperbaric oxygen if you've had a head injury.

[00:36:00] "T" is toxins. We're now living in a toxic society. A brand new study out of China: children who have the highest phthalates in their body have the highest incidence of ADHD. We need to support the organs of detoxification: your kidneys, so drink more water; your gut, eat more fiber; your liver, stop drinking and thinking of alcohol as a health food; and your skin which means sweat. New study from Finland: people

[00:36:30] who took the most saunas had the lowest incidence of Alzheimer's disease. Hit the sauna—it's not hard, none of these things are hard.

[00:37:00] There are a couple of free apps I like. My favorite is called *Think Dirty*. You can actually scan all of your personal products to tell you on a scale of 1 to 10 how quickly they're going to kill you. When I first did that, I literally threw out half my bathroom. I was like, "Holy smokes!" I've been reading food labels forever and never really read product labels like, "What's the matter with me? Do I really need to put aluminum on my body?" Yes, there's a controversial connection to Alzheimer's, so why would you put anything controversial on your body? It's your body. Don't you like yourself? That's Bright.

[00:37:30] Minds in the mnemonic Bright Minds is "M" for mental health. As we said, depression doubles the risk of Alzheimer's in women, quadruples it in men, you need to get it treated. It doesn't necessarily mean meds, head-to-head with antidepressants; fish oil, exercise, and not believing any stupid thought, have been found to be equally effective. So if you're depressed, let's do that, and oh by the way, let's check your thyroid and your toxic load.

[00:38:00] "I", the second "I" is immunity and infections which is one of the most common things we see here at Amen Clinics, whether it's Lyme or herpes or toxoplasmosis, that if your immune system is weak and you've been attacked by infections, that dramatically increases your risk. Most people diagnosed with Alzheimer's are never screened for them, which is hard. "N" is neurohormone deficiencies: testosterone, thyroid, estrogen, progesterone, DHEA. I think of hormones like miracle growth for your brain, and when

[00:38:30] they're low, you're not going to function right. Many women are going, "Well, I'm 48 and I'm pre-menopausal and should I take hormones? Will it give me cancer?" I'm just a huge fan of getting you to an optimal level.

[00:39:00] "D" is diabesity—combination of diabetes and obesity—or just having one of those is trouble for your brain, and we have seen that changing someone's diet can help so much. "S" is sleep. Sleep apnea triples the risk of Alzheimer's disease. On scans, your brain looks like you have Alzheimer's disease because your brain is the most oxygen-hungry organ in the body.

[00:39:30] If you want to keep your memory strong, you have to have a plan, and we love this Bright Minds plan because it's simple. It's not hard and people go, "Oh, it's so much to do," and it's like, "Dude, it's your brain, right?" This isn't hard but having Alzheimer's is hard. It's expensive and you'll feel deprived, right? So many people, when you nudge them to get healthy, they go, "Oh, it's too expensive, it's too hard, and

[00:40:00] I don't want to deprive myself." Like the 4-year-old inside their body is running everything and I'm like, "I've seen a lot of people with Alzheimer's over the years—expensive, hard, and everybody feels deprived."

[00:40:30] The limbic part of the brain, it's also called the emotional part of your brain, deep structures about the size of a walnut and it determines how happy or sad you are. It colors the world in a positive way or a negative way. It's also involved in bonding. It's highly-charged emotional memories. Your libido, how interested in sex you are. When it works right, people feel happy and positive and motivated and driven. When it's overactive, people tend to feel sad and blue and negative and isolated and less interested in sex. It's the part of our brain that makes life worth living.

[00:41:00] You want to feed it positive thoughts, give it good direction. Awesome smells can be really helpful like lavender and sage. Actually, sage has good scientific evidence it helps memory and when it gets hurt.

[00:41:30] For example, when you go through grief, it gets hurt. Don't let grief be your excuse to hurt yourself. That's when really great brain healthy habits can help calm that down. Don't block emotions. It's really important that if you lose something important and you feel like crying, cry because it actually helps to release the activity in the limbic system.

[00:42:00] As humans, we're a social species; we're not polar bears. Polar bears do just fine by themselves but that's not us. The more isolated we are, it's actually one of the risk factors for Alzheimer's disease. It

[00:42:30] increases our risk. When we're together, we have to work our brains, and it's like what's she thinking, what am I going to do? There's that dance that goes on and we also get feedback on how we're doing and whether or not our thoughts are helpful rationale and so on, but who you're connected to really does matter. The longest longevity study ever done found that health habits of the people you spend time with was as good a predictor as anything else as to how long you would live.

[00:43:00] I always tell people, "You want to be healthy? Find the healthiest person you can stand and then spend as much time around him or her as possible." I love this idea of being a brain warrior. When I was doing *The Daniel Plan* with Dr. Hyman, I clearly saw the war that we're in. One of the reasons I got chosen to help with *The Daniel Plan* is I went to my own church and watched them serve donuts and bacons and sausage and ice cream and hotdogs, and I was so taken aback to where I'm going to get my soul fed and
[00:43:30] these people are trying to kill me. I'm like, "It's a war."

[00:44:00] If you really want to be healthy, and that's why I love the series, you need to be armed, you need to be prepared, and you need to be aware that there are forces that will steal years off your life and your children's lives. It is really this deep sense of urgency that I want people to see the war and to have a plan to overcome it. Brain warriors, because we have thousands of them, they're happy, they're healthy. I had one, she went into one of the big box stores and she wrote to me and she said, "I walked in and
[00:44:30] saw death in every corner piled upon death. I just had never seen it before and I went in and got the few things I could get there and then I left." The fact that she's seeing it and avoiding it, she's going to be healthy for a very long time and that's what made me happy.

Dr. Datis Kharrazian:	First of all, it's really important to understand that two-thirds of the brain are actually immune cells, which tells you how important neuroinflammation is to the brain. The brain itself is really made of neurons and glial cells. Glial cells are immune cells, and we usually think of the brain as being all these neurons, but it's actually all these immune cells. So, most of the chronic neurodegenerative diseases of our time are really a consequence of neuroinflammation and immunological activity.
[00:00:30]	But when you look at the brain, it has different lobes. Each lobe has its own function. I think when you look at different neurodegenerative diseases, a lot of times people just tend to think, "I have to have multiple sclerosis or full-blown dementia to have disease." When people start to have neurodegeneration, they have consequences depending on which lobe is involved with their degeneration.
[00:01:00]	If we start from the front and go all the way back with the brain—the frontal lobe is really involved with executive function, planning, coordination, motivation. So, when the frontal lobe starts to degenerate, people will lose their motivation. People will lose their decision-making. People will lose their timelining. They're always late to events, can't plan on things, and they don't want to do anything else in life, and they really lose all motivation and drive.
	If you go back a little bit further, you get the areas of the premotor areas, and the premotor areas are really involved with motor planning and coordination. When those areas of the brain start to degenerate, people start to not be as good with sports they used to play.
	If you go a little bit further back, you hit the parietal lobe. The parietal lobe is involved with what they call somatic sensation. It's your sense of feeling where your joints and limbs are. When that starts to degenerate, people may be more prone to muscle injuries and ankle sprains because they just can't sense where their body is.
[00:01:30]	Then as you get to the back of the brain, you have your occipital lobe. And as that area of the brain starts to degenerate, you lose your blind spot or your visual field. You're more prone to miss balls if you play tennis, or get in car accidents because you don't see one side of your field as well, and those things may not be obvious to you.
	Then if you look at the brain from top down, as you go from the cortex down, you get to the cerebellum. The cerebellum is really involved with your sense of posture and your control of movement and coordination. When those things become impaired you can lose your endurance for standing for a long period of time, or lose your balance if you're going downstairs.
[00:02:00]	So, one of the things that happens in a neurodegenerative model, is people actually don't always develop a neurodegenerative disease, like Alzheimer's or dementia. They start to have degeneration in local areas of their brain, and then as those areas of the brain degenerate, they tend to lose function. Most people blame that on aging, but it's really neurodegeneration.
[00:02:30]	The most common sign of brain inflammation is really slowness in function in general. If we talk about cognitive function or recall or mental focus and concentration, we tend to see it slow down. One of the things people commonly use is the term "brain fog." They just can't find the word that they're speaking of. So, inflammation, what it does to the brain and to neurons, is that it slows down what's called nerve conductance. So, nerve conductance is how fast neurons fire from one neuron to the next. When a neuron is inflamed, the speed of nerve conductance goes down and the most common symptom of neuroinflammation, especially in the frontal lobe, is people just have a hard time finding

[00:03:00] their words or they feel their brain is slow that day. And then, unfortunately, for some people that becomes an everyday routine type of event.

Now, sometimes, we've all experienced having a sluggish brain. There are days when we're not functioning that day or something. Those are probably days where there's some degree of excess neuroinflammation that's taking place or something that's impacting brain biogenics.

[00:03:30] So, the target site for inflammation isn't really a specific lobe of the brain. There are cells called glial cells, and glial cells are—like I said before—they're found throughout the entire brain, and the goal is really to try to dampen the messenger pathways that activate the glial cells. And what the research is really showing, it's that it's really systemic inflammation that any inflammation in the body turns on brain inflammation, and for people that have chronic inflammatory diseases. Like if they have irritable bowel syndrome or some type of autoimmune disease, that chronic inflammation releases inflammatory messengers, and they actually turn on brain inflammation. So, when you look at brain inflammation, it's really susceptible to anything that triggers an inflammatory response. Whether it's

[00:04:00] chemical exposures, food reactions, an inflammatory disease, blood sugar elevations like diabetes, all those things tend to turn on the inflammatory casket in the brain.

For the most part, when you look at statistics for all types of neurodegenerative diseases, they're all on the rise. And we know that all developmental disorders are on the rise. If you look at childhood developmental disorders, I mean, there are some stats that are saying that one out of eight children in the US have some type of developmental delay, whether it's dyslexia or autism or attention deficit or

[00:04:30] hyperactivity disorder. So, it's really an epidemic, it's really growing, and we're not really doing anything to change that. I mean, really, we're actually creating this environment today where we have inflammatory foods as a normal part of our diet, we have high-level exposure to chemicals that are not being tested and they're being used in everyday products, and we have all these various factors that are then turning on inflammatory diseases and impacting the brain.

[00:05:00] When you're looking at neurodegeneration for yourself, the first question to really ask yourself is, what have you noticed change in the past 5 or 10 years? Remember, neurodegeneration can happen slowly or it can happen quickly, right? So, one of the things you can look at, for example, is your handwriting. How's your handwriting? Has it changed over the years? Has it become worse? You can look at your handwriting from a few years ago. Now, if that's become worse, then the areas of your modal cortex and basal ganglia and premotor strip are starting to degenerate. So, that's one finding.

[00:05:30] If you've noticed that you've become worse, for example, with making appointments or being motivated, those are all frontal. If your balance has gotten worse, you have to hold on to handrails, and you have to be very conscious of where you're stepping and your balance, those are associated with cerebellar degeneration. They're saying in Functional Neurology Rehabilitation, you find out what's not working, and you have the person do that. For the most part, you have to ask yourself, is your memory declining, is your focus and concentration declining, is your balance declining? Those are

[00:06:00] all the key things.

Now, unfortunately, a lot of things are hard to pick up on your own, that you really sometimes have to have an exam to pinpoint if you can discriminate if some things are not working for you or are working for you, right? Neurotransmitters are neurochemicals that allow neurons to synapse and communicate with each other; the four main neurotransmitters are dopamine, acetylcholine, serotonin, and GABA.

[00:06:30] Now, dopamine is the main motivation neurotransmitter. And your ability to want to do things, to be excited to do things, and to push yourself to do things, is associated with dopamine. So, the person who can never finish tasks or even initiate tasks, those are patterns of low dopamine activity. Now, if you look at all the research, one of the most profound ways to raise dopamine is physical activity. So, when people exercise, their brain gets flooded with dopamine. You have to have the initial motivation to start, but if that pathway gets started, then you can really flood the brain with dopamine.

[00:07:00] The other main neurotransmitter is serotonin. And serotonin is really involved with your sense of mood. And that also, please realize I'm making very strong generalizations for all of these neurotransmitters, but people that typically have low serotonin, they just ... nothing really brings them joy. So, it's not that they're depressed necessarily, it's just that the things that would normally make them happy are no longer making them happy, right? They don't really have a favorite song anymore, or they don't have a favorite food or a favorite TV show. Everything is just there, but nothing really

[00:07:30] excites them.

And then when you look at the other main neurotransmitter acetylcholine, that's your memory neurotransmitter—your ability to recall things in your life and to find words and to remember events to have photographic memory, those are all involved with acetylcholine.

And then GABA is the calming down inhibitory neurotransmitter. So that allows you, if GABA levels are

[00:08:00] imbalanced, you may have things like anxiety as a key thing or restless mind. Those are the most common patterns with those four common neurotransmitters.

First of all, the research is showing, BPA is the key chemical found in plastic products, like plastic bottles or plastic utensils. And BPA-free, research is showing, is much worse. It's much more inflammatory. So, it's probably better not to even use BPA-free stuff if you can.

I'm doing a lot of research right now with chemicals and how it impacts brain autoimmunity. And the

[00:08:30] chemicals we're looking at are not really considered toxic, because usually when you use the word toxic, you're thinking about things like mercury or lead that are known to be toxins or classified as toxins. But everyday products like TBBPA, fire retardants, formaldehyde, isocyanides, or Bisphenol A, they're found everywhere. Formaldehyde is found in carpets, fire retardants are found in all your furniture if you live in the US. And those chemicals are not classified as toxins but they may be a factor in causing a degree of neuroinflammation.

[00:09:00] Some of the research I've done with my colleagues, Dr. Aristo Vojdani and Dr. Martha Herbert—and then we've been publishing on the research—is to really understand that chemicals actually bind to our own human proteins. So, in our research we measured chemicals binding to albumin, and then that creates what's called a neoantigen, a new antigen, and that triggers an antibody response. And that antibody response has now been linked in some of our research with antibodies to brain tissues.

[00:09:30] We did research where we found BPA antibodies, so people that react to plastic foods, they have very high levels of myelin antibodies. When you do research, you do statistical analysis. So statistical analysis for these things were what they would call of p-value, which is the probability that it's maybe due to chance of what they call hypothesis is true. But our p-value is .001, so very statistically significant. So, it's not due to chance, very unlikely due to chance.

[00:10:00] We do something called the r-value for correlation if the core r-value is one, that means it's one-to-one correlation. So, if one goes up, the other goes up. In our research with BPA and antibodies to the brain, we're finding correlation values of almost one, .9, .8. So, if one goes up, the other goes up. And we've also calculated what are called risk ratios. If you make antibodies to plastic compounds, your risk for having neurological antibodies are sometimes ten times the risk. Not twice, but ten times, some may even be higher depending on which markers we're looking at. So, we tend to think that a lot

[00:10:30] of the things in our environment are safe, but they're really not—BPA being one of the key ones.

Now, research done on BPA has found that 90% of the population has high amounts of BPA in their urine, and there are studies that also show things like TBBPA, like fire retardants that are found in 90% of females breastfeeding in breast milk, so these are very prevalent. But not everyone reacts against them. Exposure alone isn't the only factor, but when you lose your tolerance to these chemicals and you start to make antibodies against them, you start to react against them, there's a high degree of

[00:11:00] neuroinflammation. In our research, we didn't check patients with autoimmune disease. We checked blood samples from the healthy population. There's a high degree of underlying brain inflammation in the population that potentially may be triggered by chemicals that is not associated with a specific neurological disease, which is really scary.

[00:11:30] I don't think limiting the exposure is the only answer, but it is part of it. So, for example if you had antibodies to BPA because you react against plastics, that means you've lost what's called chemical tolerance. Our immune systems have some degree of tolerance. Some people as they get older become intolerant to smells or to lotions or different things, but at the same time, you can be intolerant to different chemicals as you get exposed to them. When you lose your chemical tolerance—which many people do with autoimmune diseases and chronic inflammatory conditions—

[00:12:00] then everyday chemical exposures can be triggers. And then you want might to reduce your load. So, for BPA being one of the most common exposures, you know we tell patients, "Listen, don't drink out of a coffee lid." Because when they drink out of a coffee lid, that hot water releases the BPA in their fluids. Don't microwave your foods in plastic. That really increases the BPA load. Those are things we can try to do, but at the end of the day, the bigger picture is what's causing the loss of chemical tolerance in people and that goes back to the neuroinflammatory question in general.

[00:12:30] At the end of the day, all of us are playing with this game of how much neurodegeneration we get, which neurons die off and degenerate. But it's how much neuroplasticity we develop, which is neurons connecting with each other. So, in any sense, when you look at dementia, you have various triggers that cause people to have more neurodegeneration than neuroplasticity, so their function goes down. In a clinical model, if you see someone who's suffering from things like dementia or chronic decline or any type of various neurological disorder, you're trying to go, how do we switch it? How do we get

[00:13:00] them to develop more neuroplasticity and then remove all the things that are causing neurodegeneration, right? I think dementia is definitely something that happens to people as we get older, because most people have more neuroinflammatory mechanisms than they have mechanisms to develop neuroplasticity. And the goal is to try to switch that.

[00:13:30] Neuroplasticity can be activated by using your brain. But specifically, I'll give you an example. If you were a kid who never played sports, then the area of your brain, the cerebellum and motor areas, were never developed. So, then you can develop through life with having part of your brain, called the cerebellum, not really having a lot of plasticity because you never developed it, right? And then you get older and you, let's say as an uncoordinated child, your arms were flailing all over the place, and you become older and now you're considered grown out of it and it's not as prominent. But as life happens and you get inflammatory exposures—you have food sensitivities and you get environmental triggers, maybe you get a traumatic brain injury, maybe you have some diabetes, maybe you're a

[00:14:00] smoker—as all those factors add up and your glial cells turn on, you get this inflammatory cascade in the brain. Then the entire brain itself has these inflammatory spots, areas of the brain that have the least amount of plasticity to develop will be the first one to show clinical signs.

[00:14:30] So now you're back to being uncoordinated, and you have balance problems, and you know, usually those patients go in and see their doctor and go, "Yeah, my balance has really gotten worse. But I've always had bad balance. I've always had bad coordination." And if you really do the history, that's not true. They had it when they were a child, they've kind of grown through it, and then as their brains neurodegenerate, the brain that didn't have much plasticity compared to other regions is the one that shows up. You want to basically figure out what areas of the brain are involved, and then try to do things to activate those areas.

[00:15:00] Now, we tend to think that all brain degeneration is your ability to recall and focus and concentrate and think. But that's only the frontal cortex. Different areas of the brain can degenerate and they cause different symptoms. When input to the vagus nerve starts to degenerate, people have chronic constipation and motility issues. When areas of the temporal lobe start to degenerate, people can't discriminate sounds when they're in the room. If anything is going on, they can't hear the speaker or hear what's going on on TV if there's any background noise. When people's occipital lobe degenerate, things aren't as bright when they compare to other people, so neurodegeneration is very specific to

[00:15:30] different areas of the brain, and then those are the symptoms that have to be identified. There tends to be this evaluation of cognition, but cognition is only one region of the brain that's susceptible.

[00:16:00] The first book I wrote was on thyroid and Hashimoto's disease, and I wanted to add a part two to my book, which is why I wrote a book on the brain. But it was really for my Hashimoto readers. Now, people that have hypothyroidism—90% of them or higher according to research—the underlying cause is they have Hashimoto's, which is an autoimmune disease. They have antibodies to their thyroid gland and that's why it's being destroyed. It actually is an autoimmune disease, but most patients don't know that. Most patients get diagnosed that they have hypothyroid, they're told it's a genetic endocrine disorder, and that's it. And that's partly true, but in reality, genetic disorder is turning on an autoimmune mechanism that is now making antibodies called TPO, which attach to the thyroid gland and destroy it.

[00:16:30] Research is showing that TPO antibodies have amino acid homology or they have the potential for molecular mimicry, but the antibodies against the thyroid can actually attach to the brain. And when those antibodies attach to the brain, then immune cells destroy them. So, when someone has an autoimmune disease for their thyroid and they make antibodies called TPO (thyroid peroxidase antibodies), those antibodies not only attach to the thyroid gland—which then signals inflammatory destruction of those tissues—they also attach to the brain. And if this happens very acutely, very aggressively, they call it thyroid encephalopathy. But many people have it at a very subtle degree.

[00:17:00]
[00:17:30] Also, researchers have found that when people are thyroid hormone deficient—maybe they're not taking their thyroid hormones or it took years for them to get diagnosed—being thyroid hormone deficient churns on brain inflammation. The glial cells get activated and the longer it takes to get diagnosed, the more brain inflammation you have. And the autoimmunity itself for being hypothyroid churns on brain degeneration. Now, most the people that have hypothyroidism Hashimoto's have some degree of HLA-DQ genotypes for gluten sensitivity—not always celiac disease, but a gluten sensitivity. And there's also lots of strong research that shows gluten antibodies attach to brain target sites.

[00:18:00] We published a study four years ago; we looked at 400 healthy blood donors in the US, and we measured their antibodies to wheat protein and milk protein. And we found that there's actually close to 15% of the population that had antibodies to different proteins associated with casein and gluten. And of those, we found half of them had brain antibodies. So, the Hashimoto's hypothyroid person is very genetically susceptible to gluten and wheat. So when you add in their antibodies from the thyroid attached to the brain, and being thyroid hormone deficient, churns on brain inflammation ... And many of them have gluten intolerances, and that churns on brain degeneration. Brain inflammation—we see that.

[00:18:30] Now, in my clinical practice, we see, I would say about a third of my thyroid patients also have brain antibodies. One of the ways to look for neurological autoimmune disease is you check antibodies for their brain. So, these are like myelin basic protein, myelin oligodendrocyte protein, neurofilament protein. So, what we're finding is that about a third of the patients we're seeing in a private practice—mind you this is not a research study—they have autoimmunity to their brain but it's not necessarily multiple sclerosis, it's just a subtle neuroinflammatory autoimmune disease.

[00:19:00] When we see a lot of chronic patients that have hypothyroidism, their chief complaints are depression and fatigue, and most of that is brain-based in some of these patients. As their brain gets inflamed, they can't activate their brain so they have depression. Their fatigue is really brain-based because of no need to do anything, and everything they do activates their brain. So their exhaustion and depression is really all brain and has nothing to do with their thyroid. So, when they spend all this time trying to figure out the right thyroid medication dosage, they're usually unsuccessful because they haven't really addressed their brain autoimmunity or their autoimmunity in general.

[00:19:30] Not all food intolerances relate to inflammation of the brain. When you look at foods and food reactions, you don't actually react against the entire protein of foods. If you look at a food protein, each food protein has an amino acid sequence, so when you make antibodies to a food protein, you only have a portion of that amino acid chain that has a sequence that the antibodies are attaching to.

[00:20:00] So, there's a concept in immunology called molecular mimicry. If you have the same amino acid sequence of certain foods, to a target protein tissue, like brain, like myelin, then you can have cross reactivity. Gluten has gotten a lot of the attention with research recently. There's actually a neurological disease called gluten ataxia so neuroscientists have been spending a lot of time researching food connections between cerebellar degenerative disease and gluten. And the amino acid sequence of gluten has similar amino acid sequences to what are called Purkinje cells in the brain.

[00:20:30] So again, when they get exposed to the protein that make the antibody, that antibody can bind to tissues in the brain. And that creates a devastating neuroinflammatory response, so not all foods have this.

Now, we did some recent research where we purified 200 proteins and we took what are called monoclonal antibodies—those are pure antibodies with purified proteins to look for molecular mimicry. We've identified a list of foods that we have in publication and submission right now, are specific to different target sites of neurological diseases. In the future, what we'll see is certain proteins, certain food proteins, are specific to certain neurological target sites. Aquaporin is things that are found in soy and spinach and tomato. They are a protein sequence, and that has been shown to have very strong correlation to people that have what's called neuromyelitis optica, which is a form of MS that involves the brain and spinal cord. And those food proteins can trigger that disease specifically, but not gluten or dairy or other things.

[00:21:00]

[00:21:30] So, food proteins are going to be very specifically associated with which target site their autoimmune disease is. Digital dementia is basically when you use technology and you avoid using your brain. So like, you don't have to memorize phone numbers anymore, word recall or number recall is not being activated by the brain, so those areas of the brain especially in the left intraparietal or temporal start to degenerate. So, whatever you're using technology for starts to cause degeneration.

[00:22:00] I'll give you an example. In the clinical setting, we'll have patients where we evaluate what's called dyscalculia, see if they can count backwards from 100 with 7s. So, we have them start with 100 and then 93 and go all the way down to 0. Many times, when patients have dyscalculia—which is really common—we'll just have them take their phone and start memorizing all their phone numbers. And then we teach them to start dialing their phone numbers instead of just pushing the person's name, and that's actually a form of brain therapy. Because as they activate that region of the brain, they develop plasticity and connectivity, and it has far reaching impacts and other cognitive aspects of their everyday life. Everyone is specific to their own brains and everyone can have different degrees of neurodegeneration.

[00:22:30]

Now, let's say you were a person who hated math growing up and you avoid math at all cost. So, what does that do? That means as your brain develops, you don't develop enough plasticity and connections in areas of your brain that are associated with numbers and calculations—which is left parietal and left temporal. So that's the area of your brain that you've never really developed through your evolution as a human being, then as you get neuroinflammation, that's the first place to show up. So then yeah, if you're that person then math numbers would be important for you. But if that area of your brain's healthy for you, it's not the same thing.

[00:23:00]

The brain needs three things: stimulation, glucose, and oxygen. And we assume that the brain is getting oxygen because we're breathing, but that's not necessarily accurate. Our brain oxygen potential is really, first of all, dependent upon our circulation. So, if people have really cold hands and cold feet, they have white nail beds, that means they have very poor circulation. Poor circulation impacts brain function. And usually those types of people really notice the biggest change in the brain when they exercise, right? Because they exercise, they get their heart rate up, they get blood flow,

[00:23:30]

they get circulation, and all of the sudden they're like, "Hey, I can really think again. I can really focus." So poor circulation is a major issue of getting what we call cerebral hypoxia, not getting enough oxygen to the brain.

[00:24:00] Another thing is just blood pressure. So low blood pressure, for example, is a problem for brain health to some degree. Normal blood pressure is 120 over 80. If you get somewhere in the ranges of below 100 over 70 or something like that, that can actually impact your blood flow to your brain, so people who just have very low blood pressure, don't have what they call enough profusion. They can't push oxygen and blood into the brain. So, if you have low blood pressure, if you have poor circulation, those things start to show up. Most common signs of having really poor circulation is having white toenails, cold feet, cold hands. Some people that have very bad circulation end up getting fungal nail growth.

[00:24:30] Those fungal nail growths happen because the blood flow can't carry natural killer cells and immune cells to their toes, so the fungus overgrows. Those are all red flags. And in those cases, the strategy should be to look at things to improve your circulation and your blood flow.

Regular exercise is one of those things. There are lots of natural botanicals that can improve circulation and blood flow. But that's a critical thing, trying to make sure you have enough oxygen to

[00:25:00] your brain. Also, it's important to note that if you can't get blood flow to your brain, you can't carry any nutrients to your brain either. So, in a clinical model, if people have poor circulation and don't have proper blood flow to the brain, they can take all the different nutrients like essential fatty acids and fish oils and all these amino acids, but it has very little effect clinically because they can't get it delivered to the brain properly. So, it's a big deal for us when we look at clinical mechanisms and we look at a person's circulation.

[00:25:30] But the first approach when someone comes in and has any types of dysfunctional brain symptoms is to do a complete neurological exam head to toe. We evaluate frontal lobe and prefrontal and parietal and occipital and cerebellar and midline low cerebellum and brainstem and go all the way down, and try to find out what areas are not functioning well. The areas that are not functioning well, what we do is we activate them.

So, for example, if the temporal lobe is not firing well on the left, we do repetitive music and tapping. If it's right, we have them listen to jazz or different types of things. Just from functional MRI studies, we know which areas of the brain are activated by specific regions. So, the goal of the exam is to find these. Now, in a traditional neurological exam, that's not what you do. In a traditional neurological

[00:26:00] exam, you look for a disease and then there's really no treatment for it, you get labeled. But in the neurodegenerative model, you do a complete neurological exam and find what are called soft neurological signs—areas where they're not doing as well within their examination—and then try to do therapy for that, right?

But very simply, whatever they can't do is what they would do. So, if the balance is bad, they work on their balance. If their word recall is bad, they work on word recall. And then the goal from a nutritional point of view is to look at the priorities we have which are things like, glucose, oxygen, and

[00:26:30] stimulation. So, we want to make sure the blood sugars are stable—they're not hypoglycemic, they're not insulin resistant, that they're getting proper blood flow to their brain, that they're not anemic—so it really is a complete workup. It generally takes me four hours to evaluate a new patient. And we take them through EKGs and spirometric testing and do complete blood work and do a complete neuro exam and then sit back and go, "Okay, what are the things we can do that can impact most, as many symptoms as possible to make a difference?"

[00:27:00] So, for example, if someone is anemic, that's our first treatment for their brain because they have to have red blood cells to carry oxygen to their brain, right? We can't do brain therapy exercises because it can't work if they have no oxygen going to their brain. Someone else may come in and they're not anemic, they just need to activate their frontal cortex. So, we may do eye movements or different types of things to activate plasticity there. So that's our approach.

[00:27:30]

The top tips for neuroplasticity, number one, is you have to get sleep. Number two, you have to do some degree of physical exercise. And with physical exercise, the research is showing that the key thing that it releases something called BDNF; and it doesn't have to be for long periods of time, but it has to be high intensity. So, the higher the intensity of exercise, the more BDNF you release in your brain; that encourages the growths of neurons.

[00:28:00]

A lot times I'll just have my patients do what's called a seven-minute workout or something. And if they can get their heart rate up just for a few minutes, that completely changes their brain chemistry. And then the other things are, do whatever you're bad at. And this is not the trend for what people like to do. People like to do what they're good at, right? And as a kid, as you're good at some things, you get encouraged to do them—and then you don't do the things you're bad at. Whatever you're bad at, you need to do. So, if you hate learning a language, you should go learn a language. If you hate art, guess what you have to do? You have to do art. That's the best way to develop neuroplasticity.

DAVE ASPREY | Founder & CEO, Bulletproof

Dr. Mark Hyman: Dave, you just wrote a book called *Head Strong*, which is a powerful way to reset your brain—and you came upon this the hard way, which was you had a broken brain. Can you tell us about what that was, and what caused it, and what inspired you to write the book?

Dave Asprey: I weighed 300 pounds in my early 20s and I started having really good success in my career. And I
[00:00:30] started having more and more problems with my brain, where I just couldn't remember things and it wasn't working. After 20 years and $1,000,000 spent hacking myself, it comes down to the fact that I had muffin top, but also, I had muffin top in my brain.

Dr. Mark Hyman: Ah ...

Dave Asprey: And it was ...

Dr. Mark Hyman: What's that?

Dave Asprey: Muffin top is that unfortunate thing that hangs over, but it's all caused by inflammation and went into the science. Inflammation is always caused by the power plants in our body called mitochondria—and by fixing those, you fix your brain, you fix your body, you change how you look, you get new pants, you get new everything. And fat is at the center of that.

[00:01:00]
Dr. Mark Hyman: What happened to your brain? You had cognitive issues, but it was more than that: you really had brain damage.

Dave Asprey: I did. It turns out I lived in a house that had water damage, which had caused toxic mold to grow. And when I got a SPECT Scan from Dr. Daniel Amen—which looks at what parts of your brain are working— they found no metabolic activity in the front of my brain, the part that makes you human when I try to concentrate. Here I was, walking around feeling like a failure. I was fat and I wasn't eating. I would be
[00:01:30] on a low-calorie, low-fat diet, and I stayed fat no matter what I did and I was just so tired and it was the mission that says, "This is unacceptable, I don't want to live my life this way, I will do anything." It turns out the secret was, well, don't have toxins in the environment around you, and also you have to eat a lot of undamaged fat. When I did that, I made some other changes like even more vegetables than seemed sane, suddenly everything got easy.

Dr. Mark Hyman: I love that, more vegetables than seemed sane, that's the amount we should eat?

Dave Asprey: Pretty much.
[00:02:00]
Dr. Mark Hyman: When you discovered this lack of blood flow in your brain, it must've sort of hit the light bulb for you, which is, it's not an emotional problem, it's not a psychological problem; it was a physical problem that was causing your broken brain.

Dave Asprey: It was really scary, because they also said I was at high risk of stroke and heart attacks. My blood was really, really sticky, my inflammation markers were off the charts. And until then, I had felt like I'm a
[00:02:30] bit of a failure. I'd been pushing really hard, I'm succeeding in my career, but have the accelerator pressed all the way down and I'm slowing down, not going faster. All my willpower is at work, but it's not working anymore. That was the scary part, and that understanding this is a hardware problem inside me, it wasn't about how hard I tried, it was about just physical stuff. All of a sudden that's something you can hack, you can fix that—but if it's you who's weak, you're not gonna fix that.

Dr. Mark Hyman:
[00:03:00]

Yeah, and that really speaks to this phenomenon that's out there in our culture, which is that people blame themselves when they're not focused, when they're depressed, when they have no energy, when they can't sleep they go, "There must be something wrong with me."

Dave Asprey:

Yeah.

Dr. Mark Hyman:

And you had tremendous willpower. You started businesses, you're running the companies, but even though you had the foot to the accelerator, you really couldn't function, because you hadn't figured out what's really underneath it. Dave, you're really a brain expert, not by choice, but because you had to be.

Dave Asprey:

Yeah.

Dr. Mark Hyman:
[00:03:30]

And we talk about the brain, but most of us really don't have a clear idea of actually what's going on in there, and there are a lot of myths about brain and brain function. Can you talk about some of those myths?

Dave Asprey:

The biggest myth about brain power is that it's a function of willpower and trying. Different people have brains wired differently, but everything that happens in your brain—every neuron that fires, whether they grow or don't grow—comes down to something called a mitochondria. These are ancient ...

Dr. Mark Hyman:

That's a big word.

Dave Asprey:
[00:04:00]

It's a big word, but it's just ancient power plants; it's ancient bacteria that became part of our body. And they decide whether your brain has power or doesn't have power. The way to make your brain work better is to have more energy, to make these parts of the brain that support your neurons, that support all the other parts of the brain, to make them stronger. And you do that with the environment around you. By eating the right foods. These guys, they're made out of fat. You have to have the right fats in order to do this.

Dr. Mark Hyman:
[00:04:30]

Yeah, it just reminds me of one of our guests on the *Broken Brain* docuseries, Dr. Suzanne Goh, who discovered that mitochondrial dysfunction is at the root of many kids with autism. And that by optimizing these power plants in these kids' brains, you're able to take the most severely damaged brains and get these kids to wake up by understanding the mitochondria, these power plants, and actually optimizing them.

Dave Asprey:
[00:05:00]

It's not just those kids, Mark. Until my mid-20s, I had all the symptoms of Asperger's syndrome. It runs in my family. I have PhD scientists going back generations and I really can't put words to what happened when I turned my mitochondria on all the way. The reason it matters so much for our brains is that our brain has the most mitochondria in each cell – there's like 15,000 power plants per cell and the rest of you might have 1,000 power plants per cell. You feel it up here as soon as you do anything that gives you a better power system in the body, and what drives your willpower? The power system. What drives your heart? The power system. What drives your ability to love or to think or to focus? It's all about electricity that's formed by this tiny part in your cells. I wrote *Head Strong*, my book, about

[00:05:30]

what happens.

What are the things you can do to support your energy? You're feeling your head first, but it'll spread through the rest of your body. I don't have the 300-pound body anymore, and I don't have the inability to focus or make eye contact or the other things like that. It's a profound difference. 48% people

[00:06:00]

under age 40 and everyone over age 40 have a weakness in their brain that comes from the mitochondria. It is imminently fixable as long as you do the right things.

Dr. Mark Hyman:	Yeah, so what's powerful here is it's a hopeful message. We have these mitochondria—we're messing them up and we can fix them. And it's linked to almost every known disease; in fact, it's the fundamental phenomena of aging.
Dave Asprey:	Yes ...
Dr. Mark Hyman:	It's linked to Alzheimer's, to Parkinson's, to depression, to chronic fatigue, to all sorts of cognitive issues, ADD, autism, Asperger's—all these things that we think are fixed. Brain disorders? You're suggesting something pretty radical, which is they're really not fixed, that you can actually fix them.
[00:06:30] Dave Asprey:	You can fix them. The cool thing about these power plants in your cells, there's a quadrillion of them in your body and they all talk to each other, and they're designed so that the ones that are weak can die and be replaced by fresh ones. All you have to do is send them a signal. This is, "Hey, it's time to straighten up here." And when you do that they make more energy for you, and that's what I did—and that's how I can start companies that grow big, and I can be a good parent, and I can do all the things I do, because I regenerated that part of me.
[00:07:00] Dr. Mark Hyman:	It's amazing. Let's talk about the two parts of what we need to know to fix our mitochondria, which is: one: what are the things that harm them, what are the poisons for mitochondria; and two: what are the things that optimize your mitochondria?
Dave Asprey:	It's fantastic that you went in the right order there, Mark. The first thing to do is stop doing the things that make you weak. It sounds obvious, but ...
Dr. Mark Hyman:	Brain kryptonite, you call it.
Dave Asprey: [00:07:30] [00:08:00]	Yeah, it's exactly what it says in *Head Strong*, and the idea is that if you are used to carrying around a 100-pound barbell, and go like, "Oh, I'm going to get strong so I can carry another one." But what if you just set that one down—you'd have a lot of strength and that's the equivalent of getting rid of toxins. And one of the biggest toxins that affects your mitochondria is damaged vegetable oils. Fried foods and other things that are pretty common toxins, like mercury, directly impact these. What I discovered is that there are classes of compounds made by Mother Nature that impact your mitochondria as well. For instance, vegetables don't want you to eat their babies.
Dr. Mark Hyman:	Okay.
Dave Asprey:	Certain types of things like whole grains—the outer part of the whole grain has chemicals on it that directly slow down your ability to make energy. And that's supposed to tell us not to eat the whole grains, but well we might've made a few mistakes. There are definitely classes of things like that, but one that's most scary is prescription drugs. The majority of prescription drugs cause damage to these batteries in our cells. No wonder you have less energy if you get hooked on prescription drugs.
Dr. Mark Hyman: [00:08:30]	Like what?
Dave Asprey:	Metformin, antidepressants, and also all antibiotics.
Dr. Mark Hyman:	And antibiotics are basically to kill bugs, and your mitochondria are ancient bugs that you've kind of hijacked to make your energy.
Dave Asprey:	It makes a lot of sense when you put it that way, but to this very day, we're dealing with people who get cancer and diabetes and Alzheimer's disease, which are a mitochondrial problem.
Dr. Mark Hyman:	Absolutely.

Dave Asprey: And they get it after taking prescription drugs for other things.

Dr. Mark Hyman: Yes.

Dave Asprey:
[00:09:00]
It's a part of the problem, it's not the only cause. The other thing to understand is ...

Dr. Mark Hyman: There's one more drug you didn't mention, which is used by millions and millions and millions of Americans.

Dave Asprey: What drug would that be?

Dr. Mark Hyman: Statins.

Dave Asprey: I can't believe I missed statin drugs. Statins are well documented, probably the most documented to cause harm to mitochondria.

Dr. Mark Hyman: And it's not a side effect, it's an effect of the drug, which is to block your energy production.

Dave Asprey:

[00:09:30]

[00:10:00]
And somehow that's supposed to be good, because it changes a variable that doesn't cause heart disease. So, getting people off statin drugs is a very effective thing to do, but it's really scary, because we've been programmed to believe that if we eat the fat that our battery system is built out of, and we stop taking statins, that we'll die. That's a lie. It just doesn't work like that and when you get high-functioning mitochondria in your cells, what you end up with is a body that's resilient and resistant to every type of degenerative disease that we get. You also immediately reduce your cravings, you turn your brain on, you can focus ... And when you have enough energy in the power plants in your cells, we are wired as human beings to be nice and kind to each other, but you will not do that if the cells in your body are in a lacking state. You gotta be well fed, so you can be everything you can be.

Dr. Mark Hyman: That's right, most people are walking around with what I call FLC syndrome, that's when you feel like crap. And I had the same thing. I was mercury poisoned and it totally nuked my mitochondria. My muscles hurt, my brain wouldn't work, I had no energy—everything went south.

Dave Asprey: Right.

Dr. Mark Hyman:
[00:10:30]
And what happened was, I even had damaged muscles, so that my muscle enzymes increased, called CPK—which is a pretty unusual effect of it, and it was really sort of catastrophic for my health. And by fixing the mercury issue and by optimizing my mitochondria, my numbers went to normal and I got my life back.

Dave Asprey:

[00:11:00]
It's amazing, here you are as one of the big names in Functional Medicine. This happens to you. The same thing happens to me and to thousands and thousands of other people that I interact with online. I did everything I could with normal Western medicine and it had no effect on my weight, no effect on the constant muscle pain, all those things. It was only when I turned to a more holistic approach where we're looking at the system of the human body that I was able to get rid of the toxins, and then figure out what was going on, and then turn up the volume on my energy. Suddenly the things that have been life-long problems, multigenerational actually in my family, they went away.

Dr. Mark Hyman: Yeah, and there are different people who have more susceptibility to mitochondrial issues.

Dave Asprey:
[00:11:30]
Yes.

Dr. Mark Hyman: I did, I found a gene that made me more susceptible, but you can actually fix that by optimizing the way your genes are turned on or off and by dealing with this mitochondrial issue.

Dave Asprey:	You can. It's interesting that these power plants in your cells come from your mom and your grandma and so on and so forth. Only from the maternal lineage. If you look at your mom's family and there's a bunch of sick people, and you look at your grandma and there's a bunch of sick people. Well, then you know that you probably have something going on there, and you can a genetic test to see what's going on with your mitochondrial DNA—but you don't have to. What you want to do is the same thing that works for people who don't have those things. Expose yourself to less toxins; eat more of the right kinds of fat; and don't eat junk food, don't eat processed food; don't eat sugar, grains, corn syrup, artificial colorings, NutraSweet and Aspartame and Monsanto's general set of things ... You will feel amazing.
[00:12:00]	

Dr. Mark Hyman: [00:12:30]	Yeah, it's powerful, so you hit upon a lot of things that are actually poisoning the mitochondria: environmental toxins, metals like lead or mercury, persistent organic pollutants, which are all the chemicals we're exposed to—anything that drives inflammation, mostly sugar and processed food or refined oils. These are powerful things that we're exposed to every day that we have no awareness of. The sad thing is that this is the future of medicine and yet, most doctors say, "I don't know what's causing this." Or they'll say, "I don't even know about mitochondria. I don't know how to diagnose mitochondrial problems, I don't know how to treat mitochondrial problems." But there's huge science around this. You talk a lot about that in your book and you help us understand that this is not just some crazy idea. This is actually the future of how we're going to be treating patients.
[00:13:00]	

Dave Asprey: [00:13:30]	It's the future of how we're going to treat patients, because mitochondria are the uniting element that explains everything that's happening, because all inflammation comes from mitochondria. There's no other source if it. If you get to the very root of it, when you make some simple changes, everything can get better all at once instead of this ancient view, "I'll work on just the kidney. I'll work on just the knee. I'll work on just heart disease." If you fix heart disease and cause cancer—which is also mitochondrial at the same time, like some common large research organizations that we know about are doing—it doesn't work. You have to do everything and the only way to do everything is to go down to the root cause, and the root cause is your body is not converting food and oxygen into energy for you to go out and be who you're capable of being ... And we can fix that now, because we understand that system. It is hackable.

Dr. Mark Hyman: [00:14:00]	Yes that's true, you mentioned food and oxygen, which is really what your mitochondria do: they take oxygen and food and produce energy that runs every system in your body. But you talk about something very interesting, which is EOMD and that's not a form of sexual dysfunction. It's a real thing that we can actually understand by looking at little kids. The little two-year-olds are running around like crazy, never stop, always curious. Someone who's 80, sitting in a chair, not doing anything, and that's because of the mitochondria.

Dave Asprey:	It is.

Dr. Mark Hyman:	So, what is early onset mitochondrial dysfunction?

Dave Asprey: [00:14:30]	This is something that definitely affected me even since I was a kid, and it's what happens when you're old when you're young. You start making energy like an 80-year-old when you're five or 10 or 15 or anytime under 40, and half of people under 40 now have this problem. It's like when you get a new phone, you make calls on it all day and when you're ready for bed, there's still a battery left? This is so amazing, and six months later, after you've charged it a few times, it's dead by 3pm just like you.
[00:15:00]	It's the same thing, it's actually using the same kind of electrons that our bodies use. It gets them from a different source. What if you could fix that and even better yet, my goal—this is going to sound big— I believe it's possible for me to live at least to 180 years old.

Dr. Mark Hyman:	All right. I'm down with that, I'm coming to your birthday party.

Dave Asprey: [00:15:30]	All right, see, I love that. It's probably possible, and the secret to doing that is causing my mitochondria to die when they're weak, so they'll grow new ones. And giving them all the raw materials they need to make healthy, strong, amazing mitochondria and do any of the things that damage them regularly. By doing that and all the other anti-aging things that I've been doing for 20 years, maybe I'll only make 140, but I'm gonna die trying.
Dr. Mark Hyman:	That's great. You mentioned all the things you can do to actually resurrect your mitochondria. To help them work better. To build more of them. To make them more efficient. What are those things that you've learned actually that are most effective?
Dave Asprey: [00:16:00]	One of the simple things that makes me happy doesn't cost anything. Every morning you take your shower. At the end of the shower, turn the water all the way to cold and let it hit you in the face and chest. You'll last maybe 10 seconds the first time, but if you just stick with this and do it every day for about four days, after the fourth day you'll be able to do it for 30 seconds. It stops being painful and it starts actually feeling good, and the reason for that is for the first four days all your weak mitochondria are screaming, "We're gonna die, we're gonna die." And all you have to do is go, "Yes you are." And they'll be replaced with your strong mitochondria that can make heat when they need to. It sounds like a small thing, but in four days ...
Dr. Mark Hyman: [00:16:30]	Cold showers ...
Dave Asprey:	And the other thing to do is go into cyclical ketosis—and those are big words, but what that means is, occasionally eat so little carbohydrate and protein, and lots of the good kinds of fat, that your body goes into fat burning mode. This is going to sound crazy, but we measure energy in calories and fat has more calories than sugar. So when you burn fat, all that extra energy goes in your mitochondria and they dance a little party.
Dr. Mark Hyman:	They run better on fat than carbohydrates.
Dave Asprey:	Yeah, mm-hmm (affirmative).
Dr. Mark Hyman:	Which is what we need carbohydrates for fuel, for energy, right?
Dave Asprey: [00:17:00]	Right.
Dr. Mark Hyman:	Iit's actually not true. In fact, I went to Cornell and my roommate was a PhD student in nutrition, and now he's a professor at the University of Buffalo. He's studying mitochondria and he told me, "Mark, you know we discovered in athletes—in extreme athletes—that if you actually substitute fat for carbohydrates, the mitochondria work much better; in fact, they prefer fat."
Dave Asprey: [00:17:30]	The number of endurance in extreme athletes doing Bulletproof coffee is amazing. Bulletproof coffee is an oil called brain octane oil that directly turns into this fat-burning molecule that not only endurance athletes and our brains love, it's the neurons in your head. If they have a choice between sugar and this kind of fat at the same time, they will eat the fat first. It's so important, but you will never have this kind of fat-burning molecule in the body unless you go on a four-day fast, an extreme low-carb diet, or you use an external source like the brain octane oil that's part of Bulletproof coffee.
Dr. Mark Hyman: [00:18:00]	Yeah, I want to get more into that, because there are ways of tricking and hacking your body into a fasting mimicking state.
Dave Asprey:	Right.
Dr. Mark Hyman:	Right, and there was a guy who I read about recently—you might have heard about this—who was a Mount Everest guide and he'd summited Mount Everest many times. But he always needed oxygen,

and he was always using those goos and those sugar glucose things to get his energy up. He was very fit, but he was using the wrong fuel source. And he decided he would try a ketogenic diet and he was able to climb Mount Everest without oxygen for the first time.

Dave Asprey:
[00:18:30] You'll see multiple photos of Bulletproof coffee at Mount Everest base camp, because lots of climbers are doing this. When you're in ketosis, you have so much ability to burn oxygen and food, that all of a sudden it doesn't matter if there's less oxygen, because you have more capacity as a human being. I have been able to get zero altitude sickness when I do things that involve increasing mitochondrial function instead of just pounding sugar or just doing what I used to do 20 years ago when I'd go to high altitude, I'm just gonna feel like crap. You don't have to feel like crap when you're at work or

[00:19:00] when you're at the top of Everest. What you wanna do is have more energy and that's the antidote for feeling like crap.

Dr. Mark Hyman: What's interesting is that we found that calorie restriction prolongs life, but it'll make you grumpy and depressed and hungry, which doesn't sound like much fun ...

Dave Asprey: Not much of a life ...

Dr. Mark Hyman: There's a way to bypass that calorie restriction and create the same effects that lead to longevity. There was an article in the *Journal of the American Medical Association*, which talked about intermittent fasting, or time-restricted eating. Can you talk about how that works?

[00:19:30]
Dave Asprey: Intermittent fasting sounds like a technical thing and it's probably got the wrong name, but here's the deal. You eat the same amount of food every day you were going to eat, you just don't spread it out into lots of small meals. Small meals really stress out these power plants in your cells, because they need time to go into rest and repair mode. And if they're constantly in, "get food, get food, get food", you don't get to do the work. What you do is, you wake up in the morning, you don't eat anything until a late lunch, and you have a big late lunch, big dinner, and then you go to bed. You don't do it again

[00:20:00] until the next day and it turns out for 18 hours a day you don't eat. And for most people, "Not eating, I'm going to die." Except it's not like that, because you're getting enough food and enough of the right kinds of fat, and you remove the kryptonite that causes all these cravings.

What happens is you feel amazing, and the hack for that that works really well is in the morning. If you have only fat with no protein and no sugar, you can feel no hunger whatsoever.

Dr. Mark Hyman: Like Bulletproof coffee.

Dave Asprey: That's why it's so popular.

Dr. Mark Hyman:
[00:20:30] It's quite amazing. I've done it and it works. I think that it doesn't create the sense of hunger, starvation—it just makes you focused and I wrote my books doing that so it really helps.

Dave Asprey: You do, too? I've written all of my books doing Bulletproof coffee. There are special coffee beans, there's brain octane oil that converts into this fat-burning molecule called a ketone, and there's grass-fed butter instead of milk. Get this: milk protein is one of the things that can cause mitochondrial harm. Avoiding milk protein for many, many people is important, and some people handle it okay, but for me? No, you have to take that out.

[00:21:00]
Dr. Mark Hyman: Yes, amazing. There's this process that happens when you do this time-restricted eating, which is called autophagy, which basically means eating yourself.

Dave Asprey: Yes.

Dr. Mark Hyman:	And it actually allows your body to clean up all your waste, recycle all the bad stuff, and supercharge the mitochondria to make new ones ... Do all the things that help promote aging. You talk about this thing called mTor, which is quite interesting. It's a receptor, a system in the mitochondria, that, when activated, causes longevity. How do you activate it?
[00:21:30]	
Dave Asprey:	mTor is a very interesting molecule, because it causes you to put on muscle, which is helpful. But if it's chronically elevated all the time, it actually promotes cancer—so what you want to be able to do is turn mTor on and then turn it off. There are three things that help to suppress your mTor, so then you can turn it on all at once to get muscle growth without getting cancer, and one of them is exercise. So, if you exercise, it will push your mTor down so it will spring forth. Another one is intermittent fasting and the third one is coffee.
[00:22:00]	
	There's a thing called tripling down on mTor that's in *Head Strong*, where you do all three at once. You don't eat breakfast, you exercise, and you have coffee.
Dr. Mark Hyman:	Your Bulletproof coffee.
Dave Asprey: [00:22:30]	And when you're done, like okay, what just happened ... I exercised, I felt a little odd, because I didn't have any fuel except fat. But actually now I feel really, really good, and then all of a sudden you just put on muscle. But the rest of the time, this is a mistake that was made all throughout the 80s and 90s, when this low-fat mistake happened in the 70s. Everyone switched to a high-protein diet and a high-protein diet causes you to have always have high mTor, which contributes to cancer. It's a delicate balance, because your mitochondria decide whether a cell gets cancer or doesn't get cancer. They decide if a neuron in your brain will fire or not fire. They decide when a cell divides, and they even decide what genes will be turned on or turned off by the environment around you. These little guys are running us.
[00:23:00]	
Dr. Mark Hyman:	It's powerful, powerful stuff. They were discovered through some bacteria on Easter Island, right, which is a very mystical idea. Let's talk about, what you call in your book, brain kryptonite. I think everybody understands that image of Superman getting kryptonite and becoming very weak—so what are the sources of brain kryptonite?
Dave Asprey: [00:23:30]	Brain kryptonite isn't just something that comes from your food. It comes from the environment around you. You can imagine your body as having systems that look at everything around you to see what's happening so they can keep you alive. That's their job, because they think you're a petri dish for them to live in. That's okay, so one of the things that's big kryptonite for them is junk light. It's kind of like corn syrup, except it comes from lighting.
Dr. Mark Hyman:	Is that why you wear those glasses, the orange glasses, all the time?
Dave Asprey: [00:24:00]	I do. They're called TrueDark glasses and they're actually a set of filters that reduce stress on the eyes, because the eyes have the most power plants, just like the brain inside them. When you're looking at your computer screen, when you have LED lights all around you and fluorescent lights, and you're indoors all the time, it causes 23% more damage to your eyes and we're looking at a huge wave of macular degeneration. This is early-onset blindness that is caused by mitochondria weakness, that is caused by light. Junk light is a source of brain kryptonite. I use the TrueDark lenses before I go to bed to make sleep better. Another thing that's huge, that's a major cause of brain kryptonite, is simply a lack of quality sleep. And I don't mean sleeping more, I mean sleeping better. There isn't evidence that sleeping nine hours is going to make you live longer than sleeping six hours. In fact, there's evidence that that isn't the case.
[00:24:30]	
	It's about how good was the sleep and what drives how good your sleep is ... is whether you're eating junk and whether you're exposed to bright light before bed. Looking at your iPhone right before you go to sleep is something that is brain kryptonite.

Dr. Mark Hyman: [00:25:00]	Even with those different filters and screens they put on them?
Dave Asprey:	You can improve the quality of the light that comes off your iPhone, but unless you're using optical filters like the TrueDark lenses ...
Dr. Mark Hyman:	If you use those glasses you can use your iPhone?
Dave Asprey: [00:25:30]	Yeah, you can't see some colors on it, it's pretty dark. But you can at least read that way and that's actually what I do every night. I double my deep sleep—I measure this every night—and I double my deep sleep every night when I completely avoid junk light. One thing that you can do right now is you can go into your bedroom and look for every LED that's on at night and cover them up. And we make little TrueDark dots you can stick on there that do it.
Dr. Mark Hyman:	Even when they're off?
Dave Asprey: [00:26:00]	Even when they're off. There are lots of little blue lights here, green lights, they have white lights here. All of those mess with your mitochondria. And here's something almost no one knows about. Our cells make light, just like an LED light bulb. They just make little tiny bits of it, and at night, our cells talk to each other with light. And then if it's bright, though, the light from a single LED bulb can overwhelm the light that your body uses to communicate with itself. Then all the repair processes that were supposed to happen at night, they don't work, and instead of working as a system, your body works as a bunch of little things that can't talk to each other. This is why having a sleep cave is so terribly important for your mitochondrial function, for your brain and for not getting any kind of disease that you can name.
Dr. Mark Hyman:	It's true, when I go camping or in mountain, nature. And there's no WIFI, there's no EMS, there's no unnatural light. I always sleep so much better.
Dave Asprey: [00:26:30] [00:27:00]	There's a reason for that and speaking of brain kryptonite—we already talked about fried food and things like that that are obvious brain kryptonite. Another one is holding your cell phone on your head. I am a scientist. I'm absolutely not an alarmist; I've been keeping my cellphone on my thigh. I wear special pants that have a little side pocket, because my book on fertility taught me don't keep your cell phone near your junk, and I did a whole-body bone density high resolution scan. I have very high bone density because of the bio hacking I do—except right where my cell phone sits, by my femur. I have 10% less bone density right where the phone sits. Bone density is driven by mitochondria. If you are making phone calls, holding your phone up to your head, you are cooking your brain, which has the worst possible effect, because this is where you have the most mitochondria. Use the speakerphone, use the headset. If you have kids, my kid's rule is: if the phone is transmitting, you don't touch it. It's going to be on the table in front of you.
[00:27:30]	We're not allowed to hold something in your lap or hold it up to your head or hold it right here. It's just not okay to do that, because their skulls aren't thick enough to protect them.
Dr. Mark Hyman:	Have you ever looked at the iPhone "About?" If you look at the instructions in the iPhone, there's a whole section on radio frequency. I think it's called RF, you read it and it's like—this is dangerous, don't hold it to your head, has to be this far away, it's not safe—and I don't think most people realize that. This is actually the Apple iPhone. I'm sure all the other phones have it, too. It's a warning. It's like, don't do this, because it could kill you.
Dave Asprey: [00:28:00]	Just about every modern phone on the market is at the very upper limit of what's allowed for something called SAR, which is the measure for how much heat in can produce in your cells. The bad news is that your mitochondria aren't really listening to that problem; the ability to make electrons gets messed with at much lower levels. The other thing you can do to reduce brain kryptonite is put a little lamp cord control switch on your Wi-Fi router, so before you go to bed, turn off your Wi-Fi. It

doesn't cost you more than five bucks. It's a little habit. You brush your teeth, turn off the Wi-Fi, and I promise you, you won't be web surfing when you're asleep. It's okay.

[00:28:30]

Dr. Mark Hyman: That's amazing. Dave, in your book you talk about something called ATP. What is that?

Dave Asprey: ATP was a rap band from the 1990s. I'm kidding. ATP is ...

Dr. Mark Hyman: Did they have a lot of energy?

Dave Asprey: "You down with ATP, how you know me?" Remember those guys?

Dr. Mark Hyman: No.

Dave Asprey: All right. Adenosine triphosphate is the name of this chemical, but what it really is, it's the chemical
[00:29:00]
that we use to make energy in ourselves. And it's fascinating, because through something called the Krebs cycle, we make this molecule. There are only 50 grams in our big whole body. It is a tiny amount and we recycle it over and over and over as our ability to make all these electrons that let us be who we are. That 50 grams turns into 400 pounds of this chemical, because we use it, remake it, use it, remake it, use it, remake it ... Well, if every time you use it and remake it, you don't do a very good job with that inside yourselves, you get inflammation and then you run out of ATP. A lot of the hacks that
[00:29:30]
are in *Head Strong*—the things that allow you to turn the system back on—involve giving you more ATP and tiny, tiny amounts.

You're only dealing with 50 grams here ... Can completely change how much energy you have throughout the day. That's the kind of stuff that changed my life.

Dr. Mark Hyman: Essentially, when you eat food and you breathe, it goes through this power plant and out the other end comes, *plop*, ATP, and also oxidative stress or free radicals.

Dave Asprey: Yes ...

Dr. Mark Hyman: So, you have to have a balance there and when you mention light ... I don't think most people realize
[00:30:00]
what ATP actually is. It's adenosine triphosphate and when you have those sparklers on the 4th of July, that bright powerful light, that's the energy of ATP.

Dave Asprey: Exactly.

Dr. Mark Hyman: And that's what's driving our whole system, and as soon as you stop making ATP, you're dead.

Dave Asprey: You have six.

Dr. Mark Hyman: Literally.

Dave Asprey: Seconds of ...

Dr. Mark Hyman: Literally.

Dave Asprey: ... ATP in your body at any one time. It's amazing, but you're exactly right—it's all about the ATP, which
[00:30:30]
is phosphor, and your job is to take a phosphor off. And when you do that, you get lots of these electrons you can use. Electrons—the same as in your computer, your phone, your washing machine— that's what powers us. And if they don't go into powering you, they go into puffing you up and that muffin top happens. If you have that muffin top around your waist, it also means you have the inflammatory molecules called cytokines inside your brain.

Dr. Mark Hyman: Your brain ...

Dave Asprey: An inflamed brain cannot do what it was meant to do. It's when your cells are running normally,
[00:31:00]   they're like this, they're tight. When you get inflammation, because you're wasting ATP, the cells get
                    big. When they get big, now it takes a long time for chemicals and electro signals to move around
                    inside the cells, and that means that you're going to feel not as good as you can feel. It means that
                    you're going to forget why you opened the fridge. You're not going to remember where your car keys
                    are. What was that word, and you even say things you regret, because you get hypogly-bitchy and
                    hangry and all those things like that. And it's not necessary, it's just about your body making energy.
[00:31:30]   It's not about being a good or a bad person, or being smarter, dumb, or being forgetful, or anything
                    like that. It's not about being weak, it's about being powered.

Dr. Mark Hyman: Yeah, it's so true and one of the things that I want to connect the dots on here is that inflammation
                    affects almost every brain dysfunction. Depression is inflammation of the brain, Alzheimer's is, autism,
                    ADD, Parkinson's ... All of these diseases of the brain are actually inflammatory diseases and they're
                    just that person's response to inflammation. That's why you see the same cause, inflammation, driving
[00:32:00]   all these diseases and so it's really important to understand how to get the inflammation out of your
                    system ... Which is eating a whole foods diet, it's exercise, it's dealing with stress, it's fixing your
                    microbiome, it's getting rid of environmental toxins, it's actually optimizing your nutritional status—all
                    of which will help process and deal with the triggers of inflammation.

Dave Asprey: It makes a huge difference and there's something to be careful with when you say, "a whole foods
[00:32:30]   diet." Remember that some foods really don't want you to eat them. If you don't cook some foods, for
                    instance, they will have compounds in them that harm the mitochondria directly. You want to eat a
                    diet that's right for your biochemistry, and the interesting thing is that you may have evolved, Mark,
                    where you handle some foods really, really, well, because your ancestors ate them for thousands of
                    years, and someone sitting next to you, like me, may not handle those same foods the same way. It's
                    okay to have biochemical individuality, but if you eat something and then the next day your joints hurt
                    and your pants are tight, that's a pretty good sign that you don't handle that very well and you might
                    want to take that out of your diet for a little while and see if that's what's going on.
[00:33:00]
Dr. Mark Hyman: I always say your body is your best doctor.

Dave Asprey: Yeah.

Dr. Mark Hyman: Tells you exactly what you need.

Dave Asprey: It does, all you have to do is listen.

Dr. Mark Hyman: In the series, we've talked a lot about neurogenesis, which is the ability of the brain to make new brain
                    cells, which we never thought possible. But emerging science has shown that, that's actually true even
                    up to the point of death. So how does that connect back to mitochondria and what do they have to do
                    with each other?

Dave Asprey: In *Head Strong*, I read a lot about neurogenesis because I run something called 40 Years of Zen, which
[00:33:30]   is a neurofeedback laboratory up in Seattle. And we train executives to have better functioning brains.
                    It turns out the signal that causes neurogenesis is something called BDNF, brain-derived neurotrophic
                    factor.

Dr. Mark Hyman: It's Miracle-Gro for the brain.

Dave Asprey: Exactly, and it comes from things like exercise and polyphenols. There are certain types of plant
                    compounds that can raise neurogenesis four times more than exercise just by adding them to your
                    diet, which is kind of interesting, and then neurogenesis happens in two forms. There's

[00:34:00]	synaptogenesis, which is where you actually grow new synapses to be able to do things, and something called myelinogenesis, which is when you put insulation on a nerve so that it carries electro signals really fast. This is when you practice something for a while, and we found if you eat the right types of fat, you have the building blocks to insulate nerves. So not only can you cause the brain to change, you can cause it to change and become more effective and efficient, and that is powered by fat. Guess which part of the cell decides whether you're going to grow a new neuron or not?
Dr. Mark Hyman: [00:34:30]	Mitochondria.
Dave Asprey:	*Bam.*
Dr. Mark Hyman:	Amazing. You had a bad experience with a brain toxin called mold. How does mold affect the brain and how do we deal with mold? What are the mold-containing foods? What are the ways we can determine whether we have mold exposure?
Dave Asprey: [00:35:00] [00:35:30]	Mold is the single biggest source of environmental kryptonite in the world today, and when I interviewed you for the documentary called *Moldy* about this, we talked about how mold itself is an ancient enemy of bacteria. For billions of years, mold and bacteria have been fighting. That's where penicillin was discovered, because it was a mold chemical that killed bacteria. Since our power plants are bacteria, it's no wonder that mold causes this huge range of health problems. In fact, it causes so many problems that it doesn't seem like it could be one thing, because different people have different effects and it happens because of condensation. Water damage, a leak under your sink, things like that—that wasn't there yesterday, but now it's there and I just gained 25 pounds and my brain doesn't work and all these things happen. What's going on there is the mold is directly poisoning your ability to make energy in the mitochondria. At the same time, it triggers a huge inflammatory response throughout the body, so it's the mold itself and the poisons made by the mold.
[00:36:00] [00:36:30]	And how you can tell this is happening is, if you feel radically different when you go into one environment versus another, you have to pay attention. If you move or you get a new job or start working out in a new gym and, all a sudden, "Wow, I feel dizzy. I feel fat, I put on weight. I'm strangely emotional." You have to look at the world around you, because it's not just you. It's you interacting with the system of the world and you can do things like get a mold test. In fact, if you look at the science, Mark, and you look at the data, at least half of buildings in the US—particularly schools—have a toxic mold problem. This is why it's so important that you look at this. If you can smell something in your house or your workplace, you need to fix it. It's the single biggest thing you can do to keep your brain working well.
[00:37:00]	The best test out there is called an ERMI test and you can get it from a mold inspector. They'll come to your house and they'll test how much toxic mold is in the air versus the outside air. I once had 88 times more toxic mold in my kitchen, because of a leak behind the dishwasher that I didn't know about. And my dog stopped eating, I got really tired, I could sleep 12 hours and wake up feeling like I didn't sleep. Groggy, poor decision making, irritable—all these things and it just hits you and you just feel like, "Wow, what just happened?" Because you don't see the stuff, it's invisible.
Dr. Mark Hyman:	And you can't always smell it.
Dave Asprey:	No, we couldn't smell a thing.
Dr. Mark Hyman: [00:37:30]	Yeah, and it's true. It's like a chameleon because it can cause so many different issues. As a physician, I never learned about mold or mold illness or mold-damaged buildings when I was in medical school. I was seeing a patient at Cleveland Clinic last week, who is a physician, who had a horrible history of an autoimmune disease that just knocked her completely down, and she was on heavy-duty steroids, all these powerful immune-suppressing drugs. I just took her story, I listened to her history, and she said, "I was fine until I moved into this house in Virginia and it was super moldy." And they knew it was

---

moldy, because it was so obvious. It was that bad and she said, "I immediately got sick."

Dave Asprey:
[00:38:00]

It's interesting because, especially with physicians, mold doesn't affect everyone the same way. You have two people—in fact, I interviewed a husband and wife couple where they're both physicians. She got profoundly sick when they moved into a moldy trailer during a remodel, and he had no symptoms, but at least he believed her. And the problem that I had, and that most people have, and you say, "I have these 10 symptoms." And doctors are trained in med school. If someone has 10 symptoms, what are they?

Dr. Mark Hyman:

Crazy or depressed.

Dave Asprey:
[00:38:30]

Exactly. They're a hypochondriac, so then they try and put you on antidepressant. Right away, they tried to do that to me. I'm like, "Are you kidding me? Did you see my clothes?" And then they say, "Well, maybe you should eat healthy?" I'm like, "I am eating healthy, I'm working out six days a week." And then they call me a liar. This happens over and over. In fact, a substantial number of medical schools themselves have mold growing, because they're old buildings.

Dr. Mark Hyman:

Yeah, and it's true and doctors don't know what they're seeing or can't figure it out or have never seen it before. Their default is ... this must not be something real and cover it with an antidepressant. It's so sad, because millions and millions of people suffer needlessly by not getting the right diagnosis.

[00:39:00]

Dave Asprey:

Yes.

Dr. Mark Hyman:

Okay, so you talked about fat in the mitochondria, but I want to get really specific. There are bad fats, there are good fats. What are the best fats for the mitochondria and what are the worst fats?

Dave Asprey:

[00:39:30]

[00:40:00]

The best fats for the mitochondria are saturated fats, monounsaturated fats, and fish oil. This means avocados, this means macadamia nuts, and yes grass-fed butter, coconut oil, brain octane oil, which manufactures a subset of coconut oil that causes the most ketones. There's something called MCT oil that you can also get. Although it doesn't raise ketones as much, and it can cause other gastric distress issues—but it works. You'll find people who put those on their food. Olive oil, things like that. They act differently; they feel differently. Undamaged, unroasted nuts—like walnuts have some omega-6 oils—you need some of those and when you get these and you eat your fresh fish. Wild-caught fish, not the farm stuff—your brain starts to regenerate, but it takes two years in studies to replace about 75% of the cell membrane.

Dr. Mark Hyman:

Get an oil change, it takes a long time.

Dave Asprey:

[00:40:30]

[00:41:00]

It does, and cell membrane is kind of a big word, but what that really is is that each cell in your body is covered in tiny droplets of fat that push water away. Each mitochondria inside the cell—there are tens of thousands of them—are made of tiny droplets of fat. It's no wonder that if you eat the wrong fats, like vegetable oil, canola oil, corn oil, soybean oil, hydrogenated fat, or anything deep fried, even if it's fried in good oil. What you get is, you get the wrong fats built into your mitochondria cells and then they constantly cause free radicals and inflammation, and it takes a while to rebuild the system. It took me about three years of super high fat—only undamaged fats—before I finally just lost the desire. I couldn't get enough grass-fed butter, it was like it saved me. I'd been a raw vegan, I was deficient, but after three years I backed off, because I just didn't need as much as I did before.

Dr. Mark Hyman:

This is true. How do you reconcile the stats by the American Heart Association that we should reduce our saturated fat consumption—less than 10%, even 5%—and eat more of these refined oils? That's their recommendation and everybody hears that and they go, "Coconut oil is bad, saturated fat is bad."

Dave Asprey:

I almost laughed when they published that rehash of studies, the last of which was done in 1973. Every

[00:41:30]   study on fat since 1973 was rejected by the American Heart Association, so they could keep pushing the agenda of the American Canola Oil Manufacturing Association that funds the American Heart Association.

Dr. Mark Hyman: Follow the money is what you're saying.

Dave Asprey: It's a corrupt organization, and when real doctors and scientists looked at the data from the 1970s studies that the American Heart Association relies on, it turns out that the biggest of those studies, the one that ended in 1973, when you look at all the data, it actually found the opposite of what the American Heart Association says. What we're dealing with here is pure marketing propaganda from a company, a non-profit company, that is backed with an agenda and the agenda appears to be to keep people sick.

[00:42:00]

Dr. Mark Hyman: Yeah, it was interesting. There was a study that was buried for 40 years, that was done by the guy who created what we called the diet-heart hypothesis, which is that saturated fat raised LDL cholesterol, LDL cholesterol causes heart attacks. So reducing saturated fat will prevent heart attacks. That's never been proven, but it's an idea, was a hypothesis. They did a study, which they could never do now. 9,000 mentally institutionalized patients—half got butter and saturated fat, half got vegetable oil. They thought the vegetable oil group would win, but, in fact, even though the LDL levels went down on the vegetable oil, they had more heart attacks and death than the group on saturated fat. In fact, for every 30 points lower LDL, the risk of heart attack went up 22%. That study was buried in a basement for 40 years until a researcher from the NIH tracked it down, found the data, and published it just recently. And these studies could not be done now, which is a randomized controlled trial. Most of these studies on saturated population studies, they all have all kinds of confounding factors, they don't necessarily elicit the real answer, but this is a gold standard study and it's been buried.

[00:42:30]

[00:43:00]

[00:43:30]
Dave Asprey: Mark, when I started writing *The Bulletproof Diet*, when I invented Bulletproof coffee, I was doing at least 10, 12, 16 tablespoons of butter a day, which I don't necessarily recommend for people, but I wanted to see what would happen. It was my body really wanted to recover from being a raw vegan, low-fat kind of guy. I was a little concerned, being an anti-aging professional ...

Dr. Mark Hyman: Yes, you wouldn't wanna do anything that hurts you, right?

Dave Asprey: Yeah, I have kids, so I drew my blood all the time and you know what, my inflammation markers went
[00:44:00]   down. I got a calcium score, all the things like that—even after years of doing this, I am better on every measure that I know of, right, except cholesterol and my cholesterol isn't sky high. I have high HDL, the good, protective stuff and very low triglycerides, when we eat this way with all the sugar and crap like that, that actually causes heart disease. And my LDL, frankly, I don't really care as long as my inflammation markers are low. I've been inflamed all my life, because I ate margarine and soybean oil and corn oil and all the crap that the American Heart Association convinced my parents was healthy.

Dr. Mark Hyman: Margarine ...
[00:44:30]
Dave Asprey: Yeah, it's shocking and it's a ...

Dr. Mark Hyman: Better than butter ...

Dave Asprey: It's offensive, that this ...

Dr. Mark Hyman: Yeah ...

Dave Asprey: ... that they did this to us and, in fact, at this point, the American Heart Association would say a McNugget is fine. It's fried in canola oil and all this other kind of crap, but here's the deal. If I had a choice between a McNugget or a plate of french fries and smoking a cigarette, if you look at inflammation markers ...

Dr. Mark Hyman: You'd smoke a cigarette?

Dave Asprey: I would pick the cigarette. I'm not even going to eat anything fried for any reason ...

Dr. Mark Hyman: Yes, that's true ...
[00:45:00]

Dave Asprey: And I don't smoke either, but it's that bad and you have these people out there who are promoting this. I believe they probably have just convinced themselves they're doing something good. But in order to do that, you have to willfully put on blinders and keep them on and ignore all new data. Unfortunately, for the American Heart Association, there's guys like you and ...

Dr. Mark Hyman: Not just me, but researchers from Harvard and Tufts and the Dean of Tufts. I asked him, I said, "Would you eat butter or a bagel, if you had a choice?" He said, "I'd eat the butter. No bagel."
[00:45:30]

Dave Asprey: That really puts a nail in the coffin there. I'm really hoping that we cause groups like the American Heart Association, the American Diabetic Association, even the American Dietitian Association, to wake up and understand mitochondria, understand that our brains and how we feel are most important, and inflammation drives that. And that if what they're recommending for their little specific disease causes inflammation, they are not serving humans.

[00:46:00]
Dr. Mark Hyman: You know it's true, the mitochondria is so critical and it affects so many people, and doctors just have no clue how to diagnose it. I had a patient recently who was a young man, he was 20 years old in college and he had this horrible condition—probably some genetic quirk—where if he exercised, his muscles would break down. He would have sky high levels of muscle enzymes, he had severe pain, and he couldn't work out or exercise at all and I said, "Look, you've got some weird genetic thing. I don't
[00:46:30] know what it is, but let's treat your mitochondria." And, over the last 20 years as a Functional Medicine expert, I'd been studying and treating mitochondrial disorders for a long time. I gave him a cocktail of mitochondrial nutrients. Things like CoQ10, carnitine, ribose, N-acetylcysteine, and a bunch of other nutrients to help maximize his ability to produce energy. Within literally just a few days of this, he was able to exercise, his muscles didn't break down, he had no pain, he can work out again.

[00:47:00] I see this on a less extreme scale ... There are people who exercise and they kind of poop out and want to take a nap afterwards. That makes them feel good, they have mitochondrial issues ...

Dave Asprey: Every time ...

Dr. Mark Hyman: And if you give them a mitochondrial cocktail, they go, "Wow, now I can exercise."

Dave Asprey: My father, about 15 years ago, had a heart attack and a double bypass. Strangely, he had the heart attack about six months after living in a very moldy building and he had a very clean set of arteries before that, so the mold triggered some changes in his vascular system. He had a heart attack and he
[00:47:30] wakes up from the double bypass just feeling like crap. The same mitochondrial cocktail you just described—I made it for him and, this isn't new information, this is 15 years ago, we've known these things ...

Dr. Mark Hyman: Oh yeah ...

Dave Asprey: ... work, but they just haven't hit the mainstream. Within 10 minutes of drinking it, he's like, "I feel like myself again." Versus, "I just feel like nothing." So, giving your cells the power to do what they are supposed to do gives you the power to be who you're supposed to be, and that's something that everyone should understand.

Dr. Mark Hyman:	It's so powerful. So, we talked about one, brain kryptonite, which is really mitochondrial kryptonite ...
Dave Asprey: [00:48:00]	Right ...
Dr. Mark Hyman:	How to get rid of those. We talked about food and fats and how to optimize your mitochondria, and we also are talking now about some of the special "hacks" that you can use as nutrients and other compounds that help upregulate your mitochondrial function, right?
Dave Asprey:	Yes...
Dr. Mark Hyman:	It's powerful, we actually have the science of how to do this. What are some of the other things that people are doing, like meditation or exercise or dealing with other factors that might affect your mitochondria.
Dave Asprey: [00:48:30] [00:49:00]	It's really interesting. When you look at how the mitochondria sense the world around you, they look at light, they look at sound, gravity, pressure, magnetism, because they're essentially little semiconductors, which means everything in the world affects them. They don't listen to what you want very well, because, after all, they're just dumb little bacteria. However, when you change how you feel when you're meditating, or when you're feeling extreme gratitude or love or compassion or kindness, it changes how your heart beats. And when your heart beats, it makes a strong magnetic signal—the strongest signal in the entire body—and the signal is called heart rate variability. So, when you're in that place when you think about puppies or your mom or whatever it is, your mitochondria are like, "Oh, there's no threat here, let me take my precious energy and turn it towards making new proteins, towards to regenerating." And if your heart is going du dumm, du dumm, du dumm, very regularly, that's what a stressed animal does.
[00:49:30] [00:50:00]	If you're living in a state of stress—because you have a Facebook post over here and an email over here, someone is yelling at you over here, and someone cut you off in traffic, and you're not meditating—your heart sends a magnetic signal that your cells listen to, that says, "Get ready to fight." And if you're always ready to fight on a cellular level, you will never rebuild the cells, and that's why it's so important to take a deep breath, to meditate, to have a spiritual practice, and to do whatever there is. Walk in nature, whatever it is that allows you to just calm down, because it's not just you calming down. That calm signal tells the system in the body of a quadrillion cells, "Chill out and build new cells right now." That's pretty important.
Dr. Mark Hyman:	Powerful. And there are actually apps on iPhones and other devices where you can put your finger over the camera and it will tell your heart rate variability so you can actually see what happens. And the most simple heart rate, which is beep, beep, like 72, 72, 70—that's bad. And the worst one is a flat line, right, there's no variability there. And the most complex heart rate is the healthiest heart rate.
Dave Asprey: [00:50:30]	This is contrary to what a lot of people would think: it's just about a number of beats per minute. No, it's about the spacing of it, and your heart should basically be playing music, but not just playing music with the same beat all the time. The way your heart plays music is when you go to the happy place; however you go to get there, that's one of the biggest mitochondrial hacks, just telling your body that you're in a safe place full of abundance and amazingness. It changes your ability to make energy to make energy in the cells, which changes actually how you show up in the world.
Dr. Mark Hyman: [00:51:00]	Mitochondria respond to many influences, but one of the most powerful ways to access your mitochondria is exercise. Can you talk about what are the best kinds of exercise to activate your mitochondria?
Dave Asprey:	When I was writing *Head Strong*, I dug really deep in the research about mitochondrial physiology and exercise and found two distinct groups of exercise that have shown to really have a difference for mitochondria. The first is, go for a walk every day for at least 20 minutes. That's the minimum effective

[00:51:30]

dose. Just a walk. It doesn't have to be running upstairs, things like that. You can do that if it really makes you happy, but that's not going to make you a better person. Going for a walk has this effect of basically stirring the pot, and it causes your mitochondria to work better, and it causes you to grow new ones. And then, once or maybe twice a week, depending on what level of fitness you want, you do one of two heavy-duty exercises. Only for 15 minutes. This is very time efficient. One is called high-intensity interval training (HIIT). And, with this, you sprint for about 90 seconds, like a tiger is chasing you. Very few people like to do this, you do it anyway. And here is the trick that's in *Head Strong* that's never been written about, as far as I know.

[00:52:00]

Instead of walking for a minute, and then sprinting again, you actually lay on your back.

Dr. Mark Hyman: That's what you feel like doing, if you're running from a tiger.

Dave Asprey: Exactly, well, that's why you lay down, because then you're showing the body tiger, rest, tiger, rest, so the signal that your mitochondria get is, "Oh you know what, I should be ready to make a ton of energy at any time." And any one of these quadrillion cells that isn't up for that needs to step on out and I'll replace it with a better one. That's why that's important and, on the weight bearing side, which is really important, especially for women, lifting heavy stuff. I don't mean a 10-pound dumbbell. I mean as heavy as you're capable of, but you only do it for 15 minutes.

[00:52:30]

For me, I'm in the best shape of my life and in order to do that, I work out 15 minutes a week. But when I work out, I'm gonna cry, because I'm picking up the heaviest things I can do—and that's a very interesting strategy—because it also tells the mitochondria, "Those of you who can't deliver 100% energy right now to lift this heavy thing, you need to go." And it sends a signal to the mitochondria that control your bones, "Grow bigger, harder, stronger bones." And all of the other things in your body, it's all about what are the extremes. Same thing with the cold showers. It's all an environmental signal that just tells the mitochondria, "Be ready." And if you can do that in the shortest possible amount of time, that's what exercise really is.

[00:53:00]

[00:53:30]

Dr. Mark Hyman: So, what you're really talking about are little tricks that you can use to increase your metabolic function and increase your mitochondria. Most people don't realize that when they say, "metabolism", they're actually talking about the mitochondria. And people say, "I have a slow metabolism." Well, they might, if their mitochondria aren't working. And the ways to speed up your metabolism is through the interval training, through the strength training that optimize your mitochondria, and all the other hacks you talked about.

Dave Asprey: Yes.

Dr. Mark Hyman: And what's really amazing is that when you do that, you can exercise far less amounts of time and you burn far more calories throughout the day by doing nothing, just sitting on the couch.

[00:54:00]

Dave Asprey: It's very true. If you do the hacks that are in *Head Strong*—you do the cold showers, improve your sleep quality, and go for that walk, and do the other, the strength training and high-intensity interval training—you will every day burn probably 300-500 more calories without having to have a lot of extra stress to do it.

Dr. Mark Hyman: That's like running an hour. That's like going for an hour jog, right?

Dave Asprey: It is, and if your metabolism is taking your food and putting it on your hips or your legs or anywhere else on your body instead of putting it into the energy that makes you who you are, it's time to fix your metabolism. Doesn't mean you're a bad person, doesn't mean you're weak, it's just a hardware problem and it means you need to send a signal to those quadrillion bacteria that are running things and tell them, "Step up." And when you do that, they will.

[00:54:30]

Dr. Mark Hyman:
Okay so, Dave, what are the top tips that you have for becoming head strong today, and what are the top five things people can do to optimize their brain function?

[00:55:00]

Dave Asprey:
Number one, eat more good fat. That means undamaged fats that haven't been heated and fried, and none of those vegetable oils and all those other just industrial-processed things that are out there. If you do that, your brain will now have the building blocks to become a strong brain. Another thing: follow the exercise recommendations in *Head Strong*. Go for a walk every day, just a short walk, enough to stir the pot. And, once or twice a week, do something really hard for a short period of time.

[00:55:30]

It completely changes what you can do. Number three, at the end of your shower, turn the water to cold, full blast. You can curse me while you do it, but after four or five days you'll thank me. I promise, it's a brief period of discomfort and you'll burn more calories all day long when you do that and your brain will like it. It affects inflammation, it affects all sorts of things, it's very simple and easy to do. The fourth thing, stop junk light.

[00:56:00]
Consider the TrueDark glasses, go through, dim the lights at night, turn off lights you don't need. And very importantly, make a sleep cave, so that you tape over or block all of the light that you can see in your room. So that your cells, your mitochondria, can talk to each other and do the reorganization and the optimization they are supposed to do and they've done for billions of years until we turned on the electric lighting.

[00:56:30]
And the final thing is something that we talked about Mark, and it's meditation or, even more specifically, if you don't know how to meditate, it's just gratitude. Every night, before you go to sleep, find three things that you're grateful for and just think about those for 30 seconds. That's all it takes. When you do that, that's going to change your heart beats. It's gonna take you out of fight-or-flight mode, and it's going to tell your body, "Hey, were you sleeping tonight?" Maybe you should fix the mitochondria. Maybe you should grow new proteins, instead of while you're sleeping being ready to fight. If you do those things, you will be head strong; you'll turn off your inflammation and, as a side effect of all this, you'll probably need smaller pants.

Dr. Mark Hyman:
[00:57:00]
You know there's another ingredient for health and well-being that often is ignored, which there is a huge lack of in our society, which is the power of connection, love, and community. What role does that play in your health, mitochondria, your brain, all the rest?

Dave Asprey:
When I was writing *Head Strong*, I realized that there are three basic things that a bacteria does in the world that we also do. Number one is, run away from, hide, or kill scary things that might be a threat. That's our fear response. The next thing is, eat everything—bagels, cookies, whatever it is—and this is
[00:57:30]
to make sure the bacteria don't starve to death, don't run out of fuel. And the third thing, that's also an f-word is make sure that you reproduce. Fear, feed, and some other thing. Well, once a bacteria has done those things, it'll do something magic, it'll make yogurt. And, this is the fourth word that starts with "f", and its friend. What we do at a cellular level is the same thing we do as humans, and we form a community.

[00:58:00]
Yogurt is cooperating bacteria to make something bigger than any one bacteria, and your body does this to form who you are. And when you get those basic three needs met, we have individual companionship—enough of the right kind of fuel, so your cells don't feel like they're starving, we call that fat. And, when you don't feel like you're scared all the time, we call that forgiveness. When you get those in order, you're ready to go out and form a community, and the community can support you.
[00:58:30]
And we're wired to be kind, nice, and supportive to other human beings. It's our core nature, but that nature gets disrupted. When your mitochondria don't work, you just don't have the energy to be kind to other people. That's why it's so important that we fix our mitochondria and we fix our brains, because it makes us help our community naturally and that's what makes us feel best, and when we do that it creates a feedback loop.

[00:59:00]
You support your community, you have acts of kindness and you help other people, and that makes

you feel good. And when you feel good, your mitochondria get stronger, because you know you're doing the right thing and it actually pays it forward, but you always get a return on that. That's why community is so important, because community helps you and you help the community.

Dr. Mark Hyman: It's so great to talk to you, Dave. This is an amazing set of insights about how to optimize your brain, fix your power plants, and live a good, long, healthy life.

Dave Asprey: Mark, it's an honor to be on with you; your work has influenced my life and millions of people, so thanks for your work.

Dr. Mark Hyman: Thank you, Dave.

DAVE PERLMUTTER, MD | Author, #1 *New York Times* Best Seller, *Grain Brain*

Dr. Mark Hyman:	David, we have so much to talk about. Your book, *Grain Brain*, was revolutionary in its scope and the implications for how we can change our brain and how what we eat, and what we do and our lifestyle has an impact. In fact, how even our genes are not fixed, that we can modify our genes and our DNA, that has changes in our health.
Dr. Dave Perlmutter: [00:00:30]	That's right.
Dr. Mark Hyman:	Tell us more about how that works, and how *Grain Brain* explains it. But I want you to sort of synopsize it here for us, to really understand why you wrote the book, and why it's so important to understand this revolution.
Dr. Dave Perlmutter: [00:01:00] [00:01:30] [00:02:00]	Sure. Well, I wrote the book because I was extremely frustrated being a neurologist and having very little to offer patients. It really became clear that our lifestyle choices play a huge role in the fate of the brain. That we, by making lifestyle choices, change the destiny of our brain. We understood that there was a hard, smart approach, and that the foods we ate, the exercise we did, might have an effect on the rest of the body, but the brain was out of that conversation. My aim was to change that, because the data was there and my task was to gather that data, present it, package it up, and hope that the world would embrace it, and the world did embrace it—in 30 languages. So, that happened. It really is now, I think, a really well-established understanding that we have a significant role to play in controlling our genetic destiny. The brain is somewhat at the mercy of our genes, but the empowering part of the story is we can change that by our food choices, by how we live our lives in terms of stress, really leveraging the amount of exercise we get, and even something as seemingly simple as how we sleep is hugely impactful in terms of rewriting the book with reference to your brain.
Dr. Mark Hyman: [00:02:30]	Yeah, it's great. We talk about Alzheimer's as drawing a bad card. You know, your parents got Alzheimer's. You had bad genes. There are genes that predispose to Alzheimer's, you know? We know that ApoE4, which is a gene that is involved in lipid metabolism, has a big impact and can increase your risk up to 75% if you have a double four gene. What you're saying is, that doesn't necessarily predestine you to getting Alzheimer's.
Dr. Dave Perlmutter: [00:03:00]	Very good word. It is a predisposition, not a determinant, meaning that while some people have a higher risk for Alzheimer's by virtue of their genetics, that isn't written in stone. There are plenty of people who carry the Apoe4 allele who do just fine cognitively, and there are plenty of people who don't carry it and end up with full-blown Alzheimer's. I think that we're just beginning to understand that we, again, have such a huge role to play. You know, if you live to be age 85, your risk is 50/50. If you're a type 2 diabetic, which is pretty much a choice, your risk may as much as quadruple.
Dr. Mark Hyman:	Yeah, four in five.
Dr. Dave Perlmutter:	That's a lifestyle choice.
Dr. Mark Hyman:	Yeah.
Dr. Dave Perlmutter: [00:03:30]	I think genetics are important. I probably am at significantly increased risk for that disease, by virtue of the fact that my own father died of Alzheimer's, so we really have to get the word out that we may be able to cut our risk in half by doing aerobic exercise on a daily basis. That not becoming a type 2 diabetic may also cut our risk in half, and I think it's critical that these words

[00:04:00]	get out, because no one is talking about it. When you watch television in the evening, the news, all you see are advertisements for Alzheimer's drugs that do not work. I think the message is to embrace the notion of preventive medicine as it relates to the brain and that's the message everyone has to get.
Dr. Mark Hyman:	Yeah. I mean, it seems like we've done so much research. Billions and billions of dollars of research on Alzheimer's. Over 400 published studies on reversal trials on drugs, and 99.6% of them don't work, and the ones that work delay the progression of Alzheimer's such that you'll spend three months more at home before you go to the nursing home.
Dr. Dave Perlmutter: [00:04:30]	That's right.
Dr. Mark Hyman:	What you're suggesting is that this is not inevitable, that there's actually a possibility of stopping or preventing the course.
Dr. Dave Perlmutter: [00:05:00]	The cynic in me—and I'll admit it—is that this is the dirty little secret that shouldn't get out, because what has to happen is a miracle drug needs to be developed so that it can be monetized. That's how the system works, and the idea that our lifestyle choices, which don't cost anything, can prevent the very disease that's costing us, in this country $230 billion a year, that message can't get out. You know, Dr. Dale Bredesen, I'm sure he's going to be one of your interviewees, we were talking, and I said, "You know, it's the quest for the magic bullet." He said, "It isn't a magic bullet. It's magic buckshot." There are multiple factors that have to ...
Dr. Mark Hyman:	The shotgun approach.
Dr. Dave Perlmutter:	Exactly.
Dr. Mark Hyman:	Yeah.
Dr. Dave Perlmutter: [00:05:30]	But there are multiple things that come together. Lifestyle, including exercise, diet. Yes, genetics is important; medications, nutritional supplements. All of these things have to be brought to bear to keep your brain healthy, and by all means I'm here to say this is, by and large, a preventable disease that you don't have to get. Again, coming from a person who—I'm a neurologist, sure— but I'm also a primary relative of a person who developed and died from that disease.
Dr. Mark Hyman: [00:06:00]	Yeah. That reminded me of a story from Dale Bredesen, who told me that he got funding for $2 million to do research on Alzheimer's by using multiple approaches: diet, exercise, sleep, nutritional supplements; things that help support health. He was told by the institutional review board that reviews the safety and efficacy of studies, that it wasn't okay to use all these interventions, because, "How would you know what worked?" And was it safe to actually eat better, exercise, sleep, deal with stress reduction, and take a bunch of supplements? I'm like, "This is ridiculous."
[00:06:30] Dr. Dave Perlmutter:	It's the type of medicine that you and I have been practicing for years and years, and when our Alzheimer's patients stabilize or actually improve and they want to know, "Well, which part of the program do you think is doing it?" And I tell them, "I don't care. It doesn't matter to me." We're only interested in the result. Unfortunately, that's not how science in the western world works.
[00:07:00]	We want to know, "What is that variable? What is that factor?" Because then it can be monetized.
Dr. Mark Hyman:	Yeah.
Dr. Dave Perlmutter:	I just think that's ridiculous.

Dr. Mark Hyman:	It is, and we're changing that at Cleveland Clinic now. We're actually doing these multimodal interventions and then looking at outcomes.
Dr. Dave Perlmutter:	That's right.
Dr. Mark Hyman: [00:07:30]	Then we can reverse engineer. Maybe it's not important to sleep, but I think it'll be important to sleep, or maybe you don't have to exercise, but I think it will be. Then we can sort of put together, "Maybe you don't need all these supplements. Maybe you just need this one." You know? That's fair, but we need to actually be able to sort of create health by putting all the ingredients for health in. If broccoli's good for you, you wouldn't just eat broccoli and then eat that all year and be healthy.
Dr. Dave Perlmutter: [00:08:00]	Well, you know, it's funny you say broccoli. Let's just say there's a plant food that's good for you, that's associated with some great results in whatever parameter. Reduction of headaches, weight loss, blood sugar stabilization. What is happening in western culture, is they want to extract the so-called "active ingredient," and you might fail because it might not be the active ingredient, but it may be that all these wonderful things conspire to bring about a result, and it's a totally different paradigm. Turns out that it works wonderfully as it relates to the brain. Who knew?
Dr. Mark Hyman:	Right. That's true. You mentioned that diabetes caused a four-fold increase, like a 400% increase in your risk of getting Alzheimer's.
Dr. Dave Perlmutter:	Right.
Dr. Mark Hyman:	That's dramatic and they're calling Alzheimer's now "type 3 diabetes." How is this whole sugar-carb thing related? Because this is part of what your book was about.
Dr. Dave Perlmutter: [00:08:30]	Sure, and you know, I have to admit that when *Grain Brain* was written—I wrote it during 2012; it was published in 2013—the answer I would have given you, and I did give countless times, was that elevated blood sugar changes our proteins; glycates our proteins. That turns on inflammation, and it turns on the production of damaging free radicals. It works because when you see measurements of these glycated proteins, like A1c, you see it correlates very nicely to dementia risk and even shrinkage of the brain's memory center called the hippocampus.
Dr. Mark Hyman: [00:09:00]	Yeah.
Dr. Dave Perlmutter: [00:09:30]	We now understand that there is this interplay between diabetes and changes in the gut bacteria, that there's a fingerprint within the gut bacteria that identifies diabetes. We can talk about what people are doing with that in just a moment. But it's those same changes in the gut bacteria that seem to be associated with diabetes, that are also associated with inflammation in the body and permeability or leakiness of the gut, both of which are known to be turned on as it relates to the Alzheimer's brain. Now we've shifted our emphasis from just this glycation of protein, the protein binding to sugar, to the gut. I mean, here you are talking to a neurologist. We're talking about the gut, which was a book I wrote after *Grain Brain*, which dealt with this beautiful relationship that has been studied and known about for thousands of years, that we are just discovering, that the gut is playing a critical role in the health and functionality moment to moment of your brain.
[00:10:00] Dr. Mark Hyman:	It's true. I wrote *UltraMind Solution* almost 10 years ago and it was a result of nothing I read in a journal, but the extraordinary results I was seeing by accident by treating people's gut; their brain would get better.
Dr. Dave Perlmutter:	That's right.

Dr. Mark Hyman:	I was like, "What's going on here?"
Dr. Dave Perlmutter:	"That shouldn't happen."
Dr. Mark Hyman:	No.
Dr. Dave Perlmutter:	And it does happen.
Dr. Mark Hyman:	It does.
Dr. Dave Perlmutter: [00:10:30]	We work on the gut, and the brain gets better, and the skin gets better, and the joint pain goes away. These are all issues that are based upon inflammation. Guess what? Alzheimer's is a prototypic inflammatory disorder. Same sort of inflammation. Same markers, same meditators as are involved in heart disease, as diabetes, as even cancer.
Dr. Mark Hyman:	There are almost like a few common pathways.
Dr. Dave Perlmutter:	That's right.
Dr. Mark Hyman:	And depending on the person, it can hit different organs. Whether it's autoimmune disease, dementia, heart disease, diabetes, or cancer. I mean, at Cleveland Clinic, there are scientists now discovering that the microbiome plays a role in the development of cancer.
[00:11:00] Dr. Dave Perlmutter: [00:11:30]	Oh, that's right. We call these the broad strokes. There is this real push for us to be super specialized these days and to develop protocols that are so specifically targeted for the individual; we call this personalized medicine. I think that's great, but at the same time, we know that taking a step back and looking at the broad strokes, about, "What really are the general dietary recommendations? What are people doing wrong in terms of their medications, over the counter as well as prescription, that are affecting the microbiome, the gut bacteria, and are then amplifying the gut permeability, enhancing inflammation, and ultimately, in my area of interest, leading to death of brain cells?"
Dr. Mark Hyman: [00:12:00]	Yeah. You're basically talking about a revolution in our thinking because the gut microbiome, we didn't even talk about a few years ago, and we didn't understand how it's connected to all these diseases, including brain disorders. Not just Alzheimer's, but depression, autism, ADD, Parkinson's. I mean, these conditions are ... We thought were in the brain, but you're talking about the microbiome as this new organ that we have to actually investigate, learn about, treat. So, tell us more about this sort of discovery you made and how this all works in your book, *Brain Maker*, that led you to revolutionize your thinking.
[00:12:30] Dr. Dave Perlmutter: [00:13:00]	Well, again, it was because of, I think, lack of tools in the tool box. Neurologists are working on the premise of "diagnose and adios," meaning that, "Boy, we'll come up with a great name for a disease, and that sounds great. Aren't we smart?" But then there's nothing to do. We're left empty-handed and I wasn't going to spend the rest of my career doing that and having people walk out of the office without something to do. I endeavored to discover, "What were these relationships?" I mean, if we ... granted, inflammation is an underlying mechanism of Parkinson's, MS, autism, Alzheimer's; they are inflammatory disorders. Okay, then where is this inflammation coming from? Not a bad question to ask.
Dr. Mark Hyman:	Yeah.
Dr. Dave Perlmutter:	It turns out, when you look at the literature ...

Dr. Mark Hyman:	It's sort of self-evident, right? But it's not something we do in medicine.
Dr. Dave Perlmutter: [00:13:30]	Really, it's coming from the gut. Okay. That means this neurologist is going to start paying attention to gastroenterology? Oh, no. You can't go there. That's the turf of the gastroenterologist. I went to my gastroenterologist friends and began discussing this. There was no interest.
Dr. Mark Hyman:	Yeah.
Dr. Dave Perlmutter: [00:14:00]	It became very evident to me one day, when I worked on a patient with migraine headaches by changing her diet and putting her on—get this, a gluten free diet—and her migraine headaches went away. This is something she had for 25 years and was taking narcotics for her pain. She went back to the gastroenterologist, who said, "I've scoped you. You don't have celiac disease. Why on earth would you go gluten free? Go back on gluten. You need it."
Dr. Mark Hyman:	You don't need it.
Dr. Dave Perlmutter: [00:14:30]	She refused. Had she done so, we know her headaches would have recurred, but that said, there is such push-back on anything nutritional. As you well know, recently there was an innuendo based on a study that came out saying that if you go gluten free, you're going to be at higher risk for heart disease. That is not the conclusion that the authors actually reached, Harvard researchers. The conclusion was, if you go gluten free, which means likely cut back on dietary fiber, that's not a good thing. I am totally in for that. I agree with you.
Dr. Mark Hyman:	Most people don't eat gluten and dietary fiber. It's white flour.
Dr. Dave Perlmutter:	Right. But the point is that the fundamentals are that the brain is not able to deal with inflammation very well. That inflammation happens when we disrupt the gut bacteria by a diet that's inappropriate, by taking medications that are unfavorable.
Dr. Mark Hyman: [00:15:00]	What are the medications that screw up your gut microbiome?
Dr. Dave Perlmutter:	Well, the obvious ones are antibiotics. We've now seen research that indicates that antibiotics affect a type of bacterium called the mitochondria. That's got to sound like a bit of a stretch, but a new study came out looking at beta-lactam and aminoglycoside-type antibiotics. These are types of antibiotics.
Dr. Mark Hyman:	Penicillin, and ...
Dr. Dave Perlmutter: [00:15:30] [00:16:00]	Shows that these are actually mitochondrial toxins. Now, I just took a leap for your viewers. The understanding is that our mitochondria were once free-living bacteria. That's just a little tidbit, but when you disrupt the gut bacteria by taking antibiotics, understand that is a lifelong change in your microbiome that is never the same again. Antibiotic exposure is strongly related to diabetes risk—as much as a 50% increased risk from one course of antibiotics. A very large Danish study demonstrated that. The non-steroid anti-inflammatory medications are notorious for disrupting the gut bacteria, and that likely explains why C. diff (Clostridium difficile), is higher in people who generally take these non-steroid anti-inflammatories. I think the biggest issue is going to turn out to be, oddly enough, these acid-blocking drugs called proton pump inhibitors.
Dr. Mark Hyman:	Which you can buy over the counter.
Dr. Dave Perlmutter: [00:16:30]	Which are generally bought over the counter. One study out of Stanford indicated about a 16% increased risk of heart attack in people taking these PPIs, and if you have that heart attack, your risk of dying from it is increased; Is doubled, basically. That happens because of changes in the PH

of the gut. Why would you be surprised that these drugs would change the acidity of the gut? Because that's what they're designed to do.

Dr. Mark Hyman: Designed to do, right.

Dr. Dave Perlmutter: [00:17:00] When you change the acid-level/acid-based balance of the gut, it changes the environment in which the bacteria live. Certain species will thrive, certain species will be suppressed, and you have this loss of diversity of gut bacteria. That leads to leakiness of the gut and the brain, and it sets the stage for disaster.

Dr. Mark Hyman: I mean, one of the side effects of PPIs, or acid blocking drugs, is irritable bowel syndrome.

Dr. Dave Perlmutter: Who knew? And C. diff.

Dr. Mark Hyman: And that causes diarrhea, and C. diff, right?

Dr. Dave Perlmutter: [00:17:30] Well, interestingly, JAMA Neurology, the Journal of the American Medical Association's specialty journal, *Neurology*, last year demonstrated that chronic users of these proton pump inhibitors have more than a 40% increased risk of developing dementia. To the extent that the authors concluded that avoiding PPIs might be part of the program for prevention of Alzheimer's disease, all of these things that relate to increased risk for dementia. We are now looking at it through the lens of how these affect the microbiome, how they affect the gut bacteria. How does that affect [00:18:00] gut permeability? How does that reduce the production of a certain short-chain fatty acid called butyrate, which plays such a critical role in how our brain is energized, in the maintenance of the blood-brain barrier, in the change of expression of our DNA, through what's called histone deacetylase inhibition, through even the cellular functions of metabolism, that are regulated through these complex channels, that begin with what are called G protein receptors? This is what butyrate does.

[00:18:30]
Dr. Mark Hyman: Butyrate is a product of healthy bacteria.

Dr. Dave Perlmutter: Exactly right.

Dr. Mark Hyman: When you have good bacteria in your gut, it produces this compound ...

Dr. Dave Perlmutter: ... called butyrate.

Dr. Mark Hyman: ... which is this type of fat.

Dr. Dave Perlmutter: Which your brain loves, your gut loves, your immune system loves, and you nurture your gut bacteria by giving them what's called prebiotic fiber. Eating those foods, the Mexican yam, the dandelion greens, the asparagus. Foods like garlic, onions, leeks, that enhance the function of these bacteria. They're so happy, they're going to say, "I'm going to help Dr. Hyman be healthier tomorrow."

[00:19:00]
Dr. Mark Hyman: "I want more asparagus please."

Dr. Dave Perlmutter: "Because I am going to make more butyrate." The richest source of butyrate that you can eat is butter, which is in fact where the word butyrate comes from.

Dr. Mark Hyman: Yeah.

Dr. Dave Perlmutter: You know, butter is back.

Dr. Mark Hyman: [00:19:30]	Butter is back. Yes. I just reviewed an article that was a review of six million patient years, over hundreds and hundreds of thousands of patients, over many, many, many years, finding no association with butter and heart disease and potentially reverse association with diabetes. Meaning you eat more butter, you get less diabetes.
Dr. Dave Perlmutter:	Old habits die hard. You know, I was on a nutritional panel, and I think you may have been on it, in New York a year or two ago. There was another individual who just ... It was all about how butter will kill you. It'll make your children born naked or some terrible thing.
Dr. Mark Hyman:	That it will.
Dr. Dave Perlmutter:	And low fat is the way to go. Hey, I'm all for listening to other people's opinions, but let's look, like you say, at, "What is the research telling us?"
Dr. Mark Hyman: [00:20:00]	Yeah.
Dr. Dave Perlmutter:	The research is telling us that sugar, for example, isn't necessarily a good thing. Well, you need sugar to help the medicine go down, but sugar will destroy your brain and it does so through its effects on the gut bacteria.
Dr. Mark Hyman: [00:20:30] [00:21:00]	Yes. I just want to pause for a minute, because most people I don't think understand the impact that it actually has on our health. I was recently thinking about it. We have 10 times the number of bacteria in us than our own cells, and we have probably 100 times as much bacterial DNA as our own DNA. What our DNA does is produce proteins, information molecules that govern the function of our body. When you think about it, your genes maybe make a hundred, a couple hundred thousand chemicals or proteins. Your bacterial genes are making literally millions of proteins that are getting absorbed that are interacting with your biology, so your microbiome metabolome, in a sense the metabolites that are produced by the microbiome, are probably more influential in your health than your own cells.
Dr. Dave Perlmutter:	No question.
Dr. Mark Hyman:	That begs the question I'm going to ask you, which is how do you make sure you cultivate the healthy inner garden? What are the things people can do and take away that help them actually fix that, taking away the drugs that are gut-busting drugs.
Dr. Dave Perlmutter:	Good point. That's a great place to start. What are the things, first of all, that are bad for your gut bacteria? And then we can talk about, okay, what do we do that's good?
Dr. Mark Hyman: [00:21:30]	You mentioned sugar.
Dr. Dave Perlmutter:	Yeah. Well, just to recap, really important: medications. Everybody's got to review their medications, especially antibiotics, the non-steroidal anti-inflammatories, and the proton pump inhibiting acid.
Dr. Mark Hyman:	Then the birth control pill, I hate to say.
Dr. Dave Perlmutter: [00:22:00]	Even the birth control pill, or how we were born, by caesarian section versus vaginal birth. There are a lot of immune-related issues, like type 1 diabetes, celiac disease, autism, ADHD, even adult obesity. Issues that are dramatically increased in terms of risk in kids who were born by c-section. Why? Because they didn't get the seeds. They didn't get the anointment of bacteria that they would have gotten by passing through their mother's birth canal, by virtue of having been born by c-section. Chlorinated water, lack of sleep, stress. We're now seeing data that correlates higher levels of diversity of gut bacteria, correlated with max VO2. Meaning the more ...

Dr. Mark Hyman: [00:22:30]	Exercise.
Dr. Dave Perlmutter:	... cardiorespiratory fitness you have, it correlates with higher levels of diversity of gut bacteria. That is not to say that getting in shape will increase your gut diversity. I think it does, but extrapolating from that article doesn't allow me to say that, but you allow me to say that.
Dr. Mark Hyman:	Say it.
Dr. Dave Perlmutter:	To rebuild, though, the microbiome, I think we've got to be really super diligent about the diet. The diet has to be very high in fiber, so missing from the standard American diet, western culture.
Dr. Mark Hyman: [00:23:00]	Yeah.
Dr. Dave Perlmutter:	I think that the issue about fat is really important. We have to welcome good fat back to the diet, that others have been castigating for such a long time. Fat is fundamentally important.
Dr. Mark Hyman: [00:23:30]	Let me stop you there, because there's evidence that high fat diets can negatively affect the gut microbiome, and when I looked at the data, it was, "What kind of fat?" And omega-3 fats seem to optimize gut flora, whereas omega-6 fats, inflammatory fats like soybean oil, may actually negatively alter gut flora.
Dr. Dave Perlmutter:	That's right. When you emailed me about fat and the microbiome last year, the article that I sent back to you, as I recollect, was ... The article you had sent me talked about the possible detrimental effects of fat on the microbiome. I said, "Mark, look at it, though." The study actually was high fat and high sugar.
Dr. Mark Hyman:	Sugar diets. Right.
Dr. Dave Perlmutter:	That's a take-home message.
Dr. Mark Hyman:	Yeah.
Dr. Dave Perlmutter: [00:24:00]	If you're pounding sugar ... Everybody wants to eat more fat now, because we've heard that it's good for you. But if you're eating sugar, all bets are off. You're just paving the way for disaster.
Dr. Mark Hyman:	Yeah. I call it "sweet fat." Whatever you want to call it. Bagel and butter.
Dr. Dave Perlmutter:	Yeah, but if you're going to bring fat back to the table, and you should, A: it has to be good fat; Healthful fat. We'll talk about that in a moment. But B: you've got to simultaneously cut the sugar. Got to go. And what are people now doing? They're getting the low sugar message, and they're drinking and eating artificially sweetened foods. Well, that is about the worst thing you could do.
Dr. Mark Hyman: [00:24:30]	For your gut microbiome.
Dr. Dave Perlmutter: [00:25:00]	For your gut microbiome. We didn't understand why artificially-sweetened beverages were associated with diabetes, for example. More so than drinking sugar-sweetened beverages. People who drink artificially-sweetened, no-calorie, no-sugar beverages, yet they're more than doubling their risk for diabetes. How in the world could that be? It's counterintuitive. We came up with all kinds of ideas, but now Israeli researchers have shown us it is straightforward because of changes in the gut bacteria. Last month, a study came out showing a dramatic increased risk, over 44% increased risk of getting Alzheimer's disease, becoming demented, in people drinking artificially-flavored and sweetened pop or soda. Again, what could be the mechanism? The authors hit it on the head. It's because of changes in the gut bacteria, which then code for increasing

inflammation, the cornerstone of every brain disease that you don't want to get.

Dr. Mark Hyman:
[00:25:30]

Mm-hmm. Speaking of the brain, we're talking about, in a sense, a bacterial brain that lives in your gut. But there's also kind of a second nervous system, called the second brain, in the gut. Talk about how that influences your health, and Alzheimer's, and brain function, and what people can do about it. What causes it?

Dr. Dave Perlmutter:

You know, the notion is that there is a gut-brain, or brain-gut, as I prefer to call it obviously, connection.

Dr. Mark Hyman:
[00:26:00]

It's the most important organ in your body.

Dr. Dave Perlmutter:

I'm not going to go there. But that said, it doesn't really make sense anymore to differentiate between the gut and the brain, because they really are functionally very, very similar, and they're connected. There are large channels, like the vagus nerve, which is a superhighway connecting the gut to the brain, and interestingly, it looks as if the vagus nerve is transporting all kinds of things these days, beyond just electrical impulses, that are having a role to play in brain health or disease. For example, a recent study demonstrated that in people who had what's called a vagotomy years ago ...

[00:26:30]

Dr. Mark Hyman:

Where they cut the vagus nerve.

Dr. Dave Perlmutter:

... where the vagus nerve was cut, which is what they used to do for ulcer treatment—vagotomy and pyloroplasty—that their risk of Parkinson's is dramatically reduced. It turns out that what the research now is revealing is that misfolded proteins that have their genesis in the gut were being transported through the vagus nerve into the brain and may relate to the risk for Parkinson's. That's pretty exciting. But more importantly, I think that the relationship of the gut to the brain is both physical, but it's also chemical. We talk about serotonin and dopamine, and so-called neurotransmitters, failing to recognize that the lion's share of these chemicals are not made in the brain. They're made in the gut. They are made at levels that lead to mood stabilization when the gut is healthy. Dr. Emeran Mayer at UCLA wrote a wonderful book about this relationship between the gut, the gut health, and mood regulation, for example.

[00:27:00]

[00:27:30]

Intriguingly, we now look upon, for example, depression (an inflammatory disorder) as possibly having its genesis in the gut. How do we know that? Because markers of gut leakiness, or permeability, are dramatically elevated in correlation with depression, as they are in Alzheimer's disease, autism, and even Lou Gehrig's disease. Again, we mentioned earlier that we've got to pull away from being so cerebro-centric and look at the body as a whole, and particularly the gut, for reasons that you well-described. The number of organisms. Their bacterial, rather their metabolic products, and not the least of which, their genetic compound, in terms of being hugely relevant, in terms of health and longevity.

[00:28:00]

Dr. Mark Hyman:
[00:28:30]

Yes. It's pretty stunning when you think about the way we sort of missed the boat, and blamed all sorts of other factors, like bad parenting, or emotional trauma, or stress, or mental illness on the brain, as opposed to the gut. I'm not a researcher, although now we're doing research at Cleveland Clinic. For most of my career I've been a practicing physician, and I just noticed this phenomenon. I wasn't even trying to treat the brain and it would get better from all sorts of conditions by simply fixing the gut.

[00:29:00]

Dr. Dave Perlmutter:

Well, as we often learn as of late, these issues are oftentimes two-way streets. When you mentioned early life trauma, for example, there are now signature gut bacterial changes that are seen in association with people who had trauma during their early lives, and that these changes in the gut bacteria correlate with measurable changes in brain areas. Certain areas of the brain are less functional in correlation with those changes in the gut bacteria that correlate with early life trauma.

Dr. Mark Hyman:
[00:29:30]
That's amazing. What you're saying, basically, is your thoughts and your feelings and experiences talk to the bacteria in your gut, and change them in ways that are harmful.

Dr. Dave Perlmutter:
And then the gut also communicates back and alters our feelings, alter our gut.

Dr. Mark Hyman:
Yes.

Dr. Dave Perlmutter:
Alter how we perceive the world. Dr. Emeran Mayer, I mentioned his work earlier, he took a group of 21 women and divided them into three, or actually I think 22, and cut them in ... They didn't cut the women in half. They cut the group in half.

Dr. Mark Hyman:
[00:30:00]
It's a magic trick.

Dr. Dave Perlmutter:

[00:30:30]

[00:31:00]
Part of the group got a yogurt that had no probiotics. The other group got a yogurt that was enriched with probiotics, and after a period of ... I think it was a couple of months, he measured brain activity, and found that those individuals who were consuming higher levels of probiotics had changes in their brain functionality. Now, that's breathtaking, because that tells us that gut bacteria can change the function of our brains; that gut bacteria can change the expression of our 22,000 genes that we got from Mom and Dad and from all of our forebears. That tends to make our gut bacteria assume a much higher, I think, place in terms of respect, and in terms of where we are today, and certainly where we need to go in the future. When we are confronted by things like Alzheimer's, and cancer, and autoimmune conditions for which we have really very little to offer. Except for in the case of autoimmune issues, the so-called biologics, which work at the very end of the cascade of immune problems, where we now understand that the problems actually begin further up the line. By paying attention to the gut and manipulating the microbiome with specific probiotics and even groups of probiotics, we finally get to the beginning or the origin of these issues.

Dr. Mark Hyman:
[00:31:30]
David, in your practice and in your book, you've identified ways to optimize the gut flora, as a way of treating the brain. Could you take us through the strategy and the practical application of, how do you tend your inner garden, and what are the steps you take to transform your gut?

Dr. Dave Perlmutter:

[00:32:00]
Sure. I think that, having mentioned what we did in terms of what makes a good microbiome go bad, those steps are, again, favorite prebiotic foods like I mentioned. The jicama, the garlic, onions, leeks, the dandelion greens, the asparagus. Those are foods that are really important because they nurture the gut bacteria. They help the gut bacteria reduce inflammation, produce more butyrate. These prebiotic fibers have actually been shown to increase what's called BDNF, and therefore play a role in growing new brain cells through this intermediate of the gut bacteria.

Dr. Mark Hyman:
They're like fertilizer for the good bacteria.

Dr. Dave Perlmutter:
[00:32:30]
They're fertilizer for the gut bacteria, to do what they want to do, and that is keep you healthy. But beyond that, there is a place for probiotics, that's for sure. There are some very good probiotics on the market. We look for products that have a large number of different strains, that have been studied. 10, 12, 14 different strains, 15. Many billions of bacteria, but you really want to look for products that have a guaranteed shelf life. I think that's really very important. Beyond that, some of the things where we push the envelope a little bit in the clinical practice is giving probiotics not just orally, but giving them through enemas. I know that sounds strange. We've had terrific results with it, and you know we have.

Dr. Mark Hyman: [00:33:00]	Yes.
Dr. Dave Perlmutter: [00:33:30]	Putting probiotics in an enema bag and administering them, and even beyond that, going as far, in some cases, as doing what is called fecal transplantation. This is not something that everybody who's learning this information needs to take home, but there is a time and a place to consider revamping and reestablishing healthy gut bacteria by taking fecal material from a healthy individual and transplanting it into somebody whose gut bacteria has been really disrupted. We know that more than 500 hospitals in America today are doing fecal transplantation, as crazy as that sounds, in the treatment of a life-threatening diarrhea illness called Clostridium difficile, which now still kills 30,000 Americans each year. Most hospitals don't do it, and yet it is by far and away the most effective treatment known to man.
Dr. Mark Hyman:	I mean, half of the regular treatment fails.
Dr. Dave Perlmutter: [00:34:00]	Yeah.
Dr. Mark Hyman:	And then 98% of fecal transplants work.
Dr. Dave Perlmutter:	Right.
Dr. Mark Hyman:	Immediately.
Dr. Dave Perlmutter:	That's right. I mean, the standard of care for treating C. diff is, of all things, antibiotics.
Dr. Mark Hyman:	Antibiotics. Right.
Dr. Dave Perlmutter:	Which likely produced the C. diff in the first place.
Dr. Mark Hyman:	Mm-hmm.
Dr. Dave Perlmutter: [00:34:30] [00:35:00]	It's about 26% effective, in terms of putting a person in a position where they will not have a relapse. As you well mentioned, 96% to 98% cure rate with fecal transplant. Is it icky? Is it bizarre? Yeah, I get that. Of course it is. But I get through that when I see an autistic child speaking for the first time in his life and I see University of Arizona doing a trial of fecal transplant in 20 autistic children. When I see a researcher in Amsterdam, Dr. Max Nieuwdorp, reversing diabetes by doing fecal transplantation. Is it bizarre? Sure it is, based upon our upbringing about poop. But you know, we could put that aside and recognize this is a powerful modality based upon recalibrating what's going on in the gut, and hoping for improvements throughout the body, including in the brain.
Dr. Mark Hyman: [00:35:30]	That's huge. You mentioned sugar, and you mentioned sugar in the brain. We talked about Alzheimer's, type 3 diabetes. It's such a manifest problem in this country, with the average person having 22 teaspoons of sugar, where the American Heart Association says, "Eat six." For some, it's much more, including children. We eat 152 pounds of sugar and 146 pounds of flour. That's a pound of sugar and flour a day for every man, woman, and child in America. How is this impacting the brain and what should we do about it? Also, I'm going to touch on the title of your book, which is *Grain Brain*. Are grains included in this or is it just sugar? And should we be eating any grains?
Dr. Dave Perlmutter:	Well, there are a lot of questions there.
Dr. Mark Hyman: [00:36:00]	Yes, there are.
Dr. Dave Perlmutter:	First of all, there are some grains that I think are not necessarily threatening, and I think that if

[00:36:30] you can find a non-GMO corn, or you want to eat some quinoa, which by definition is not necessarily a grain, but everybody talks about it as if it were. The issues with grain are two-fold: it's their carb content and the fact that they contain gluten, in my opinion. There are other issues as well. We know that wheat is, although it is not genetically modified in America, is still sprayed with an herbicide called glyphosate, which is powerfully threatening to the gut bacteria, as the work of Dr. Stephanie Seneff has made very clear to us.

Dr. Mark Hyman: Roundup.

Dr. Dave Perlmutter: Roundup. You got it. We understand that this ... Going tangentially here, but that's a powerful threat to the microbiome. It has insinuated itself into so many foods. It is the largest global

[00:37:00] herbicide in terms of its use. 1.35 million metric tons being sprayed on our food, and our animals' food, around the globe. Threatening the soil microbiome, threatening the microbiome in you and me, and it needs to stop. The World Health Organization has characterized glyphosate, the active ingredient in Roundup, as a probable human carcinogen. That was published in the well-

[00:37:30] respected journal *The Lancet*. As it gets to sugar, you're right. I want to just take a step back a little bit on sugar, because as we've learned from one of our mentors, Dr. Jeffrey Bland, food is information. It means that the foods we eat are changing the expression of our DNA. That's a heady notion, but the food we eat changes the expression of our DNA from moment to moment.

[00:38:00] Our DNA has been honed to make us the best we can be, over a couple of million years, to make us the most able to respond to changing environments, smartest, or some might argue these days how smart we really are. The point is, though, we have this wonderful relationship with our genome, with our DNA. When I say we get our 23,000, or 22,000, 23,000 genes from our parents, yeah, but who did they get it from? It's been passed down generation to generation. Food is

[00:38:30] information. Suddenly, 200 years ago, we developed a technology to overwhelm this information paradigm with sugar. We're now sending signals to our DNA, the likes of which it has never seen, and our genome is freaking out and doesn't know what to do with the signal that's coming into the body. There are many things we can talk about. Diabetes, dictation protein, leakiness of the bowel, inflammation, with reference to sugar, but I think it's good to every once in a while take a

[00:39:00] step back to look at the genetics of what this has done to us. We know that diets higher in sugar enhance that very process that we've got to do everything to avoid, and that is inflammation.

You're right. The statistics on what we're doing in terms of sugar consumption are overwhelming, and what so many people don't recognize is that they're consuming sugar, though they don't spoon it out into their food, but yet, you know, the glass of orange juice. The 12-ounce glass of

[00:39:30] orange juice is nine teaspoons right there that you didn't even add in. That's before the croissant or whatever wonderfully-languaged something arrives. "It's okay because it's a croissant. It's from France. It's got to be good for me." Or the bagel, you name it. More sugar, more carbs. The problem is that we're in this mindset that fat was what we should have eaten, but we stopped the fat in favor of the sugar and it has amplified diabetes, cancer, heart disease, you name it. The

[00:40:00] good news is that through books like the ones you've written, that fat has been really validated as an integral part of our diet, and it's the sugar, it's been the sugar, like Gary Taubes and Robert Lustig have talked about, and Mark Hyman. It's the sugar.

Dr. Mark Hyman: "It's the sugar, stupid," right?

Dr. Dave Perlmutter: You know, old habits die hard. We have a sweet tooth. It's a survival mechanism.

Dr. Mark Hyman: Of course.

Dr. Dave Perlmutter: We love our sugar. There's no one who's going to watch this who doesn't like sugar. I would eat
[00:40:30] sugar if it wasn't harmful. What did we do? We said, "Well, sugar's bad. I'll take the diet drink." Now we look at the data I talked about on the diet sodas, and we're digging the hole even deeper.

Dr. Mark Hyman: [00:41:00]	The flip side of this, of the sugar being a driver of a lot of the health issues, including Alzheimer's, including depression, including ADD, autism, all through the ways that we described, the flip side of that is, fat has been exonerated. You wrote a lot about that in your book, and even saturated fat, which still is demonized. I think that you talk in your book about ketogenic diets as a strategy for brain health, and we see this being used in Alzheimer's, in epilepsy, in brain cancer.
Dr. Dave Perlmutter:	That's right.
Dr. Mark Hyman:	Tell us about that flip, and also the kind of extreme version, which is eating, like, 80% fat.
Dr. Dave Perlmutter: [00:41:30]	Right. Well, first I'll say that when *Grain Brain* was written, did I ever take the heat for that, for saying we should be eating less carbs and more fat. I mean, that was back in the ancient times of 2013. The Amazon comments, "Oh, this is a diet that's going to kill you." And I'm not dead yet. Monty Python, "Not quite dead yet." And so, I took my lumps, and continued to do so, which is good because if you're not an outlier, no one's going to say bad things about you, so that's a good thing.
Dr. Mark Hyman:	The pioneers have arrows in their back.
Dr. Dave Perlmutter: [00:42:00] [00:42:30] [00:43:00]	Yes. Just the basics of, "Do we choose to power our bodies with fat versus carbohydrates?" was looked at in the *Journal of Alzheimer's Disease*. The study was published by researchers at the Mayo Clinic, and they demonstrated that those individuals who favored a higher fat source for calories for their bodies had about a 44% reduction in risk for dementia. As opposed to about an 87% increased risk for dementia if you chose to go the carb route, eating more healthy carbs and healthy grains that, you know, as you say it, that's been debunked. Taking it to the extreme, when you really restrict your carbs and sugars and really add in not just dietary fat, but other unique types of fat like coconut oil, or even more effectively, what is called MCT, medium-chain triglyceride oil, you ultimately shift your metabolism to a point where your cells begin saying, "You know what? I'm not going to be burning sugar all the time, because it's not around." We are flex-fuel organisms. We can burn other things. We can shift, we can adapt to burning fat. Not just dietary fat, but fat that we harvest from our own bellies or wherever we're storing fat. Through the liver, these free fatty acids then are metabolized into what are called ketone bodies. These ketone bodies are an incredibly efficient, power-fuel ... powerful fuel.
Dr. Mark Hyman:	They're a power-fuel.
Dr. Dave Perlmutter: [00:43:30] [00:44:00]	Power-fuel. I've got to get the dot com before you do. The URL, "PowerFuel.com." But that said, it's a terrific way to power your brain. Pharmaceuticals have known this for a long time, to the extent that they actually developed a powdered product years ago that they were marketing, and still market, as a way to power the brain and get results in terms of memory. It turns out that powering your brain with fat is a better way of augmenting brain function, preserving the brain, preventing brain decline. It's been used therapeutically since the late 1920s to treat epilepsy. In 2005, in the journal *Neurology*, was a powerful article showing incredible improvement in Parkinson's patients by going on what we're describing, a ketogenic, a diet that makes ketones. A ketogenic diet. More powerful than any medication, in terms of reducing the rating scale that's used to rate how bad Parkinson's patients are doing.
Dr. Mark Hyman:	That's amazing.
Dr. Dave Perlmutter: [00:44:30]	Just dietary, and yet all that neurologists do generally is treat the symptoms of Parkinson's. I think there's merit to using those drugs. I write the prescriptions, but you've got to treat the fire, not just the smoke. We do that by, in Parkinson's, by giving things like coenzyme Q10. By giving things like NAC, and putting patients on a ketogenic diet. Why? Because it makes sense, but beyond that, it's what the science tells us we should be doing.

Dr. Mark Hyman: [00:45:00]	Yet it's almost absent from medical care, right? Doctors treat patients with Alzheimer's and Parkinson's never mention diet. Never talk about it.
Dr. Dave Perlmutter: [00:45:30] [00:46:00]	It's true, and I'm not going to curse the darkness, but my mission is to light the flame, and that is, for any people who want this information, that's what this is all about. That's why we do these presentations. For those people who want to learn that there's more out there, I'm here to say there is a lot more out there, and there are a few people who are going through the literature published in the most well-respected peer-reviewed journals. What did I just quote? *The Journal of Alzheimer's Disease.* What did the *New England Journal of Medicine* tell us in September of 2013? They made a very simple statement. Here's the study. They took several thousand individuals. They said, "Hello, how are you? We're going to do two tests on you today. We're going to measure your blood sugar, and we're going to measure how well your brain is working." They followed these people for about seven years. They came back and they only did one test, "How's your brain working?" They did an examination of brain function. Didn't even measure the blood sugar at that examination. What they found was a dramatic correlation between their original blood sugar, and whether or not they became demented. What they found was really quite startling. That is that even having a blood sugar of 105 ...
Dr. Mark Hyman:	Which is normal.
Dr. Dave Perlmutter: [00:46:30]	... which is so-called normal, was dramatically associated with risk for dementia. You just put the word "normal," and these are quotes for those who don't know, in quotes, because we need to challenge that. That is, not go with what is the normal value, but what is optimal. A blood sugar of 100 is ...
Dr. Mark Hyman:	Not optimal.
Dr. Dave Perlmutter: [00:47:00]	... not optimal, and yet go to the doctor, you'll get a pat on the back, or who knows where, but they'll say, "It's fine. You're in the normal range." For people like you and people like me, who are helping to get better information out, we want optimal range. We want the best information. Blood sugar 85 to 90, for example. That's what you want. You want your A1c not at six, because you're still not diabetic. You want your A1c at 5.3, 5.4. That's ideal. That's what's associated with brain preservation, and these are things that are based upon sugar versus fat.
Dr. Mark Hyman: [00:47:30]	We talked about saturated fat, and I want to sort of help get that debunked, and I also want to talk about statins, because you write a lot about statins, which are ubiquitous, and prescriptions. I met a 39-year-old woman who was given a statin, who exercised all the time, had normal triglycerides and HDL, who really was healthy and took care of herself, and normal weight, not diabetic, and their doctor was giving her a statin. How does this affect the brain and should we be worried about saturated fats?
Dr. Dave Perlmutter: [00:48:00] [00:48:30]	Well, these I think are two different topics. Let's first start with saturated fats. The brain loves saturated fats and the body loves saturated fats. We've been eating saturated fats for as long as we've been walking the planet. You know, when you realize that 50% of the fat in breast milk is saturated fat, who would you say got that wrong? Mother nature or God? I'm not willing to take that position and accuse either by taking either of those two positions. We need saturated fat. Why is it so good for us? Because by virtue of the fact that saturated fat is saturated, it means by definition it cannot be oxidized. That's the beauty of saturated fat, why we incorporate saturated fat into our cell membranes, and our brain cell membranes, our neurons, is because they can't then be oxidized.
Dr. Mark Hyman:	Or damaged.

Dr. Dave Perlmutter: [00:49:00]	Or damaged by these crazy chemicals called free radicals, which we actually need, but which everybody seems to be mounting a war against. I think that it gets back to something that we talked about earlier. In the context of eating a diet that's got a lot of sugar in it, then we begin to wonder about having high levels of saturated fat and total fat in the diet. Now, as it relates to cholesterol ...
Dr. Mark Hyman:	Ice cream, fried ...
Dr. Dave Perlmutter:	All those good things. Yeah, a fried ice cream would be about as bad as you could get. It's not just fat, but it's got trans fats too.
Dr. Mark Hyman:	Yes.
Dr. Dave Perlmutter:	But the notion of cholesterol being our enemy is ... you know, somebody's ...
Dr. Mark Hyman:	That's the whole thesis of saturated fat, is that it raises your cholesterol, so it's bad, because cholesterol is bad.
Dr. Dave Perlmutter: [00:49:30] [00:50:00]	Cholesterol is bad, and there is something, believe it or not, that somebody has called, "bad cholesterol." LDL. It's breathtaking ... I don't know if it's Don Draper, but somebody on Madison Avenue came up with the idea, "We're going to call it LDL. Bad cholesterol." It's not bad and it's not cholesterol. It's neither of those two things, and yet everybody wants their LDL as low as possibly they can get it and their cholesterol as low as they can get it as well. You know, when you realize, for example, that those elderly individuals who have the lowest cholesterol have the highest risk for dementia, you should take a step back and say, "Gee. Therefore, does it make sense that we should declare war on cholesterol?" No. We need cholesterol. Why? It's a critical part of cell membranes. It is a brain antioxidant. It is the chemical from which your body makes testosterone, estrogen, progesterone, cortisol, and even vitamin D. We wonder why it is that people who have the lowest level of cholesterol have such issues.
[00:50:30]	There are plenty of factors that we can read about on a lipid profile that do relate to cardiovascular risk. One of them is a damaged form of this LDL that we call oxidized LDL and what does it mean?
Dr. Mark Hyman:	They say, "rancid LDL."
Dr. Dave Perlmutter: [00:51:00] [00:51:30]	Rancid. Rancid LDL. What does it mean? It means it became oxidized. It became damaged by free radicals. Now, more and more laboratories are demonstrating that, because we can reduce the oxidation of our LDL by—believe it or not—reducing our sugar. How does it work? Oxidized LDL correlates with the level of glycated LDL, the level of this protein that has been bound to sugar. The less our level of our blood sugar, the less that process happens. Reduce the glycation of LDL, it reduces the oxidation of LDL. That's why that's important; If you don't know your oxidized LDL, you can infer whether it's high or low by looking at your A1c. That's a blood test that far too many Americans are very familiar with, because 28 to 30 million of Americans are now diabetic, and estimates are that as many as 100 million of us may be what is called "pre-diabetic." It's not a surprise, when you look at the numbers, you look at people in general, that that's happening.
[00:52:00] [00:52:30]	Diabetes is happening because of our diets being higher in sugar, but it's also happening—and this is really important—because of changes in the microbiome, as is obesity. There are plenty of people who aren't taking in very many calories, and are now on low carb, low sugar, and eating a little bit of fat, and still can't lose weight, and they will not lose weight until they first reprogram their microbiomes, their gut bacteria, that right now think their body is starving, and hold onto every calorie as if they are starving. That scenario sets the stage for diabetes. It sets the stage for Alzheimer's disease as well. Diabetic? You quadruple your risk of Alzheimer's.

Dr. Mark Hyman: [00:53:00]	What about statins? Because you were just saying that cholesterol is important, that it's not the enemy we thought. That it's damaged cholesterol that's the issue, and that's worsened with sugar in your diet and other factors. Millions and millions of Americans are getting statins. People who don't have heart disease, who have low risk factors, normal blood pressure, normal blood sugar, who exercise, who don't smoke, but their LDL is high. They're getting statins. What is the risk of those drugs, and what is the future of this?
Dr. Dave Perlmutter: [00:53:30]	You know, it's what greases the skids. These simple ideas that cholesterol is bad and will kill you, that a diet high in fat is bad and will kill you. They take traction, and they are tenacious, and it takes a long time and a lot of work, for forward-thinking, progressive health care practitioners to reverse those wrongs. By and large, people who have elevated cholesterol without other risk factors, in my opinion, do not need statins, and yet they're prescribed left, right, and center, as you well characterized. Are there people with multiple risk factors, with familial hypercholesterolemia, genetically elevated cholesterol, who should bring their cholesterols down to a more reasonable level? I think there's an argument in favor of that.
Dr. Mark Hyman: [00:54:00]	Yeah.
Dr. Dave Perlmutter: [00:54:30] [00:55:00]	But not overdoing it. It's not, "the lower, the better." But at the same time that cholesterol is being lowered with a statin drug, ask yourself, "What are the downsides of statins and is there anything we can do to offset those downsides?" Yes, we understand that taking a statin drug has a detrimental effect on coenzyme Q10 level, a nutritional supplement that people can buy in the health food store. The idea of taking a statin drug without adding CoQ10 will not be considered malpractice, but in the world of integrative medicine, if we ever could influence that, it would be. We need CoQ10 on board, I think all the time, but certainly in the presence of a statin medication. I think many, if not most patients on statin drugs, shouldn't be taking them. They are dramatically overused in patients with stroke, who have no heart disease, because of the correlations of stroke, and maybe the patient does have some heart disease hiding in the background. The data is very sketchy on reduction of a next stroke by taking a statin medication. There are researchers trying to squeeze the use of statins into an Alzheimer's treatment protocol, which makes absolutely no sense whatsoever.
Dr. Mark Hyman: [00:55:30]	Mm-hmm. Amazing. For people reading, they're both probably enraged and enthused about what they can do, and what's been happening to them. What would be the things you'd want to say to them to help them become empowered about their brain? What are the take homes?
Dr. Dave Perlmutter: [00:56:00] [00:56:30]	I love the word "empowered." That is having the knowledge to make change, and let me just say that we live in a world where we are told to live our lives come what may, and when the shoe drops and we are given a diagnosis, we hope there's a magic pill. There is no effective treatment for Alzheimer's, and yet, Dr. Hyman, it is, as you well know, a preventable disease. That's the message. It's a dietary issue. Exercise is fundamentally important for growing new brain cells, and staving off Alzheimer's. The diet has to restrict sugars dramatically. I think vitamin D is critically important. These are things that we're covering in this series. I'm sure that many of your other speakers are going to cover these issues, but the message is: embrace this information and make these changes. Don't wait for a cure because once the diagnosis happens, it happens very, very quickly. The changes happen quickly and those changes happen far more quickly than there's going to be any pharmaceutical intervention that's going to cure Alzheimer's.
Dr. Mark Hyman:	Yeah. Yeah. It makes me think of that Leonard Cohen song, *There Ain't No Cure For Love*. It's like, "There ain't no cure for diabetes." I mean, for diabetes or anything—for Alzheimer's—in a pill. It's all the things that we can do ourselves to change our biology, to affect our brain. Thank you.

Dr. Dave Perlmutter: The word doctor doesn't mean "healer." It means "teacher." That's exactly what we're doing, and I've always praised you for that.

Dr. Mark Hyman: Thank you, Dr. Perlmutter.
[00:57:00]

Dr. Dave Perlmutter: Thank you, Dr. Hyman.

BROKEN BRAIN

DAVID MUSNICK, MD | www.peakmedicine.com Bellevue, WA

Dr. David Musnick:

[00:00:30]

I originally got a Masters in Public Health at UC Berkeley, and I somehow got into a little bit of the holistic medicine arena through a course I took there. It opened my mind up a little bit, and then I just got into more internal medicine. Then I got into sports medicine. But what was really interesting was I wanted to help people heal any musculoskeletal injury. And so, I started opening up my horizons to acupuncture and scar injections and something called prolotherapy, which heals loose joints. And then frequency-specific microcurrent and basically anything that would heal the musculoskeletal system.

[00:01:00]

[00:01:30]

Then around 1996, I was working at a sports medicine clinic and I went to the American Holistic Medical Association meeting and I met Dr. David Perlmutter. I talked to him a little bit and then it just opened up my whole world. I was interested in anything that would help people. I realized I didn't know everything, and I also realized the model where you just take a list of symptoms and label, "You've got this and then you need that," that didn't make much sense to me anymore. I wanted to expand. I saw a lot of complicated patients and I didn't like saying to people, "I don't know what to do." I wanted to say, "I have ideas for you," so I started literally going to any lecture, going to any seminar. And I started teaching for the Institute of Functional Medicine around the year 2000 or 2001.

[00:02:00]

Well, the conventional approach is basically if someone hits their head as a kid or an adult—let's say it's a kid, because I have a lot of compassion for children that hit their heads—so they usually go to the children's hospital in their area. They're seen by an emergency room doctor or someone like that. And they basically just tell them, they try to determine if they could have a bleed in their brain. They often will do a CAT scan. The CAT scan often doesn't show very much or doesn't show anything.

[00:02:30]

And then they tell them to go home, and often tell them not to go to sleep or make sure you can wake this person up every couple hours. And so, these people get completely exhausted or sleep-deprived. Then they basically tell them about what symptoms they could have called post-concussion symptoms, and then they have some follow up with a neurologist possible then the neurologist, if they don't find any really gross, really bad thing on the exam, that's it.

[00:03:00]

[00:03:30]

And these people might actually have headaches, dizziness, brain fog—the kids or the adults—have all kinds of symptoms, and then they might go to a primary care provider. If they're a kid, they go to the pediatrician, otherwise they go to their adult doctor. And they just don't have an approach to it. Because they don't have something they can match to it like, "Okay, you need this drug." There's no drug for it really. And so sometimes they're sent to a speech therapist if they're having problems with speech or if they're having problems with memory. But there's only a certain percentage of speech therapists that are actually trained to do much work with what we call cognitive rehab. They're almost never put on any vitamins or supplements at all. They're almost never given any advice regarding exercise.

[00:04:00]

The conventional approach really is very deficient, and will often leave people with cognitive deficits, or what we call a decline in brain reserve, because we all have a certain amount of brain reserve whether we're a kid or an adult. But if there's brain injury, and if it's not taken care of appropriately, then the person's brain reserve can go down. If it goes down enough they'll start having symptoms. So, the conventional approach is very, very limited. And I'm very concerned about it.

That's even true in the NFL, with the National Football League. I mean, the conventional approach there is more like: do initial testing on the field and on the sideline to determine whether the person can go back in. Make sure that someone doesn't go back in when they still have any type of cognitive problems, because there's something called the second-impact syndrome where the brain can go

---

[00:04:30] through a part of the skull and the person can die. So, the approach in the NFL is much more sort of, "Let's make sure you don't have second-impact syndrome," as opposed to healing the brain. And that's pretty much, in most places, the conventional approach to treating a head injury.

[00:05:00] One thing a lot of doctors don't realize is, there's a lot of people that have hit their head or had a head injury, and they just don't even find out about it. So, a doctor needs to ask questions like, "Have you ever hit your head? Have you ever fallen down and hit your head? Have you ever fallen off a horse or a mountain bike? Have you ever hit your head while you were skiing?" And oftentimes people will say, "Yeah." And they'll go, "I didn't even realize that I actually did have a head injury." Like they slipped skiing and they smashed their head, and then they hurt their knee and they forgot about their head.

[00:05:30] So, the first part of this is sort of discovering more that it happened. Then also realizing it can happen without someone actually slamming their head. Like someone can be in a motor vehicle accident and they can have enough force so that their head moves back and forth and their brain moves inside their skull. They can actually have a traumatic brain injury without actually hitting their head, like hitting their head on the steering wheel or the windshield or something like that.

[00:06:00] And so then getting some more information like, "Well, how did it happen?" And what the forces were. Like I had a personal experience that I can talk about later in a mountain bike accident, and the forces were pretty significant. "What kind of protective gear were you wearing?" That actually affects the head injury. And you could ask me later on about that because there's definitely better protective gear now, and people need to know how to choose it.

[00:06:30] Basically, what I did was, I've been treating head injuries for a long time and I get head injuries referred to me from the local emergency room and from other doctors, chiropractors, other doctors. And I decided that an approach needs to happen, which is figuring out what stage the head injury— like acute, like the first week, the first few days—and figuring out, okay, is there anything serious going on? Like real brain damage, severe brain damage, then figuring out what stage they're in and what's going on in that stage.

[00:07:00] For instance, it's been found that even in football players, if they draw their blood within one or two hours of slamming their head, they can start having antibodies in their own blood-brain barrier, which is actually the lining of the brain with the blood vessels. So, one of the things that I'll frequently do, is get a blood test to see if this person has antibodies to their own blood-brain barrier, because the blood-brain barrier is supposed to keep things out of the brain. And if it's increasingly permeable, it

[00:07:30] will let toxins in the brain and things in the brain that just should be getting in there that can damage the brain. So, one of the Functional Medicine approaches that I've developed is assessing whether the blood-brain barrier has been damaged or there can actually be antibodies to the blood-brain barrier. Then having a treatment program to heal the blood-brain barrier.

[00:08:00] Then, in terms of the functional medicine approach that I've developed, it's looking at, "Okay, is there a lot of neural inflammation?" And there almost always is. So how do we find the sources of neural inflammation like in the GI tract, in the gut, and actually treat the gut when we're concerned about the brain? And then also treat the brain. Like there are some things that can actually pass into the brain. There's a form of curcumin that passes in the brain better than some other forms, that can actually decrease neural inflammation, and there's some other things that can do it too.

[00:08:30] And then we want to look at what stage they're at, because there could be all this congestion in the brain. Then we want to think at some point, "Okay, do we need to stimulate nerve stem cells? Like new nerve cells—how do we do that? How do we create brain-derived nerve growth factor, how do we increase it to get more nerve stem cells going? How do we increase synaptic connections in the brain?" Because that's the thing that helps create memory and that's the thing that's going to help learning.

[00:09:00] So, I've sort of devised a program that incorporates the right supplements to do these things based on the research, as well as brain training, because brain training is the main thing that will create the synaptic connections. Also incorporating exercise to increase brain-derived nerve growth factor, as well as using some modalities like frequency-specific microcurrent that is applied that can actually

[00:09:30] heal areas of the brain. And also other things, because when someone has a brain injury the hormones can be affected, so I want to look at all the hormone levels and make sure they're tuned up, because sometimes the actual pituitary gets damaged and all the output from the pituitary can go down, and the person may not have the hormones that they need. So, that has to be addressed.

And then stress management is very important because often people are very stressed after this type

[00:10:00] of injury. It's important to treat the pain that they have, because the pain can drive cortisol levels up and cause all kind of problems. Oftentimes there's a head injury, neck injuries and musculoskeletal injuries at the same time that need to be treated so they're not in constant pain. So that's a long answer and there's a lot more detail to it.

One of the things that's really important after any kind of head injury—whether a kid slips skiing or

[00:10:30] falls off their bike, or an adult falls off a horse or whatever it is, or an auto accident—is we want to decrease inflammation in the diet. How do you do that? Well, you decrease fried foods and breaded foods and eliminate all trans fats in the diet. And also, have people eat a low glycemic index diet where they're not eating a lot of starches and breads.

[00:11:00] But there are some other things they can do. They should go on a gluten-free diet even if they don't have antibodies to gluten, because there's information that some of the molecules in gluten can create an autoimmune process in the brain if the blood-brain barrier is having a problem. So, there are some molecular sequences in gluten and in dairy that can damage the brain after a brain injury. Everybody needs to go on a completely dairy-free, gluten-free diet for about eight weeks. About eight

[00:11:30] to ten weeks is what's called the critical period after a brain injury, when we need to do this kind of dietary intervention in a big way. But there are a lot of these things you can still do after that period.

Then I put everybody on omega-3 fats, especially the DHA part of it. With kids, they won't take

[00:12:00] capsules. There are some liquid forms of DHA and fish oils that taste like lemon or mango, and so I know which brands these are, and I just tell the parents to give these kids like a teaspoon or a tablespoon twice a day. That will get them the fatty acids that they need.

Then I put everybody on wild blueberries. What's really interesting, is that there are biochemicals in blueberries that help heal the brain after brain injury that are even also good if someone wants to

[00:12:30] prevent dementia and other things. But wild blueberries have this purple pigment. What's funny is if you're even unwrapping a pack of wild blueberries and you get some on your fingers, it stains your fingers purple because this pigment in there is so strong. But wild blueberries have many times that pigment than a regular blueberry, because what's really interesting is that the more stressed out the plant is, the more of this protective pigment it produces. So, these wild blueberries are often from Canada and some other places, Vermont and New Hampshire, different places where they can get

[00:13:00] wild blueberries.

And I have people mix like a third of a cup, something like that, fourth to a third of a cup, and create a protein smoothie with them twice a day, because I want a lot of this, they're called anthocyanins. They're a certain type of phytochemical and they're a pigment that helps to heal the blood-brain barrier in the brain. So, I put everybody on these blueberries and of course if they want to eat blueberries they can eat blueberries. But I have them go to places like Trader Joe's and Whole Foods

[00:13:30] that have these in bulk, the wild blueberries in bulk, and then just mix them in their smoothies or put them on foods like oatmeal or other things. But I often want them to put protein in their smoothies too, a little bit, but not dairy, because I don't necessarily want them to be getting a sugar rush with these blueberries, I want them getting some protein too.

[00:14:00]

So, if you're doing this with kids, if I'm doing this with kids, the kids actually like it because they get smoothies twice a day and they're getting this flavored fish oil. But adults seem to like it too because it tastes good. It's a basic way that people can eat. I mean, I also put them on a regular diet of a lot of cruciferous vegetables, and just a really healthy diet in general. Like if they're going to eat meat, grass-fed meat. So, an anti-inflammatory diet, high in certain phytochemicals, high in omega-3s to help heal the brain.

[00:14:30]

You can think that in many systems of the body we have reserves, so let me give you an example that might make this a little bit easier. Let's say the lungs—let's say someone's normal in their lungs, then they don't even think about their breathing, and they could go on a hike or workout and they often don't feel winded or short of breath, unless they do interval training. So, they have a lot of reserve in their lungs, right? Well, let's just say someone gets a cold and then gets temporary asthma. They lose reserves in that system, and they start getting winded and short of breath with basic exercise or walking. That's the concept of ... symptoms start when someone gets below a level in terms of a reserve of function.

[00:15:00]

[00:15:30]

So, in the brain, if we have a certain level of reserves whereby a person's memory is good, their organizational abilities are good, their word finding is good, their ability to do complex work is good, then they won't notice any problems. But if a head injury affects their brain reserve, they'll start having symptoms. Like they'll complain, "I go in a room, I don't know why I went in there." They might even say, "I left a pot on the stove with the burner going." You know, they're forgetting all kinds of things, they're having trouble with organization, stress is affecting them too much. So that if the reserve gets too low, they start having brain symptoms. And so everybody starts with a certain amount of brain reserve before the head injury, and if they're having symptoms by definition, their brain reserve has gone down. One of the goals is to increase it to a place where they don't have symptoms anymore.

[00:16:00]

[00:16:30]

Hyperbaric oxygen can be a good treatment after a head injury, especially within the first 12 weeks. But it can also be used after that. It's usually used in groups of 10 to 20 treatments at like 1.3 to 1.5 atmospheres. It's kind of a commitment on the part of a person or a family, because people are going like five days a week. Hyperbaric oxygen increases the oxygenation level in the brain. And one of the theories is that there's some decrease in oxygenation in the brain because of the damage to blood vessels and the decreased ability to get oxygen in the brain. Oxygen functions in cells to help create energy—that's one of the biggest ways it functions. So, what I would say is, I don't recommend hyperbaric oxygen to everybody, but if it's a more moderate injury, or they're really having some significant symptoms, I'll say, "You can do this. And it's probably a good idea because studies show that it can help, it can be effective."

[00:17:00]

[00:17:30]

So, here's a concept: Most people in their homes have Wi-Fi 24/7, it's going and it's strong. And you know, if you ever turn on your phone and say, "Okay, let's find out where the Wi-Fi is," it's often not just your house, it's like you're receiving Wi-Fi from other people's houses. I know when I do it at my house there's like five Wi-Fis available and most of them are locked. I don't even have Wi-Fi at my home because it's all wired. But I can turn it on if I want to. There's information that electromagnetic fields can actually damage the brain.

[00:18:00]

They've done studies with children that, when a cell phone is held near their head, they've done studies that show the pattern of penetration into the brain. And they've done studies with rats in which it's shown that electromagnetic fields from cell phones actually cause immediate brain damage. One time I was at Sea-Tac Airport literally going to give a talk at a Functional Medicine meeting, this was like five years ago, and this news came out that cellphones held near the brain could cause brain damage. Everybody went like this for a second, "Oh my God," and texted somebody. And then right back up to it.

[00:18:30]

So, one of the things I do and I recommend, is to decrease electromagnetic fields after a head injury. I

[00:19:00] recommend everybody turns off Wi-Fi at night, because you don't need Wi-Fi when you go to sleep. A lot of brain healing occurs while we're sleeping, but it appears that brain healing occurs better if there isn't a strong Wi-Fi field. And then I ask everybody to turn off their cell phones. A lot of people have their cell phones next to their bed. These cell phones are constantly receiving emails and text messages, there's this going on all the time. I ask them if they do that to try to please turn it off, or get it way away. Then some people have clock radios that are plugged in, and there are huge electromagnetic fields from that. So, I basically want people to decrease the electromagnetic fields for

[00:19:30] about 12 weeks afterwards. Or if it's a person that has a traumatic encephalopathy, like a football player that's had multiple hits to the head and I tell them, "You're going to be doing this for a long time." I see a fair amount of kids with head injuries, I tell the parents, "Look, just turn the Wi-Fi off at night. Your whole family will benefit."

[00:20:00] So, Wi-Fi and cell phones, we absolutely do not want kids putting cell phones to their head either after a head injury or even before a head injury we don't want it either. But afterwards it's even more critical. It's better to use the speakerphone function, have it farther away from the person. Bluetooth is not that much better; Bluetooth is still electromagnetic fields. There is something called Bluetube; there's a Bluetube that plugs in that actually does not have the wire right up here, it's just a Bluetube and it's safe. They measure the fields for that, almost nothing. And I've had one for years and it's very

[00:20:30] clear. It's called Bluetube. I recommend that if people want the headphones.

But the concept of electromagnetic field protection is basically: protect the brain after injury. Because one of the things we want to do is, we want to do active healing, but we want to protect the brain and the nervous system while it's trying to heal, because we don't want to damage it either.

[00:21:00] So CTE stands for chronic traumatic encephalopathy. It's much more common in people that do sports, high level sports. It's very common in football players, because many football players get multiple hits to the head. It's common in hockey players, like ice hockey, soccer, any sport where people have gotten multiple concussions. It became popularized a number of years ago because the

[00:21:30] symptoms of CTE are like a football player, let's say they were playing actively in their 20s. Well around in their 40s or early 50s, they're having trouble remembering things. They're acting like they have initial mild cognitive impairment and mild dementia. And then they have severe anger management problems, irritability, personality changes, headaches, and progressive dementia. A lot

[00:22:00] of them commit suicide because the problems are so bad. So, it needs to be evaluated and treated.

Now, a doctor that knows about this can figure it out clinically, and it can pretty much be diagnosed with what's called a SPECT scan, which is a type of imaging. It's said in the literature, that it can't be diagnosed without a brain biopsy, but there's something called functional MRI that actually can show

[00:22:30] in traumatic encephalopathy that parts of the brain are smaller, the hippocampus is smaller, there's other parts, there's brain shrinkage. So, it can be diagnosed, and it can be treated with a Functional Medicine approach. What I would say is, it's a very comprehensive Functional Medicine approach with diet, supplements, exercise, brain games, and hyperbaric oxygen. There's a study at the Amen Clinics where they worked with a number of football players with this, and got them significantly better, so it

[00:23:00] can be evaluated and treated and people's lives can be saved.

One of the major genes is the ApoE4 gene, and so if someone has that pattern, that genetic pattern, they're more susceptible to more serious head injury after the same head injury than say somebody else got. But I don't think anybody should be necessarily barred from contact sports, unless they had a head injury and they're still suffering from all kinds of symptoms. Because then they're at risk for this

[00:23:30] thing called the second-impact syndrome, where their brain swells and they die. But I don't think that we should use screening and say, "Well, you shouldn't participate." Because with this Functional Medicine approach I've developed, virtually anybody can be helped significantly after a head injury. I mean, it's one thing if they had some massive, really, really, really serious head injury. You know, you hear about these people in high velocity motor vehicle accidents that got thrown out of a car and

[00:24:00] landed on their ... I mean, those are God awful and these people can be in wheelchairs and have all kinds of problems. But still, in terms of sports, I don't think anybody should be screened from a sport.

[00:24:30]

What I would say is, that after a head injury there's a role for blood testing and most doctors don't do any blood testing, but all the hormones need to be checked to screen for pituitary problems. I think the APO gene type should be screened to evaluate for that. There are a number things—cortisol should be checked. There are a number of things to be checked because all of those things need to be tuned up. You can't really tune up the ApoE4, but you can address the issues much more comprehensively. Like if I got someone who has that I'm going to say, "Look, you have to follow all these things." Because they might say, "Doc, that's a lot of things to do and it's a lot of things to take and it's a big change in my diet." I might say, "Yeah, but you got the ApoE4, it's even more important." I don't use it against them, I use it for them.

[00:25:00]

There are some sports—you know—where they don't wear any protective gear. So, I think, I'll tell you what, if someone's going to do boxing I think they should wear protective gear, at least some type of protective gear. But they don't, because they're actually looking for ... they want to have a concussion. I mean, the person who's boxing doesn't want the concussion, they want to give somebody else the concussion so they're lying on the ground, and then they go like this. So, I don't think that that's a great outcome. But I don't think that they should be banned, I think there should be more protection being used in terms of the brain.

[00:25:30]

I'm an avid cyclist, mountain biker. I got into this about four years ago and really got into mountain biking and even downhill biking. I got to the point where I would go up to Whistler, Canada, and put my downhill bike on a lift. The bike would go up and then I get on the lift behind it. Then when you get up there, and you get all your armor on, like you're motocross, and you go down. You go over all kinds of crazy stuff. So, I've had to look into this for myself, because I had a concussion two years ago and then I really looked into it.

[00:26:00]

[00:26:30]

The average bicycle helmet is inadequate for a head injury. It doesn't protect the head enough. It protects the head better than if there was no helmet, but it's not adequate. So, there's some technologies that have come out to absorb rotational forces. One of them is called MIPS, M-I-P-S. I always tell people, "Look, at least get a MIPS helmet." I say, "It's not the best, but it's better than a non-MIPS helmet. And get it for their kids." And they go, "Oh wow, that costs $25 more." I go, "The brain is worth a lot more, and if you have a head injury or your kid gets ... Oh, you're going to spend a lot more than $25; how about $25,000 to take care of that brain injury?" It's like, spend the extra money to get the protective helmet.

[00:27:00]

Then a level up from that is 6D. 6D is a company that's been working on protective helmets for motocross and for bicycles. I believe they have the most protective technology for bicycle helmets. And yeah, my 6D helmet for mountain biking cost $250—and it's worth every cent. I don't even want to see if it works, because I know it works. But it's worth every cent. They have two shells, not just one shell, and there are these rubber grommets in them that can move in any direction and absorb impact if there's a head injury. They're not that heavy.

[00:27:30]

And then there's a company in Seattle that just came out with a new football helmet. They just came out with this, apparently 24 teams are going to be trying these helmets out. I've just been looking at the research on this helmet, and it is miles above the helmets that are being used right now, so I'm hoping that basically every NFL player gets one of these things. They're football helmets.

[00:28:00]

Now ski helmets—I think ski helmets have a ways to go. I think 6D should start making ski helmets because the same technology needs to be used in ski and snowboard helmets. Because some of these people fall, slip, smash their head on crusty stuff, and the ski helmets are not adequate. They're just a little bit better than the standard bike helmet, but I'm just hoping that someone's going to come up with some better design for these ski helmets to absorb head impacts.

[00:28:30]

[00:29:00] What can happen is, that someone gets a traumatic brain injury or a concussion and things in here can change almost overnight. To having the wrong kind of bacteria growing in here, which is called dysbiosis. And the microbiome, which is all the combination of all the bacteria, and everything in there can change so that it can become much more inflammatory. Then, actually, it can contribute to further brain injury. So that's why it needs to evaluated and what I would call tuned up.

[00:29:30] So, you asked about how can a traumatic brain injury affect the gut? It appears that there's so much stress, and then because of the stress and the pain, people don't sleep very much. They can get depressed. There are so many things that can happen that can affect the pure sympathetic and the sympathetic nervous system. Then people's appetite changes, they eat differently afterwards. So, there are all kinds of things that affect with diet and stress and lack of sleep that affect the microbiome.

[00:30:00] I find it fascinating that there are actually some studies where they took mice and rats and put backpacks on them or something. How do you overload a rat or a mouse? I don't know how you do it, but they did it. They looked at every form of exercise, whether it was just stretching, or aerobic exercise, or resistance training. How do you have a mouse do resistance training? You know, go to the gym and tell them to do bicep and tricep curls? But they figured out how to do resistance training with

[00:30:30] rats and mice. What's been found is, it's primarily the aerobic exercise, and it's a duration of 45 to 60 minutes a day that's important. It increases brain-derived nerve growth factor, which increases neuronal stem cells, and can aid in synaptogenesis and more synapses, which is the biggest stimulus, but we don't want people exercising with headaches. I also have them do resistance training, because

[00:31:00] there's some doubt on resistance training but it's primarily the cardio-aerobic stuff that really does the trick. And also, it's good for anybody to do that to keep their brain healthy, even if they haven't had a head injury.

Sleep is incredibly important. So, one of the things that happens after head injuries, people often have neck injuries with their head injuries, they're in pain, they don't sleep as well. What happens is, if someone doesn't sleep that well and goes below six hours of sleep, they have all these inflammatory mediators. Like I've got inflammatory mediators in my body right now because I didn't get as much

[00:31:30] sleep last night because I flew into a conference and got, I don't know, five hours of sleep. So, the studies show for three days, inflammatory mediators from less sleep. So, I want people to have eight or more hours of sleep. And I encourage them to get more, because some people will say, "Oh, I just wanted to sleep," and they'll sleep for 10 hours. I go, "That's fine." So, we actually want people sleeping more because sleep is very regenerative for the brain.

[00:32:00] Part of what you have to do is get people, you know, start people off and say, "You have to have a bedtime and it's got to be reasonable. So, it has to be before 11pm." I have a whole program that I do to enhance sleep, because I've been working with sleep for a long time. I tell people to actually set a sleep alarm clock half an hour before they want to go sleep, then all the electronic devices are off. And before that, I have them decrease the blue light that they're getting in the eyes. But half an hour before, the TV goes off, the Internet goes off—whatever—and they turn down the lights, because

[00:32:30] that's a stimulus to produce melatonin. Then I want them to make sure there are no bright lights in their hallway into the bedroom. What I do instead of active relaxation techniques, because if they want to stretch or do some yoga —that's great—is I have them read in bed. Like with a Kindle app with the black background and the white font at the lowest level of light, and for most people that will put them to sleep.

[00:33:00] I often use melatonin with my patients, because melatonin actually increases brain, nerve stem cells, so I want to use that anyway. But what a lot of people don't know, they think they should take melatonin right before they go to sleep. If they want to go to sleep at 10pm, they should take it at around 6pm at night. So, melatonin is actually used inappropriately by most people because they take it like, "Okay, I'm going to sleep, I'd better take my melatonin." Which is okay if you want to stimulate brain stem cells, but if you want to go to sleep at a reasonable hour, and some people turn into night

[00:33:30]   owls after a head injury ... There are a lot of night owls anyway, which isn't good. What I mean by that is they go to sleep after 11pm, or they just wake up after 10 or 11pm. It's not good for people, so I'll often dose them with a melatonin, like 1.5 to 2 milligrams around 6:00pm and just experiment with it to get them to sleep.

[00:34:00]   And depending, I might have them do stress management techniques. There's a tapping technique I might have them do called EFT to work on pain and stress, but decreasing stress and increasing sleep is important.

[00:34:30]   I think people should set up the pattern of exercising whether they had a head injury or not. I usually recommend to my patients that five to six days a week, I want them doing something active. Cardio, aerobics, getting into their target heart rate zone, or just walking. I want the average person eating the blueberries, wild blueberries if they can. Getting the omega-3s; having an anti-inflammatory, brain-healthy diet. I want the average person decreasing electromagnetic fields. Because I'm not just trying to treat everybody after a head injury, I'm trying to preserve people's brain function so they have the best brain reserve no matter what age they are. I'd recommend a whole combination of

[00:35:00]   those things to the average person. They're just healthy lifestyle things for people to do.

Dr. Deborah R. Simkin:	I was a professional dancer—a ballet dancer—but my story sort of predates this. I was an A-student until about sixth grade and then things sort of fell apart. By the time I got to high school, I was actually told by my counselor I was too stupid to go to college and if I ever went I should only go part-time. I believed her. When I finished my professional career as a dancer, I went to college.
[00:00:30]	I only had a 2.6 average. I struggled in a lot of things. Then when I found out ... When I was about 27, I found out that I had four learning disorders and just didn't know it, but a very high IQ. So, I realized that if you know what the learning disorders are, then you can overcome them.
[00:01:00]	I went to grad school and got a 4.0. I didn't apply to med school until I was 32. I ended up with a Chancellor's Award and then ended up going to Harvard for my residency. I don't think any of that would have ever happened to me had I not been able to discover those things about myself. When I was at Harvard, one of my mentors, Charlie Popper was, believe it or not, the editor for the *Journal of Child and Adolescent Psychopharmacology*. We began to work together at The Academy. What happened with Charlie is he switched from using psychopharmacological drugs to micronutrients to treat disorders like bipolar and depression, ADHD. He and I started this bond. At
[00:01:30]	that time, they were going to start a committee on Functional Medicine for The Academy of Child and Adolescent Psychiatry and they enlisted me. We put on a whole day institute and I was asked to do a presentation on meditation and neurofeedback, of which I knew very little.
[00:02:00]	That really opened the door for me. I then became very interested in looking at elimination diets. I found out myself, I was sensitive to four different foods. Then from there, actually was asked to become co-editor for textbooks on Functional Medicine or complementary and integrative medicine in child and adolescent psychiatric disorders. Then finally, it led to what I'm doing today, which is I'm one of the first child psychiatrists to set up a Functional Medicine curriculum for Emory School of Medicine for child and adolescent psychiatric residents. That's my journey. That's how I got here.
[00:02:30]	Your question to me is, "How does the brain-gut axis play a role in psychiatric disorders?" I think it's a little bit more unique because what we do know is when lipopolysaccharides are given off in the gut, that's going to cause an immune reaction. What happens is that particular entity is presented on a dendritic cell, which goes to a T lymphocyte and causes the T lymphocyte to start
[00:03:00]	to differentiate. It produces something called TNF kappa beta, which then causes a lot of cytokines to be produced. Now, what does that do? That then signals the vagus nerve, the afferent end of the vagus nerve, to the brain. What's unique here in psychiatric disorders is that that is going to cause a glucocorticoid resistance in the hypothalamic-pituitary axis. You might ask, "What does that mean?"
[00:03:30]	Whenever your hypothalamus is excited and you give off something called corticotropin-releasing factor, it goes to your pituitary that gives off a CTH and goes to your adrenal glands. That gives off adrenaline and cortisol. Normally, there's a negative feedback loop. In other words, when cortisol goes up, it tells the HPA axis to shut down. When these increased cytokines are produced because of the stimulation with the vagal nerve, that causes the glucocorticoid resistance, which means
[00:04:00]	the cortisol can no longer turn off the HPA axis. In psychiatry, that's extremely important to post-traumatic stress disorder, to depression, to making all those symptoms worse.
[00:04:30]	There are two other things that happen in the brain with psychiatric disorders. One of these is that we get an activation of microglial cells. These microglial cells will then start attacking normal neurons instead of cleaning up debris, which is what they normally do in the brain. A third thing that happens is that we actually get the cytokines themselves, the pro-inflammatory molecules

cause something called tryptophan, which is a protein that normally is converted to normal neurotransmitters like serotonin, norepinephrine, and dopamine, and instead it's converted to a glutamate agonist, which really plays a role in psychiatric disorders and making them worse. In fact, we've been able to identify certain cytokines that are found in certain disorders.

[00:05:00] For instance, with PTSD and depression, you will find increased CRP. You will see increases in TNF. You will also see IL-6. Bipolar is very different though. Bipolar has very different cytokines. So now psychiatry is starting to look at the identification of cytokines or proinflammatory molecules to identify which ones are more likely to be associated with certain disorders. There's also another

[00:05:30] very important thing here. I just talked about the afferent loop of the vagal nerve. But there's also an efferent loop. You can try to correct everything by healing the gut and doing all the things we normally do in Functional Medicine, but you also have to find a way to stimulate that efferent pathway, so that your parasympathetic stimulation increases. That actually heals the gut. There are many ways to do this, but one of the best ways is through meditation, believe it or not.

[00:06:00] We use a lot of these things in psychiatry. We do the traditional things in healing the gut that I'm sure every Functional Medicine doc has talked about, but our aim is looking at other ways in which that influences psychiatric disorders in particular. The child who came in with extreme vitiligo: she had asthma. She had rheumatoid arthritis. She was having rages that made her look

[00:06:30] like she was having bipolar disorder. She had been hospitalized literally eight times within the last ten months before coming to me. We found out she had a lot of food sensitivities and we eliminated those, of course. I gave her some supplements like quercetin and curcumin. We did some meditation. Of course, we did some family therapy. There were some chaotic things going on in her life. We needed to reduce the stress in her life. Put her on omega-3 fatty acids, put her on probiotics and prebiotics, and gave her some L-glutamine to heal her gut. Her vitiligo

[00:07:00] disappeared. Her rheumatoid arthritis is no longer there. She doesn't have these rages anymore. She's not been hospitalized since.

In regards to the post-traumatic stress disorder, I think the best example I have there is ... First, I should start by saying I treat a lot of veterans for free, because I feel like I have to give back to the community. I had this one veteran who was formerly with MI6 in England. He had fallen off a tank and hit his head. He couldn't walk or talk for nine months. He did rehab and recovered. He then

[00:07:30] had a horrible experience with PTSD, because his best friend was shot next to him in the head when he was in the Falklands. He was a very resilient guy though. He came to the United States. He worked for the CIA, the FBI, and he was teaching special ops at the Air Force base near me. He was at the top of a staircase and the next thing he knew he had fallen. He was in the hospital.

[00:08:00] Something happened here that was different with this traumatic brain injury. He went into his daughter's room and he was tearing up everything in her room; just destroying everything. He got very fearful that he would hurt somebody. He started crying. He would leave the house. His wife called me in desperation. I said, "Well, just come in." Of course, we did an MRI to make sure there were no gross problems. What I did for him, because I couldn't do an elimination diet at that time, but I wanted to sort of calm down his gut, I gave him a meditation to learn. I had to settle

[00:08:30] down his brain a little bit with some Lamictal, which is an anti-seizure drug, so that it could be calm enough to try to take on some of the things I was going to ask him to do. After that, we did LORETA neurofeedback on him. After 13 sessions, he's back to normal and he is no longer on the Lamictal and doing very well. We've now since put him on an elimination diet and he's lost about

[00:09:00] 30 pounds, and feeling much better. Look at, again, all the things we do with Functional Medicine. I think that neurofeedback is going to probably be the one thing in psychiatry that's going to change the way we approach what we do.

Neurofeedback is traditionally something that's ... The way that we talk about it is in terms of

[00:09:30] operant conditioning. So, what is that? Basically, it started because Sterman had this cat—this is one of the researchers who did this originally—and had an electrode in the cat's head. There was

[00:10:00] this traditional thing where the cat would hit a bar and food would come out. Well, he paired a noise with that. The cat knew, as long as the noise was one, if he hit the bar, nothing was going to come out. So, he would sit there very still. He observed through the electrode that when the cat was sitting still and focused, this certain brain wave pattern came up, which was interesting to him because it was a 12 to 15 hertz brain wave pattern that basically kept the cat very still and focused. So, he wanted to see if he could get the cat to produce that brain wave pattern on his own without the noise. Lo and behold, the cat learned how to produce the brain wave on his own so the food would be delivered.

[00:10:30] That's actually what we're doing in neurofeedback. We put on a 19-channel cap, which has several electrodes on it, and we will record all the brain wave patterns with eyes closed and eyes opened. Then we will compare it to a normal database. For instance, in what happened with the veteran who came in with PTSD and traumatic brain injury, we targeted the areas of the brain and the symptoms that would be abnormal for those conditions. Then when he came back in, we decided we were going to just program it to look at those areas. He would look at a car on a racetrack, for instance, and every time the right brain wave occurred by chance, the car would [00:11:00] move. So, the brain gets excited and goes, "My gosh, where did that come from?" So, it looks for it again. Eventually, the patient is learning how to make that car move. Once they've done that, we can extend the amount of time that they're holding it until the brain wave patterns go back to normal.

[00:11:30] What's different about LORETA neurofeedback is that old traditional neurofeedback, which we called surface, had two to four electrodes and under each electrode, all the frequencies of these brain wave patterns were mixed. What LORETA does is it scrambles all of these frequencies and finds the deep source location in the brain of it. We can actually translate that to a 3D picture of the brain that corresponds to a functional MRI of the brain. It's basically called the poor man's functional MRI. Because of that, we can watch changes in brain wave patterns. The evaluation [00:12:00] where you're looking at the differences between what's going on in someone's brain that has in some particular area that's abnormal to a normal database is called a quantitative EEG. In fact, when you look at some of the disorders that we're targeting—not really the disorders, the symptoms associated with the disorders—your FEC sizes in many cases are better than medication.

[00:12:30] Now the Research Domain Criteria and National Institute of Mental Health has basically set forth a whole objective now that is aiming to not just treat symptoms, but to cure. One of the sub-analysis that they want us to look at besides genetics, which I also look at, is circuits. What you really can do is change all of these circuits in the brain and get them to go back to normal.

[00:13:00] One of the problems out there is that the FDA has approved a lot of equipment and so a lot of people are buying it who don't really know what they're doing. I'll give you an example of this: I had a parent come in with her child and she said, "By the way, I'm doing neurofeedback." I went, "That's interesting. So, where are you doing it?" She told me. I said, "How many sessions have you done?" She said, "45." Well, LORETA takes 10 to 20. Old traditional neurofeedback took 40 to 80. But I asked her, "After 45 sessions ..." It wasn't old surface that she was doing. Supposed to be a [00:13:30] formal LORETA. So, I said, "Well, after 45 sessions is there any change?" She said, "No."

[00:14:00] What I did was I went and found out what was going on. Someone had bought some equipment, made up his own database, which was not scientifically valid, was telling people to put a cap on these children, and then do a quantitative EEG. He would send the quantitative EEG to this particular person. He would set up a protocol and send it back without even knowing what was going on in this child's life, not even doing an appropriate evaluation. That's one of the things I would strongly suggest, that no one ever try to go out there and do this without making sure you're using someone who's board certified and someone who does a very, very thorough biopsychosocial before they do neurofeedback. For instance, if I have a vet come in and he's using illicit substances or he's drinking 12 beers a night, I'm going to take care of that first before I'm going to do neurofeedback.

[00:14:30] So, I think that, yes, can anyone use it, but I worry about people hearing about this, getting excited about it, and then just going to someone who, in my mind, may be seen as a fly-by-night in terms of offering these services. We're trying to educate people about this to know who to look for, what to look for, and to make sure they don't waste money on something that's not going to work.

[00:15:00] There has been a lot of research on micronutrients. Unfortunately, for me, I think there are a lot of companies out there right now selling a lot of products. Some of these products aren't very pure and they're supporting a lot of research and saying that, "If you buy, this micronutrient is going to help." But it's very clear, particularly in ADHD research, that the only time you should treat with a micronutrient is if you have a micronutrient deficiency. Absolutely, if you have zinc

[00:15:30] deficiency, which helps with production of neurotransmitters, if you have a magnesium deficiency, if you have a ferritin deficiency, which is your iron stores in your body, that is going to make your ADHD symptoms worse. You do want to treat when there's a deficiency. It's not going to necessarily cure it, but the symptoms will be less severe.

[00:16:00] We have a lot of people going out there and buying micronutrients and giving it to their kids. In some cases, for instance, if you give too much ferrous sulfate for a low iron storage deposit in your body, you can start having hemochromatosis, which is iron deposits in your organs. That can cause organ degradation. So, I think we have to be very careful with what's going on out there. There are some broad-spectrum micronutrients that are also on the market, which are good, but you have to be trained in it. You have to know how to use it. For instance, if you ever use these broad-spectrum micronutrients in someone who was taking lithium, the lithium dosage would be

[00:16:30] increased by 100 times and might become toxic, and literally knock out your kidneys. You really have to know what you're doing and I think training is extremely important.

[00:17:00] Media and ADHD—well, there some wonderful studies out there. There's one study that looked at 1,300 children, and looked at the amount of exposure to TV they had early in life. The best predictor of ADHD at age seven was those who were exposed to a lot of TV early in their life. In fact, greater than five hours of TV a day almost put you at 100% risk for developing ADHD by age seven. There's something going on. We're over-stimulating the brain in many cases. There was another particular study, which was very interesting. They compared four-year-olds who had been exposed to SpongeBob, educational TV, and drawing. What happened was, the kids who

[00:17:30] were exposed to SpongeBob, because of the overstimulation there, actually had decreases in executive function on psychological testing.

[00:18:00] It does play a role. We do have to watch what's going on. I have kids who can get addicted now to video games, in the same circuitry—I'm a specialist in addiction medicine as well—the same circuitry that's involved in chemicals, which caused addiction, those circuits can be utilized with video machines and they can actually become addicted to video machines. They get what I call the three Cs. They're preoccupied with wanting to use them, then compulsively have to use them. They have this loss of control. They cannot stop. It's the same pattern you see with addiction.

[00:18:30] Do I think there's more ADHD today than there was in the past? I think we're better at identifying things that may be ADHD or look like ADHD. I can remember being in sixth grade and I had a 16-year-old in my class who was trying to make it, who wanted to graduate from school, but he couldn't. So, he just dropped out. A lot of people who were not identified with learning disorders or ADHD just left school. So, we didn't see them. We didn't see them as productive in educational realms. But, on the other hand, we've also had an increase of problems with, as we just talked

[00:19:00] about, with the media. We've had problems with environmental toxins in the environment, which we know there's a direct link to this as well as autism. We have a lot of problems with food sensitivities.

[00:19:30]

I think really the foods we're eating, even though we're a modernized society, what it's led to is causing a lot of problems in terms of how that affects the developing brain. On one hand, the Individualized Disability Education Act allowed us to identify children earlier, but are we seeing more because we're identifying them earlier or we seeing more because the influence of the environment? I think it's both and what's going on and what we're doing.

[00:20:00]

If you suspect your child has ADHD, you want to have a good evaluation. You want someone who knows what they're doing. You want somebody to come in and evaluate everything that can be going on. For instance, I've had several cases where we've had teachers and parents reporting that they think the child has ADD. By asking just a simple question about staring spells, the kid had temporal lobe epilepsy. That would have been a mistake to give that child a stimulant. You also will have, for instance, food sensitivities; you can sometimes find out if kids are sensitive to foods. The hyperactivity component particularly goes down in somebody who truly has ADHD.

[00:20:30]

Another component of this in terms of evaluation is, is this really an anxiety disorder that's going on? There are some people who can do continuous performance tests and they're nice. They're looking to see your ability to pay attention. I may score abnormally on that if I have an anxiety disorder. That doesn't necessarily mean I have ADHD. I think that one of the most missed things today is learning disorders. I think there are way too many children being given stimulants who in fact have a learning disorder. Yes, they may be paying attention better, but it is in fact not identifying the learning disorder. That's important to me because of what happened to myself in terms of learning disorders.

[00:21:00]

[00:21:30]

A good evaluation is very important. Unfortunately, an evaluation in my office takes an hour, an hour and a half. If you go to somebody for 15 minutes, even if they've gotten information from teacher report forms, I don't think that's a thorough evaluation. I think that there are many other things out there, for instance, LORETA neurofeedback, that can really be helpful in ADHD, and looking again at the gut and the supplements that we use for this. People have to seek out people who have good training, and not necessarily just a psychiatrist, but somebody who has some Functional Medicine or an Integrative Medicine background as well. Because I think that's going to bring us to the forefront.

[00:22:00]

[00:22:30]

Oxidative stress and autism—that's a very, very loaded question. Of course, oxidative stress can influence mitochondria and there are a lot of mitochondria problems in some children with autism. But also, there has been some recent research that is looking at the ratio of glutathione to oxidized glutathiones; GSH over GSSH. Glutathione will help with oxidized stress. It will really ... It's one of the things that prevents it or helps to prevent it more than anything else out·there. You can get that up by taking N-acetylcysteine. There's one study that's looking at that ratio. When that ratio is low, they've been looking at those children in terms of giving them methylated B12. Why? Because methionine is changed into homocysteine, and then that become glutathione. Then that's oxidized. If you have a low ratio there, then obviously you're going to have a lot of oxidized stress. But when you convert from methionine to homocysteine, you also are using a methylated B12 there.

[00:23:00]

[00:23:30]

Now, in autism, not only does oxidized stress cause problems with mitochondria, but it also may play a role in defining or regulating how DNA (which is wrapped around a histone, like a sphere) will unravel. If it's unraveling, the DNA is not changing, but it's unraveling inappropriately so it's being read wrong. In those kids with low GSH to GSSH ratios, they've been giving methylated B12 and they've seen some great improvements. In fact, there was a study that it didn't really look at the kids for GSH over GSSH ratio, but it did look at giving N-acetylcysteine to kids with autism. They started out with 900 milligrams the first month, 1,800 milligrams the second month, and then 2,700 milligrams. What they found is there was a tremendous decrease, a significant decrease, in not only irritability but the stereotypical behaviors.

[00:24:00] One would wonder, though, how many of those children are slow metabolizers of 2D6. 2D6 is a P450 enzyme that is responsible for breaking down pesticides in the environment. If you have that, then you need to be given N-acetylcysteine (NAC) so we know that you're taking care of the oxidized stress. What I would wonder in that study is, one, how many of those kids had a low GSH to GSSH ratio and/or how many of those children were slow metabolizers of 2D6. I think we're just starting ... It's really exciting for me right now, but we're starting to peel the skin off the onion to see what's going on.

[00:24:30] There are really five types of meditation. I just finished writing a chapter on this. Basically, there is focused attention, where you're focusing on one thing over and over again. There is open monitoring, which is where you sort of teach yourself to be objective and look at a situation without emotion. There's transcendental meditation. There is mind-body, which is meditation with some relaxation or breathing techniques or relaxation techniques. There's body-mind, which [00:25:00] is things like meditation with yoga or tai chi movement. Those also can be subdivided into how they affect the brain, and they do affect the brain differently. For instance, focused attention really will decrease the amygdala, the activity of the amygdala, which is fight-and-flight syndrome. We find that with focused attention or mindfulness, we're really decreasing anxiety a lot.

[00:25:30] With transcendental meditation, it's very, very different. Transcendental meditation basically is where you're given a mantra and these mantras have been mathematically analyzed to see which ones really help relax the brain. The difference is that when you're doing transcendental meditation, you start out by focusing on the mantra, but eventually the mantra goes away and your brain is completely blank. Under those circumstances, what happens is a circuit called the "default mode network" turns on. It just so happens that the default mode network in your brain [00:26:00] only turns on when your mind is completely at rest and still. It also increased the coherence between connections in the brain, improves them. We also see a theta beta ratio, which is you want high betas so you attend more and theta to go down, because when it goes down, it allows you to attend and focus better. All those things are influenced by transcendental meditation. In [00:26:30] fact, transcendental meditation is the number one meditation that's recommended by the American Heart Association right now for decreasing blood pressure.

They're all different, and you have to sort of look at what's going on for your patient and decide what's best. For instance, autistic kids really do well with body-mind because they like to watch what you're doing. That seems to improve what we call mirror neurons in the brain. Mirror neurons in the brain actually increase empathy and your ability to connect. That's what we use, say, with autistic kids.

DREW RAMSEY, MD | Assistant Clinical Professor of Psychiatry, Columbia University, Eat Complete and Eat to Beat Depression E-course

Dr. Drew Ramsey: My background began in rural Indiana. I grew up on a really small farm, which actually, my family and I, I just moved back to. I'm a farm boy and became a New York City psychiatrist. I came out to Columbia after med school at IU and I got interested in food mainly, as a lot of the medications I prescribed as a psychiatrist caused changes in weight, changes in appetite. I'd have patients whose symptoms were getting better on a medicine but they gained 20 or 30 pounds, and so it felt like I really needed to give [00:00:30] them a set of tools on how to deal with that. As I started to give the standard nutritional advice that so many of us in medicine were trained: don't eat fat, don't eat cholesterol. First of all, it doesn't work. Secondly, it just isn't helpful advice. I really began an exploration around food and brain health, and how I can add this as a tool for my patients.

[00:01:00] Personally, I've really been interested in health. It's one of these fascinating things where, as a physician, in your personal life a lot of us are so interested in wellness, but just really recently, it feels like we're now starting to be able to integrate that into our professional work. I think that's what happened to me. I was fit, trying to eat lots of plants and super healthy, and I wasn't incorporating that into how I evaluate and work with my patients. I radically changed that, and I would say it's been some of the richest information I get to learn about people. This little secret move I have in my interview, that now I get to teach to the residents at Columbia, which is, how do you engage a patient around [00:01:30] food and how do we shift our stance to help people really find joyfulness, and use food to feed their brain and improve their outcomes?

I do a simple food evaluation, and it's what we've been teaching at the American Psychiatric Association for the past five years. It's simple. It's really about moving through the life of an eater and the day of an eater, and understanding more of the details.

[00:02:00] A lot of people will say, "Well, I eat a pretty healthy diet," and then what they describe is not that healthy. They'll be focusing on low-fat food, or they'll be really proud they're eating a lot of chicken. What's missing are some of the most nutrient-dense foods—those foods that are supercharged in nature, where there's an incredible number of nutrients and concentration of nutrients for not a lot of calories, like a mussel or an oyster. The bivalves are incredible.

[00:02:30] I like to walk through each meal, snacks, preferences. It's been really important for my clinical work to understand people's cultural background. I have a patient who grew up in Morocco and is separated from their food. One of the ways to really both understand their dynamics, but I think really help them passionately and joyfully connect, is to help them reconnect with more of the traditional foods that they find in their culture. Those types of questions, and then a lot of people have different rules and [00:03:00] morals and ethical guidelines for how they eat, and so I'm really a believer that I'm here to help you feed your brain no matter what tribe of dieter you are or eater. Whether you're a vegan or vegetarian, or you're eating gluten free, or you're eating paleo, or whole 30—it's my job to help make sure you're getting all the nutrients that you need for great mental function from your food.

Let's talk about some of the statistics. When you think about the health epidemic in America, we don't talk enough about the mental health epidemic. The reason that's so important is it really takes a lot out [00:03:30] of our bottom line as a country, but also, these are disabling illnesses. If you look at what's called a "disability-adjusted life year," which is a measurement of how much does an illness disable an individual, the top causes for sure are mental health disorders because they hit us when we're younger. As opposed to heart disease that you get in your 60s, when you get depression, or an anxiety disorder, or schizophrenia, that strikes you when you're young, usually 15 to 18. The statistics are grim no matter which way you slice them.

[00:04:00] We see that right now between 10 to 25% of Americans are on an antidepressant. And part of me thinks that's great—which is not maybe a very popular view—but at least, people are engaging in getting treatment. I think it's something that we, in mental health and in psychiatry, we're constantly working to improve the efficacy of our treatments.

[00:04:30] In terms of disability, depression is the top cause of disability worldwide. It is going to be, or already is, the top cause of disability in America. When you look at some of the most common mental health disorders in America, it's been like 40 million Americans have a diagnosable anxiety disorder. Just look at things like, what? There are now 60,000 overdoses in the opioid crisis. There were 40,000 suicides last year. These numbers are growing.

[00:05:00] When I look at those numbers, I feel like there is a wave that is crashing on our country, and it's a wave of mental health disorders, which are rooted in brain health. When you take the mix of really not a lot of parity, we don't reimburse and value mental health in the same way medically as we do medical health. And when you think about the stigma, even my patients who do great and do wonderfully in treatment, they're completely ashamed that they've ever done what so many of us do, which is to spend time with a mental health professional understanding ourselves and the complexity of emotions and who we are.

[00:05:30] I think the most exciting statistic that's come out about mental health actually was from a trial that came out in January 31, 2017, which is the first ever randomized controlled clinical trial using diet to treat depression. A real, randomized trial. That's what we've been missing in some ways in the data. There's been a lot of correlation. A modified Mediterranean diet was found to get 31% of patients into full remission. These are patients who had pretty severe depression and were already on meds and in

[00:06:00] psychotherapy. That's a statistic I like, people getting better using food.

How do we combat stigma and what does it take for us to feel comfortable sharing this very personal part of ourselves? I think in my training, one of the first things I realized, I was just so ashamed when I was scared. I remember being in the ER with somebody who was really psychotic. I was an intern, a

[00:06:30] second-year resident, and I just remember being frightened. It makes, I guess, sense. You're watching someone that was a young man. He looked like me. We were in the same drawer as it were, and his brain was just not working. Completely psychotic, terrified, paranoid, hearing voices.

[00:07:00] I think we have to confront that mental illness scares us, and it scares us for a very good reason, which is that we're all vulnerable to it. This isn't something that you get in your genes. Depression is nearly ubiquitous in the sense that, unlike something like heart disease and cancer, which you've not really ever experienced. I think everyone has experienced sadness and a low mood. Everyone's experienced crippling anxiety. Everybody's had a touch of insomnia. It's sort of striking that even though we have this shared experience of struggling with having a human brain, which is a fragile thing ... I mean, human brains and psyches are very complicated. They break kind of easily. Sometimes for all of us, they

[00:07:30] don't make perfect sense. I think what it takes for us to have that frank conversation is increasing conversations. And all of us who are in the mental field or who have mental health disorders, doing the brave thing and being open about that. That's a hard thing for us to do.

[00:08:00] I think the tide is turning. What I love is hearing of all the wonderful, amazing, gifted, successful people who also are telling us, "Yeah. I have depression. I have ADHD. My family has bipolar disorder." That's been a really exciting development I would say in the last 10 years where we're talking about it, and I think that that's the only way we save lives. If we agree it's not something that you have, or like she has. It's like something we all have. I don't know a single family in my personal or professional life who

[00:08:30] doesn't have some stuff going on, that when they see me get a function will kind of be like, "Hey. I got this cousin ..."

[00:09:00]

[00:09:30]

I think one of the things in the American Psychiatric Association that we're quite concerned about is there's this gap between great treatment and getting people better. I think that's one of my main messages is that people get better. I'm not in the business of not getting people better. We really want that message getting out to the public more and shifting from, I think, a traditional view of psychiatry—that we push meds, and we just want to talk about your mom, and want to put you on the couch for a million years—to what we actually are. We're experts in brain health. We are the medical specialty that focuses on emotional health, and we take that very seriously. There's a lot of, I think, great science coming out and a new revolution about to happen where we're going to begin to use genetic data to better tailor treatments.

Man, the reason I went into psychiatry is I thought, "Gosh, a lot is going to happen in this field, because we don't really know anything about the brain." I feel like that's paying off much earlier than I thought it would, because it's getting really nuanced and interesting in how we understand how the brain works and how we help people fix their brains.

[00:10:00]

[00:10:30]

The MAD diet is the modern American diet. You also hear it called the SAD diet, but I prefer MAD because it makes me personally mad that we got here. As I grew up on a farm, I was standing out back in one of our big gardens with one of my buddies. Actually, it's the photographer from *Fifty Shades of Kale*. Ian looks out, and he's like, "Man, how is it people go hungry in this country with all this food growing?" It's an incredible amount of food. I left the farm on Monday, I dropped in a bunch of sunflower seeds, a bunch of squash, I came back on Thursday. Friday, we eat sunflower sprouts. The squash is up. That's not the MAD diet.

[00:11:00]

The MAD diet is not food that we grow in the ground on our great small American farms and share with each other. The MAD diet is a diet that got created for efficiency, and it got created on bad, bad science. That now is 100% clear. We moved from living in rural America, and eating food from small farms, and eating a lot of plants, to eating highly processed foods that really consist of very few ingredients. They get mixed together all kinds of different ways, but you're talking about cheap vegetable oil, soybean oil, corn oil. Lots and lots of sugars, every single way you can say it: sugars from corn, sugars from sugarcane, sugars from beets ... And then a variety of things to make that more palatable, fake colors, fake flavorings. What then gets created is a diet that is missing the most important nutrients for the brain.

[00:11:30]

If you look at what happened, for example, long-chained omega-3 fats. These are really a great example of one of the most important things that I tell my patients to focus on eating. That's what I focus on. I look at my week. How do I judge it? Did I eat fatty fish that has long-chained omega-3 fats? One of my top criteria for eaters who are looking to support brain health, omega-3 fats just got entirely stripped from our diet. We actually moved from having an omega-3 fat-based diet, a grass-based diet, to a diet that's based much more in seed oils and what are also essential fats, but are thought to be much more inflammatory.

[00:12:00]

[00:12:30]

The MAD diet is a diet that is very clear in the data. It increases your risk of depression between 50 and 100%. It increases your risk of dementia. Some studies show that it's doubling the rate of dementia. It doubles the rate of attention deficit disorder. These are strong correlations we see across the board between modern diets, or the Western diet, that consists of empty calories, which is the opposite of eating for brain health where you're getting nutrient density. Lots and lots of nutrients per calorie.

[00:13:00]

When we meet eaters in our Nutritional Psychiatry here in New York City, we do our eater evaluation, and we see eaters fall into a few categories. There's the beige diet, or we call it the "12-year-old boy diet," where it's people like, "Ah. I eat pasta, pizza, chicken fingers, and martinis. That's my diet." It's like the 12-year-old diet plus alcohol. That's some New Yorkers. We look at that, and what we really work to do is create a method where we help people find joy in their food.

[00:13:30] That's really our goal and to do that through enjoying real whole foods, enjoying them in a simple way, and focusing not on singular foods like kale or wild salmon or blueberries, but to focus on food categories. Food categories help people really think more broadly and more creatively about their diet. If you're only eating kale, what about that great Swiss chard or those amazing sunflower sprouts or some parsley? Those are all wonderful leafy greens, and they all have great health benefits. That's really the hope is that the MAD diet will be undone by this new movement we're seeing where, by last count, there were 8,144 farmers markets in America. I don't think there's better medicine for our country.

[00:14:00] If you think about what happens there, right? These local communities that are just being ravaged, absolutely ravaged, in America, have a new source of income. There's food being grown, which means there's food being passed around. You have a feeling of being part of a community as opposed to dependent on all these outside sources bringing your food. The MAD diet is an anathema of, I would say, bad agriculture, bad science, and bad choices—all packaged in an absolutely delicious, heavily [00:14:30] branded and marketed way, that has created a set of habits for a lot of eaters that it really leads them to a bad place in terms of their overall health, but specifically in terms of their brain health.

[00:15:00] Our brain runs on sugar. If you think about blood sugar, that's very important stuff. 99% of the brains on the planet are running on blood sugar, on glucose. If you think about primal society, there were periods of fasting. There were periods of plenty. Sugar naturally triggers us to lay down fats in the sense that we eat sugar, we have an insulin spike, and then we lay down some fat stores. You can see that kind of worked when we were more seasonal. Happens to me. In the winter, I eat a little differently. I get a little puffier. I sleep a little more. I eat more carbs. In the summer, super lean, super fit, eating differently. We really lost that natural rhythm of our foods.

[00:15:30] We're addicted to sugar for a number of reasons. One, it's in everything. A second reason that I think is overlooked is we've shifted our palate. I haven't eaten simple sugars. Haven't had them in my house for a long time, and when I get something, boy, it's so sweet like a candy bar, it's out of control. It's super saturated. We've lived in this milieu of very salty, very sugary, very powerfully flavored foods, and so people's palates have shifted towards craving and desiring that. It's ubiquitous. It's everywhere. You [00:16:00] can't pick up anything without sugar in it. Toothpaste has sugar in it. It's in everything. There are a billion names for it, and the reason that we like it is our brain responds to it.

[00:16:30] If you think out there in the natural world, so go to my farm, where is the sugar? There's only one place that there's actual, concentrated sugar, and that's in my beehives, and that's hard sugar to get. When you do get it, I don't know if anybody out there has tried to eat a teaspoon of honey, you don't. It's too much. All the other sugar on my farm is in all my rainbow vegetables and in the plants, because I love sugar in the sense that that's the basis of our food supply. Every single molecule of our food, if you think, starts with a very simple chemical reaction of photosynthesis, by which our lovely friends the plants turn sunlight into sugar.

[00:17:00] There's a way that as we talk about sugar being toxic, part of me feels that people have gotten quite confused. Sugar is a nutrient that our brain is quite dependent on and uses every day, and maintaining healthy blood sugar is absolutely critical. Cutting out simple sugars from your diet is one of the most important steps, I think, for people to take to reclaim their eating. At the same time, when you eat a plant-based diet, you're eating a lot of sugars, but they're a slower-burning, lower-glycemic-index sugar, and they come with all these nutrients. What's really hurting us are the sugars, the empty [00:17:30] calories, that don't come with any nutrients. It's like having lots of gas and no way to deal with the exhaust.

Low-fat diets and vegetarian diets are interesting in the sense that some of the ideas behind them are great. We, overall, eat too many calories. I tell my patients, "I never want people to trim calories," because I think it's a really big waste of good food to turn it into a complicated math equation. You know whether you're eating too many calories or not based on one simple factor: whether you gain

[00:18:00] weight or not. I have actually eaten the exact same number of calories every week, year in, year out, since I was 18. I know that because my weight's been stable. There's no other measure that in some ways matters.

[00:18:30] Vegetarian and low-fat diets focus on helping people reduce calories, getting more plants. Those are great. The problem becomes when you exclusively eat plants or when you cut all fats out of your diet. First of all, we only eat about 15% protein so if you cut all of the fats out of your diet or many of them, you're just eating carbohydrates. Again, most people are getting in a trend towards the simpler starches and sugars, because they're the easiest and the cheapest.

What happens clinically, what we see is people, first of all, they get depressed. Your brain is made of fat. It needs fat. It needs certain fat-soluble nutrients. Certain fats, like the long-chained omega-3 fats, are highly correlated with depression. We actually have a reasonable data signaling you can use them [00:19:00] to treat depression. Most recent meta-analysis by the Cochrane Group found that there was a statistically significant improvement if you pull all the studies. Not hugely clinically significant, but statistically significant.

Again, a really important signal that while this is a fat that we want people to eat, I think the thing I had about all this messaging that has gotten me really frustrated, is it's not nuanced and it focuses on the [00:19:30] wrong things. When we think about the average knowledge base of the average American eater ... A lot of patients sort of sheepishly look at me on the couch, and they're like, "Where do I find protein? What's a fat?" If I'm honest, if I think about even after medical school when I started really intensely studying nutrition, I didn't know that stuff either. I talked to some of the smartest doctors I know, and it's like, "Hey, what's the top source of folate?" They're like, "I don't know." I really hope in my work to help people focus more on nutrients and foods. You know it's a good choice without knowing all the [00:20:00] numbers behind it.

If you eat an oyster, you get a massive dose of zinc. If you eat six oysters, you get 500% of your daily need of zinc. What does that mean in my life as an eater and what we've prescribed? It means we want you eating bivalves on a regular basis. Again, not a recommendation I think a lot of people get. They get a recommendation like, "Eat fish. Don't eat meat." Again, I don't think that's a very joyful way to [00:20:30] present food. Around the same thing with the cholesterol argument. If you look at the science behind dietary cholesterol, it's not in any way conclusive. As a clinician, I see patients all day every day. When you tell people not to eat cholesterol, that leads to zero action. The only way to do that is to stop eating animal products, and there are lots of ways to eat animal products and eat seafood that are very, very healthy and correlated with lots of positive health outcomes.

[00:21:00] Quality of food is something that people don't focus on enough. The idea that we talk about beef, like beef is one thing. That's not true. Meat, red meat. You talking about venison that we've killed in our woods that's lived wild and is some of the leanest meat around, or are you talking about grass-fed beef? One of my buddies Jim Fiedler, who dedicates his life to having 1,000 acres of beautiful pasture and raising grass-fed cattle. If you think about a grass-fed steak versus a grain-fed steak, the grain-fed [00:21:30] steak, first of all, has a third more calories. It's a fattier cut. There are more fats in it, and they're not exactly the fats we hope for. Whereas, if you look again at a cut leaner, some more omega-3 fats, about eight times as much vitamin E, about six times as much beta-keratin. More nutrients in that beef.

[00:22:00] As a quasi-farmer, if you look at what happens on a farm, it's clear where you want to spend your food dollars. You go to a grass-fed farm, usually you see a happy farmer, you see pasture. You usually see a kind of dynamic rotational system where we're really restoring the land, caring for that topsoil like it's our mother because it is. You go to a traditional cattle operation, or go out to the feed lots, and mainly it's sad. I drove out to Dodge City, Kansas, when we were researching the happiness diet, and there are [00:22:30] tears in your eyes because it's so much gas and methane and stink. It's not like meat packing is a particularly happy industry.

[00:23:00] It's where quality makes a difference. If you think about salmon, there's a difference between farmed salmon, which is fed soy and corn and then given a pink dye so it looks like wild salmon, and then real wild salmon. Just a huge nutritional difference. Farmed shrimp and wild shrimp. Really, I think focusing on helping individuals spend their money wisely and pick foods that are good for the planet—good for their brains, and good for their family, in the sense of creating a lot of joy around the dinner table. That I feel is a really important intervention. An intervention that we feel is increasingly happening in mental health.

[00:23:30]
[00:24:00] It's important to eat locally for a number of reasons. One of the things that causes people to struggle with their mood and to struggle with their emotional health is isolation. The world is very isolating now. We feel connected on social networks, but we don't look each other in the eye nearly as much. Living here in New York City was actually the first time I went to a farmers market a lot. I was living down in the West Village. We were about to have kids, and I didn't even know. I moved into this cute little place and opened my door one Saturday, and there was like 10 farmers and a seafood monger. Suddenly, I'm really far away from our farm, but I'm eating more farm-fresh food than I ever have before. I start to love that Saturday morning. I'd go out and I'd shake Farmer Dave's hand and talk with him, and I get some seasonality back into my diet. There are new foods that he's excited about growing.

That's actually where *50 Shades of Kale* came from: the Abingdon Square Farmers Market. Muddy Farm. Farmer Dave had six shades of kale. *50 Shades of Gray* was going up, and I just thought, "Well, I could put those things together."

[00:24:30]
[00:25:00] The reason local communities should support their local farmers is it's a dying profession, and it's a noble profession. There is no feeling I've ever had like planting seeds on my farm and harvesting that food. I'm always overjoyed to spend time with people who haven't done that, because if there is a very clear visible miracle on Earth for me, it is that you take this tiny, tiny little seed—the tiniest little seed, a speck—and you put it in the ground. Literally days later, you have a sprout, and 50 days later you have a giant plant. It's just giving you a plethora of food. That is wild. Farmers markets help people enjoy that, they help you connect with their community, and they help us eat the right foods.

[00:25:30]
[00:26:00] If you think about it, what's in a farmers market? If you're eating whole, fresh, local produce as the base of your diet, supplementing that with really, really well-chosen seafoods—mainly bivalves and the wild fatty fish, some good grass-fed meat occasionally, and some other things, nuts, lots of beans ... I grew black beans for the first time. We have this jar of black beans, like this big. We literally just put some plants in the ground. I have more black beans than I could eat in a year. That's what I think a farmers market gives you is that window into what's happening in your community, and a place to come together and keep our food dollars local. That's, I think, the saddest thing for me is to be seeing so many small farms in America disappear just because there's nothing that can be done. I think our local food movement is changing that.

[00:26:30] A colleague of mine, Laura Lachance, and I have created the first nutrient profiling system called the mood food scale. We looked at all of the scientific literature that's out there related to food and depression, and tried to find the nutrients where there was substantial epidemiological data, looking at populations—people who don't eat zinc get more depressed, for example—and then looking at clinical data. We gave some people zinc when we gave them an antidepressant, and they also got better. Saying, "Seems like zinc has some antidepressant qualities. What are the foods that have the most zinc?"

[00:27:00] We went through this and found eight to ten nutrients. Really the evidence supported that those nutrients play a significant role in the pathophysiology of depression. When we think about mood foods, when I really focus on what's missing in most people's diets and the long-chained omega-3 fats in the fatty fish. There are lots of other ways to think about mood. If we think about mood, a good mood, as not just an emotional state but as a state of brain growth, there are six nutrients that have a

[00:27:30] clear role in promoting BDNF, brain-derived neurotrophic factor. One of the reasons zinc and omega-3 fats and some of the phytonutrients—the flavonols—come up in a lot in our work is that in the science, it looks like they promote the molecule that really helps the brain grow and be resilient and recover. When I think foods like that, I think those are we call them brain foods or mood foods.

[00:28:00]
[00:28:30] In terms of eating for other specific symptoms or conditions, there are a lot of different moves that we have in our clinic. For example, when people have anxiety, there are a number of foods that we really want to add that surprise people, like eggs. Eggs have a lot of choline, which is a B vitamin. Choline is actually one of the only nutrients that is highly correlated with depression. Even though anxiety disorders are one of the most commonly diagnosed disorders, there's actually almost no science when it comes to how food and anxiety relate. Again, one thing we tend to see a lot is people have anxiety disorders getting anxious, not having regulated eating, and beginning to get a little hypoglycemic. Oftentimes, people with panic disorders and anxiety disorders, they have a kind of heightened sensitivity to somatic and bodily sensations. As they feel that rumble in their tummy, their anxiety gets tweaked in their brains differently than people without anxiety disorders. That's where a food intervention can be very helpful in terms of helping people really be mindful of what they're eating and thinking about. The structuring of their intake is really vital to their mental health.

[00:29:00]
[00:29:30] I would say the strangest thing for me in all these years is the number of smart people that I've met, doctors even, who don't in their mind have any connection between brain health and food. I'll be asking. They're like, "Why are you asking me about all this food stuff?" I didn't start talking about food with my patients until maybe a few years into my career. There's this natural gap I think we have to help people bridge to think about not our food as something that is just about weight gain or cancer risk or heart disease risk, because those messages have just really been given to us wholeheartedly, but to really think about depression risk.

[00:30:00] If you think about it, the most dangerous illness for you and your family, isn't cancer and heart disease. The most dangerous illness for you and your family is depression by far. It's more prevalent. It's easier to get, and, unfortunately, it's more lethal. The good news in that is the science is really clear that the biggest factor under your control to influence your risk of depression, is in what you eat. We've just launched an e-course called *Eat to Beat Depression*. It revolves around this idea that by focusing on a few foods and a few nutrients, you can radically and rapidly shift how someone eats. That's very satisfying to see.

[00:30:30]
[00:31:00] I think all of us who are talking more with patients about food, one lovely part is how much people engage when you partner with them when it's not a set of rules—don't eat all this bad stuff, you can die—and it's more like, "Let's have fun together. What kind of salads do you love?" I had a patient show me a picture of her sunflower sprouts she bought in the farmers market. That was her homework, and it's a really rewarding medical experience to have there be more in the conversation than just therapy and meds and coaching—to really have this piece very focused on food.

[00:31:30] I'm a general psychiatrist. I do lots of psychotherapy. I do med management for people. Increasingly over the years I've gotten to be a real nutritional psychiatrist where an individual will have their med person, their psychopharmacologist, and someone doing their therapy, and I just get to run the show on food. We actually had a woman who came in just about a month ago really struggling. She told me she ate 14 cookies the night before she saw me just to make sure I got it, and she was just really dealing with a lot of emotions from emotional eating, leaning towards those very satisfying carbs. We look at the fastest way to boost serotonin in the brain is to eat pure glucose. There's something physiological about that kind of carb craving that happens to people.

[00:32:00] She was living on a very beige diet—simple carbohydrates, a lot of treats, a lot of soothing herself, and struggled in terms of didn't really know how to cook. She had someone in her home helping her cook she sort of guiltily admitted to me, and I think, "That's great. Have them cook more of the foods that we know you should be eating." She started keeping a food journal. We went through a few simple

BROKEN BRAIN

[00:32:30]	food categories, and like a lot of people, what I love about this work is you know what a good brain food is. If I held up a plate of beautiful rainbow vegetables and a nice piece of fish versus a hamburger and fries, everybody knows that's brain food. What's really fun is, it's almost like helping people discover these foods that they hadn't thought about.
[00:33:00]	I said, "What about avocado?" She's like, "I love avocados. Can I eat avocados?" It's like, "You should eat an avocado every day." Now, every day she starts with an avocado, eggs, some mushrooms. Look at her food journal, and—sure—there's the occasional brownie, a little chocolate donut here and there, but mainly it's real food. What's happened is we've also given her some cooking instructions. Something that we do that I think is a little unique to our practice is, we take people to the farmers market.
[00:33:30]	We have a great food therapist, Samantha, who's a chef and a social worker, and she diagnoses what the problem is. It might be like, "You don't know how to cut vegetables very well. You don't know how to chop food. Let's help you with that." Or, "You have anxiety that any time you cook fish, you're going to get food poisoning. Let us help with you that. Let us help you feel safe and fearless and joyful about your food." This woman is now—she's about a month in, and you look, and man she is just eating differently.
[00:34:00] [00:34:30]	Part of it is the foodcebo effect wherein we care for ourselves, we feel better about ourselves. Everybody knows that. You go to the gym, doesn't matter how you feel going in. You come out, you just feel better. You know you did something for yourself. Along with all of the nutrients, there's this very powerful factor when we care for ourselves, we care for our families, we care for our table. That is a very powerfully antidepressant. Think about the last time someone cooked you a thoughtful, caring meal and said, "Oh hey. Come over. I remember you love fish. I made this for you." Boy, we feel so nourished and cared for. I guess my hope is that we increasingly see more of that. We see local food, meals together, and the idea that it's not a million miles away. It's not this heavy lift that you have to eat all these specific things. It's really simple. I'm not a great chef, but I love cooking simple food.
[00:35:00]	This is something I think that is attainable to everyone. All the times we hear, "Ah. The brain food costs too much." Nah. That's not true. Look at a can of wild salmon. Three bucks. Lot of wild salmon in there. "I'm a little scared of canned fish." Well, you take that out. Put on some pickles, celery, little touch of mayo, some mustard. All the sudden you get that amazing, instead of tuna salad, you get amazing salmon salad. Make a little salmon burger. $3.50. There are, I think, all kinds of ways to make it quite affordable to eat right.
[00:35:30]	The exercises that I really encourage in all of my patients struggling with emotional health and really wanting to improve their brain health. Certainly there's the food part, which is, I tell people, "It's simple. Seafood, greens, nuts, and beans." It's not a complex equation. At the core of behavioral change for all of us is being mindful. Part of changing your food is looking at your plate and thinking with intention, "What am I putting in my body? Where did it come from? How does it line up with my values?" It doesn't always, right?" You're stuck at an airport somewhere, you've got to eat, but as much as possible, can we be more intentional?
[00:36:00]	Increasingly over the years I really have focused on helping people be more mindful and more present with themselves. I think communication skills are a big thing that improve brain health when you look at the catatoxic effects of stress. And stress often have a root in people struggling to have authentic communication, and be clear with themselves about who they are and own that, and be clear with others in terms of what they need.
[00:36:30]	Of course, we all like to exercise. I'm a little bit of a stickler. I think a lot of people are out there jogging away, not doing very much for their brain health. I think that as we understand more about how you're ultimately healthy, I increasingly feel that I do a lot more interval-based training where I'm

really ... A lot more just regular daily activity. It's one of the perks of living in New York. I love all my farm work, but boy, you're always doing 10,000 steps in New York.

[00:37:00] I guess to summarize, my brain prescription for people starts with food. It includes a healthy serving of mindfulness. I really love working with people on how you say things and how you connect with the people in your life both using food, but also simply to decrease stress and improve the clarity of your relationship and the quality of those relationships. Then I hope everybody spends more time moving. I think when we can think about the joyful moments in our life, moments when we transcend the angst

[00:37:30] of being human. For many patients I treat and people I know and for myself, that's when I'm in a full run or I'm sitting at a table with a set of good friends laughing and enjoying the food. I think that those really are the keys to a solid emotional health. They're something that we all have to work to build and work together to build.

[00:38:00] Food can be used in all kinds of ways. One of the patient populations that I work with are people who are struggling with addiction. If you think about addiction and how it relates to food, they're very related. Especially people struggling with alcohol and alcohol abuse. Actually, we're beginning to understand some of the genetic changes that drive those individuals towards simple sugars, alcohol being a simple sugar. Food is great for people struggling with addiction because it helps you care for

[00:38:30] yourself. It gives you something to do that is meditative and thoughtful. It gives you structure. Where people with addiction struggle, once we help get them into a period of sobriety, is filling their time and managing stress. Filling their time with productive activities.

This is where I love using food. The notion of, "What do you feed yourself when you're stressed? What do you feed yourself when you're craving? What do you replace alcohol with?" Some of our patients who aren't going to go towards sobriety and they want a more harm-reduction model, "How can we

[00:39:00] help you? Instead of having like eight drinks, have a drink and then some kombucha." That we can reduce the load. Food becomes a really big part.

Look at what a lot of people struggling with addiction eat. It is the MAD diet. Simple carbs. Cheap food. Easy food. Being wrapped up in addiction, you don't have the kind of time, mindfulness, and focus to really engage with the self-care. It's a very handy tool.

[00:39:30] Chronic fears—thinking about in terms of phobias or anxieties or past trauma—what we often see is this influence how people eat and care for themselves. Again, one of the ways that food can be used is something ... I like it because it's very concrete. If you think about as a mental health professional, as a psychiatrist, I've got meds. I've got my interpretations about your parents and your life and your dynamics and your unconscious, but in terms of something to go home and do today, we don't do such

[00:40:00] a great job sometimes in mental health. That's where food can help. If people are really having a lot of trauma, to make a meal that soothes them, that's the type of recommendation increasingly that I've been doing.

Then, really following up. Saying, "Send me a picture of that special dish your grandma made. Tell me about it. What does it evoke for you? What was it like cooking it? What was it like sharing it with your

[00:40:30] family?" It's, in some ways, the food becomes a vehicle for people's self-expression, for their ability to grow and enhance their own self-care. And, I think, most importantly, the part that I really love about food is it gives us the ability to concretely love and nourish people. The idea that, "I want to care for you in a cellular way. I want to help your cells. That's how much I love you." Again, that's part of the excitement of this food movement that we've seen in America over the past 10 years. Everybody's

[00:41:00] thinking about it. Everybody's talking about it. I think that's eventually going to lead to better mental health for all of us.

Epigenetics is this very exciting concept, and I think about it a little bit like a card player. Your genes are the cards. You get dealt your cards, and you're sitting there with your little hand of cards. But a skilled poker player, no matter what they get dealt, they're going to beat me. They're better at me than poker.

[00:41:30]

[00:42:00]

They're going to win. It's how they play the cards. I think about epigenetics like that. Epigenetics is the idea that your genes, the expression of your genes, are controlled by environmental factors. If we put in environmental factors like lots of zinc, B12, omega-3 fats, a dietary pattern that is based in plants and the right fats and good, healthy seafoods—we turn on genes that lower inflammation. When we eat lots of plants, we turn on genes that help us fight chronic disease. That's how food works at the most fundamental level. It's powerful. It is the factor that is under your control that really has a very, very powerful genetic and cellular impact.

[00:42:30]

What's nice is you're already doing it every day. You're already influencing your genes, and so can you help each decision that you make be a little bit better of a decision? I'll sometimes look, and I'll think, "What is the best thing for me to eat?" It'll be both the nutrients, and also like, "What's going to give me the most pleasure?" Having a pleasurable experience, I think is ... I guess it's horrible, but as a doctor I'd much rather people have a really joyful, rich, delicious life and die at 70 than have a horrible, low-fat-eating, miserable, angst-ridden existence where they're counting calories and they die at 85. I just feel like I'm about quality of life I guess.

[00:43:00]

[00:43:30]

The most important piece of advice I would want people to hear is my message of hope. I've treated thousands of people with clinical depression, and I am shocked at how much people can transform of being on my couch ready to kill themselves with nothing to live for—tearful, not able to sleep, right about to head into the hospital—and some weeks later, months later, be there as a bright, vibrant, loving, human being with all of what a human can offer. I think people are frustrated because I don't perfectly know how to get from A to B, but I do know through engagement, through good clinical treatment, through good alliance, that you can get from A to B. I think the first thing I would want people to hear is a message of hope, which I know when I've struggled with my mood, that's hard to believe.

[00:44:00]

[00:44:30]

The next part, because I'm a nutritional psychiatrist, is I think people need to incorporate food into their plans. What are you eating tonight? What are you eating for lunch? To focus on what I think most people already know. Let's eat whole foods. Let's think about where your knowledge gaps are. A lot of people don't know how to cook vegetables. Brussels sprouts for most people is like, "Oh", like a bad PTSD experience from the high school cafeteria. That is not what Brussels sprouts are like in my house. They're like, "Wow. Amazing, crispy deliciousness." Figuring out where those knowledge gaps are around food and pushing yourself.

[00:45:00]

I didn't eat or cook seafood at all until I was 30. That's kind of late. It smelled yucky and fishy to me. I cook everything in the sea now. That notion that you can evolve as an eater, and specifically if you're struggling with depression, if you're struggling with anxiety, there are a core set of foods that you should be eating as part of your treatment, as part of you caring for your brain. That, I think, is the message I want people to hear. I've tried to spread that far and wide both in the books, but also to other psychiatrists and mental health professionals, to utilize this very simple tool. We are what we eat. Your brain certainly depends on you having a healthy gut and a healthy diet. Your brain is made of food.

[00:45:30]

Think about it, every molecule in your brain, besides oxygen, starts at the end of your fork. Period. It's how it gets there. That's a lot of control at the end of that fork, and so I would encourage anyone struggling with depression or anxiety too, who has that in their family and is nervous, to feel hopefulness and to start feasting on brain food. Know that you are nourishing your most important organ, and all of the science tells us, and all of my clinical experience tells me, that it works. It really helps.

[00:46:00]

Eat to Beat Depression is an e-course that I created to help people get these fundamental tools. It's a modular video course that goes through the latest science relating to neuroplasticity and brain growth and food and depression. The course really focuses in on depression, and then it really works with individuals for them to assess their own diet just as we do in our clinic, and walk through the important food categories, and help people set small, weekly attainable goals. *Eat to Beat Depression* is really aimed to be a resource for individuals to get some of this knowledge and then to get encouragement.

[00:46:30]   We've run a number of people through the course, and our first group, it was interesting. About 80% of those individuals were already using food to treat their depression, but 0% had ever been talked to by a mental health professional about food. That's the gap that I'm hoping we really see shrink. That this is increasingly viewed as something that can help individuals and empower our patients. The course is my first effort to have there be a product other than a book to really give people another set of resources.

ELIZABETH BOHAM, MD, RD | The UltraWellness Center

Dr. Elizabeth Boham:	My undergraduate and graduate degrees were in nutrition and exercise physiology and I loved nutrition. I loved working with people on changing their diet and realizing how powerful food is, so I wanted to learn more about how the body worked. I decided to go back to medical school, which was really a wonderful experience, but it took me a little bit away from prevention. When I got out of medical school, I learned a lot about Functional Medicine at Canyon Ranch when I met Dr. Hyman and Kathie Swift. It was wonderful. It was this amazing experience for me because I realized that I could incorporate my nutrition background with my medical school training and really learn how to have this map to use nutrition as medical therapy. Functional Medicine really gives me that map to incorporate my nutrition education and use nutrition as medicine.
[00:00:30]	
[00:01:00]	There was a lot of time during and right after medical school where I was really questioning my decision. I was doing a lot of acute care medicine, and we weren't really focusing on nutrition and prevention, and I was frustrated. I was absolutely frustrated with medicine and questioning significantly what I got myself into. When I found Functional Medicine, it was great because I could say, "Okay, I can do this type of medicine. I really appreciate this type of medicine. I see how this type of medicine works." It was that great map so I could continue to practice medicine in a way that I felt fulfilled.
[00:01:30]	When I was 30, I was diagnosed with an aggressive type of breast cancer, and that came as a real shock to me because I was really interested in nutrition and prevention and had no family history of cancer. When, at the age of 30, I was diagnosed with breast cancer, I was completely shocked as many people could understand. It was a time where I had to step back and say, "Why did this happen to me? What was going on in my body that allowed this to occur?"
[00:02:00]	That's when I started to learn more about Functional Medicine and it really helped me answer that question of why. I was able to step back and say what sort of shifts had occurred in my body that maybe had an impact on how well my immune system was working or my digestive system, and therefore, the ability for my body to detoxify from toxins that I was exposed to, and how that influenced my risk of getting cancer. It really helped me figure out what sort of things led to that cancer developing in me and how I could prevent it from maybe happening again.
[00:02:30]	
[00:03:00]	Patients always come to me and say, "Oh, my doctor said it doesn't really matter what I eat," whether they're having problems with their memory or their mood or their digestive system. It's really because physicians have not been trained in the importance of nutrition, so they just don't realize, they don't know that there's such a connection with nutrition and our health. We know that food is really powerful medicine, so there's a tremendous impact. Of course there is, in terms of what we eat and the health of our body. We're really working hard with the Institute for Functional Medicine to get that message out there and to train physicians so they can recognize that there is this important connection, and they can start to use food as medicine.
[00:03:30]	There's absolutely an increase in brain disorders that we're seeing and we know that, for example, with autism. Now, one in every 68 children are on the autistic spectrum and that's a huge increase. It's a big concern. There are multiple reasons for this increase. There's an explosion of toxins in our environment, excessive use of antibiotics, and our really processed food supply. There's a whole range of reasons why we're seeing this explosion in brain disorders.
[00:04:00]	It's important that we look at all these different aspects so we can really decrease the explosion of brain disorders that we're seeing and have a good impact on people's brain health. The gut-brain connection really shows us that there's an absolute connection between all the different systems in our

body, so that our digestive system is impacting our brain health and our brain is impacting our digestive system. We know that. When we get anxious, we have digestive symptoms—maybe some people get more constipated or other people may rush to the bathroom more frequently.

[00:04:30] We also know that our digestive system is impacting our brain health. When there are imbalances in our gut flora or all of those bugs in our digestive system, that really impacts our mood and our brain health. When there are imbalances in this gut flora, people can have more anxiety. We see that often. When we treat it—those imbalances with changes in diet—with good bacteria like probiotics, with fiber, sometimes even with medications to lower those imbalances, we see improvements in brain health like we see improvements in anxiety. It's pretty exciting.

[00:05:00]

Nutrients have a huge impact on our brain health. Some of the most important nutrients for our brain health are omega-3 fats. Omega-3 fats are those essential fatty acids that make up a good portion of our brain and are critical for adequate brain health. Unfortunately, we are seeing a decrease in our omega-3 fats in our diet. That's happening naturally because our food supplies are becoming more and more deficient in omega-3 fats.

[00:05:30]

Another really important nutrient for brain health is vitamin B12. Vitamin B12 comes from animal protein and has a huge impact on our brain health. When there are deficiencies in B12, we see many disorders like depression, numbness and tingling, difficulty with walking, dementia, and changes in memory. B12 is critical for brain health. It's really important that we check B12 levels. We can do a serum B12 but that's not that great of a test, so we'll often look for other markers of B12 deficiency, such as the methylmalonic acid or homocysteine. B12 deficiency occurs as people get older. We need to have enough acid in our stomach to digest our protein and pull our B12 from our food. As we get older, our stomach acid often decreases and that results in B12 deficiency.

[00:06:00]

[00:06:30] In addition, many people are on acid blockers. Acid blockers decrease the acid in our stomach. People take them for heartburn, for example, but what ends up happening is that we don't digest our protein as well and we don't pull our B12 from our food as easily. So many times, when people are on acid blockers, over time, they'll develop things like B12 deficiency. And B12, as we talked about, is critical for our brain health.

Healthy fats are critical for our brain. Our brain is made up mostly of fat and so it's really important that we get enough fat in our diet.

[00:07:00] Some fats, though, you want to avoid. Those are the trans fats or hydrogenated fats. They've been largely pulled out of our food supply but they're still there. When you look at a label, you want to look for two things. One, you want to make sure there are no trans fats in that food. It'll say 0% trans fats but sometimes, foods can say 0% trans fat and still have some trans fat in it. You want to look at the ingredients to make sure there's no partially hydrogenated oil in there. If you see the words partially hydrogenated oil, you want to stay away from that food.

[00:07:30]

There are some fats that, if they're not stored properly, can be unhealthy for us. So, for example, some fats are very delicate—fish oil or ground flaxseed, those are high in omega-3 fats, but it's really important that we store them properly. You don't want to keep your ground flaxseed on the shelf. It will get rancid or oxidize, and that's really not good for us. Keep your flaxseed in the freezer. Take some out every week or two, grind it in a coffee grinder, and then use that up within a week or two, and then you can replenish your stores from your freezer.

[00:08:00]

Coconut oil has a lot of wonderful properties in it. It's a wonderful fat full of medium-chain triglycerides, which is easily digested and absorbed into the body. There have been many studies showing that those medium-chain triglycerides are good for our digestive system health, our brain health, and can be incorporated into a healthy diet. I feel coconut oil is a wonderful food to incorporate into your diet.

[00:08:30]

[00:09:00] There are a lot of new therapies out there that can be really helpful for some people with brain disorders. In autism, we've been using—for some children—helminth therapy. Helminths are a worm that are parasites but they are non-parasitic to humans. People will consume these helminths and they impact their brain health. For some children, the helminths will decrease the immune response in their body, will lower inflammation in their body, and they can have improvements in their symptoms. That's kind of an interesting treatment that some people will benefit from and, really, it causes no harm to try.

[00:09:30] There are a lot of reasons why conventional medicine isn't always open to some of these alternative therapies. Some is just where the money is and, unfortunately, that impacts how we're trained in medical school and what therapies we are taught to use. Sometimes, it just takes time for us to realize how helpful these other therapies can be and how much they can help people. I think over time, more and more people will incorporate them into their practice.

[00:10:00] Another area we've been really excited about are looking for and detecting these folate receptor antibodies. A very high percentage of kids on the autistic spectrum have antibodies against these folate receptors. Folate receptors are in your brain and you need folate, which comes from foliage or leafy green vegetables. You need folate to bind to these receptors for proper brain development to occur. Unfortunately, a lot of children with these folate receptor antibodies are having changes or decrease in brain development. When we check for folate receptor antibodies, we see a high percentage of children on the autistic spectrum with these antibodies. There are ways we can treat that. We can treat

[00:10:30] that by giving higher doses of folate, and also by removing dairy from their diet because dairy often will cause these folate receptor antibodies to occur.

[00:11:00] Sleep is absolutely underrated especially in our current culture. Sleep is critical for brain health. Sleep deficiency has been seen time and time again within multiple studies to be linked with decreased cognition, lower mood, mood disorders, and having a harder time with memory, focus, and attention. Sleep is really critical for our brain and we need to focus on it all the time. As our children—as all of us are using more and more technology, unfortunately, that often leads to less and less sleep and a lot of issues in terms of attention and focus and ADHD and memory problems. It's critical.

[00:11:30] Many times, people feel that, "Okay, I can get by with four to five hours of sleep at night." Or over time, they just shortened their sleep cycle a little less, a little less, a little less, and they think they're getting away with it because they're not realizing how much it's impacting how they feel, so it's critical. I work with sleep with all of my patients. That's one of the first things I ask them. How many hours are they getting? How restorative is their sleep? Are they waking up in the middle of the night? Are they feeling rested when they wake up?

[00:12:00] When I was 30, I was diagnosed with an aggressive type of breast cancer. It was triple negative and so I needed to go through chemotherapy and radiation treatment. Like many people who are dealing with a life-threatening illness, I went through those five stages of grief. First, it was denial and then, it was anger, and then bargaining, and then depression. Prior to the fifth stage, the acceptance, depression definitely set in. It did for me as well. There were many things that helped me through that process. One was a gratitude journal. My gratitude journal was critical for me. It helped me change my thought

[00:12:30] process and how I dealt with having this illness and changed how I thought about things, and really helped with my mood and realizing the good things that came from having gone through this process, this unfortunate diagnosis.

[00:13:00] I really paid attention to exercise. I focused on exercising every day. Even on days where I really didn't feel up to it, I did something. I remember with my radiation treatments, I would walk every day to the hospital to get them done and the exercise really was helpful. We know that when people exercise through their treatment, they often will do better. If you're not feeling up to going for a run, at least go for a walk or do some yoga. Exercise really is helpful for our mood. We know that, and it helps when going through a difficult diagnosis.

[00:13:30]	When I went through chemotherapy, I definitely got chemo brain. That is a hard thing to deal with. I had to learn how to be gentle with myself and to recognize that my memory changed for that period of time. There were some things that really were helpful. Glutathione is a wonderful antioxidant and detoxifier. I use it all the time in my practice. It helped me and it helps many of my patients. We can give glutathione as a liquid that gets absorbed through the cheek in your mouth. There are other ways you can give glutathione as well—IV and in creams. It's a really great antioxidant and detoxifier that works well after you've gone through chemotherapy.
[00:14:00] [00:14:30]	NAC is also something I recommend all the time to my patients, about 600 milligrams twice a day. It helps the body with the production of glutathione. As do all of your cruciferous vegetables—your broccoli, cauliflower, cabbage, kale—they help with glutathione production. We call junk food "junk food" because it's really devoid of all the nutrients that are necessary for our bodies to work well and our brain to work well. It has the calories but it doesn't have much nutritional value. It's important for all of us and especially for our children to really be watching, keeping the junk food away. Junk food is also high in additives and food coloring, and there have been multiple studies to show that these food colorings and additives can have an impact on our children's attention and focus. We can see good improvements in kids' attention and focus when we take them off of these processed foods and foods that have food coloring added to them.
[00:15:00] [00:15:30]	Some of the most important things for improving your children's diet is, first of all, just having good healthy food available. We know that when there's good, healthy food around, kids will choose healthy food. You want to get the junk food—get the processed food—out of the house and have healthy food around. Have vegetables cut up so kids can snack on them. Have fruit available. In addition, get your children involved in cooking and get your children involved in the food that you provide for the family. When children are involved in cooking and food preparation, they're much more excited to try new and different foods. It's really a great thing that you can do for your kids, get them involved in the kitchen. Get them cutting up the vegetables. Get them preparing the foods because they're more likely to choose and eat them.
[00:16:00]	We all recognize when our blood sugar gets out of balance that we don't feel good. When our blood sugar drops, we all notice that we feel more tired, have a harder time focusing or concentrating, so that's critical for all my patients and for our children. It's really important that we work to balance our blood sugar. What that means is that at every meal, you want to have some fat, some good healthy fat, some good fiber, and some protein. Those three things together will help keep your blood sugar balanced and help you feel better, have more energy, and have an easier time with focus.
[00:16:30]	Often, we're eating foods that don't help our body balance the blood sugar. If we're feeling tired, we might reach for a piece of candy or a piece of fruit. And that might help bring our blood sugar up for a short period of time, but then it may crash again afterwards. If you are going to have an apple, have some almonds with it or some nut butter with it, that the fiber and the fat in the almonds will help balance your blood sugar and help you feel better for a longer period of time.
[00:17:00] [00:17:30]	In addition, for breakfast, so often, we're giving our kids cereal. There are not a lot of good healthy fats in that. There's not a lot of protein and sometimes, there's not even a lot of fiber if it's a sugar-filled cereal. Their blood sugar may go up quickly afterwards and then an hour or two later, they're going to be feeling tired and have a harder time focusing in school. It's critical at breakfast time that you have some good protein, good healthy fats and, again, that fiber that can come from your vegetables and fruit to help keep your blood sugar balanced for a longer period of time.
[00:18:00]	We react to gluten and dairy in many different ways, but one way that many people react to gluten and dairy is because of these gluteomorphins and casomorphins found in gluten and dairy. These are the peptides. Gluteomorphins and casomorphins are these peptides that can cross the blood-brain barrier and impact our mood, concentration, focus, and our energy. Many times, when people come in with fatigue or problems with focus, concentration, problems with their mood, or depression, we can check

for these and gluteomorphins and casomorphins. We can do a test to look for them. But often, we'll just remove gluten and dairy, and see if that helps with their energy and their focus and their mood—and it often can.

[00:18:30]

[00:19:00]

We see the power of food as medicine in this practice all of the time. I had a patient the other day. She was about 50 years old and she came in with symptoms that we see all the time. "I feel tired. I'm just having a hard time with getting up in the morning. I want to take a nap in the afternoon. I've put on about 20 pounds over the last couple years or so, and I just don't feel good anymore." We always start with diet. It's amazing to see how much people can improve just with dietary shifts. For this woman, it was amazing. We took away the junk. We took away the processed food that she was eating and helped her with balancing her blood sugar, and we took away gluten and dairy. For her, it made a tremendous impact on her brain health. She started to feel better. She had better energy. Her mood improved and she lost that excess weight she was struggling to lose.

[00:19:30]

[00:20:00]

I had a boy who was four years old when he came to see me, and he was diagnosed on the autistic spectrum. We did some simple blood tests. We found that he was really deficient in B12—and B12, we know, is critical for brain health. We also found that he was low in vitamin D and that he had a reaction to gluten. He had these gluteomorphins that were having an impact on how well he could interact with people and focus. With this child, there were just three things that we did. We replaced his vitamin D, we replaced his B12, and we took gluten out of his diet and it was amazing. He started interacting more. His communication came. He had better behavior and he actually is not considered autistic anymore. Sometimes, it's amazing to see how simple changes can have a huge impact on a kid's health.

[00:20:30]

[00:21:00]

The most important things to do to improve your brain function are, first and foremost, exercise. Exercise is critical for brain health and you want to get some exercise every day, really important for prevention of dementia but also for just improving brain health today. The second thing you want to do is really eat from the rainbow of colorful plant foods. You want to choose foods from every color of the rainbow every day. These phytonutrients that create the color in our plant foods have a tremendous impact on our health. They have anti-inflammatory properties. They can prevent dementia. They can decrease risk of cancer. You want to reach for a plant food from every color of the rainbow every day. Then, the third and probably one of the most important things we can do, is to get adequate sleep every night. You really want to reach for those seven to nine hours of sleep every night and give your body time to rest.

EMILY FLETCHER | Founder of Ziva Meditation, Creator of zivaMIND.com

Emily Fletcher: I first became interested in meditation during my 10-year career on Broadway. My last Broadway show was *A Chorus Line* and I understudied three of the lead roles, which means that you show up to the theater and you have no idea which character you're going to play. Sometimes, I would start the show as one character and halfway through, they would switch me to a different character. I would just be chilling in my dressing room doing my taxes and someone would get on a loudspeaker and say, "Emily Fletcher, we need you on stage." I would start panicking because I wouldn't know which costume to put on, so I would just grab all three of them, run down seven flights of stairs. Sometimes I would be on stage before I knew which character I was going to play.

[00:00:30]

Now, some people are very good at this job, I am not one of them. I was living my life in this constant state of anxiety and overwhelm and I started going gray at the tender age of 26. I started getting sick all the time, I was getting injured. It was really confusing to me why I was living my dream, doing the thing I had wanted to do since I was eight, and I was miserable. Then thankfully, the girl sitting next to me in the dressing room was a meditator, she had a harder job than I did, but she was crushing it. I was like, "Lady, what do you know that I don't know?" She said, "I meditate."

[00:01:00]

This is a decade ago so no one was really talking about it then like they are now, but I thought, "No, come on. She can't be this good at her job just by sitting in her chair and doing nothing." I just kept having insomnia, I kept going gray, I kept getting sick, I kept sucking at my job. Then finally I was so embarrassed about my performance that I thought, "Well, let me try it." I went along to this intro to meditation talk. I liked what I heard. I signed up for this course and the first day of the first class, I was meditating. To be honest, I had no idea what that meant, but I was in a different state of consciousness than I had ever been in before and I liked it. Then that night I slept through the night for the first time in 18 months, and I have every night since, and that was 10 years ago.

[00:01:30]

Then I stopped getting sick, I stopped going gray, I stopped getting injured. I started enjoying my job again and I thought, "Why does everyone not do this?" I left Broadway, I went to India and started what became a three-year training process to teach. Then I opened up Ziva five and a half years ago, and it's been the best thing I've ever done. When I started to see how dramatically meditation improved my performance and my life, I felt really inspired and actually compelled to be able to share it with others. I was like, "This thing is so good. Why is everyone not doing it?" I'm the kind of person that when I find something that works for me, I really want to share it with as many people who are interested.

[00:02:00]

To be honest, when I started my diaphragm meditation, I thought it would just be a side interest or I was just going for my own benefit. Then when I got to India I realized, "I'm going to teach this." I didn't know when or why or how, but I knew I was going to. Then I sort of arrogantly thought that I could keep acting, and keep teaching acting, and teach meditation. There was this one week where I was in final callbacks to play Velma in Chicago on Broadway. I was starting the world's first online meditation training and I was teaching six people to be acting teachers at my studio. I was like, "Nobody wins here." That was when I made a very conscious decision to stop teaching acting, to stop acting, and move into teaching meditation full time—and then Ziva has just grown exponentially since then.

[00:02:30]

[00:03:00]

Really, the desire to teach came out of how dramatically meditation improved my performance. I tend to work with a lot of high performers. I teach Broadway performers and athletes and CEOs and hedge fund managers, and they all say the same thing to me. All these types of high performers say in their own way, "Emily, I need my stress. My stress is the thing that gives me my competitive edge." My actor or my artist clients will say, "Emily, I need my stress, I need those hurdy-poohs. That's the thing that I create from." The reality is, stress is not doing us any favors in the performance department; stress actually makes you stupid. We don't like to hear that, but it's true.

[00:03:30]

[00:04:00] Yes, there is such a thing as good stress. Yes, there are saunas or cryotherapy or high intensity interval training, but that's not what I'm talking about. I'm not talking about good stress—I'm talking about chronic stress that most of us are suffering from. Doctors are calling stress the black plague of our century and I don't think that that's an over exaggeration. If you want to understand why the human body reacts to stress in the way that it does, we have to cut back in time a few thousand years. Say we're hunting and gathering in the woods, and let's say that a sabre tooth tiger jumps out at us with the intent to kill.

[00:04:30] The first thing that's going to happen is that our digestion will flood with acid to shut down digestion because we need all hands on deck to fight or flee this tiger. That same acid will seep onto the skin so that we don't taste very good if we get bitten into by that tiger. Our bladder and bowels will evacuate so we can be light on our feet. That's what the nervous poos are before you have a big thing to do. Your immune system goes to the back burner because who cares if you're going to get cancer if you're about to be killed by a tiger? Your adrenaline levels increase and your cortisol levels increase. Those are actually acidic in nature and that can actually accelerate the body's aging.

[00:05:00] We all know this intuitively. If we're working too hard, not sleeping, we look in the mirror and we look 10 years older than we are. And we go on vacation, we're like, "Uh, I look amazing." That's sort of real-time feedback of what stress is doing to the body. That series of chemical reactions is very useful if your demands are predatory attacks. If your demands are in-laws or kids or deadlines or text messages or emails, then these fight-or-flight stress reactions become maladaptive and they're now disallowing us from performing at the top of our game.

[00:05:30] This is where meditation really comes into play. Meditation goes in and it gets rid of that adrenaline and cortisol, and it actually starts to flood the brain with dopamine and serotonin, which are bliss chemicals. That adrenaline and cortisol, they're acidic in nature, accelerates aging; whereas, dopamine and serotonin—they're bliss chemicals. They feel amazing and they actually can reverse body age. This is some of the cool new neuroscience that is coming out around meditation. Not only does meditation feel amazing and improve your performance but it also can reverse your body age by somewhere between 8-15 years, which I think is nuts.

[00:06:00] When I first heard about this I thought, "Well come on, it's not magic. It's not a fountain of youth, it's not a miracle." And it's not. What it's doing is that meditation is actually lengthening your telomeres. The way I like to think about telomeres is that they're like the little plastic thing at the end of your shoelace. If that plastic thing unravels, then your shoelace unravels. Well, similarly, if your telomeres unravel then that can impact your actual DNA, it can impact how quickly that unravels. We know that now over time, the more you meditate the longer your telomeres become, which is pretty rad.

[00:06:30] There are lots of different styles of meditation. I think it's important to clarify because as meditation becomes increasingly more popular, I think we want to be really specific with our vernacular. A lot of people are using the term mindfulness and the term meditation as synonyms when they're actually not synonyms. Mindfulness is a derivative of styles of meditation that were made for monks and it's more of a waking-state practice. Like, I'm going to bring my awareness to my breath, I'm going to bring my awareness to the body. I would call mindfulness the art of bringing your attention to the right now, which is really beautiful and incredibly powerful.

[00:07:00] If you actually look at a brain scan of someone practicing mindfulness, then a very small part of the brain lights up very, very bright. Now, there's this whole other category called meditation. I'm admittedly a meditation snob but how I would define meditation is when you're accessing a verifiable fourth state of consciousness, something different than waking, sleeping or dreaming. In this fourth state of consciousness, the right and left hemispheres of the brain actually start to function in unison. Meaning that if you were to hook your brain up to an EEG machine in waking, sleeping, and dreaming states of
[00:07:30] consciousness, right and left hemispheres are functioning separately.

[00:08:00]

In meditation, all 16 leads of EEG rise and fall in unison, which I think is pretty cool—that sitting quietly in a chair could actually change the signature of your brain. Cool party trick but who cares, why do I want that to happen? I think everyone should because the left brain—and that's sort of an over simplification for the prefrontal cortex—the left brain is the critical mind. It's in charge of math, language, navigation, balancing our checkbooks—all really important activities for most of us who've been taking our left brain to the gym for a very long time.

[00:08:30]

Now, our right brain is the piece of us that's in charge of the right now. It's in charge of creative problem solving, intuition, color, music, connectiveness, creative problem solving. For most of us, our right brains have been atrophying for a while. We've just been thinking, taking action, achieving, making money so we can be happy in the future. Meanwhile, our right brains are like, "Hey, I have a creative idea. I have a suggestion." You're like, "Shut up, right brain, I have to think and take action and achieve and make money so I can be happy in the future." If you look at a human brain it splits right down the middle, 50-50, and I don't think that nature makes mistakes. I don't think that nature would have given us 50-50 if it wanted us to use 90-10.

[00:09:00]

In the style of meditation that I teach at Ziva, we're actually using a mantra. And a mantra is not a slogan, it's not an affirmation. The mantras that we use, they're meaningless primordial sounds, and those mantras actually help to de-excite the nervous system and help us start to take that right brain to the gym. That pendulum swings for a little while but over time the whole brain lights up. In mindfulness, it's a smaller part of the brain that lights up very bright versus the style of meditation that I teach at Ziva, the whole brain lights up but not as bright.

[00:09:30]

The whole brain lighting up leads to a level of neuroplasticity, brain cohesion, and over time it actually strengthens something called the corpus callosum. Now, the corpus callosum is quite literally the bridge between the two hemispheres of the brain. We've known for a long time that meditators have thicker corpus callosums than non-meditators but we weren't able to prove if it was causal or correlated. Now we know that the longer you meditate the thicker the corpus callosum becomes, which again, cool party trick but why do I want a fat corpus callosum?

[00:10:00]

Well, everyone should because it is the bridge between your critical mind and your creative mind. It is the thing that allows you to come up with all those creative problem solving ideas when it's go time. Let's say you get into a fight with your partner and it starts to get pretty heated, and then after a while you just shut down and you retreat to the bedroom. A few hours later, once you're calm, you start to come up with all these amazing witty comebacks and you're like, "Why? Why couldn't I have thought of that in the moment?"

[00:10:30]

Well, my hypothesis here is that the longer you meditate, the thicker your corpus callosum becomes, the easier it is for you to come up with those witty comebacks when it counts. For sure, the number one misconception around meditation is that people think that they have to clear their minds. People think that the point of meditation is to give the mind a command to be silent. If you're judging yourself at how good you are at meditation based on how good you are at giving your brain a command to shut up, then you're always going to feel like you're failing and you're definitely going to quit. None of us will do anything for very long that we feel like we're failing at.

[00:11:00]

While there are different styles of meditation that are good for different use cases, the reality is what most people need is some training in how to meditate. Really truly, meditation is like any other skill, but because it's simple, people assume that they should already know how to do it. They think, "Well yeah, I should just sit in a chair and close my eyes and be like, okay brain, stop thinking." Then it looks like this, "I sure would like a snack. I love snacks, snacks are delicious. I got a whole ring called snacks. Wait, now I'm thinking about snacks. Right now, I'm thinking about how I'm thinking about snacks. I suck at meditation and I quit." That's the beginning and the end of most peoples' meditation career. Really,

[00:11:30]

they're only quitting because they're judging themselves based on misinformation.

[00:12:00] I feel like there's this one dude going around telling everyone that in order to meditate, you have to clear your mind. And I wish I could find him and teach him how to meditate because it would make my job so much easier. The analogy that I like to use here is, let's say we were going to do a 21-day Portuguese challenge. For 20 minutes a day for the next 21 days, we're all going to speak Portuguese. Now, if you don't know how to speak Portuguese I think that's kind of a silly challenge to take and yet that's what everyone is doing with meditation. Like, "I'm going to have a 21-day challenge. I'm just going to sit down and close my eyes and shut up rain," but it doesn't go all that well.

[00:12:30] I think if you have a little bit of training, if you have a technique that's designed for you, the meditation can be so simple and so beautiful, and then it becomes something that you actually crave. Something that you look forward to versus a torture device or something that your parents used to do to you when you were a child. Ziva Meditation is a beautiful trifecta of mindfulness, meditation, and manifesting—the three Ms, if you will. I'd like to think about mindfulness as the appetizer, meditation as the main course, and manifesting as dessert.

[00:13:00] The way that I use mindfulness is really as a runway because we tend to work with a lot of high performers, hyper achievers, people who really like to go. It's hard to go from 60 miles an hour to zero right away. I feel that people like to use that mindfulness as a little bit of a runway. In the mindfulness techniques that we use, it will be breath work or sensory work, just tools to help ground you in the right here, right now. Then the meditation is where you're accessing that verifiable fourth state of consciousness. You're also giving your body rest that is five times deeper than sleep. That's not an insignificant point because when we give the body the rest that it needs, it knows how to heal itself. One of the things that it heals itself from is stress. The less stress we have in the body, the better able we are to perform at the top of our game.

[00:13:30] Then finally, we end the meditation with some manifesting tools. I know that that word manifesting gets a bad rap because we think of *The Secret* back in the 90s. Manifesting just means consciously creating a life that you love. It means intending the things that you want to have happen. I give people some tools to utilize that juicy time at the end of meditation to help visualize a life that they dream of. Honestly, I think the single most valuable piece of advice that anyone could take with them as they start a meditation career is this: the mind thinks involuntarily just like the heart beats involuntarily, so trying to give your brain a command to be silent is as effective as trying to give your heart a command to stop beating.

[00:14:30] Just to drive the point home, on the count of three try and give your heart a command to stop beating. Ready? One, two, three, and please don't die. We see that that's so silly. We can't command the heart to stop beating or our nails to stop growing, that's not up to us. Similarly, we cannot command the brain to be silent. Instead, you will develop a technique. You learn a technique. You get a bit of training—you get a technique that was designed for you and then you move towards the technique, not away from the thoughts.

[00:15:00] People ask me sometimes if I miss performing on Broadway and the answer is decidedly no. Selfishly, why I do what I do is that every single day I get to wake up to emails from people saying, "Emily, my anxiety went away, my depression's gone," "I was able to finally get off my meds with the help of my doctor," "My insomnia's gone, my IBS is gone," "My skin cleared up," "I broke up with that guy," "I started writing that book." Every day I get emails like this and it's so rewarding to feel like I played a role in that transformation.

[00:15:30] It's not me—it's them, it's the practice. But I'm really happy to help facilitate that. Some stories that stand out to me: I taught a gentleman once and he was in his late 60s. We were doing a private and he had Parkinson's and it was pretty advanced. I could tell that he was a bit self-conscious about it, he was holding his hands. When he first learned, I gave him his mantra and his tremors got very, very pronounced. Then he closed his eyes and he started doing his mantra silently and his tremors stopped immediately. It was very dramatic. I started crying because I'd never seen it happen before, it was very moving.

[00:16:00]

Then afterwards when he opened his eyes, I didn't want to make a big deal about it but he said to me, he said, "Did you notice that my tremors stopped?" I said, "I did notice that." Then the next day we meditated again and for the whole 10-minute session his tremors stopped, and afterwards about five minutes later they came back. The next day we meditated for 20 minutes, they stopped. Afterwards, about 15 minutes later tremors came back. The next day, in 20 minutes they came back. The next day it took 30 minutes for them to come back. I can't claim that meditation cures Parkinson's but I did see firsthand that that dopamine and serotonin that the brain produces when you're meditating seemed to give him a bit of a reprieve. That reprieve lasted longer and longer. That was the first time I'd ever seen

[00:16:30]

anything so visceral and so instant.

The reality is, our bodies are very fast. When you have the brain of fear, within 10 minutes you have the marrow of fear. Similarly, when you start meditating, if you have the brain of bliss, within 10 minutes you have the marrow of bliss. That's how long it takes from a stimulus to something to go to the most viscous fluid in our body, which is the marrow in our bones—10 minutes. Really, every action that we

[00:17:00]

take, every time we get stressed, every time we meditate, every time we eat food that's nourishing or food that's toxic—it's impacting every cell in our body within minutes and so that was really exciting for me to see.

I had a woman tell me that she got a $120,000 scholarship to a nursing program that she didn't even apply for. I said, "I totally attribute this to meditation." The people finish their books, finish their films, book TV shows, win Oscars, win Tonys, win Grammys. My goal is to have the EGOT of meditation. So far,

[00:17:30]

they have Grammy, Tony, and Oscar award winners but I think it'd be fun to have the EGOT of students. Almost every day when I tell people I'm a meditation teacher they say, "Oh Emily, I really want to meditate. I know there's some fascinating neuroscience coming out telling us how good meditation is for you, but I'm busy. My life is crazy, I don't have time to meditate." My favorite thing to say to that is, "Okay, do you have time to feel like crap? Do you have time to have insomnia? Do you have time to

[00:18:00]

have anxiety? Do you have time to get sick? Do you have time to not perform as nature designed your brain to perform?"

I think that we really, very urgently need to move meditation out of this "spa day for your brain" category. Meditation is not a pedicure for your brain. This thing is not a luxury item; this thing is the single most important act of mental hygiene that you could perform. You're not going to leave your house without brushing your teeth. My goal is to make leaving your house without meditating as rude as

[00:18:30]

it would be to leave your house without brushing your teeth. If you start to understand that meditation is not wasting your time, it's actually optimizing your brain performance, then you can't really imagine your day without it.

People who develop a daily routine, they report this again and again and again that that second meditation is like a supercharged power nap. If you schedule in the time to do it, afterwards you have this hit of creativity and productivity and energy, even more so than if you took a coffee or a nap or had

[00:19:00]

some chocolate. It's this self-sufficient sustainable means by which to optimize your brain performance instead of being dependent on chemicals to do it for you. My top tips for enhancing brain health, aside from meditation, we're going to assume that meditation's my number one. Other than that, it's sleeping, for sure. I used to be very much a night owl, 10 years on Broadway leads to late nights so making your sleep earlier.

[00:19:30]

According to Ayurveda, the optimal times are 10pm to 6am. It's not just how much sleep you're getting but it's when you're sleeping. The sleep that you get before midnight is actually better for you than the sleep that you get after midnight because your body's running a whole host of cleansing operations. Sleeping and the timing of your sleep, and eating a ton of raw fat. I eat so much raw fat. People are like, "But Emily, you're so thin." Fat doesn't make you fat, rest doesn't make you lazy. Fat is actually fueling

[00:20:00] your brain. The brain runs almost exclusively on EPAs and DHAs. If you're not getting that in your food, then your brain is actually going to suck that up from your body, and it will create dry skin and a feeling of dehydration. Eating lots and lots of raw fat has really helped my brain performance.

[00:20:30] Then, taking the right supplements, figuring out what you're deficient in, what you have too much of, and then supplementing around that. Yes, ideally, we're getting all of our nutrients from the food that we're eating. The reality is that our soil has been depleted and a lot of our food isn't food anymore. Even if you're eating a healthy diet, sometimes you need to supplement to bring us back to baseline. If you don't yet have a meditation practice but you're having a high-demand, high-anxiety moment. I call them an OMFG moment. I actually have an OMFG technique and that is simply inhaling through your nose for two and exhaling through your mouth for four. You're just doubling the length of the exhale from your inhales, which is in through the nose for two and out through the mouth for four.

[00:21:00] When we do that, when we double the length of the exhale, we actually strengthen and ease the vagus nerve. The vagus nerve is really the biggest connector between the mind and the body. As we soothe that, it's easier for the body to move out of that fight-or-flight, and start to move into what I call stay-and-play. It's really quite simple and it's a simple thing that you can move towards, versus a lot of people [00:21:30] when they start having anxious thoughts or sad thoughts or angry thoughts; they try to move away from those. They try to say, "Well, don't think about my ex, don't think about my taxes, don't think about these terrible things," but then you're pushing against those thoughts. Then they're going to push back and they're going to win. Instead, if you move towards this two x breath or the OMFG technique then it's a way to move toward the positive instead of away from the negative.

[00:22:00] It's interesting, in the west, we spend a lot of time naming and analyzing the different flavors of anxiety. You have anxiety, we have depression, we have ADD, ADHD, PTSD. Not to diminish or oversimplify but when I was training in India, they would just call all of this stress. These are different symptoms of this underlying imbalance, which is stress. What we do with meditation is we start to bring the body back into balance and that can start to let some of those symptoms fall away. Now, the reality is if you're dealing with very intense anxiety or very intense depression, then I really think it's important to make sure that you're working with someone one-on-one, face-to-face. Even though I have an online [00:22:30] meditation training, I recommend that people who are dealing with severe PTSD or severe depression, that if they do it, they make sure they're working with a therapist because there's nothing that can replace that human face-to-face contact.

The reality is that when people start a meditation practice we want it to be this spa day for the brain. We want it to be this magical cure-all. It feels a little magical, it feels a little miraculous, but it's not. It's actually just taking all of the old stress that we've been accumulating our whole lives and it starts to [00:23:00] bring it up and out. If you're dealing with depression, it's very possible that your symptoms can get more intense before they get better. No one's really talking about this in the meditation world. Then it can be confusing or challenging when people start a meditation practice because they think it should just be sunshine and roses, and instead they have a lot of sadness or anger coming up and out.

[00:23:30] I think it's important to educate people that when you start a meditation practice, you can expect some degree of an emotional and physical detox, and that that's okay. That's actually part of the healing. My theme song for that is better out than in. Better out than in, better out than in. This is my nerdy dad joke, is that you want to have that stuff in your tissues versus in your tissues. It's better to cry that stuff out than let it stay in the body for decades and then we have to cut it out years later. I really think that we have an opportunity to learn our lessons on the spiritual plane, and if we don't learn them there, then we have to learn them on the psychological plane. If we don't learn them there, then we have to learn them on the physical plane.

[00:24:00] Really, it's faster and easier and cheaper to learn it on the spiritual plane and meditate. If not, then we've got to go to the therapist for a few decades—and if not, well, then we have to go to the surgeon. I just think it's a way to re-frame, but then I really just want people to know that if they start a practice and things get a little messier before they get cleaner, that that's okay—there's nothing wrong with you. It's just like you've got to let your house get a little more messy before it gets cleaner if you're cleaning out your closets. That's part of the process.

[00:24:30]   The beautiful thing is that the stress is finite. If you're really meditating twice a day and eating well and getting good sleep, there is an end date. There is a moment where you've eradicated the entire backlog of stresses that you've ever accumulated in your entire life. Then on the other side of that you're able to be so present, so conscious, so mindful, you're able to enjoy each moment, and so your whole life really becomes a celebration, and that's why I think we're here.

[00:25:00]   My favorite raw fats to eat would be definitely avocados, I love me an avocado. I probably eat at least one avocado a day. I'll put cold-pressed organic olive oil in my smoothie, just like a teaspoon or tablespoon. I'll put olive oil on almost anything that I eat, a soup, a salad.

I will eat sometimes a raw nut butter. I love an organic, raw nut butter. Sometimes, if I'm feeling fancy,
[00:25:30]   I'll even do some raw dairy. I know that's super controversial but I have a dairy dealer that comes to my house and I pay them in cash like a drug deal.

FRANK LIPMAN, MD | Functional Medicine Practitioner, *New York Times* Best Selling Author and Founder of Be Well

---

Dr. Frank Lipman: I was trained as a Western doctor, and there we actually don't have an idea of what health is. We have a disease care system, not a health care system. I never was trained as a doctor to promote health; we were trained in drugs and surgery. We have few to no tools to get people healthy or to keep them healthy.

[00:00:30] To me, "healthy" is way beyond just eliminating disease, it's teaching people to create healthy habits, it's teaching people how to eat properly, teaching people how to exercise, getting them to sleep properly. There are so many ways you can support someone's health, but I didn't learn that at medical school.

Gut bacteria are really interesting because they affect much more than the gut. One of the areas they affect is the brain. There's this direct highway between the gut and the brain; it's the vagus nerve.

[00:01:00] What's going on in the gut is going to affect your brain. Gut bacteria are affected by so many things that we do in our lives. Even the water we drink. We have chlorinated water, that's going to affect our gut bacteria. The antibiotics in our food are going to affect our gut bacteria. What we eat is going to affect our gut bacteria. How you treat your gut bacteria is going to affect not only your gut, but your brain and the rest of your body. I'm obsessed with our gut bacteria.

[00:01:30] What's interesting is we have more gut bacteria in our gut than we have cells in our body. We're actually more bacterial than human. We, as a culture, are obsessed with killing bacteria. We see bacteria as bad guys. Even in the holistic world, or the Functional Medicine world, we see it as good and bad. I see it a little bit differently. I see it as this inner ecosystem. We have an ecosystem in our gut, and we have to balance it. In that ecosystem, in certain areas, good bacteria can be bad, and bad bacteria can be good.

[00:02:00] It's all relative. I don't believe there's such a thing as good and bad bacteria; it's about the balance of all of these things. How you balance your bacteria is going to affect your health.

How do we optimize our gut bacteria? It's much more than just taking probiotics or taking antibiotics or antimicrobials to kill the bad bacteria. It's about how you feed the bacteria in your gut. The more diverse

[00:02:30] your bacteria in the gut, or the more types of bacteria in your gut, the healthier you're going to be. How do you create a diverse bacterial gut? By eating many different foods. Different bacteria are going to feed on different foods, so it's important to eat different types of vegetables. I always tell my patients, "Eat the stalks and the stems, because that's the fiber, the fiber that your body doesn't break down properly. The bacteria love that." Eat lots of different types of vegetables. Eat lots of different types of

[00:03:00] foods. The more diverse your diet, the more diverse that food is going to be for the bacteria. What you feed your bacteria, how you treat your bacteria, is going to create a more diverse microbiome.

I have a slightly different view on detox. The way I see detox is, how do you optimize your body's own

[00:03:30] detoxification systems? The brain actually has a detoxification system. We now know we have a system called the glymphatic system. The glymphatic system is sort of like a garbage disposal system in the brain. If you have a party one night and you don't clean up, the next night you have another party and you don't clean up, after a couple of nights, the garbage builds up and up. This is what happens with the glymphatic system. If you don't sleep at night, the garbage builds up. If you don't sleep two nights, it

[00:04:00] gets worse and worse. We have this natural system in our brain where we're clearing out toxins and we're clearing out byproducts all the time. The brain actually is detoxing all the time and it's mainly detoxing when you're sleeping. So, if you don't sleep properly, you're not going to detox the brain.

I think it's important to view the detox system as this comprehensive system that works throughout the body. What's going on in the gut is going to affect your brain, what's going on in your liver is going to

---

[00:04:30]   affect your brain. I believe a lot of the toxins that we're exposed to come from our internal mechanisms—from the bacteria in the gut, from the waste products of our own body systems. If your gut is not optimized, if your liver is not functioning properly, you're going to get a buildup of these toxins and obviously it's going to affect your brain as well.

[00:05:00]   What is brain fog? That's a really good question. I'm not sure exactly what leads to it, but I can tell you clinically what helps it. I have so many patients who come in complaining of brain fog. They can't focus properly, they can't remember things properly. A lot of the time, when you clean out their gut, when you help balance the ecosystem in the gut, the brain fog improves. A lot of time when you get people to sleep properly and get their glymphatic system working properly, the brain fog improves. A lot of times when you get them to deal with the stress, the brain fog improves.

[00:05:30]   I think, like everything in the body, everything works together—how you sleep, how you think, how you deal with stress, what you're eating, how you're moving your body—this all affects our detox systems and our brain. Whether you have brain fog or joint pains, I often treat it very similarly. Change people's diets, get them to move, get them to meditate, get them to watch where their thoughts go. Everything works together. You can't really separate the brain from the body. It's one big ecosystem. Same as we

[00:06:00]   have an ecosystem in the gut, our body is one big ecosystem. Everything works together.

The biggest challenge with our medical system and the way they see brain disorders is they think brain disorders are a separate department. You go to the neurologist or the psychiatrist in his own separate category and its own separate department in the hospital. You can't separate what's going on in the brain with what's going on in the body. In fact, most of the problems I see that affect us emotionally, psychologically, or in the brain per se; the problem is actually not coming from the brain. The problem is

[00:06:30]   often coming from the gut or somewhere else. We have a system where a symptom affects one organ system and you go to that specialist for that particular organ, when the problem is not originating with that particular organ system. You are given a drug for that particular organ system, but you're not treating the underlying imbalance or dysfunction, and ultimately, you're not treating the cause, which is usually not where the problem presents.

[00:07:00]   When someone comes to me with anxiety or depression, the first thing I think of is: is this a typical psychological problem or emotional problem, or are there other factors that are going on that are presenting as anxiety or depression? Anxiety and depression are often just symptoms of some other

[00:07:30]   underlying imbalance. As with most disorders, I usually look at the gut. If someone comes to me with anxiety or depression, the first thing I'll do is try and ascertain is there a problem in the gut, is there a problem with the gut bacteria? That's always what I look at first, and obviously one needs to look at is someone stressed out, how are they sleeping, how are they exercising, what's going on in their life? Are they having problems at work? A lot of the time, I find with anxiety and depression, the problem is

[00:08:00]   actually not a psychological or emotional problem and can be corrected by changing someone's diet, getting them to exercise, getting them to go to some yoga, and always getting them to sleep better.

I see this as this ecosystem out of balance. I think we all have some parasites, we probably all have some yeast, there are these viruses, these bacteria, and you have some which are providing a positive function and some a negative function. How they all live and survive together and function together is very

[00:08:30]   interesting. I used to think that it was as simple as you had an overgrowth of yeast and you kill the yeast and everything would be fine. Or you have a parasite, an external pathogen like a parasite, you kill the pathogen and everything is fine. Over years and years of doing this, I've realized that it's not as simple as that. It's how all these bugs works together. Some people can have a parasite or some yeast in their gut and be perfectly fine with it.

[00:09:00]   It's really about how you create some balance; how do all these bugs work together? That can be tricky. The way you treat this is very individualized, because everyone's different. I've seen the same type of presentation or the same type of problem, where one person will do well on an antifungal drug and the next person won't. One person will do well on antimicrobial herbs, the next person, it can cause more

[00:09:30] problems. One person will do well on a probiotic, the next person will get bloated and gassy and get diarrhea. It's a very tricky area and we don't really know that much about it.

[00:10:00] What I explain to my patients is you're measuring this amount in this huge room full of our microbiome. We have very limited tests to work out what's going on in the microbiome, so a lot of the time it's a clinical diagnosis and you're guessing. Literally, it's a crap shoot. Even when you give probiotics to someone, you're guessing. Some people do fine with a probiotic, the next person won't do well with the same probiotic. We're really in the infancy of our understanding the microbiome.

[00:10:30] What foods are good for one and bad for the other? I have some generic ideas about foods. Some foods I think no one should eat, but once we go beyond that, it becomes very tricky. Some people do really well, for instance, on a paleo diet; other people do fine on a vegan diet. I think as we get older, the majority of people do better on a low-carbohydrate diet, but I have patients who do well on a vegan diet, so it doesn't really fit into my philosophy on food except that there's no one right diet.

[00:11:00] In terms of what foods no one should eat, well, that's pretty simple: sugar is the devil. No one should eat sugar. We all know that. I'm a big believer in gluten being a problem for a lot of people. I'm starting to believe that most grains tend to be a problem for a lot of people, too. Not everyone, but I'd say at least 70-80% of my patients do better when they take grains out of their diet. I think soy and corn are a problem for most people in America, maybe because it's genetically modified. I think genetically modified foods are a problem for most people. We don't know for sure, but I'm not going to take a chance, and I generally see people do better when they take corn and soy out of their diets. Having said **[00:11:30]** that, I see people doing perfectly well eating that, too. If I had to pick some generic foods to take out of people's diet, it would be sugar, all processed foods, gluten, soy, and corn.

[00:12:00] What are healthy foods for the brain? Probably I would choose, number one: healthy fats. When I talk about healthy fats, any fat made by God is probably healthy and any fat made by man is probably not. The healthy fats are fish oils, olives, olive oil, coconut, coconut oil—I love coconut oil, despite what the American Heart Association says—nuts and seeds, pasture-raised eggs, grass-fed meat, wild fish. There **[00:12:30]** are lots of sources of good, healthy fats, and I encourage my patients to eat healthy fats. I think those would be probably one of the most important nutrients for the brain.

Every week, I see probably at least two or three patients who come to me complaining of anxiety and depression, and they've been put on antidepressants or anxiolytic or drugs for their anxiety. When we correct their gut, which is probably the most common thing I do, and we get them into healthy habits, their anxiety and the depression gets better. I just saw someone this week—a young woman who had **[00:13:00]** taken a lot of antibiotics for acne when she was younger—came in with actual autoimmune problems from that, and was really anxious and depressed and had no reason to be anxious or depressed. She obviously went to the psychiatrist, she was given an antidepressant, and actually some Klonopin. After **[00:13:30]** being put on four or five drugs, started questioning, "This is not right. This can't be right that every specialist I go to gives me a drug for this particular organ."

[00:14:00] She came to me and I did what I normally do: I change people's diets, I get them off the foods that I think are a problem, I start correcting their gut. She came back a month later, her anxiety and depression were completely gone. They hadn't been helped by the drugs that she was put on, and her autoimmune symptoms in her gut started getting better. The first thing that actually cleared up for her was her anxiety and depression and all we did was clean out her gut.

[00:14:30] I'm a big believer that the little things we do on a daily basis have huge effects on our health. How do we spend time with our family and our community —do we spend time in nature? Are we listening to music? All these little things that you can do on a daily basis make a huge difference to your health. We get hooked on drugs and surgery, and then we get next level to diet, exercise, sleep, and stress reduction, which are all hugely important, but we ignore the little things that can be done on a daily **[00:15:00]** basis, which I believe make a huge difference to one's health being passionate about something, having meaning in one's life, the community around you. Isolation and loneliness are really bad for one's health.

[00:15:30] I'm a huge believer in spending more time in nature. If you think about this, this is all going back to the way we used to live. Now, I'm not suggesting people go back and live in their huts the way we used to live maybe 100-200 years ago, but we've lost that connection to nature. We've lost that connection to our community. We've lost that connection to music. I grew up in South Africa. Music is such a part of the local culture. Music isn't entertainment. There's music for weddings, for funerals. Music is just part of the culture.

[00:16:00] Here's an interesting point on music: you know that your heart or your body entrains to external rhythms. Everyone knows when they sit at the beach, you start relaxing and your heartbeat slows down. If you're in the traffic of New York City, you start getting hyper and your pulse gets more rapid. Same thing happens with music. Your heart and your body rhythms are entraining to the external rhythms of life. If you listen to Bob Marley, which usually beats at about 60 beats per minute, your heart starts [00:16:30] beating at the same beat. If you're listening to hard rock, your pulse starts beating faster. You can use music and entrain to the beats of music. I find reggae extremely relaxing—it doesn't have to be reggae—but any music with a slow beat, your body will start entraining to those rhythms. Rhythm is one aspect of our health that we completely ignore. How you entrain to external rhythms is going to affect your [00:17:00] health, and music can do that, being in nature can do that, having love around you can do that. The little things that we can change in our lives or do in our lives make a huge difference to our health.

What do I do to keep my brain sharp? Now that I'm 62 years old, I have to start worrying about it. I don't really think about keeping my brain sharp, I just think about keeping healthy. I basically practice what I [00:17:30] preach. I eat a low-carbohydrate diet, I exercise, I try and meditate every day. I need to get back to doing it every day. I did yoga until I broke my wrist. I try to spend as much time as I can in nature. Luckily, I'm passionate about what I do. All these little things, I do the same thing, and I'm hoping it's [00:18:00] going to keep my brain sharp. In terms of keeping my brain sharp, probably eating a low sugar diet is one of the most important things you can do. Getting enough sleep, and dealing with all the stress in your life.

What is my advice for anyone suffering from anxiety, depression, or any what we call brain disorder? Start thinking about your issue as less of a specialist problem and more of a whole-body problem. If [00:18:30] you're driving your car and the oil light goes on, you don't just put a band-aid over the oil light. You see why the oil light is going on. Do the same with your body. See why the oil light is going on. The oil light is telling you something is off balance in your system. See why you have anxiety. Anxiety, depression, brain fog are just symptoms of a system out of balance. Look for why that system is out of balance.

[00:19:00] In Western medicine, we look at the body as a machine. If a body part isn't working properly—in other words—if the brain isn't working properly, we give it a drug or we take it out. We don't take the brain out—we do it for other organs—but we treat that particular organ. In Chinese medicine, I was taught to see the body as a garden. If the leaves are going brown or the plant isn't growing properly, you don't just paint the leaves green. You look to see, is the plant getting enough water? Is it getting enough sun? Are [00:19:30] the roots impinged? How is the soil? You have to look at the whole ecosystem. I encourage people, look at the whole ecosystem. Don't just look at the body part, look to see why that particular body part is having a problem.

Expert Interviews – Frank Lipman, MD

© 2017 Hyman Digital. All Rights Reserved.

168

GABRIELLE LYON, DO | www.ashcenter.com

Dr. Gabrielle Lyon:	How I got into the field of Functional Medicine, I was actually raised in it. I moved in with my godmother, Liz Lipski, at 17, and she's one of the founding Functional Medicine nutritionists. From that point on, my trajectory was set. I knew that nutrition was where I was going to go, so I went to the University of Illinois and studied human nutrition, vitamin/mineral metabolism. Then after that, I went to medical school and did two years of psychiatry, three years of family medicine, and then a postdoc at Washington University in nutritional sciences and geriatrics.
[00:00:30]	
[00:01:00]	Brain health is dependent on muscle health because muscle is the organ of longevity. When you think about brain health and you think about the issues with brain health, it rides on obesity. It rides on inflammatory conditions, creating a leaky blood -barrier. and the wider your BMI, the higher your BMI, the lower the brain volume. If that's the case, you need to have an ideal body composition. What does an ideal body composition mean? It means being under fat and more muscled.
[00:01:30]	The issue isn't over fat. Everyone focuses on obesity and diabetes. That is a huge problem, but the real problem is being under muscled. You really need to change the ratio of muscle to body fat. Being under muscled is because we're sedentary. We're not moving the way that we used to, we live in a very domesticated way. 10,000 years ago, we were hunters and gatherers. We were moving 10 to 14 miles a day. We're not doing that anymore.
[00:02:00]	Metabolism is important for brain health, because a healthy metabolism is really the metabolic sync, and the metabolic sync is your muscle. Muscle is the organ of longevity. The healthier your muscle is, the more glucose that you burn, the more carbohydrates that you burn, the more fat that you burn. So, it's the site of fat oxidation, and it's responsible for your resting metabolic rate. When you're thinking about brain health, you need to have a healthy metabolism because you don't want excess calories, you don't want pro-inflammatory states. You really want a body that's in balance.
[00:02:30]	When working with my patients, one of the things we really focus on is optimizing body composition. It's really about optimizing lean muscle tissue, and we do that through diet, exercise, really targeted nutritional training programs that augment the muscle. I see a lot of patients with Hashimoto's and thyroid disorder, as well as hormonal imbalances. The first thing we do—and there's one patient in particular—she came to me with Hashimoto's, and her antibodies were through the roof. Her metabolism was just really wrecked. She had gone through years of yo-yo dieting, and so we know when you yo-yo diet, each time you lose weight it's not quality weight.
[00:03:00] [00:03:30]	What I mean by quality weight, it's usually muscle. You do lose some fat, but the integrity of the muscle changes, and when the integrity of the muscle changes, you have a trajectory of gaining weight. We worked really hard; we worked over eight months, and we reduced her antibodies. She was on a very anti-inflammatory diet, but interestingly, what we did is we really increased her protein intake. She started at around 160 pounds, so what we did is we actually augmented her diet with mostly proteins. She was eating about 140 to 150 grams of protein a day, divided into meals that had 30-40 grams per meal, in addition to really heavy weight training. She's lost a tremendous amount of weight. Her body fat has come down, and her muscle tissue has improved, and her Hashimoto's has gone into remission.
[00:04:00]	I get this question a lot. Are Americans under-eating protein? Because you hear actually that people say we're eating way too much protein, and that's not true. What's actually happening is the distribution of the way that people are eating protein is absolutely incorrect. The standard distribution of eating, for example, for breakfast they have maybe 12 grams of protein or a vegan protein shake, or maybe two eggs. We know that you need 30 grams of protein or 2.5 grams of leucine—which is the amino acid that triggers muscle protein synthesis—per meal.

[00:04:30]	What happens is that if you undershoot that at breakfast—breakfast is the most important meal for setting up your metabolism—you have to compensate for something else. If you are low in protein, you're typically high in carbohydrates. If you're higher in carbohydrates and fat in that balance, then four hours later we know that you're going to be starved. FMRI imaging definitely shows that the first meal that you have is the most important because four hours later, reward centers are all lit up. When it comes to Americans eating too much protein, it's that they need to distribute it over time.
[00:05:00]	Each meal should have around 30 to 40 grams of protein per meal to trigger that muscle protein synthesis, but what Americans typically do is that they have two meals with low protein amounts. Breakfast is the two eggs, lunch may be a small turkey sandwich, and then dinner is a big steak. You reach that threshold one time and that's in the evening, and a lifetime of doing that destroys your metabolism because it does not augment your muscle.
[00:05:30]	So, for breakfast, I do one of two things. I often fast and if that's the case, then I don't have anything. If I'm having breakfast, I'll have either ground chicken, I'll have about four ounces with MCT oil. I tend to not have carbohydrates in my first meal even if I'm training in the morning. I tend to back load my carbohydrates or have it later on in the evening because insulin sensitivity goes up later on in the day. Your body is more sensitive to glucose later on in the day, as opposed to having toast in the morning and these higher carbohydrate meals. You end up storing body fat all day if you're not a competitive athlete, or you're really training.
[00:06:00]	Carbohydrates, in general, are not bad. If you are burning carbohydrates and you're not, say, on a ketogenic cell diet, the body's maintenance dose, you need about 90 grams a day. Everything other than 90 grams is earned, so that's earned through physical activity. Every hour of physical activity—running, weightlifting (which is my favorite), resistance training—you earn that carbohydrate. So then, you're talking about between 20 to 60 grams an hour, if you're really training intensely.
[00:06:30]	The other aspect of carbohydrates is if you can plan it around your training schedule. If you really want to burn it, I actually tend to use protein before a training session, and I recommend my patients do the same unless they're elite level athletes, and then they can have carbohydrates while the muscle is primed. You don't need more than 30 to 40 grams, really, of carbohydrates. And then protein also, the muscle is primed to then turn over muscle protein synthesis after you train.
[00:07:00]	Exercise is important for the brain in a number of ways. Number one, we know that when it comes to dementia, Alzheimer's, and aging brain, we know that optimal body composition is number one. So, having lean muscle tissue, low body fat, is number one for protecting the brain, because you want to have low inflammatory issues, you want to have a healthy metabolism. What controls your metabolism? The organ of longevity, which is muscle.
[00:07:30]	I practice something called "muscle-centric medicine" and, really, the focus of everything is the organ system of muscle. You keep your muscle health, then you have your brain that's healthy. The other important aspect of exercise and the brain is that muscle as an endocrine organ. When you use resistance training, it actually secretes things like growth factor. It secretes things like BDNF. All these things help rejuvenate the brain and they actually cross the blood-brain barrier. You're not just training your muscles, but you're also regenerating your brain.
[00:08:00]	The patients that come to me when it comes to a sedentary lifestyle, by the time they get to me they're really ready to change. and of course, as in the military, there's a crawl, walk, run, so we first crawl. We just begin, we talk about movement, we talk about the difference between exercise and physical activity. A lot of people do physical activity, which is just movement-based, and not a lot of people do exercise. Exercise are really planned, executed programs with progressions, and typically you train with somebody. Exercises that are good for the brain target large muscle groups.

There has been a lot of study on cardiovascular health in the brain and I think one of the reasons that

[00:08:30]	is, is because it's really easy to measure. That was the big thing, was endurance training in the brain in BDNF. However, emerging data is really looking at resistance training, and resistance training is lifting weights. Lifting weights actually stimulates the muscle and creates things and situations that are healthy for the brain, like those growth factors that we talked about. It also helps with mood and cognition. Some examples of great exercises are really heavy compound movements. To be very specific, you're thinking about the squat, the deadlift, the bench press.
[00:09:00]	Another important aspect is that it's typically 70 to 80% of someone's one-rep max, and what that translates roughly to is 8 to 10 reps. So, you pick 12 to 16 exercises, and you really have to put in energy. You need to go to fatigue. You have to work hard. There are two parts of being able to really stimulate muscle, and that's having the mental fortitude to really be able to work hard, and challenge yourself because that is required for the positive effects of muscle. You do that, and of course, tai chi
[00:09:30]	and those wonderful relaxing types of exercises, but, really, what I think, people are doing not enough of is the resistance training, and having a really good resistance program is key.
	What occurs in brain health and muscle—that's a very interesting question because they kind of ride along together. What happens is as we age, there's sarcopenia and that's the loss of muscle that ends up happening. When that happens, by the time you're 80, you have had 50% of the muscle that you
[00:10:00]	had when you were 30. These issues with sarcopenia—and that's poor muscle mass, function, and strength—they actually begin in the 30s and 40s. Interestingly, that's the same time that Alzheimer's, dementia, and cognitive impairment starts. Dementia, type 3 diabetes—that starts in your 30s and 40s, alongside with the declining ability to use your muscle, and the quality of your muscle.
[00:10:30]	How can you treat obesity? Obesity is much easier to treat than sarcopenia, or sarcobesity. The most important thing is prevention and I think a lot of physicians talk about that when we talk about having a collaborative effort—to be creative with our patients is really prevention and finding protocols that work for them. The way to protect your muscle is ... There are really three things I talk about with my patients, and that's protein quality, quantity, and distribution, when you're thinking about protecting your muscle. So, it's the quality of the protein you're eating that's very important. Plant-based protein
[00:11:00]	is not the same as animal protein, that's not the same as collagen or bone broth protein.
	Getting the right amino acid profile, all proteins are not the same, so you have the quality of the protein, the distribution of the protein, which is distributed over three to four meals, with four to five hours in between if you'd like, and then the timing. So, when are you having your protein? When are you having your largest protein meal? That's really key, so the nutrition is one aspect. The other aspect
[00:11:30]	is training. Really training their muscle, getting them on a good program—a three to four, even five-day program of resistance training.
	If a patient is vegetarian or vegan, it's really important to incorporate branched-chain amino acids and typically move them to a much lower carbohydrate load. I don't think being vegan or vegetarian is bad. Everyone is entitled to what works well for their body. I found that patients have a very specific phenotype. Everybody is different. If they are vegetarian or vegan, they have to add in branched-chain
[00:12:00]	amino acids to their meals, and they have to time it appropriately. So, for example, if you're eating quinoa for your protein, that's not actually enough, as you need six cups of quinoa to equal one chicken breast. If you do that, then the carbohydrate and caloric load is way too high, so then you're driving up inflammation.
[00:12:30]	In order to avoid that from happening, I tend to switch vegetarians or vegans to a higher-fat, lower-carbohydrate diet, augmented with branched-chain amino acids. Branched-chain amino acids are amino acids that are essential, meaning you have to get them from the diet. Out of the essential amino acids, primarily the branched-chains, you're thinking about leucine. Leucine is required for what we spoke about before, which is muscle protein synthesis. What's interesting about leucine is that it's required in a bolus amount, so you actually have to reach two and a half grams of leucine to get a muscle triggering effect.

[00:13:00] Anything less than that counts as calories and you don't actually get the stimulation to your muscle. What would an example of that be? That would be your two eggs. Your two eggs have maybe one gram of leucine. Your breakfast of two eggs and then your lunch of a small turkey sandwich is, maybe, 20 grams of protein, so you've now undershot your leucine amount and you don't stimulate your muscle protein synthesis. Then dinner, you've got your five ounces of steak, which is perfect, but now you've only stimulated your muscle protein synthesis one time.

[00:13:30] Branched-chain amino acids must be ingested and they are necessary for metabolic functioning. They have to be targeted, so it has to be a certain amount that you're getting at one time. For example, a branched-chain amino acid, you can't sip it. So, if you're sipping the branched-chain amino acid, you're never actually triggering your muscle. Collagen powder is very interesting. Collagen is not high in the branched-chain amino acids, but it is high in glycine and proline and other amino acids. Recent evidence is emerging that it does help with body composition. It is still questionable as to why that is, because it doesn't stimulate muscle protein synthesis.

[00:14:00] I do not have my patients count the bone broth or the collagen as protein. It's not a complete protein, but there are some really amazing effects that we're starting to see in sarcopenia and body composition. So, you take an untrained elderly person and you start training them with resistance weight, and then you add collagen, it's been shown to improve their body composition. That makes no sense when it comes to the science.

[00:14:30] My personal opinion is grass-fed organic is the best. The amount of protein is different in, say, fish than it is in beef. For every one ounce of animal gravity-bearing protein—that means if you have to kill it, and it runs around, it's a gravity-bearing protein—that has seven grams of protein per one ounce. You need five ounces per meal. You need between four and five ounces per meal, which will get you to 28 to 35 grams, somewhere in that range. Fish, for every one ounce, it has five grams of protein. You need to have a six-ounce piece of fish to be able to trigger that muscle protein synthesis.

[00:15:00] That's not all or nothing, right? The older you are, the more protein you need at once, because of this concept called "anabolic resistance." The muscle tissue becomes resistant to the amino acids. You actually need more protein as you age, which is a really important topic because right now, the recommendation is 0.8 grams per kilogram, and that is creating a huge issue with sarcopenia in our population. 0.8 grams per kilogram is incredibly too low. It came from nitrogen studies that were from

[00:15:30] 18-year-old college students. The truth is the emerging evidence and everything that is coming out is saying 1.2 grams per kilogram up to 1.6 to even 2 grams per kilogram. That's almost a gram of protein per pound. For example, my dad—my dad is 160 pounds. He eats about 60 grams of protein to maintain his muscle tissue.

[00:16:00] Do I recommend tracking your meals? I think in the beginning it's really important and I think that what happens is you become very good at building your meals around protein. So, you build your meals around protein, you decide how much carbohydrates you're going to have based on how much activity you're doing, or where your metabolic flexibility is. For example, if you have Hashimoto's, or if you have hormonal imbalances, I tend to lower the carbohydrates and increase the protein. Then, the fat is wherever that is. I'm not crazy about adding too much or taking it away. Fat is essential for the body,

[00:16:30] but to track, they can use FitPal or write it down. I like to write it down. But it's important in the beginning to be able to eyeball it and really see what you're getting. And then after that, don't worry about it.

[00:17:00] Fasting is amazing. Research shows that by eating in a time-restricted feeding manner, it has incredible effects on blood markers as it relates to obesity and diabetes. And we know that obesity and diabetes create major issues in the brain, right? You've got type 3 diabetes, which is Alzheimer's and dementia. Fasting can really help with that when you're younger. It becomes much more difficult for more elderly patients to fast. I personally fast, I think that it's amazing. I think that it's not ideal for muscle health, so if you're going to fast, you need to train more, you need to lift weights, because there are only two ways to stimulate muscle, and that's either through diet or exercise.

[00:17:30] So, if you're fasting, your body starts to become in a catabolic state, which is why you see yo-yo dieters lose muscle tissue and gain fat. I tend to fast 16 hours a day. I'm experimenting with fasting 24 hours twice a week. We'll see how that goes. I'll keep you posted. But I use the fasting protocols for my patients, especially patients that have weight to lose and hormonal imbalances, depending on where their adrenal status and everything is.

[00:18:00] The fats that I recommended first and foremost: you need omegas. Omega-3—and I recommended EPA and DHA—in two grams per day. You can go up, certainly there are some benefits. They're starting to show benefits in the much higher doses. MCT oil is fantastic; it's a flavor enhancer, it's also burned more like a carbohydrate and less of a fat. There's some good data to suggest that it helps thermogenesis and body fat. Mono and saturated fats are great—olive oil, avocado oil, coconut oil— saturated fat. I tend to not use a ton of that personally.

[00:18:30] The patients that come to me, none of them hate to exercise. They're going to the wrong physician, but okay, so let's say a patient was really resistant, I would ask them what's their why. "Why are you doing this?" We have to have a commonality in terms of what we're promoting for health. I think that if someone comes to me and hates exercise, it's because there's some emotional or experience that they've had that is really preventing them from having the opportunity to be optimal. Because the body was designed to move. People were designed for physical labor and movement.

[00:19:00] Top tips for staying sharp. Number one, most important, optimizing body composition. The issue is not over fat, it's really about being under muscled. Optimize your body composition. Number two, stay active in your brain processes. Always be learning, stretch your brain, think about things, really don't get comfortable. Number three, exercise. Resistance train, pick 12 to 16 exercises, lift heavy, put in the effort. It will pay off.

GARRETT HALWEG, MD | Amen Clinics

Dr. Garrett Halweg:	Initially, I got involved in a holistic approach because I realized that the traditional method of training someone in psychiatry to be a brain doctor involved looking at lists of symptoms and matching them with a diagnosis that insurance companies were happy with and then pairing that diagnosis with a
[00:00:30]	standard treatment, which typically involved medication. This was somewhat dissatisfying as I realized that individuals are different and vary greatly. So, I became aware of a practice opportunity that is more in line with true medicine, which is developing a relationship with a patient that doesn't necessarily involve a list of symptoms. It involves making a hypothesis about what that person is
[00:01:00]	suffering from and then testing that hypothesis with different tests.
[00:01:30]	At the Amen Clinic, we do things like SPECT imaging and this tests out those theories of diagnoses and confirms them or refutes them and gives you an idea of the diagnosis with better accuracy. Then it also allows for treatment outside of the standard treatments, which typically are just medication. It pulls from a range of things you can do. I also noticed a disturbing trend within medication and that was that
[00:02:00]	many of the medications I used made patients fat and cognitively dull. There was another alarming group that lumped all medications together. So, for instance, a class like benzodiazepines, this is an unsustainable class of medication. Once you get a patient on it, you end up just increasing the dose for less and less effect. Patients were lumping all medications with these medications that were not sustainable. There was a lot of discernment that was needed in prescribing medications. Alcohol is very
[00:02:30]	effective for anxiety, but it's not something sustainable.
[00:03:00]	I wanted a practice environment that included a wide of range of holistic treatments. I do an interventional technique called transcranial magnetic stimulation and I remember one patient, in particular, who was on psychotropics—several psych meds. I used this technique and was able to not only get them into remission but after they wanted to get off their medications, we used exercise, diet, different life style modifications, and brain training, and through these techniques, they actually achieved remission, which means an absence of symptoms. They remained that way for the entirety of the time that I followed them.
[00:03:30]	Exercise is paramount in providing the nutrient factors of the cell to stimulate a healthy garden of receptors. The brain neuron grows receptors. These receptors are watered by different
[00:04:00]	neurotransmitters and that signal signals the cell of the neuron or the nucleus of the neuron to grow these healthy brain receptors. Exercise produces the fertile nutrients of the cell. How does it do that? It does that through energy metabolism. Now, of course, exercise is only one factor. Nutrition, which I'm also very passionate about, is important in fertilizing that cell, in growing that healthy garden of
[00:04:30]	receptors. One of the factors in improving brain-derived neurotrophic factor is through a healthy diet. What is a healthy diet? Very simply, it's whole plant foods and not too much. And how do you figure out not too much? Well, I love the technique of limited-time feeding.
[00:05:00]	What is limited-time feeding? Limited-time eating or limited-time feeding—some people call it restricted-time feeding—limited-time feeding is a technique used to eat during five hours and fast during 19. So, all your daily intake is taken in five hours of the day. It isn't important what five hours those are. If you're a breakfast person, you can start the clock with breakfast and eat for five hours and
[00:05:30]	then stop and fast for 19 hours and then you start up again after you sleep. Or if you like dinner, and you have a family meal plan, then you can start your clock and have your first meal at noon. So, you're taking in your daily intake over the five hours.
[00:06:00]	I also like to eat a healthy mix of all the nutrients provided in plant-rich sources, so a rainbow. You have the anthocyanins from anything purple. My favorite are Okinawan sweet potatoes. 65% of the calories of the Okinawans who are a centurion Blue Zone group—they live healthy into their hundreds. 65% of

[00:06:30] their calories come from these Okinawan sweet potatoes. I also encourage people to eat green leafy vegetables at each meal. It's very important for antioxidants.

Also, cook with curcumin. This is an active ingredient in turmeric, so if you're using turmeric root or cooking with turmeric spice, it's a great way to decrease inflammation. All of these factors lead to building those healthy receptors—the healthy garden of receptors that make neurons so healthy.

[00:07:00]
[00:07:30] I always encourage people to use a high-intensity interval training; it's the most efficient. I have one up on the wall in my office that is a simple exercise to follow along. It takes 21 minutes and it's very effective. High-intensity interval training, for people who don't know, is a system of exercise where it's a burst of exercise with a phase of recovery. So, if you exercise really hard to your maximum effort for 30 seconds and then recover for about a minute and then again 30 seconds as hard as you can with a recovery for a minute. If you do this for enough cycles for 20 minutes, you can have a very efficient workout that will provide long lasting results.

[00:08:00]
[00:08:30]
[00:09:00] I'm glad you asked about weight because fat tissue—many people think as this inert tissue that just stores fat. In fact, fat sends its own signals. It has chemical messengers to the brain and the body. These chemical messages can send a message that says, "Hey, you don't need to repair. You don't need to build new cells. There are plenty of nutrients or plenty of energy around and we don't need to go into this repair mode." I was speaking earlier about a time limited feeding strategy. That drops insulin levels and sends this opposite signal. It sends signals that say, "Hey, this is a time of repair. This is a time that we need to send out signals and tip off the brain-derived neurotrophic factor." Adipose tissue is not this inert tissue that just sits there and stores fat; It's actually sending chemical messages to the brain and the body.

[00:09:30]
[00:10:00] Kill your television: it turns your brain into mush and it's really toxic. We need to engage with people. We need to come back together for conversation and understanding each other. It's really bothersome that we live in such an age of access to information and yet we don't take the time to understand each other. To listen to each other. Media is a double-edged sword; it's a mixed curse and a blessing. On the one hand, I'm very passionate about getting out the message of something like IV Ketamine and media can be a source of information that we can access to maximize our health, the health of our brain, and our body. But there's a sinister side to it. For instance, many people on Facebook are looking at the highlight reel of other people. This is like putting your brain on a treadmill of envy. It's as if you're training your brain to be envious.

[00:10:30]
[00:11:00]
[00:11:30]
[00:12:00] What we've learned about the brain is neurons that fire together, wire together. So, if you're firing the neurons that are exercising the envy circuit, then you're going to train your brain to be envious and dissatisfied. The other thing is we're so distracted by technology today. If we're confused about what each other is saying, or the point of view that someone is coming from, we need to stop, turn off your phone and put it away, and engage in conversation. I find myself so often clarifying with my wife, who I know very well and I have a very good relationship with, but I am flabbergasted by the fact that sometimes we misunderstand each other. It's at that point when I ask very important questions. I say, "What do you mean by that?" And, "How did you come to that conclusion?" And I find that I learn that someone that I think that I know, either I or she might be distracted by the phone or some technology and we don't hear each other. We don't listen. We don't understand. I think it's very important that as people, as community, we come together, and we listen to each other, and we clarify, and we do one thing at a time with our deep sustained focus and give it all of our attention.

[00:12:30] It's the way that our brain was made. We have neuronal circuits that were designed for deep focus and deep concentration. Accessing and resourcing all our brain to put forth and solve a particular problem or understand or connect with another person. If we're depriving ourselves of that, we're depriving ourselves of the human experience and anything less is something I don't want to experience.

[00:13:00]

[00:13:30]

So, it's important to find community that supports good brain health. The first thing to know is good social connectedness. When you experience a positive social interaction, that increases oxytocin in the brain. Oxytocin is the anti-stress hormone; it actually combats the effects of cortisol in the brain. This is revolutionary because this is natural medicine. This is a medicine that's accessible to everybody today. But we need to be careful. We need to foster good relationships. Sometimes, this means facing the fact or acceptance of people in our lives that are detrimental. People in our lives that bring us down and facing them with necessary endings, limiting our exposure to these people. And sometimes that means a job change and sometimes that means just minimizing our exposure as much as we can.

[00:14:00]

[00:14:30]

Other times, that means being vulnerable to new situations and putting ourselves out there; it's really uncomfortable. It can be very challenging to risk ourselves or engage with someone, but I think the benefits far outweigh the risks because when we learn to become vulnerable to one another, we learn that those other people have the same vulnerabilities, and we break down walls. We start sharing a lot of similarities that make us feel more and more connected and more and more like each other. We find similarities more than dissimilarities.

[00:15:00]

[00:15:30]

Some of the other tips that I would say is don't eat out; cook for yourself. There can be a lot of things that can come from that. My wife and I cook every meal together. We shop together. We call our kitchen my laboratory because I like to find foods and recipes that ... Nutrition works as medicine, and it's really satisfying to have a rich plant diet that is both nourishing but can also cure many things. My wife has experienced gastrointestinal problems that we actually diminished to a degree of about 95% of her symptoms simply through diet alone. This can truly be medicine.

[00:16:00]

[00:16:30]

My wife had irritable bowel syndrome, it's what they classified it after being scoped and getting many tests, and she was just simply dissatisfied. She could not accept the fact that her doctors, her gastroenterologist, did not know what was going on. One day, in frustration in driving to work, she just told me, "Hey, I do not accept the fact that I am still suffering with this, and I want an answer, and you need to give it to me." I'm a brain doctor, so I'm used to dealing with the other end.

Of course, this was a daunting task, but I took it on and started digesting the journals and looking into what changes can we make in our own life. What changes can we make in our diet and the way that we do things? I found out some fantastic things. The first thing we did was we eliminated any processed foods.

[00:17:00]

[00:17:30]

[00:18:00]

Anything in a can or a bag or a box got thrown out. We also had to realize that going out to restaurants often involved foods and preparation methods that were very harmful and that would give her instant feedback; she would have symptoms right after that meal. So instead, what we did was we went to a whole plant diet; mostly vegan. This diet did include some fish; mostly wild salmon. Wild salmon is very expensive, so we have experimented with many other aspects of nutrition in getting the nutrients, the macronutrients, the micronutrients that we need, but after a sustained regiment of this practice, she actually saw an incredible amount of relief. There wasn't 100% of relief and, admittedly, she would say there wasn't 100% compliance. Occasionally, she'll come in, admit that, "Hey, I had a bite of this and it made my stomach turn."

[00:18:30]

[00:19:00]

The better that she does with compliance, the better results we get. These are much like exercise. If you're consistent with exercise, it really doesn't matter what you do. Many patients ask, "Hey, what's the best gym? Should I get a gym membership? Should I have a home gym? What should I do?" And I always tell them, "The best gym is the one that you use." I have gym equipment in my office. I have it at home. If you consistently do something every day, you're gonna see changes and your body is no different. It has the genes it needs to repair the cells and it knows what it wants to do. You have to just provide the right environment for it to heal. When we gave my wife proper nutrition and healthy food, she started to see a difference and those symptoms went away.

[00:19:30]

[00:20:00]

[00:20:30]

[00:21:00]

For those patients that hate to cook, there are prepared meal plans that you can sign up for. They will be specific, custom-tailored to diet needs. You can look for these online, but they involve getting your meals delivered. They can be expensive, but I would say don't be afraid. I would say experiment. Try one meal a week. So, on the weekends say, "Okay, I'm going to try this meal out." Trust me, I've had tons of errors. I've tried meals out that just taste bad or are too costly or too hard to make. I would say have fun with it. Make it a project that you can include people. If you're not good at it, talk to your neighbors and ask them for help. Or take a cooking class. Make sure that it's one that puts an emphasis on health rather than taste, but I would say experiment and get to know what cooking food is all about and cooking healthy food. Get to know what you're putting in your body.

I think the greatest motivation in getting people into the kitchen and to start cooking is to turn over the box of what you're eating and look at the ingredient list. It should cause you panic because there are so many things in there that we don't know what they are and so many chemicals and dyes and things that are toxic to our brains and our body. We don't need it. You can just throw it out and use whole foods. It's so simple.

HYLA CASS, MD | Integrative Psychiatrist and Author of *8 Weeks to Vibrant Health*
& The Addicted Brain and How to Break Free

Dr. Hyla Cass: I've been involved in an integrative approach to psychiatry probably for 20, 25 years. I'm a doctor's kid, and my father had his office at home, and he was a family practitioner. I would actually greet his patients—I was like 3, 4, 5 years old, I would open the door, talk to them. And he would actually talk about, not specifics about people, not real personal things, but he would explain how he approached

[00:00:30] people. I would just see people came in really distressed, having medical issues, and they would leave happy. I got that the relationship was really important. He would also explain what he was doing.

That was my first orientation to being more integrative—to being more relational and how important

[00:01:00] that was in the therapeutic relationship and in the healing process. Then, after I went to medical school, internship, residency, I was really interested to see how people's lifestyle affected how they felt. I never was a big fan of medication when I trained; by the way, I trained at Cedars-Sinai at a time when it was more psychoanalytic and psychodynamic, so the emphasis then was not on medication.

[00:01:30] I had a very good grounding in psychodynamics, also in systems, family systems, because I studied family psychiatry. That was so good as a background for the systems approach that we do in Functional Medicine. There are family systems, but there's our system within and how the different aspects relate. That's all preamble.

[00:02:00] Then, we get into being actually in practice. I've seen so many people having terrible, terrible side effects from medication—and they can't get off the medication, but staying on it is not helping them either. I've always looked for ways to work differently so that they would be able to work and play and be healthier without all the effects of medication, the unwanted effects. Unfortunately, conventional psychiatry is built on treating symptoms. That's just not how it works. We have to go to the root cause. I

[00:02:30] love Functional Medicine because we are always looking for the root cause. We have the ability as a human being— as part of nature—we have the ability to heal ourselves when we're given the right materials.

I think in a way the use of medication is kind of a lazy way. Just treating symptoms is lazy. It's not going

[00:03:00] to look for what's really going on. Is it a B12 deficiency? Is it an MTHFR defect? Is it a genetic defect? Is it a hormonal issue? These are the things we really, really need to look at as physicians. I'm so glad I went to medical school, I'm a physician, and I can write prescriptions if I have to. People trust me because they know I'm not just saying that because I can't write prescriptions, but I really choose much of the time not to.

[00:03:30] Many side effects to the medications – one of the ones that's particularly bothersome – is people may lose, for example, they may lose the depths of their depression. But, at the same time, they also lose their joy. They may not be hideously depressed or with anti-anxiety medications. They may not be really, really anxious, but they also—instead of having the ups and downs of life, of feelings, of emotion, of

[00:04:00] experience—there's kind of a flat, chemical brain. They're not thinking right. They're not feeling fully, and it really affects relationships, also sexual side effects.

Another really bad effect is weight gain. I've seen, particularly with young women, because it affects them so badly psychologically. You get a girl—16, 18, or a young adult—put on an antidepressant and some of the psychotropic meds, she'll gain 10, 20, 30 pounds in no time. It's horrifying. Men, too, but I'm

[00:04:30] just saying it's particularly devastating to the girls. It's just not a good thing.

[00:05:00] It's interesting to note that one of the big side effects of medication is something called acataphasia. Acataphasia is defined as "motor restlessness." It's a kind of a feeling like you're crawling out of your skin. They have to do something about it. People become very irritable and they do some really bad things. They start to imagine. Because it is their imagination, they start to think that they're getting messages to do harm to someone or to themselves. It's almost like it's outside themselves, but it feels like it's them and it's hard to explain unless you talk to someone who's experienced it. It's so distressing.

[00:05:30] I remember speaking to one woman who said she couldn't believe it; she'd been on an SSRI, an antidepressant, and was having these weird thoughts of hurting someone. It was actually someone in her family, and she said, "That's not me, this is crazy." So, she stopped the medication. She's someone who had some awareness. She had worked in the health field and had some idea and had the courage to stop the medication. And immediately, immediately, that very distressing and very dangerous symptom went away.

[00:06:00] When people have these bad reactions to medications, all kinds of things are really going on, and there's a lot we don't understand about the brain. What we do know is that some people, genetically, are more prone than others to have these side effects from medication. Some people are more prone to become very agitated. If you can do some genetic testing in advance, you actually can tell who's going to be [00:06:30] better suited to a particular medication. My preference is really not to medicate in any case. Let's work with nature whenever we can.

I get a lot of people coming to me specifically because they're dissatisfied with their medication. It's not working, they're having side effects, they just want off it. But they know—and some of them have tried—when they go off too quickly, they have very bad side effects. Really bad effects. With some of [00:07:00] them, people become suicidal. It's so scary they go back on the medication.

The doctors are actually complicit about that because when a patient says, "I want to go off the medication," they'll usually say, "No, you really should be on it for life because you have, blah, blah, blah." Whatever—you have depression, you have bipolar disorder—you need to be on it for life and you should not go off it. But then, okay, you wanna go off, do that, and the doctor knows they're going to have terrible withdrawal.

[00:07:30] The way to do it is very different. I'll tell you how I approach it. First of all, I approach it like I approach any other patient: what's going on in them, what is the origin of the issue that made them be on medication. They could be depressed and they're on an antidepressant, but if they have an actual thyroid issue or an adrenal issue, let's address that. So, I address that. I look at their diet. I look at their nutritional status. I look to see if they're, say, B12 deficient or have a genetic disorder having to do with [00:08:00] how they methylate, which is an important aspect. It's a chemical reaction in making your neurotransmitters or your brain chemicals.

I'm looking at a lot of different things and as I treat them—this is even before we start going off meds— I'm building up their body. I'm building up their own resources. Then, we very gradually start to [00:08:30] withdraw the medication slowly, really slowly, and reinforcing or supporting the system—the neurotransmitter system—with targeted, very specific nutritional supplements.

If somebody wants to get off their medication, the first thing you do is talk to your doctor because they're in charge of the prescription, and just see what their attitude is. It's also very useful to either find a doctor, and it doesn't have to be a psychiatrist, but some sort of a doctor, MD or ND, who can help to [00:09:00] support you in the process to support your biochemistry. For example, if you're getting off a stimulant, you want to be also on some specific amino acids like tyrosine, phenylalanine, B vitamins, and so on. You want to either see somebody like that or have your doctor work in conjunction with a more holistically-oriented practitioner. Or, have him or her—the psychiatrist or the prescribing doctor—take care of the [00:09:30] medication, the prescription. And at the same time, see someone else who really understands the process. It's better if they're actually talking to each other, but that's not always possible. That doesn't always happen.

[00:10:00] In order to know what specific supplements you need, if you're doing this by yourself—let's say you have a psychiatrist who's helping you withdraw slowly, and I mean really slowly. At the same time, for example, in *The Addicted Brain and How to Break Free*, I actually discuss in one of the chapters how to get off medications and then what supplements to use ... What particular targeted nutritionals to use for the specific medication or type of medication or class of medication that you're on.

[00:10:30]

[00:11:00] Hormones are very influential on our brain and our brain health. Hormones like the thyroid, which is a butterfly-shaped gland in the neck that really runs our energy system, as do our adrenals. Our adrenals are back here above the kidneys. These are all really tiny glands, but they're very important, very influential. The adrenal glands put out adrenaline and cortisol, and other things too, but they're our fight-or-flight glands. If we've been, for example, really stressed for a long time, we're putting out a lot of fight-or-flight chemicals. We get worn out. We get tired. What happens is, the brain kind of dials down the adrenals because it's like you just can't keep going full bore all the time.

[00:11:30] What ends up happening is you get really, really tired and depressed, and so that depression may not be clinical depression. That's an interesting term, clinical depression. To me, clinical depression just means you're depressed, let's find out why. I take a history. If they've been through a stressful time, a court case, a divorce, something really big, a job loss, and they're feeling that way. You could say, "Oh well, yeah, you're depressed because that happened to you," but let's look at the level of stress that's gone on. Let's have a look at the adrenals. Let's look at adrenal function. You can check that with a saliva test, which is pretty simple.

[00:12:00] Then you give some adrenal nutrients. We also check the thyroid. We check for Hashimoto's thyroiditis as well. Then also, sex hormones; testosterone, even in women. Estrogen, DHEA, progesterone—all of these really do make a difference in how our brains are working.

[00:12:30] When a woman has PMS, it's generally a sign of an imbalance in her female hormones. The progesterone is a problem. There's usually an imbalance in progesterone. One of the things I do, I test progesterone levels, but that doesn't mean you need to take progesterone. Although you can get it over the counter—and sometimes I will recommend it—but even before that, you need to just check out and see if you're "toxic." And that's a whole can of worms—like what's toxicity, what does that mean? What that means is you're eating bad food. Probably too much sugar, chemicals, all of these things really affect our hormones. In affecting your hormones, it's going to affect your mood. It's going to affect PMS, it's going to affect everything.

[00:13:00] First of all, I say get on a clean diet. Stop the Diet Cokes, the sugar, the junk food. And very often the PMS will clear up, which means your hormones are actually becoming balanced. Then, the other thing is, I will sometimes just add in some progesterone. It's great. There are also some herbs you can use that help to balance hormones.

[00:13:30] One of the big issues I deal with is women who come to me who are perimenopausal. They're having hot flashes, depression, anxiety, trouble sleeping. And how they're treated—and this is sort of the standard of care—they're being treated with antidepressant medication or anti-anxiety medication, or both. That's just not treating the root cause. The root cause in this case is an imbalance of hormones. Treating the symptom of depression, anxiety, and sleep problems just doesn't cut it. What you really want to do is let's look at why there is an imbalance of hormones. Well, obviously, if somebody's perimenopausal, it's their age, but also let's look at the gut.

[00:14:00]

The gut may not be detoxifying and recirculating the hormones properly. It's more complex than that, so we look at all levels of hormones, how they're being metabolized by the liver. We want to look at liver function. We want to look at gut function, and then treat accordingly. We treat the liver. We treat the gut. We may add in some bioidentical hormones, and I've seen women just thrive that way and get off

[00:14:30] their medication because the medication is just making them feel kind of blah, gain weight. That's the last thing they want. I mean, really? I'm really happy to see women like that because I know what to do.

[00:15:00] There are a lot of foods that are toxic to the brain, and mostly the Standard American Diet (SAD) is very distractive to the brain. Sugar—we need to avoid chemicals and preservatives. So much of the "frankenfoods" people are eating contain these chemicals that really do affect the brain. So, very important to eat a clean diet. It makes a world of difference.

[00:15:30] Rather than eating the chemical-laden Standard American Diet, it's very important to eat well—to eat fresh, organic, natural foods. To eat a good balance of fats like natural fats because our brain cells are actually made from fat. If we're not ingesting good fats like in salmon, avocados, certain other foods, flax oil, and omega-3 fatty acids, then we don't have the materials to make brain cells. We need enough protein because we're making neurotransmitters, which are made out of amino acids, which are the
[00:16:00] breakdown products of protein. We need sufficient protein, fish, chicken ... But don't eat fish that has mercury in it and don't eat farmed fish. This a whole story in itself, what we should be eating, so I'm just covering this very briefly. This is what I tell my patients.

[00:16:30] In terms of carbs, the best source of carbs is actually in the vegetable kingdom. Don't eat a lot of the standard carbohydrates. Avoid gluten, very often there's gluten sensitivity. Even if you don't have celiac disease, or even if you don't have specific gluten sensitivity, gluten itself is inflammatory. All of these things, gluten included, and all these chemicals cause inflammation in the brain. An inflamed brain is a brain that is not working properly.

[00:17:00] For mental focus, I think it's important to have a good lifestyle. To eat an appropriate breakfast. To eat good food, healthy food, not avoiding breakfast or skipping it all together. It's important to exercise because that's going to keep your brain really sharp and focused. Meditation is really good, although it's hard to meditate if it's hard to focus, so it works both ways. But if you keep up your meditation practice, it actually will help enormously for your focus.

[00:17:30] Then, what I do, specifically for my patients, is I'll give them targeted nutritional supplements that have tyrosine, phenylalanine, ginkgo, ingredients like that. My Focus products have those in it just so people don't have to get one of these; it's all in one product. There are others on the market, so sometimes it's just taking something. Taking a good nutritional supplement formula to get you started in your day, and then you can take it from there.

[00:18:00] Ginkgo is great. I put it in my Brain Cell Support Plus product because it enhances blood flow, and we need really good blood flow in the brain in order to bring the nutrients and oxygen and take away the waste products.

[00:18:30] It's kind of interesting about when somebody is too sick for a natural approach and really needs drugs. It doesn't even work that way because sometimes people can be pretty sick and what they really need are nutrients, not drugs. At the same time, if somebody is having a bipolar episode, a manic episode, or if somebody's severely depressed, and you need to get them out of it quickly for their own protection, as much as anything, then use medication, but use it wisely. Use it minimally and for the shortest amount of time possible.

[00:19:00] I think addiction is being treated pretty badly, which leads to the revolving door that we have. It's just expected people are going to relapse, and they'll be back and keep coming back over and over and over again, which is great for business, you know, the addiction facilities. The staffers are usually really very dedicated, caring people, but the business of the whole addiction business, is a little scary. They're not using the information that we actually have. My point of view, in which I really emphasize in *The*
[00:19:30] *Addicted Brain and How to Break Free*, is that addiction isn't a moral issue. It's not about willpower. It's not about white knuckling it. It's a biochemical imbalance. When you can deal with it with nutrition, lifestyle, supplements, you actually can get your brain back and you can make the right decisions.

[00:20:00] When you're in a craving mode, you don't even have your prefrontal cortex. You don't have your frontal cortex. You don't have your thinking brain on at all. You have your primitive brain operating. You know, you're like a two-year-old. So, what are you going to do? You're not going to have proper thinking, proper willpower, so forget it. What you really need is something that's going to keep your brain working on all cylinders all the time, then you'll make the right decisions. You'll make the right choices. You'll be able to use the psychotherapy that you get because I think it's important.

[00:20:30] I think that people who have been addicted do need support and therapy, but when their brain is not working properly, because: A) they've been using; and B) the standard of care in treating people who are withdrawing from addiction in these facilities, or as outpatients, is to give them medication. Unfortunately, they become as hooked on the medication as they were on the drugs of abuse. I don't know if you've really solved the problem, except that you're now patronizing the pharmaceutical industry and they're happy, but I don't know if it's in the best interest of the patients.

[00:21:00] I have a lot of cases of people getting off medications successfully. One woman who heard me speak about getting off of SSRIs (Prozac, Zoloft, Celexa, Paxil, and so on) did it herself.

[00:21:30] There's actually help to be able to do it yourself. She, with the help of her psychiatrist, began to lower her dose of Zoloft, and at the same time began to take 5-HTP (5-hydroxytryptophan), which enhances serotonin, which is what the Zoloft was doing. Over a period of three months, she actually got herself totally off the Zoloft that she'd been on. Here she was, a 50-year-old woman. She'd been on it since she was 18, and she said, " Oh my God, I got my brain back. I hadn't been able to think this clearly, and feel this fully." Since then, she'd forgotten. She said it was miraculous. I run into her once in a while. She's

[00:22:00] still doing great because she got off of a medication that just becomes a habit, an addiction, and you can get off it.

[00:22:30] In terms of addiction to substances, very simply, I had this woman. She was an alcoholic, and there was no way she was going to stop drinking, but she wanted to stop drinking. But she was so under the control of it that it was really difficult. I had suggested glutamine. Glutamine is an amino acid that goes right to the brain and actually acts the same way as a substance would—as alcohol would—but in a good way, a healthy way. Glutamine is an amino acid that works on the brain in a healthy way to cut cravings.

[00:23:00] She was totally amazed. She said, "I was about to go to the liquor store—it was late at night—I was going to go to the liquor store, and I remembered what you said, and I had this glutamine from you. I did what you said, I opened up the capsule, I put some of it under my tongue, and I could not believe it. I suddenly had no more urge to go. I put down my keys, and that was it. I did not need to go to the liquor store." That's pretty amazing, and she said, "I've been doing that ever since. I just take glutamine and

[00:23:30] now I'm not drinking." Not all cases are that simple, but you actually can do something. You can do something on your own.

When JJ's son was injured, it was just so horrifying. I still remember going to the ICU at Harbor General and just being like, what can I say, it was just so painful to see. Because here's my friend, anyone looking at him with all the tubes and he was in a coma, it was so painful. I wanted to do anything I could. We

[00:24:00] were limited because he was in ICU at a regular hospital, but what I was able to do is help him to get fish oil and progesterone.

[00:24:30] Now, progesterone can be used topically as a skin cream, so I don't think we asked permission, but progesterone helps to rebuild brain cells. Pregnenolone does as well, and so when you take progesterone, you can just rub it on. He had so many IVs ... You actually can use IV progesterone, but that was not going to happen there. We just put it on his skin, and I think that helped. Everything helped. So many people came and did their magic, so it was really a combination of everything. And it was just beautiful to see how everyone came together and how well he recovered.

[00:25:00] What I want to tell somebody with anxiety or depression, feeling really hopeless, first of all—there is hope, there's always hope. And, to really check out the biochemistry of what's going on. Yes, there are situational things, yes, bad things happen that make you feel depressed and anxious. But, very, very often once you address the biochemistry, whether it's hormonal, vitamin deficiency, an adrenal burnout

[00:25:30] issue, thyroid issue, once you've addressed that and you're supporting the biochemistry, very often that anxiety and depression will clear up.

If there are remnants, if there are things to still deal with because we're human beings—and I think therapy's a good thing—then you can really have therapy and you can apply it. But when you're just painfully anxious or painfully depressed, it's really hard to absorb the information and therapy, or really

[00:26:00] apply it because you're just so out of it. You're not working on all cylinders, and the advice is always to go see your physician. I don't know ... Unless it's a holistic physician, or Functional Medicine physician, it's a little tricky because you're going to be prescribed a medication, be told you need to be on it for a very long time. And then, once you're on it, it's really hard to get off, and you're in this vicious cycle.

[00:26:30] First of all, do a lot of the things that I've been talking about, and all of us have been talking about. I think the simplest approach to getting off medication is in my *The Addicted Brain and How to Break Free*, which talks about how to do it stepwise and what nutrients to take. Also on my website, I talk about the brain and what the neurotransmitters do, and what the different amino acids do to support the different neurotransmitters. I have information available.

IZABELLA WENTZ, PharmD, FASCP | Pharmacist, Researcher, & Patient Advocate

New York Times Best-Selling Author of *Hashimoto's Root Cause & Hashimoto's Protocol*

Dr. Izabella Wentz:

I wasn't always interested in thyroid health. In fact, in pharmacy school, I never thought that thyroid disorders were really what I was going to focus on. In fact, it wasn't until my own diagnosis in my mid-20s when I really became interested in the thyroid gland. My symptoms started off with being fatigued all the time. I was sleeping for 12 to 14 hours, not really knowing why I was so tired all the time. I used to be this bright-eyed and bushy-tailed kid, and all of the sudden I was missing classes in undergrad and even missing exams. That continued on even in my studies during pharmacy school where I was just so tired all the time. I continued to have more and more symptoms with every passing year.

[00:00:30]

What started off with fatigue ended up being irritable bowel syndrome. Then, I started having acid reflux. Then, I started having panic attacks, anxiety attacks, brain fog, and carpal tunnel in both of my arms. It wasn't until almost nine years from the beginning of my symptoms until I was finally diagnosed with Hashimoto's at age 27, when I had already been a practicing consultant pharmacist for three years.

[00:01:00]

When I was struggling with Hashimoto's, it was really, really scary for me because I had anxiety attacks and panic attacks that I had never had before. I started to have new onset anxiety disorders, and I started to have social anxiety. One of the worst things that happened with Hashimoto's was that I started to have brain fog. The brain fog that comes along with thyroid disease is quite scary, because you don't know what's happening to you. You can go from being this really intelligent person that's on top of your game, can tell jokes very quickly, can study things and remember things very quickly—to, all of the sudden, walking into rooms and forgetting how you got there in the first place. That can be very, very scary when you feel like your mind is slipping away from you, where you're slowly losing parts of yourself. I became less funny. I became less outgoing. I became less interactive with the world around me, and this was all related to Hashimoto's.

[00:01:30]

[00:02:00]

People with thyroid disorders can exhibit a lot of symptoms that affect their brain. Some of the things that I've seen are going to be fatigue, brain fog, apathy, irritability, anxiety, and panic attacks. We're also going to see times of depression. I've seen people who were misdiagnosed with bipolar disorder, and I've even seen people who were hospitalized for psychotic disorders as a result of Hashimoto's. Hashimoto's encephalopathy is also a commonly undiagnosed condition where thyroid antibodies can actually cross-react with brain antibodies, or, perhaps, there's a mechanism where thyroid antibodies cross through to the brain. What can happen at that point is a person can actually have a lot of challenges. We might see them having struggles with their gait, with their balance. They may have seizures. They may have symptoms like dementia, delusions, and even hallucinations. There's a big spectrum of how Hashimoto's can affect the brain.

[00:02:30]

[00:03:00]

There are so many different root causes of mental health issues, brain deterioration, and brain fog. The thyroid is actually one of these causes that is fairly resolvable. Whenever you have these symptoms, you may have heard that there's nothing you can do about your brain function—that you're just getting older, that this is what happens when you're a mom—but actually, the thyroid condition can be a root cause of a lot of your brain symptoms and a reversible reason for them too. Unfortunately, there have been many times where people were misdiagnosed and told they have X-condition, whether that was a mental health condition or sometimes a type of dementia. And the conventional medical approach was that this condition wasn't really reversible, and that this person either had to wait as they deteriorated or take lifelong psychiatric medications.

[00:03:30]

[00:04:00] What we've been able to find is that when you actually address somebody's thyroid condition, in many cases, these symptoms can be reversed. Then, many cases, there are things that are commonly misdiagnosed such as bipolar disorder, even seizure disorders, panic attacks, anxiety attacks. All of these things can stem from thyroid disease and are fairly easily reversed when you get the proper thyroid treatment, and when you address the autoimmune component of your thyroid condition.

[00:04:30] Some of the most common root causes of thyroid conditions include food sensitivities, nutrient depletion, an impaired ability to handle stress, an impaired ability to handle toxins, chronic infections, as well as digestive challenges which oftentimes present with intestinal permeability. This whole spectrum of various types of root causes and triggers will set off an autoimmune cascade

[00:05:00] where the immune system no longer recognizes the thyroid as a part of our own body and launches an attack against the thyroid gland. Eventually, this is what leads to an underactive thyroid, and this is something that can also lead to an overactive thyroid. Most cases of thyroid disease are actually autoimmune in nature.

[00:05:30] The microglial cells are the brain's immune cells. They respond to different threats against the brain. What happens with Hashimoto's is an inflammatory response. Whenever we have Hashimoto's antibodies that perhaps cross-react with brain tissue or cross the blood-brain barrier, what we'll have is the microglial cells will produce an attack. An inflammatory attack on this can lead to inflammation in the brain as well as damage of the surrounding brain tissue.

[00:06:00] There's a really important connection with what's going on with our gut, with our thyroid, and with our brain. Gut health plays a very important role in thyroid health. Whenever we have an autoimmune thyroid condition, one of the key root causes associated with autoimmune thyroid disease is going to be intestinal permeability or a leaky gut. Whenever we have a person with a thyroid condition, it's really, really important to address the state and health of their gut and figure out why it's permeable. Some of the causes may be infections, food sensitivities, nutrient deficiencies, or deficiencies in digestive enzymes.

[00:06:30] When we have this gut inflammation, that's going to eventually lead to inflammation in the thyroid gland where the immune system will start attacking the thyroid gland. Once the thyroid gland is compromised, there are many consequences of not having enough thyroid hormone, as well as consequences of having too much thyroid hormone. Some of these consequences may be seen in early fetal development. Children who don't have enough thyroid hormone—they can actually have higher rates of developmental disabilities, intellectual disabilities, higher rates of autism. We also see

[00:07:00] this in adults whenever we have people who have an underactive thyroid or even an overactive thyroid. This is almost always resultant from an autoimmune attack. They're going to have struggles with brain function. They may have more irritability, they may have more depression, they may have more brain fog, they may have panic attacks.

[00:07:30] In some cases, thyroid antibodies and Hashimoto's antibodies may also cross-react with brain antibodies and brain tissue and brain cells. We may have a whole other cascade of thyroid disease progressing into brain disease. It's really, really important to make sure that if you have a person who is struggling with impaired brain function, impaired cognitive function, we really look at what's behind that. Is the thyroid contributing? Is the gut contributing? A lot of times it's going to be both that are going to be contributing to the picture.

[00:08:00] Every case of autoimmune disease, there's an inflammatory component present in that. Whether that is going to be Graves' disease or Hashimoto's thyroiditis, we're going to see inflammation. Inflammation in the brain can lead to degeneration of the brain. It's really important to figure out the source of the inflammation in the body. The biggest challenge with the conventional approach to thyroid treatment is that the conventional approach doesn't recognize thyroid disease until we're in the late stages of Hashimoto's.

[00:08:30] There are five stages to Hashimoto's. The very first stage—for all intents and purposes—we just have the genetic predisposition, but all things are normal. The second stage is when we start seeing an attack on the thyroid gland. This is also the stage where we might start seeing some brain symptoms such as anxiety, fatigue, irritability, perhaps even depression. Conventional medicine, when they identify thyroid disease at that stage—and most of the time they don't—won't have a treatment for it. Oftentimes, patients will be referred to psychiatrists, or told that it's all in their head, or told that

[00:09:00] they need to get more rest, or perhaps that they're hypochondriacs.

In the third stage of Hashimoto's, the condition continues to progress with more symptoms in the body and more symptoms in the brain, more destruction of the thyroid gland. But yet, most conventional medical doctors are not willing to do anything at that point. The fourth stage is where we actually start seeing that a significant portion of the thyroid gland has been damaged. At that

[00:09:30] point, the body is no longer able to compensate and make enough thyroid hormone. At that point, the conventional approach is to give the person more thyroid hormone. The challenge here is that the condition continues to progress after that point.

The fifth stage of Hashimoto's is going to be progression to other types of autoimmune disease—multiple sclerosis, lupus, rheumatoid arthritis—and the thyroid hormone doesn't stop the progression. Thyroid hormone is basically like giving somebody a little bit more water to put into

[00:10:00] their bucket that has a hole in it, rather than plugging up the holes of that bucket. Additionally, the medical conventional approach doesn't individualize thyroid hormone therapy. Most people with a thyroid condition with an underactive thyroid are just placed on T4-containing medications, which may not be properly activated and utilized by many people with thyroid disease.

Now, what I would really, really like to see is to have an early diagnosis where a person is diagnosed

[00:10:30] at the very beginning stages of Hashimoto's, in that second stage when the immune system starts to attack the thyroid gland. And I would love to see some interventions at that point, where we would be thinking about what can we do to stop this attack on the thyroid gland, what can we do to reduce and dampen the attack on the thyroid gland, and, hey, can we start supporting the thyroid gland at this point with some bioidentical therapies?

The conventional medical approach only looks at thyroid conditions in a vacuum. It's like, okay, the

[00:11:00] thyroid gland is either producing enough thyroid hormone or it's not. They have a one-size-fits-all approach, which is to give one medication—Synthroid synthetic hormone—for that person, only if they meet the threshold of not producing enough thyroid hormone. There's so much going on on this other side. There are so many other things that can be addressed. There are so many pathways, inflammatory pathways, nutrient deficiencies, and food sensitivities that are actually causing the body to attack the thyroid gland. All of that is, unfortunately, ignored by conventional medicine.

[00:11:30] The answer is we don't have enough studies, we don't have enough data. There's not really good evidence that food can cause reactions against the thyroid gland, or that selenium should be utilized. We've seen time and time again clinically, that when you take a person with Hashimoto's off of specific foods, they actually start feeling better and their thyroid antibodies go down. In some cases, their thyroid function comes back on board. We've also seen really positive results with various

[00:12:00] nutrient therapies where that can help dampen the autoimmune response, and people feel a lot better. I really feel like conventional medicine needs to take their head out of the clouds and look at the patients, at the patient experience and see what they're going through, and help them get better doing whatever it takes to get that person better. We know there are so many solutions out there, and it's just a matter of picking the right ones, and individualizing them for each patient.

[00:12:30] The TSH test is a standard of care test for figuring out if a person has a thyroid condition. Unfortunately, this test—while it's very, very good in the late stages of Hashimoto's and thyroid disease—can miss thyroid disease in the first five, ten, sometimes 15 years that we have it. Yes, do the TSH test, but also look at your thyroid antibodies. TPO (thyroid peroxidase) antibodies and TB

[00:13:00] (thyroglobulin) antibodies will show up in the very early stages of Hashimoto's when the attack on the thyroid gland starts and when a lot of the brain symptoms start. We know that there's an immune system imbalance and that we can do something about it. TPO antibodies, TG antibodies, TSH—three most important tests.

[00:13:30] I also like to look at free T3 and free T4. This tells us what amount of thyroid hormones we have available in our body to interact with thyroid hormone receptors. Make sure that you ask your doctor for all these different tests and not just look at the TSH. Because many times that test can be "normal" for many years while you have this attack on your thyroid gland, and you can just be not knowing that part of your body is under attack because you're not getting the right testing.

[00:14:00] In many cases, we'll see that there are objective markers we can measure in the blood, where we see that thyroid antibodies are elevated, or we see alterations in TSH, alterations in T3 and T4. Sometimes there's something called reverse T3 that may also be altered. But beyond that, I also encourage clinicians to really look at their patient's symptoms because there are instances where a person can have something like seronegative Hashimoto's, where they have the attack on their
[00:14:30] thyroid gland but it may not show up in blood work. Doing thyroid ultrasounds can also be very helpful to determine if a person has an attack on their thyroid gland—that can be visualized on an ultrasound. In some cases, those can also miss Hashimoto's, so I do advise really looking at the person as a whole and considering what their labs look like, what their ultrasounds look like and what they feel like, what they're telling you that they're going through. This will help figure out what is going on with the person.

[00:15:00] In some cases, utilizing thyroid hormone therapy, as well as all of the lifestyle interventions that I'm a a big proponent of, can help a person feel like themselves again. That's really the most important thing we're aiming for.

What I like to do with people with Hashimoto's is, I want to look at getting them back into balance. We're going to be looking at, first and foremost, of course, their thyroid hormones and see if those
[00:15:30] hormones are in balance and how do we individualize their therapy. We may utilize T4, T3 medications. We may utilize natural desiccated thyroid medications or even compounded thyroid medications to meet that person's needs. Then, also very, very importantly and not to be ignored, we're also looking at what's the root cause of their condition. What's causing their body to attack their own thyroid gland? A lot of times it's going to be related to the foods they're eating, so we're going to be thinking about what foods can we remove from their diet that can be causing cross-
[00:16:00] reactivity or inflammation within their thyroid gland. We're going to be thinking about what nutrients they're going to be missing.

These are going to be two of the cardinal things that we oftentimes will just start a person on and they feel significantly better. Once we remove the inflammatory foods—gluten, dairy and soy are the most common—and once we add some nutrients to the mix, like selenium, vitamin D, the B vitamins,
[00:16:30] especially thiamine and B12, as well as magnesium, we start seeing big improvements in how a person feels. Beyond that, it kind of can be a little bit like peeling back the layers of an onion. I like to focus on addressing toxicity by supporting the person's liver. I like to focus on addressing their stress response. I like to focus on addressing the health of their gut, and then also dialing in and seeing if they have any kinds of chronic infections that can be cross-reacting with their thyroid tissue.

[00:17:00] When a person has an infection within the thyroid gland or, perhaps, even somewhere else in the body, the immune system may attack that infection and either where the infection lives, which may be the thyroid, or anything that looks like the infection. In some cases, some infectious organisms can resemble the thyroid gland when you look at them in tiny, tiny pieces, which is how the onion system recognizes what's a friend and what's an enemy. It's a really comprehensive whole-person approach to try to figure out how do we get the person back into balance, how do we establish
[00:17:30] safety in their body, how do we get their immune system to start recognizing the thyroid gland as a

friend and part of us once more.

The approach is going to vary for each person. For some people, it may be as easy as just removing one food from their diet. And within two to three months, they're going to see that all of their symptoms melt away, their thyroid antibodies go away, and in some cases, they can even wean off of thyroid hormones. Sometimes it happens in two to three months. In other patients, we may have to go deeper. We may have to pull out a whole bunch of different foods. We may have to address various nutrients. We may have to address various infections, various traumas, a whole host of toxins, and it really varies on the individual to see what are their unique triggers, what are their unique root causes to bring them back into balance.

[00:18:00]

[00:18:30]

Gluten, dairy, and soy should absolutely be avoided if a person is dealing with a thyroid disorder. We've seen 88% of people with thyroid conditions feel significantly better off of gluten, about 80% feel significantly better off of dairy, and somewhere between 60 and 70% feel much, much better off of soy. A lot of times we see miracle stories happen when they just get off of those three foods. Some of the most common thyroid toxins we're going to have fluoride in our water supply. This can be potentially problematic. We're going to have BPA in our plastics and triclosan. This is going to be present in our antibacterial soaps. Flame retardants in our bedding. These are all potential triggers and toxins that can contribute to thyroid disease.

[00:19:00]

[00:19:30]

I recommend doing a cleanup of your environment; get rid of some of those low-hanging fruits. Get a reverse osmosis fluoride filter to try to get some of the fluoride out of your tap. You're going to want to go green on your personal care routine, so you're going to start getting rid of the antibacterial soaps. You're going to get rid of the heavy chemical-based products like shampoos, lotions, potions, and perfumes. You're also going to be thinking about not utilizing as much plastic, especially for cooking your food or microwaving your food or storing your food, so you're going to go to all glass. We see that when you stop adding in toxins to the mix, we can start to finally get rid of them. Another component of addressing toxicity is to support your liver with nutrients, as well as some herbs, which can help it detoxify and get rid of some of the toxins that you've been building up in your body.

[00:20:00]

[00:20:30]

What I'd really like to recommend for people with Hashimoto's and for thyroid disease is to focus on eating a whole foods-based diet that's minimally processed. The diets that I've seen the most benefit from are going to be the paleo diet, as well as the autoimmune paleo diet. We've actually been able to see and measure improvement in people's symptoms, as well as in their thyroid antibody markers, which can tell us how aggressive the thyroid condition is. We see symptoms like headaches, panic attacks, palpitations, waking, fatigue—all of these symptoms begin to melt away when we get rid of the reactive foods and we focus on having organic, wild-caught, real foods within our diet. I love to see people eating bone broth. I love to see them eating good fats. I love to see them eating organic and wild-caught meats.

[00:21:00]

As far as nutrients go, one of the most important nutrients that we want to address is selenium. Selenium deficiency has been recognized as an environmental trigger for thyroid disease. We find that 200 to 400 micrograms of selenomethionine can reduce the attack on the thyroid gland by about half. We also see that it reduces anxiety. It reduces hair loss and a whole host of other thyroid symptoms. I also really love to see people with thyroid disorders on thiamine, especially when they have any types of fatigue or brain fog. Thiamine around 600 milligrams has been clinically shown to reverse thyroid disease in as little as three to five days. I love the benfotiamine version as well. This has been very, very effective for many of my clients and readers.

[00:21:30]

[00:22:00]

I recently got a letter from a woman who was on disability because of her brain fog and because of her fatigue. She started utilizing benfotiamine 600 milligrams a day, and within a few months she was able to go back to work full time. If you give the body what it needs, it can absolutely heal itself. Some of the other additional very helpful nutrients that can support thyroid health include magnesium, vitamin D, as well as B12.

[00:22:30] When we really think about all the different root causes of thyroid disease, we're thinking about food sensitivities, nutrient depletion, and infections. When we get to the bottom of it, all these things send a signal to the body that we're not safe, that we're not going to survive. The body always wants us to survive. The body always wants to help us. One of the best ways to survive times that are very stressful is by withdrawing and by slowing down our metabolism. Really, that's what thyroid disease does.

[00:23:00] Anything that really sends a signal to our body that we're not safe can have an impact on the thyroid gland. There's actually research that shows that the thyroid gland sends out safety signals and danger signals, so the thyroid gland is actually an environmental sensing gland. Whenever it senses that we are in danger, it's going to send out messages to the rest of our body to help the body survive. The body does that by attacking the thyroid and slowing it down. From an adaptive physiology standpoint, whenever we have stress—whether that's in the form of physical or mental—that's going to put our bodies in a conservation mode. The best way to conserve energy and resources is to slow down the metabolism by attacking the thyroid gland.

[00:23:30]

[00:24:00] A key component of addressing thyroid disease is to address the stress response. If you're dealing with a thyroid disorder, I really, really encourage you to be your own health advocate, to learn as much as you can about your thyroid condition so you can take action on getting yourself better. Some things you can do in your very own home include going on a gluten-free, dairy-free, and soy-free diet. We see transformation sometimes in as little as three days where people's symptoms will melt away once they do that. Make sure you're eating blood-sugar balanced. Get plenty of good fats and proteins in your diet. Reduce your carbohydrate intake. You're going to start feeling a lot better. The fatigue is going to melt away, the anxiety is going to melt away, and your brain is going to be functioning much better as well.

I also encourage you to take on some stress-relieving hobbies. Whatever you can do to put your body into more of that rest-and-digest state is going to really, really help you in the long term.

Dr. Jay Faber:	Medicine, like any other industry, has gone through its evolution over the last 25 to 30 years. I've seen some great things, and I've seen some things that I've not seen as great. One of the areas I saw where there were true opportunities to help people focus on health, live healthy, breathe healthy, was Functional Medicine. Henceforth, I decided to make some commitments with my time and my thinking to go into Functional Medicine to a much greater depth so that I could not only use medications but use supplements that help the brain and the body to think, feel, and behave better.
[00:00:30]	
[00:01:00]	Medicine, from my perspective, because of some of the changes with HMOs and the whole insurance industry, has gone to more of an algorithmic approach to taking care of people. Now when I say that, what exactly do I mean? You come in with a problem with depression and so I say, "Okay, here. Try this antidepressant." It doesn't work, so what do we do? "Well, here's the next antidepressant on the list. If that doesn't work, well, let's try the third or the fourth or the fifth or maybe after the fourth time it's not working, maybe we switch to a mood stabilizer or something else."
[00:01:30]	There's not so much a lot of thinking about what's going on and what's causing this person to feel or think the way they are. It's more if something doesn't help, then try the next medication on the list. In contrast, the functional approach really asks deeper, probing and, from my perspective, thinking questions, which most doctors have spent a lot of time learning, and we might as well get the best out of their brains to help people get better.
[00:02:00]	A good example would be last week. I had some gal come in who thought she may have had a history of trauma in past abuse. She was having all these memories that would pop up in her mind, for no reason, of people traumatizing, hurting her, yet she'd never really been depressed. In fact, she'd never been irritable, and so her whole history didn't really flow with your classic picture of depression, anxiety, or post-traumatic stress disorder. What in the Lord's name is going on with this gal? That's why she came to see us. By the way, she'd been on several medications already (no change) and she was very frustrated.
[00:02:30]	This gal's 51 years old, okay? She's starting to have hormonal changes and menopause and she actually had a head trauma in her past. When we looked at her scans here at our clinic (we do SPECT scans, by the way), which looked at blood flow to the brain. Her temporal lobes had shown some decreased blood flow. I asked about past head injuries and she said yes indeed, she did have a past head injury. It happened when she was probably about 13 or 14 years old.
[00:03:00]	Now, it got interesting with this gal, these thoughts she was having that kept popping up. Actually, it stopped for about 15 to 20 years by practicing some simple brain exercises and dieting correctly. It was around 50 when all these really started. After speaking with her and hearing some of her hormonal changes, my hunch with her is this, "You know what, I could give you another medication for your temporal lobes, like a mood stabilizer. We could try another antidepressant, but I don't think that's the problem. I think the issue is this—as we age, we all lose neurons, and as we age, we all lose estrogen."
[00:03:30]	
[00:04:00]	Now, for females, their brains love estrogen. My hunch is, as she lost estrogen, she also lost more brain cells in her temporal lobe, or they're not working so well. Rather than just starting out with another mood stabilizer, we actually used some supplements to help her temporal lobes. I've ordered her estrogen and progesterone levels, which are going to be low because she's 51, and so we're going to use some, what I'd call brain trophic agents—estrogen, progesterone—to actually help her brain work better. That's going deeper. It's asking more personalized questions. It's digging more into what

is the real cause and what can we really do in 21st century medicine to help this person have a youthful and healthy life for the next 25, 30 years.

[00:04:30] Some of the key hormones we think of—thyroid hormone, estrogen, progesterone for females, testosterone for males, but also for females, too; insulin, cortisol—are huge. Which one? I'd say all of them. They all can affect brain functioning and how we think, feel, and behave. What does that mean?

[00:05:00] It means that I, as a psychiatrist, now have to understand the physiology and pathophysiology of how these hormones are produced, how they're excreted, how they're metabolized, so I can help those individuals with hormonal problems think, feel, and behave better.

Let's say we have somebody who's 35 years old, a male, who's unhappy, depressed, he's stressed, he's got low energy, he's got low concentration, he's gained 40 pounds over the last year and a half, and

[00:05:30] he's actually exercising every day. Time out. Something's going on here. Now, what might be happening? His thyroid levels might be off. His testosterone levels might be off or, what we're really seeing a lot more of, his cortisol levels might actually be low.

I won't go into other details. We did not check thyroid or testosterone first because his symptom presentation pretty much coincided with someone who was having low cortisol level. So what did we

[00:06:00] do? We went and got a salivary cortisol level test and we light-tuned the salivary test because our salivary or our cortisol levels don't flatline all day like most of our hormones. We wake up in the morning, we get this huge surge of cortisol, and then throughout the rest of the day it decreases.

Now, we could get blood levels, but that would mean going to the lab four times during the day to get blood and we find that if we have you just, for the lack of better words, spit in a little test tube at 8am,

[00:06:30] 12pm, 4pm, and 8pm, and watch those levels, we can see if they're too high or too low. Now, this individual who I'm talking about, his levels, rather than being here, were actually done here and throughout the day, and they were lower than they were supposed to be.

In addition to treating his depression, we started to treat his weight by using supplements that help

[00:07:00] support the adrenal glands. He's feeling better and he's losing weight. Now, if you're feeling better and you're not losing weight, how are you going to end up being? This is where we're finding it really important. If we're really, truly doing 21st century health, we want to help the brain, but we also want to help the whole body get better.

There are a couple of amino acids—in specific called tryptophan and another one called

[00:07:30] phenylalanine—which our bodies just don't produce. We have to digest them in order to get them into our system. Tryptophan helps produce a neurotransmitter called serotonin. Phenylalanine helps produce several neurotransmitters including dopamine, norepinephrine, epinephrine, which all help us focus and feel better.

If we're not digesting food properly or, what we've seen a lot of times, we're not eating the right types

[00:08:00] of foods, we might not be producing enough serotonin, epinephrine, norepinephrine or dopamine, which leads to people just not feeling very happy. One of the things I've really seen in the last couple of years is that we'll have people coming in, maybe eating one meal a day, and that meal is typically in a fast food restaurant, soda and some carbs, and they're just not feeling good. They don't feel happy. We look at their scans and we notice the areas of the brain, for example, the anterior cingulate, which

[00:08:30] help produce serotonin, aren't working so well. We see the thalamus, which really thrives on norepinephrine, isn't working so well. We look at the whole cortex and it looks a bit more bumpy than it should be. It's not working so well.

The problem isn't even really an antidepressant issue. It's a diet issue. One of the first things we're going to do is help them get on the proper protein-rich foods so they get the tryptophan and

[00:09:00] phenylalanine they need to have their brain work better. The most helpful foods are your proteins that are low fat—so chicken, fish, low-fat beef, vegetables—which produce and help make a lot of enzymes to produce neurotransmitters and fruits. It's not rocket science, to be honest. It's just eating the right foods.

[00:09:30]

The things we really want to try to stay away from are our trans fats which, by the way, are illegal in some countries. A lot of our food companies now use trans fats because they help foods stay fresh and preserve them, which is great for the food. The problem is they're not so healthy for our bodies. Those types of foods, carbohydrates, breads, pastas, cookies, chocolates, as much as we love them, they're not necessarily so healthy for our body. They help create more of an oxidized state in our body, and by oxidized, think more acidic. When our body is more acidic, the cells just don't work as well.

[00:10:00]

We really want to eat more, I'd call it, a Mediterranean style of diet with lots of fruit, vegetables and protein. How many fruits and how many vegetables? If you go by the American Academy of Anti-Aging, they're recommending six vegetables and four fruits a day, *a day*. Now, how many of us do that? We have people coming to see us that are eating three vegetables and maybe four fruits a week. You can see where there are the challenges and the opportunities to create behavioral change.

[00:10:30]

The simple stuff, all right, is just what we're kind of talking about here to build brain resilience. Good diet. I mean, I can't emphasize that enough. High protein, low simple carbs, more of a Mediterranean style diet, exercise. We're recommending now—and this isn't me, this is from other medical foundations—six days of exercise per week for 55 to 60 minutes per day as long as your other health is in shape. We don't want someone with a cardiovascular problem to be necessarily exercising that much unless a doctor recommends it, three days a week doing cardiovascular exercise. That could be running. It could be biking. It could be a Precor and in three days a week, doing resistance exercises with weights.

[00:11:00]

[00:11:30]

I tell my 30 and 40-year-old males that they don't necessarily have to go to the gym and put three 45s on each side of the barbell and watch the bar bend to show off to all the young kids. It's more low weights and lot of reps to keep our shape and our form and not damage our tendons or muscles. There's that piece. Then, one of the big factors, I think, is continuing to grow and develop. How do you do that? I personally find reading and journaling as a great way to start to think, create, and develop oneself. The nice thing about school is it really gives us the ability to set structure and time learning specific topics, but once you're done with school, how do you keep developing yourself? Reading and journaling is one great way.

[00:12:00]

[00:12:30]

The other thing I'd say is just keep thinking youthful, stay on top of trends, stay on top of music, stay on top of what's going on in entertainment, stay on top of what's going on in politics. Keep your brain vibrant and young. Learn new things, reading, journaling, you really want to journal because it's one thing to read it, but reading it here and having it go from here to here, that's where journaling challenges your brain to think at the deeper level really helping and then, staying on top of trends, what's going on in the real world.

[00:13:00]

Are the lifestyle changes I recommend across the board the same for every individual patient, whether PTSD, depression, ADD? My answer would be, "No." We do SPECT scans here at our clinic. One of the beauties is, we can see parts of the brain that are overreacting or underreacting and we know that certain foods are used as medications to help those parts, hopefully, work better. Now, for example, one part of our brain, called the anterior cingulate cortex (which is located maybe about an inch down from one of my frontal lobes right here) if it's overacting, it's telling us we don't have enough serotonin. What do people do? They start finding ways to get serotonin.

[00:13:30]

[00:14:00]

Where's a good place to get serotonin? All of your simple carbohydrates. Junk foods, hamburgers, cookies, cakes all help increase serotonin. Now, here's the problem. Those foods increase serotonin, but not very much. What it does do is increase our girth size, and our weight. We start self-medicating with carbohydrates to get that part of our brain working better.

[00:14:30] Another part of our brain really deep down in the center, called our thalamus, if it's overactive, if it's demanding norepinephrine and it also, when it gets that hot, is craving sugar. You can eat sugar. The problem is you get all the problems that sugar creates, and your thalamus still doesn't work that well. You can look at different parts of the brain and start to give more target-focused diets, depending on what parts are overworking or underworking.

[00:15:00] Yes, the sugars are an interesting issue in terms of what actually happens to the brain when we eat a lot of sugar. There are probably a few things going on. The way I kind of reckon it is, it's like looking at clocks or watches. I mean, most of us, and again, this gets back to my medical training, there's more of a linear approach and really, our bodies are more like watches. They've got all these little wheels going at the same time and you have to keep all of them working well.

[00:15:30] Back to glucose (sugar). Sugar, if we eat too much, has to go someplace. What does it do? Well, one thing it does that's not so healthy is it will bind to other fats. That will then eventually get lodged in our arteries, which will then eventually be told by immune cells that this isn't healthy. It's not supposed to be there. All of a sudden, we get all this inflammation in our arteries. What happens next? Our arteries start to narrow because of the inflammation. We get less blood going to those vital organs or body parts that need it.

[00:16:00]
[00:16:30] Sugar: there are a lot of theories as well in terms of if you eat too much, your insulin levels will go up. If your insulin levels go up, then, all of a sudden, your blood doesn't have enough glucose. If you don't have enough glucose, then our cells might not have enough energy to function well. All of a sudden, all of your cells aren't getting as much energy as they should and they start to produce what we call reactive oxidative species. It's sort of a big fancy word for basically saying the breakdown products in your cells are increasing and when they increase, your cells don't work so well. Sugar is really inflammatory. I mean, the more we see it, eating too much especially, it's just not healthy for our body.

[00:17:00] Sleep and neural plasticity—this is a huge, huge topic right now, especially concerning the immune system. Research is starting to show that our brain actually has an immune system in it. Some of the cells surrounding our neurons, called astrocytes and glial cells, actually get rid of toxins in our brain. The question is, when do they do it? What we're starting to see is that these toxins are removed from our brain when we go to sleep. Sleep is not only a time to get refreshed, but it's also a time for our brain to get rid of all the pollution it created throughout the day.

[00:17:30]
[00:18:00] Now, if we're not sleeping, then all of those toxins stay in the brain. When all of those toxins stay in the brain, what happens? One, our cells don't work so well. Two, they create more inflammation. Three, the ability of those cells to grow their axons like roots from a tree (be able to extend out), is reduced, because the environment they're in isn't as healthy as it should be. Sleep is becoming a real important time to get our brain's environment back to what's considered a more healthy, homeostatic place for neurons to function well.

The sleep issue really depends on the patient and what problems they're having. For example, we might have an adolescent come in who's going to bed at 10pm but he's not sleeping until 3am, and then the poor mother or father can't wake their kid up in the morning. You have to kind of go deeper to see what's going on. He's going to bed at 10pm. Is he lying in bed trying to sleep that whole time or is he doing other stuff?

[00:18:30] Now, for most teens, they're usually doing other things. They've got their new best friend, the cell phone where they're texting all their friends. They're back up on the computer playing all sorts of online games or they're talking with their friends. You start with the simple things. Now, some people actually do, I think, have some biochemical problems with sleep, so then you have to start asking, biologically, what can be done?

[00:19:00] Now, ideally, I like to start with melatonin first, and see if that doesn't help. The interesting thing about melatonin is we used to use pretty low doses (three milligrams). We're actually starting to give 5 to 10 milligrams a couple of times at night. We're also finding out melatonin is doing other things to help the brain besides just sleep, in terms of repair. It's another whole unique topic. Valerian root, we
[00:19:30] can use that a lot for sleep, theanine, another supplement. If those don't work, then we can start looking at maybe some medications like Trazodone or Belsomra to help patients get a deeper, richer—stage three or four—non-REM sleep.

I am at a point where I want to write a book, and there are several ways I can go with that. My first
[00:20:00] one I would do strictly for free. I thought, "Well, who's the group that really needs a book and it can help the most?" My first thought was prison inmates. Unbeknownst to most people in terms of data, 85% of people in prison have substance abuse problems—*85%*. That's huge, which means if you were able to solve the substance abuse problem, what would that do to tax dollars spent on our country's prisons? Where else could we use that money?

[00:20:30] There's a seven times higher rate of traumatic brain injuries among people in the prison system than outside, so are these people who've been jailed really bad people? Or instead, do they just have bad brains? If they do indeed have bad brains, which perhaps means, if 85% of them have substance abuse problems, that would certainly lean towards maybe having a bad brain, would it not be in our best
[00:21:00] interest to try to help them rehabilitate their brains to get them healthy?

Hence, that's where the book, *Escape*, came from. The book can be downloaded for free from my website, in case anyone wants, **www.drjayfaber.com**. I wrote it *pro bono* because the people who need it the most can't afford it. It's there for those patients to use or anyone to use, for that matter.
[00:21:30] Families have found the book helpful, as well. There are basically five principles, nothing rocket science about them in terms of their ideation. In terms of implementation, that's sort of where everything is.

We talk a lot about your peer group, who you hang around with, who your friends are, your
[00:22:00] environment, socially. We talk a lot about substance abuse and the need to stay sober. We talk a lot about self-esteem and how to start feeling good about yourself and challenging yourself to feel good about yourself. We talk a lot about self-improvement, how to develop and grow each day to make yourself a better person. We take all those concepts and put them in one book. We used stories that are, from my perspective, more culturally relevant and trendy. There's a story about, for example, Elon
[00:22:30] Musk and how that Tesla battery was made, which is fascinating. We talked about "Man in the Mirror," the Michael Jackson song, and how that was created. We then take entertaining stories, and go deeper, penetrating people's brains, and, also, I think, their hearts, to make them better people.

I think the prisons are starting to get it. The California Department of Corrections just commenced a
[00:23:00] $103 million plan to help do intervention work to help these individuals. The big question is: "What's the biggest bang for your buck?" The prison systems are getting individuals coming at them with all sorts of really good ideas. I think the question is, "What makes the most sense? How can you implement the most effective plan at the cheapest dollar rate?" We'll see where that unravels.

[00:23:30] With stem cells and where medicine is going, it's really exciting. Twenty years ago, we thought if you lived till 75, 76, you've had a good life. Well, with all the things coming in medicine, the likelihood of you living to 95 to 100 and having a great quality of life has gone way up. I would encourage you to
[00:24:00] optimize your body, and for my specialty, your brain, to get it to work at its best so you can have all the great experiences as you get older that perhaps people two decades ago couldn't do.

Some of the principles I talked about earlier—diet, exercise, thinking youthfully, thinking diversely—can really help so that when you're 85 or 90, you're still having a blast with life. A parent, and this was when I was living at Atlanta, brought her 30-something-year-old kid who'd been using drugs, selling
[00:24:30] drugs, living on the streets, having all sorts of problems trying to stay away from the cops, to our

office. In general, the prognosis for someone who's not very motivated to get better is pretty poor.

[00:25:00] Well, this kid came in, and it was kind of like what I expected. He was more what I'd call in a pre-contemplative state of change, which is fine. We'll take people where they're at and accept them and we kind of walk them through a process. I got to know him. I showed him his pictures. From all this drug use, the surface of his brain was really bumpy, and he got it. He's like, "Oh, my gosh. There is something here I can finally see that's not necessarily right."

[00:25:30] We put him on a brain plan. He went home, came back to see me a month later and he said, "Well, I didn't use drugs or alcohol for a month." I said, "That's pretty dang good." I was, to be quite honest, pretty surprised, and he said, "I went on the diet. I've lost 15, 20 pounds." I said out of curiosity, "Of all the things that got you motivated, what was the most motivating?" He said, "Well, losing the weight. I could actually see some changes." I go, "That's interesting." So, if they can see something, it helps.

I had him come back a month later. He was continuing to work out at the gym. He's doing better. I said, "Come back and see me in three months." He came back in three months, still sober, going to meetings, and he was taking a training seminar to become a certified fitness trainer at the local gym. Fantastic. Patted him on the back. He stayed away from drugs, was growing, moving forward. Then, I said, "Come back and see me in six months."

[00:26:00]

[00:26:30] Six months, and this is where it gets crazy. He says, "I'm working at a gym. I'm a certified trainer and now, I want to go on the Navy SEALs." Now, this is a kid, six months before, who was living on the streets selling drugs, and by following a brain plan, for just that short period of time, wanted to join the Navy SEALs. This is powerful. This is special. Now, I didn't see him for a while. He came back about a year later and he's back in college. He hadn't joined the Navy SEALs. He was having a few struggles, but he was off the brain plan. We got him back on. Last, I know, he's doing fine.

[00:27:00] The scoop is this: if we can take a kid off the streets selling drugs and get him motivated enough by following a structured brain plan to be a Navy SEAL, what persons or what parents would not want their loved ones to get involved with a program like that? There's hope and there's optimism and there's change if we do the things that help us feel, think, and behave better.

JEFFREY BLAND, PhD, FACN | Founder, Institute for Functional Medicine

Dr. Mark Hyman: Jeff, you've been described as the father of Functional Medicine. We are going to talk about this incredible model of brain plasticity, which is how the brain can respond differently to different inputs, and actually change the structure and function of the brain. The idea of Functional Medicine and brain

[00:00:30] plasticity has been around for a long time. You mentioned that 25 years ago, you presented the first Linus Pauling Award at the Institute for Functional Medicine to a man who demonstrated the reversal of severe brain damage in children, which was unheard of before. How do you see the Functional Medicine movement and brain plasticity movement sort of coming together, and changing the way we think about the brain function and how we practice medicine?

[00:01:00]

Dr. Jeffrey Bland: Well, Mark, I think you just really put your finger on one of the greatest and most important advances that we're seeing in the whole of health sciences. You know, when we went to school—certainly when I did, which was a few years before you—we learned about neuroanatomy as the brain had these fixed places for speech, vision, and hearing, and we have these brain maps where, supposedly, specific functions were located.

Dr. Mark Hyman: That whole Broca's brain model, right?

Dr. Jeffrey Bland: Exactly, yes. And if a person with that brain got injured you would supposedly lose that function,
[00:01:30] right?

Dr. Mark Hyman: If you took too many drugs in college you were in trouble.

Dr. Jeffrey Bland: Or too many fraternity parties, or whatever. So, it was a very kind of what you would call deterministic model of the brain, so there was nothing you could do about it. The brain didn't repair itself, it didn't heal itself. If you lost so many neurons on a Friday night you weren't going to get them back the next week, and that was a very kind of discouraging model about the way the brain functioned.

[00:02:00]

Dr. Mark Hyman: Sort of a fatalistic model, right?

Dr. Jeffrey Bland: Very much so. Neurology kind of grew up with that as a paradigm shift, I mean a paradigm concept saying the best we can do is to take these people that are injured, and we'll make them comfortable, and we'll keep their symptoms suppressed, and we'll try to make their life as good as possible, but there's nothing we can really do once the brain is injured. Now what has happened since?

Dr. Mark Hyman: It's unbelievable.

Dr. Jeffrey Bland: It is just unbelievable because now we're saying, no, actually the brain is plastic. It's able to respond to
[00:02:30] trauma. It can heal itself. It can move stuff around that was in one place that has been injured to another place that's still well, and it can improve its function, but it has to be in the right environment to do so. This is a very key concept, right? That the function of the brain like the function of the whole body is dependent upon the environment of the enrichment of that environment. What does enrichment mean?

[00:03:00]

Dr. Mark Hyman: I want an enriched brain.

Dr. Jeffrey Bland: That's right. It's use it or lose it, isn't it?

Dr. Mark Hyman:	Yeah.
Dr. Jeffrey Bland:	We think if we want to train our muscles to be strong or fast or endure then we have to have certain kinds of training. We didn't think of the brain that way. But now suddenly with this plasticity model, we're saying, no, hold it, we can design specific tailored therapies for individuals to exercise their brain in a certain way to generate neurogenesis.
Dr. Mark Hyman:	That's like create some brain cells.
Dr. Jeffrey Bland:	Exactly, right.
Dr. Mark Hyman:	So, we can actually create new brain cells.
Dr. Jeffrey Bland: [00:03:30] [00:04:00]	Which was thought of to be impossible when I was in medical school, and I think this is so uplifting. Now you might say, "Well, that's a great little concept, but is there any proof of the concept?" This is where we get into some really exciting stuff because for the first time, we're starting to see proof in clinical practice of what were considered irreversible brain injuries and it goes back really to what you talked about 25 years ago when we gave Glenn Doman the first Linus Pauling Functional Medicine Award. He and his group worked at the Institute for the Achievement of Human Potential in Philadelphia with over a million families of brain injured children teaching their brains how to heal—just unbelievably important stuff.
Dr. Mark Hyman:	I was reviewing the presentation you're giving at the annual conference for Functional Medicine and I was amazed to see the number of recoveries in terms of walking, speaking, writing, reading, lack of seizure ... just tremendous changes that we don't even see in conventional medicine; they're absent.
[00:04:30] Dr. Jeffrey Bland:	Absolutely, and you know it's interesting. There are no coincidences in our lives, as you and I have grown up together, what we've witnessed are meeting people that we think is coincidental that we've met them that have changed our view of the way that the body works and how it functions.
Dr. Mark Hyman:	And meeting you.
Dr. Jeffrey Bland: [00:05:00]	Well, vice versa, right? Then we say, "Hold it. Was that really a coincidence, or was I on a guided path because maybe I'm just seeking out the kind of people that will help me to understand?" When I met Glenn Doman, which was a coincidence, we were both speakers at a meeting in Philadelphia and he preceded me on the program. I listened to this 70-year-old senior wise-sage-talk about the reality of dealing with a million brain-injured children over the course of 50 years, and I sat there thinking, "I'm going to be speaking next. I have nothing to offer."
[00:05:30]	I mean this is like paradigm-shifting incredible revolutionary stuff, so I then was fortunate enough after that, and he must have liked my talk because he came up, and he said, "Jeff, you need to be on our Medical Advisory Board." So, I spent 20 years being on the Medical Advisory Board of the Institute each year going to what they called their Graduation to Life ceremony. The Graduation to Life was where these children that had come in as infants often not speaking, no muscle coordination, serious injuries by the time they were 15 ...
Dr. Mark Hyman:	This wasn't just because of reading about diet or stress.
[00:06:00] Dr. Jeffrey Bland: [00:06:30]	Oh, no, this was super intervention where the parents were actively involved in the Institute's program, which was physical, mental, and nutritional intervention. I would see them at 12, 13, 14—these infants that were supposed to be institutionalized were doing complex gymnastics who are doing Shakespeare in Old English by memory, who are playing instruments—high-level musical instruments—in concert style. Of course, every year we would go to this we were in tears. I mean it was just like the most emotionally uplifting experience. The parents, obviously, had worked tirelessly with their kids to introduce these programs to get neuroplasticity to be real, so when I saw this I said, "There is very little that's impossible if we open our minds to the possibility." What the body is

capable of doing if it turns the genes on so that they can express their full function is beyond anything I think humans actually have previously understood, so that's the threshold where we find ourselves today.

[00:07:00]

Dr. Mark Hyman: It's extraordinary and just to kind of touch on your personal experience, your son Justin had a brain injury.

Dr. Jeffrey Bland: Yes, absolutely.

Dr. Mark Hyman: You saw it firsthand ... the impact of this.

Dr. Jeffrey Bland: Yes.

Dr. Mark Hyman: Tell us about that and how you came to work with Glenn around this and what actually happened.

Dr. Jeffrey Bland: Here again, there are no coincidences, right? I'm at this meeting, Glenn Doman speaks, I'm totally
[00:07:30] overwhelmed. I get on their medical advisory board, and my youngest son—I have three sons—had been told about him by his neurosurgeon that he probably would never go to school normally. He would probably not speak because he was born with a corpus callosum injury on birthing. He had an intraventricular bleed. He ended up having a shunt put in at three months and his prognosis looked very guarded.

Dr. Mark Hyman: So, he had a bleed in his brain that damaged his brain.

Dr. Jeffrey Bland: Absolutely.

[00:08:00]

Dr. Mark Hyman: He also had hydrocephalus, which is fluid on the brain.

Dr. Jeffrey Bland: The hydrocephalus was a secondary consequence of the fact he had scarring of the brain, so he couldn't filter his cerebrospinal fluid effectively and had brain pressure, so this was not a good outlook at all. He, fortunately, had a very good pediatric neurosurgeon, had an excellent shunt placement, but then the question is how is he going to respond because there is probably a very mixed response to
[00:08:30] infants that get shunts relative to their development. Well, to make a long story short as a consequence of me being introduced to Glenn Doman, and getting the institute's knowledge, we were able to get Justin to be involved in that program over the course.

Now he's 35 years old, just to give you a kind of context of time. He graduated from college with high marks. He worked for state senator Patty Murray in Washington, D.C. as a legislative aide. He's
[00:09:00] finishing his Masters in psychology because he wants to work with developmental issues in children. He is a model speaker for parents and families that have hydrencephalus, trying to help them understand that there's a potential for their children moving forward. He's going to be speaking with me at the Institute for Functional Medicine about his own experiences, and how he's been able to use brain plasticity to create his future.

Dr. Mark Hyman: That was an incredible story about your son, but I'm imagining there were specific things that had
[00:09:30] impact that were the most important and I'd love to hear about those.

Dr. Jeffrey Bland: The program that we're talking about this neuroplasticity approach is just like any kind of training program. It's not so easy. If you want to build strength and endurance, you have to be in a rigorous training program for your musculoskeletal system and it's the same thing for the brain, so this is not a casual program. The way Justin really entertained this, and he was supported by his family very
[00:10:00] significantly, and also through the Institute was a rigorous nutrition component.

Dr. Mark Hyman: Which was what?

Dr. Jeffrey Bland: Well, it was basically the things that we talk about in Functional Medicine all the time getting rid of sugar is eating closer to the earth. More plant foods, more phytochemicals, making sure that you get

[00:10:30]

[00:11:00]

the low glycemic index and staying away from additives and preservatives. It's all the stuff that we talk about in the Institute for Functional Medicine. Then the movement part of the program was really designed to pattern your brain starting with creeping and crawling, which seems very strange when you're talking about someone that's already walking to go back and start creeping and then crawling to re-pattern the physical movements of your brain because the construct of the Institute's program was that there's an interrelationship between movement and function that goes beyond just musculoskeletal that you're really patterning the brain to be more plastic to accept and to collateralize things into parts of the brain that are not damaged.

[00:11:30]

[00:12:00]

This creeping and crawling and then strength building ... a lot of cardiopulmonary because the concept is that a brain that has been injured is probably oxygen deprived and is the reason it's been injured, so you want to deliver as much oxygen to the brain. Remember that the brain, although it's 6% the body weight approximately, it consumes over 25% of the blood sugar and probably something like 30% of oxygen that the body processes because it's so hungry for oxygen and food nutrients. This program is designed to improve cardiopulmonary function getting more oxygen to the brain, getting better vascular function so there's a lot of conditioning that goes on, and then there is the last part of it, which is the mental conditioning working with various kinds of tools to improve. Justin had strabismus, which is the ability almost not to be able to see 3D. You see everything in 2D; it's flat. Could you imagine living in a flat world? I mean, it really makes things very complicated.

[00:12:30]

[00:13:00]

There are ways to train the brain how to be able to start to see in 3D, so he practiced that with these various tools they had and it was an "aha" for him. In fact, I remember the day that he first said, "Oh, my word, I didn't recognize I wasn't seeing in 3D. Now there's so much depth to the world. I'm actually now being able to see that there are things within the context of the field of vision that I didn't even fully understand before." I think these are the kind of things that go on with intent. They don't happen overnight. It progresses for a while. It's like almost isometric exercises you don't think you're doing anything, and then all of a sudden—boom!—you breakthrough and you get to the next level. The brain is a tough critter. It doesn't change easily, but it will change with the appropriate amount of conditioning and training.

Dr. Mark Hyman:

That's extraordinary. We just heard about a dichotomy between how traditional/conventional medicine approaches the brain, and Functional Medicine. Can you explain that difference, and what are the features of Functional Medicine that are the most different, and how do they work so well for the brain?

Dr. Jeffrey Bland:
[00:13:30]

[00:14:00]

Well, I think you and I have shared collaboratively this extraordinarily robust enrichment of this model that we came up with in the early 1990s called Functional Medicine. I want to credit you with putting a huge amount of the real, what I would call, sophistication and clinical understanding of that concept that we had kind of birth without really knowing whether it was going to prove clinically to be as successful as we thought it might, so what is the concept? The concept is that every disease that medicine deals with has a preclinical phase that's associated with altered function that you cannot have any disease in the absence of some altered function. Even an infectious disease has something to do with the function in the immune system because we know if you expose a classroom of kids to a flu virus you might have three-quarters of the kids who get the flu virus, but a quarter of the kids don't.

[00:14:30]

[00:15:00]

What was the function of their immune system that allowed them to prevent getting the flu when all the other kids did, so we know that there are across all conditions crisis diseases as well as chronic diseases there's a functional component that ultimately arrives at a state of dysfunction that we can finally put a name on it, and call it a disease, right? It's a number, it gets reimbursed and it gets a specific protocol for its treatment, so if you really want to deal with understanding the origin of disease you must understand the function we felt, and you just don't deal with the pathology, which is the end stage. Well, that was then requiring us to say where does the function start, or where does the dysfunction start? The dysfunction doesn't start just in one organ. The dysfunction may start at a place that's distant to where you ultimately diagnose it.

Dr. Mark Hyman:	Right, so the headache doesn't start in your head.
Dr. Jeffrey Bland:	That's exactly right. That's a good example.
Dr. Mark Hyman:	A joint thing doesn't start in your joints.
Dr. Jeffrey Bland:	Right, so you might even say a problem with sleep disturbances is not just your sleep center or your brain is off if your gut is having a problem it's sending signals to your brain, right?
Dr. Mark Hyman:	That's right.

[00:15:30]

| Dr. Jeffrey Bland: | I think this construct that we're a system of biology, we're not just a set of collected organ parts that get stuck together like plumbing gets done. I would call it at the time was a fairly novel concept because we all learned medicine in a differential diagnostic way about each organ by itself. We'd study it, we're good at that, we'd close the book, we take a test, and then we move onto the next organ, right? |

[00:16:00]

Dr. Mark Hyman:	I always say if you know the name of your diagnosis you don't necessarily know what's wrong with you.
Dr. Jeffrey Bland:	That's right.
Dr. Mark Hyman:	Or what's causing it.
Dr. Jeffrey Bland:	Functional Medicine was really to try to ask the question not what you call what you get, but where it came from, which seems very simplistic to say, but quite honestly, we had all studied so much how to recite on demand what the name of the stuff was you got, but we didn't really know much of where it came from.

[00:16:30]

| Dr. Mark Hyman: | That's the evolution of medicine is our deeper understanding of the causes, but we haven't applied that clinically, right? |
| Dr. Jeffrey Bland: | Exactly right. Thank you for saying that because I think that's an important point. This sounds a little bit like "holier than thou" like we designed, or developed, something in the vacuum all by ourselves, and that wasn't the real case. What was going on when I was in premed, and then medical, and then my PhD work in the 60s. Basically, if you asked did we know the cause of most chronic diseases, heart disease, diabetes, cancer, arthritis, the answer is no. We could describe them very well. We had good diagnostic criteria for them, but we didn't really understand their origin, so it was hard to be functionally based say in the 60s because we didn't have the biological explanations for these. |

[00:17:00]

| | Things changed quite dramatically from 1970 to 2000, in which the biology of many of these conditions started to be understood and we call that the etiology of the cause, so we started to be able to understand where things like heart disease arose from alterations in vascular function. The word function started to slip more and more into the lexicon of the medical world in which by the time we founded the Institute for Functional Medicine in 1991, we had a foundation of good biological sciences upon which we could say, "Here are the ways that dysfunction can arise ultimately to produce a disease." That was then understanding the cause rather than just the effect. |

[00:17:30]

[00:18:00]

Dr. Mark Hyman:	Functional Medicine is medicine by cause not just symptoms, right?
Dr. Jeffrey Bland:	Exactly right.
Dr. Mark Hyman:	It's the medicine of why we get sick instead of just what disease do we have that we can describe.
Dr. Jeffrey Bland:	When you think of a disorder like type 2 diabetes—let's say we had 100 type 2 diabetic patients.

They had all been diagnosed, and they all had undergone the proper assessment, and all the docs agreed these had type 2 diabetes. Would they all be the same patient?

Dr. Mark Hyman: No.

Dr. Jeffrey Bland: [00:18:30] Of course they wouldn't; it would be 100 different variations on the theme, so then you say, "What are these variations?" We have to understand the journey that each of those patients were on relative to their function, so that we could treat them individually, and that's precise, personalized health care, which is where we're going right now.

Dr. Mark Hyman: In the brain, you've got Alzheimer's or Parkinson's...those are just named after the guy who described the symptoms.

Dr. Jeffrey Bland: That's exactly right.

Dr. Mark Hyman: [00:19:00] It doesn't tell you the differences between patients with Alzheimer's or Parkinson's. It doesn't tell you the cause. It doesn't give you any map to navigate how to fix these patients because it's simply descriptive of the cause. We talk about basal ganglia, and the Parkinson's being damaged, and not able to produce dopamine in mitochondrial injury, but we don't ask what's causing it or why. The same thing with Alzheimer's. After I got into Functional Medicine, I went back and read *Robbins and* [00:19:30] *Cotran*, which is the pathologic basis of disease that all medical students read in their second year of medical school. Chapter one said, "Every pathologic change is preceded by a biochemical change."

Dr. Jeffrey Bland: Yes.

Dr. Mark Hyman: Functional Medicine is reinvigorating. We learned, for example, in medical school that we should study the Krebs cycle as part of our initiation, but it would never be meaningful clinically, and yet it's one of the most important things I look at when I'm treating a patient now.

Dr. Jeffrey Bland: Exactly.

Dr. Mark Hyman: [00:20:00] We've changed our whole approach to this and I think it's particularly applicable to the brain because I always say the brain has only so many ways of saying ouch. You get fatigue, you get brain fog, you get memory issues, you can get diseases like Parkinson's, depression, anxiety, ADHD, autism. These are sort of the ways the brain manifests, but the question is: what is driving all that? That's where Functional Medicine gives us a roadmap to start clinically treating these people. Based on what you said, and what you taught me, and the movement has taught me is that I can apply this with patients even if I've never seen that type of thing before I can actually create a roadmap to fix the things that [00:20:30] could be causes without even knowing if it was going to work, and it has worked.

Dr. Jeffrey Bland: Now you're talking about what David Deutsch, the Don at Cambridge, said in his book *The Fabric of Reality*—which is so powerful—in which he pointed out that medicine is a young science. As a [00:21:00] consequence, it's still fairly descriptive. It hasn't yet got into being so predictive because it doesn't understand the first principles of this case, but he said, "What is going on right now is a revolution in understanding the principles that underlie what we call disease." As it evolves over the course of the next decades, we will then become like all other sciences, a predictive science based on first principles, and when so doing we'll do exactly what you said, and we'll be able to predict the outcome of therapies that were never before tested based upon first principles and understanding of the mechanisms.

[00:21:30] That is what systems biology, and what Functional Medicine, is all about. It really is harnessing and accessing this new knowledge that we have that allows us to understand the aggregating principles that lead to what we later call disease in the individual. You actually said something very interesting, I think, when you were talking about the Krebs cycle, so I want to go back there for a moment if I can— to the origin of Functional Medicine back in 1990. At that point in time when we were thinking about [00:22:00] the brain we were saying, well, how does a brain produce its energy? It produces its energy principally by the metabolism of sugar of glucose, right? It's what's called a glycolytic organ, meaning it breaks down sugar to produce energy. How does it do that? It does it in the neurons in cells that possess an energy powerhouse called the mitochondria. All cells have mitochondria, but those cells that are undergoing a lot of energy production have more mitochondria.

[00:22:30]

Dr. Mark Hyman: The brain has the most, right?

Dr. Jeffrey Bland: The heart has the most, actually. 75% of the cardiocyte is occupied by mitochondria because the heart has to be working all the time, but the brain is right up there, too. It has a lot of mitochondria in the neurons, so then in 1990, we started to say, "If the brain has all these mitochondria, and those mitochondria are fed by different kinds of things including all the nutrients that are necessary for support of the Krebs cycle and the glycolytic pathways that produce energy, then maybe some of these brain problems are a consequence of the alteration and nutritional status, or the way that certain individuals process energy." We started looking at mitochondrial, or neurological disorders. Lo and behold as it turns out now—some 27 years later—we were right on target. Now the big revolution is mitochondrial diseases as it associates with encephalopathies and brain chemistry.

[00:23:00]

Dr. Mark Hyman: From autism to Parkinson's.

Dr. Jeffrey Bland: That's right.

Dr. Mark Hyman: Alzheimer's.

[00:23:30]

Dr. Jeffrey Bland: Here's a first principle concept that underlies many different named diseases, so you study the concept because you want to treat the cause not just the effect.

Dr. Mark Hyman: I had a personal experience with this with a broken brain really, because this is really how I got into Functional Medicine. I got very sick and ended up with chronic fatigue, which is an energy problem based on the mitochondria, but it also affected my brain. I couldn't focus, I couldn't sleep, I couldn't remember anything. I had depression, anxiety, all these things that were really new to me that all of a sudden happened as a result of it turned out to be mercury, which is a very potent neurotoxin, mitochondrial toxin. I got it from living in China and being exposed to huge amounts of pollution and cleaning out an air filter everyday plus tons of fish and fillings, and a whole array of things that really had an impact on my biology. It affected my immune system, gut, brain, and the mitochondria involved in all of those things.

[00:24:00]

[00:24:30]

I was actually recently speaking with a guest from Harvard—they're studying mitochondria and inflammatory bowel disease, so it's sort of an underlying concept of Functional Medicine we've been doing for years. By applying this model, I was able to recover my brain function. I was able to write 14 books after. I was able to lead many initiatives and build my practice and clinic and speak around the world. I felt like I had to share this because it was something that wasn't fixable. Chronic fatigue is not fixable. Memory issues usually are not fixable. The cognitive impairment I had was so great that I always thought I was destined to this, but I realized this wasn't destiny. I didn't understand the science behind how to fix it and that's really what Functional Medicine provides is a roadmap to do that.

[00:25:00]

Dr. Jeffrey Bland: [00:25:30] Yes, I think that the experience of life is a great teacher if we're willing to learn, right? We have to be a receptive student, and it's always interesting to me how some people like yourself are really good students of life both from what they observe, and the patients, and other people around them, and what they observe in their own life. They access that, and they use that as tools to gain greater wisdom and move forward. Other people make observations and it doesn't seem to be encoded at all in their learning experience.

[00:26:00] I'm always amazed at the practitioners we have in Functional Medicine—they seem to be very good students of themselves. They're really listening, they're conscious, they're out there, and they're saying—now—hold it. This doesn't all make sense what I was told here, because my personal observation and experience says something different; let's see if I can rationalize that. This whole new field of what I would call functional neurology—again—I want to take a sidebar and say when we developed the term "functional," I had a lot of pushback actually from my colleagues about that term because they said, "Well Jeff, you really don't want to call this Functional Medicine."

Dr. Mark Hyman: It's all in your head like functional valency, right?

[00:26:30]
Dr. Jeffrey Bland: Yes, it's really psychosomatic or it's geriatric; it's related to parts of our body that are broken down. It's not a very enlightened term, but what I recognized was in the late 80s, early 90s was that we started to see the medical literature, functional neurology, functional radiology, functional cardiology, functional endocrinology. People were using the term in a different way, and I said, "Maybe we ought to be skating where the puck is going, and maybe we will find over the years to come that functional is actually a really redefined term."

[00:27:00]
Dr. Mark Hyman: That's what we all want is optimal function.

Dr. Jeffrey Bland: That's right. Exactly.

Dr. Mark Hyman: We don't want the absence of disease, we want enrichment, as you said.

Dr. Jeffrey Bland: When I started looking at functional neurology, which was really coming out of new radiological technologies like SPECT scanning and PET scanning, so one could actually start examining the brain's function in ways we never had access before, and starting to see certain portions of the brain would light up with certain kinds of stimuli, and we could actually start doing studies to see how you would alter brain function in intact human beings without having to take out their brains and do surgery.

[00:27:30]

Dr. Mark Hyman: That's how they used to do surgery—they'd poke a needle in the brain, trigger it, and see if the arm moved, right?

Dr. Jeffrey Bland: Precisely.

Dr. Mark Hyman: Crude.

Dr. Jeffrey Bland: Now we have an ability to do roadmaps and brain mapping, basically, using these technologies. What happened was the consolidation or convergence of that with genomic testing, now we start to see people that have certain genes maybe have different ways that their brains function. The first way we made an exciting breakthrough there was with Huntington's Disease. It was a major Nobel Prize-winning discovery that there was this specific mutation of this gene that would lead into Huntington's Disease.

[00:28:00]

Dr. Mark Hyman: Which is a movement disorder with sort of weird strange movements, right?

[00:28:30]
Dr. Jeffrey Bland: Exactly, and ultimate death that's right. I think it gave people, unfortunately, the Huntington's example—the thought that all of these brain things were single genes and that we all just had to find the gene that was mutated and we'd be able to understand brain disease. Well, it turns out that, yes, there are some of these monogenic neurological disorders that is true, but they're very infrequent, and very rare in the population at large compared to depression, anxiety, schizophrenia, autism, and conditions that are related to dementia, so where are those diseases coming from? They're coming from polygenic multiple genes working together in ways to interact with the environment to create the outcome that we later call these diseases, so they are functional disorders, right? They're not pathologic disorders to the same extent that you would see with Huntington's Disease.

[00:29:00]

[00:29:30] I think we're seeing a transition right now from where genes are thought to be the cause of mental illness to where genes are part of the way our body responds to its environment to give rise to the function of our nervous system. Now, that to me is a very big shift in thinking because now it opens up the door for all sorts of new studies, new therapies, new optimistic ways of saying, "Well, hold it.

[00:30:00]	You didn't get a death certificate with a kind of gene that's just telling you how you're going to die." It's really genes that are telling you how you're going to live and what are the environments that will optimize your brain's function, so that you won't have early-stage-loss of whatever function you are concerned about.

Dr. Mark Hyman: This reminds me of a patient I had early on where I took the principles of Functional Medicine, applied them, and I studied his genetics. We looked at genetics of detoxification how do you get rid of

[00:30:30] environmental toxins, glutathione genes. We looked at genes that regulate methylation, which is a critical pathway in the body that's responsible for almost every function from gene regulation to neurotransmitter function to detoxification, and it's the B-vitamins, basically folate, B6, and B12; mostly methylation issues. We found all these things in this guy that we actually used to treat him, so

[00:31:00] we found he had a high load of toxins from years of fish and fillings, living in Pittsburgh. I mean, everybody from Pittsburgh at my practice is mercury toxic because they use coal ash in the steel plants to cover the farms and to cover the streets in the winter from ice.

I applied the principles. He had gut issues and inflammation, so all these things were compounded. I found the clinical expression of his genes and I just treated everything. We literally reversed his Alzheimer's. He went from basically drooling in a corner to running his company again, and I was like

[00:31:30] "What?" I mean it was the principle like David Deutsch I'd never done that before and I just apply these concepts. The recovery was extraordinary. Same thing with Parkinson's—we've seen arresting, or even reversing of Parkinson's. We've seen reversal of autism. We've seen reversal of depression, anxiety, even schizophrenia an enormous impact just applying these principles. I'd never seen a schizophrenic through the lens of Functional Medicine before. I tried it and it worked, so I began to realize that combining this idea of functional genomics with functional neurology and psychiatry was

[00:32:00] really the future of how we have to deal with the brain.

Dr. Jeffrey Bland: Thank you. I think you really said it beautifully. As you're speaking, I'm thinking about the incredible work that's been done by Moshe Szyf and his group, and his colleague Dr. Meaney at McGill University up in Montreal, Canada, looking at the epigenetics of brain patterning because this concept that you're talking about of how the brain genes are influenced by the environment often leads to

[00:32:30] what are called these epigenetic marks. It doesn't change the genes. It changes how the genes are marked with specific things including methyl groups that come from the methylation patterns you're talking about that then alter the way the genes are expressed, so what they have found in these studies are just remarkable. In fact, one that's been most recently talked about are the so-called ice babies ... maybe you're familiar with them.

[00:33:00] The ice babies were babies that were born after this huge ice storm in Canada that caused power outages and families couldn't leave their homes for some time. Women that were pregnant at the time were subjected to very high stress. They couldn't get to the store. It was weeks of isolation, so they had a very high stress experience at a time of critical development of their infant in utero, and what they found is that these ice babies—that were born after this situation—were those that had a

[00:33:30] very high-stress-prone archetype, and they started looking at the methylation patterns on their white blood cells. They found that they were epigenetically marked probably as a consequence of the in-utero psychological stress experience of their mothers that then created in the infant a change in the patterns of their neurochemistry.

[00:34:00] Think of the implications of that, right? We're not talking just about nutrition or about exercise. We're talking about the psychosocial environment, high stress, traumatic. Think about posttraumatic stress syndrome, so they've done extraordinary numbers of controlled studies in animals showing that stressful environments can actually modulate how brains are expressed in terms of their function. Now that opens up the door for us again to think about how do you repattern these epigenetic ...

Dr. Mark Hyman: You can modify those.

Dr. Jeffrey Bland: That's right, because the scientists call these Metastable epialleles.

Dr. Mark Hyman: That's a mouthful.

Dr. Jeffrey Bland:
[00:34:30]

That really is, meaning that they are not stuck on permanently. They can be put on and taken off based upon the environment and the experience that the individuals confronted. Now, they may be fairly stuck, so you might have to work hard like I was talking about with my son Justin, or they might be simply stuck, and you can make a change in the function by just changing diet.

Dr. Mark Hyman:

That's not a pause for me because what you're saying is so revolutionary that you can actually modify your gene expression.

Dr. Jeffrey Bland:

Yes.

Dr. Mark Hyman:
[00:35:00]

That if you've been dealt a bad hand by your environment, by stress, by other factors, that by strategic interventions using nutrition, lifestyle, exercise, and stress reduction, sleep and even detoxification, and optimizing nutritional status you can literally shift your genes into a health pattern instead of a disease pattern.

Dr. Jeffrey Bland:
[00:35:30]

[00:36:00]

That's exactly right, and this is the revolutionary concept I believe in the 21st century that we're talking about because in the brain where we have thought for so many decades of its rigidity, of its determinism to now see that actually these brain functions can be modulated based on environment by enriching the environment and practicing the right things. This is a hugely uplifting optimistic opportunity to recreate the whole field of neurology, the whole field of neurosciences because it's now recognized that maybe many children who are brain injured that we thought, "Well, they're just destined to be that, and we'll give them a good environment that makes them comfortable," so we kind of had this laissez-faire attitude that was really not appropriate at all. They needed to be put into an environment with extraordinary enrichment to get dendritic branching, to get synaptogenesis. What does that mean in English? What it means is you can actually increase the cortical thickness of the brain, the executive center of the brain, by enriched environment.

Dr. Mark Hyman:

You grow new tendrils or new neurons.

Dr. Jeffrey Bland:

Grow new neurons. That's exactly right.

Dr. Mark Hyman:

Increase the connectivity between them.

[00:36:30]
Dr. Jeffrey Bland:

Precisely, even in damaged tissue, and they've demonstrated this beautifully. Dr. Marian Diamond, maybe you're familiar with her work at UC Berkeley, just extraordinary pioneering work in controlled studies and enriched environment with animals showing with neuroanatomy brain synaptogenesis, and increased cortical thickening. In fact, she was the one that did some of the neuroanatomy of Einstein's brain and got sections of his brain to do studies on showing this thing about complexity of the neurogenesis and how it influences brain plasticity.

[00:37:00]
Dr. Mark Hyman:

Einstein had a lot more connections.

Dr. Jeffrey Bland:

That's right. He didn't have a bigger brain, but he had a more connected brain, right? You can make more connections by practicing the right things. So, these are like extraordinary, empowering opportunities to recreate the whole field of neuroscience, and neurology, and get away from this deterministic model that once damaged is forever there.

Dr. Mark Hyman:
[00:37:30]

What about the genes that make the most difference that we can modify? What are the nutritional genomics, if you will, or lifestyle genomics, or environmental genomics that can actually start to shift the brain into a different pattern recovery?

Dr. Jeffrey Bland:

[00:38:00]

I think you already started alluding to it. The first gene seekers with brain disease were those that were seeking the monogenetic diseases like Huntington's, so if you go into the genetic literature you will find literally hundreds of papers in which the gene seekers were looking for a gene that was connected to a neurological disease. As I said, there are literally hundreds, probably, of different neurological diseases that are very uncommon, but are associated with a specific gene, but they as a

[00:38:30] whole represent but a small fraction of the overall neurological problem. So, then the next level, which is where we are now, is to say, "What is it that actually controls the brain function?" We recognize that the brain is made up of two principle types of cells what are the so-called neurons, which we think was the business end of the brain.

[00:39:00] Then the other were the glue-like cells called the glia and when I learned neuroanatomy we were thinking that the glia, the microglia, in the brain were just to glue the neurons together, so that they could do the work. Now we recognize that the microglia is the brain's immune system. The brain's immune system is very important in determining its function, so some of the genes that regulate brain function are related to glial function related to the brain's immune function, neuroinflammation, neuroimmunity, so now we're starting to look at families of genes that regulate function, genes that regulate the insulin sensitivity in the brain, genes that are related to inflammatory signaling the brain, genes that are related to synaptogenesis, and neurogenesis in the brain, right? Brain-derived neuro factor, BDNF, these particular genes now are becoming the center of the complex understanding of [00:39:30] how the brain functions. Rather than just looking at single genes that cause small diseases, we're looking at the families of genes that regulate brain function.

Dr. Mark Hyman: The more you have of these altered genes the more likely you are to get in trouble.

Dr. Jeffrey Bland: That's right.

Dr. Mark Hyman: I mean I had this patient I was telling you about he had ApoE4—which is the Alzheimer's gene, which is not a fixed gene; not everybody with ApoE4 gets Alzheimer's. So, the question is, "What was triggering it?" He had this huge exposure to mercury and we know that this gene on the protein chain [00:40:00] is missing an amino acid that's important for detoxification called cysteine, so you can't clear the mercury from your brain, so I had to, based on knowledge of this gene, and how it functioned I was able to support him with the amino acids and the nutrients to build up glutathione, which is the main detoxifier. We know that if you look at a cohort of people with ApoE4 they have much higher levels of metals.

Dr. Jeffrey Bland: Yes.

Dr. Mark Hyman: Let's talk about metals for a minute because I think in medicine we sort of ignore it like unless you [00:40:30] have an acute toxicity, whether you're poisoned by lead, or you have heavy metals that you're exposed to in an occupational way, you know, you're in an occupational environment that has other metals then, okay, we acknowledge it, but we don't have a great way of treating it except avoidance. In Functional Medicine, we understand that there's a low-level impact of these things that can happen over decades for smaller levels.

[00:41:00]
Dr. Jeffrey Bland: Let's talk for a moment about this neurotoxicology area because this is a really important additional advancement in our understanding. In the 1980s and the 1990s, neurotoxicology was principally related to acute toxicity where the brain cells would be killed as a consequence of the exposure to some kind of a drug or traumatic toxin, however, what was growing up in the late 80s and 90s and [00:41:30] into the 21st century was this other view of chronic neurotoxicology just like chronic immune problems as kind of a concept. We started to see chronic neurotoxicology growing up as a field, and the reason it was growing up is that people finally had the ability to measure in the laboratory the effect of low levels of toxins on neurological function, so here's another example of where Functional [00:42:00] Medicine started to get some scientific support.

As people started looking at the effect of sometimes part per million levels of certain things, which were not actually killing a cell directly, but were altering its function, they started to say, "There may be a whole other level here of activity of these compounds that are floating around in our body that [00:42:30] we never recognized that are injuring how a person functions and producing complex symptoms not just a disease." So that then led people to say, "What are the families of substances that might be low-level neurotoxicants that are altering neurological functions at a low level of impairment." Heavy metals came up as one of those important families. We know that acute exposure to mercury produces Mad Hatter Disease from Alice in Wonderland.

Dr. Mark Hyman: Because they used mercury to make the hats stiff.

[00:43:00]
Dr. Jeffrey Bland: Of hats, yes, so we know that the chronic exposure now as we started to study how neurological cells actually respond to part per million even part per billion levels of these we started to say, whoa, hold it. Much lower levels than we ever expected are altering function, and it's a sensitivity that might be also dependent upon certain genes. Certain genes may be more sensitive than other genes to these

[00:43:30] low levels, so that then led to a very interesting change in the medical legal world, because before toxicity was only related to acute toxic effects.

Now suddenly you could start saying patients were injured by exposure to some industrial chemical, or some pollutant at levels that were below acute toxicity, and those people that were throwing this in the environment could be considered liable for these symptoms. Now the field started to grow up with a whole different medical legal kind of interpretation of what toxicity is, and how people were

[00:44:00] impacted in negative ways. Heavy metals, not just mercury, but lead, cadmium, and arsenic, which is really not a heavy element, but is a toxic element that at low levels produces chronic symptomatologies, and have neurotoxic effects that are very complex that are often missed as you're pointing out.

Dr. Mark Hyman: They don't even know how to test for it.

Dr. Jeffrey Bland: That's exactly right, so what we're starting to see, in fact, I met a woman by the name of Vera Stejskal
[00:44:30] a number of years ago. I'm not sure if you know Dr. Stejskal, but she was at Astra, the Swedish large pharmaceutical company. She's an immunologist, and she actually was able to save one of their important drugs from being not approved because she found a way of studying its toxicity, and showing that it was actually not toxic to the immune system as some people thought. It wasn't going

[00:45:00] to get approved, so the leadership of the company was so pleased to have her make that discovery that they said, "Dr. Stejskal you can study whatever you want. We're going to give you your own laboratory in Stockholm at Karolinska, and you can do whatever you want."

She said, "I want to study heavy metal low-level toxicity." They said, "Go for it. We're giving you millions of dollars you can do whatever you want." So, she developed methods using whole white cell assays to evaluate different individuals low-level toxicity to cadmium, mercury, lead, arsenic, and it

[00:45:30] was unbelievable what she found. She found that the level that was producing adverse effects on the immune system in some of these individuals, and she also looked at nickel, palladium, and platinum. Some of these things that are found in Dell materials were found even in replacement joints that were considered inert were not inert at all. In some individuals at part per trillion levels they were producing immunological adverse effects in these individuals.

[00:46:00] She published a whole series of papers on this over the course of 10 years, and she developed a laboratory method for assessment using white cell analysis for looking at heavy metal toxicity that's revolutionized the concept of chronic immunotoxicity from heavy metals well below a million or more levels lower than had ever been previously recognized to have adverse effects. She showed that this effect could vary from person to person by orders of magnitude. One person might have no adverse

[00:46:30] effects. Another person at a much lower level had a significant effect, so this is a whole new frontier as to where Functional Medicine would see itself versus pathological toxicology.

Dr. Mark Hyman: Yeah, I think this is a very great point. I just want to bring it clinically for a minute because the idea that your immune system is driving brain dysfunction was really never a medical concept. We're seeing the neuroinflammation being a central concept now as so many diseases across the spectrum—from Alzheimer's to Parkinson's to autism—have tremendous amounts of inflammation in

[00:47:00] their brain to depression, which we thought was more of a psychological issue maybe driven by inflammatory factors from your gut, from infections, from toxins, so it's revolutionizing our way of thinking about it, but it hasn't really revolutionized our practice of medicine.

[00:47:30] [00:48:00]	In Functional Medicine, I treat all those conditions with extraordinary success by using this concept of neuroinflammation and neurotoxicology from this sort of emergent research. It's pretty compelling. I think we don't really understand and genetics are really critical, too. I mean we know that they did a study looking at the cohort of patients who were given fillings, kids, and plastic fillings, which is mercury fillings, and they followed these kids for a long period of time in a study. When you actually tested the genetics of these kids, the ones who had good detoxification genetics weren't really impacted by the mercury. The kids who had poor detox genetics, they had a seven-year developmental delay in their brain function compared to the kids who didn't have the mercury fillings.
Dr. Jeffrey Bland: [00:48:30]	You're making my brain just go wild because Dr. Michael Maes, who is a neurologist, psychiatrist, M.D., Ph.D in Belgium, has published a whole series of papers. It would be more than 30 now looking at the effect of chronic immunological activation on neurological function in his patients, and he is absolutely a believer that fibromyalgia, chronic fatigue syndrome, multiple chemical sensitivity, a whole series of different neurological conditions are really associated with neuroinflammation driven through the immune system, so you treat as you're saying the source of the inflammation, which could by the way, start in the gut as we well recognize.
[00:49:00] [00:49:30]	This also leads me coming back to heavy metals to one of the most extraordinary chapters I believe in understanding the brain the sensitivity to these heavy metals. You're probably familiar with the work that was done on lead and intelligence in children. That particular work, which started at Harvard Mass General with, I think, it was 2,146 children back in the 70s that were followed by the lead in the dentin of their deciduous teeth, so these are teeth that fall out and are replaced by adult teeth. They measured the lead in the dentin level, and they found that their ability to stay at task and to stay performing, meaning not ADHD, was inversely related to the level of lead in the dentin of the teeth.
Dr. Mark Hyman:	So, we have lead out of gas, and lead in paint.
Dr. Jeffrey Bland: [00:50:00] [00:50:30]	That's right, but through that process you're probably familiar that the individual who unfortunately recently passed away, the individual that did that work, that original work was under such pressure by the lead battery and lead industries that he lost his position. He ultimately went to Case Western and continued his work and published many more papers. Eventually, he was vindicated. They said, "He falsified his data." He hadn't falsified his data. He went up against four different times over a 20-year period of different people that were courts evaluating his data. It was always proven to be correct, but it was such resistance to accept the fact that lead could actually induce such a problem in children without producing anemia, and then the classic symptoms of acute lead toxicity, so this was all chronic. Ultimately, as you said, it did lead, by pressure, to the removal of lead from gasoline, which was a major source of lead exposure to children at the time, so I think that these are historically very powerful concepts that sometimes meet very great resistance in change.
Dr. Mark Hyman: [00:51:00]	You've got leading figures we'll be interviewing in the series like Suzanne Goh looking at autism and the role of toxins. You've got Dale Bredesen looking at toxins and the role in Alzheimer's, so we're seeing these concepts start to emerge in literature. But when you go to a doctor for autism or for Alzheimer's, they don't ask you what your toxic exposure is. They don't ask you what your risks are. I mean I had a patient last week with Parkinson's disease who had tremendous exposures as a kid to pesticides and insecticides coming out of the back of trucks working in industries where he's exposed to toxins, working in environments, occupation that exposed him.
[00:51:30] [00:52:00]	No one asked him about it. No one is looking at how to treat it, and that's the beauty of Functional Medicine. We actually have tools. It's not just, "Oh, you have this, too bad." It's, "Actually, we can do something about it to remove the toxins." I think the thing that strikes me as being just almost unbelievable is that we did prove that low-level lead is highly toxic. We saw the level was 50, then it was 40, then it was 20. Now data shows that between 1 and 10 are at risk. Even it's an incremental risk from 1 to 10, so we don't apply that understanding to any other toxin whether it's mercury, or pesticides, or flame retardants, or phthalates, or BPA; all these things have been linked to the same issues.

Dr. Jeffrey Bland:

[00:52:30]

I'm really pleased that you brought that up because I think that this is a concept of total load, right? What's the straw that broke the camel's back, that analogy? I was at a seminar in Hawaii recently in which one of the state Hawaii agricultural research experts was talking about pesticides and organic farming. There's a big battle in Hawaii as to do they want to be an organic-focused state. What she was pointing out is that there is application without regulation of sometimes six pesticide treatments a day, or herbicide treatments a day that are given to some of these crops.

[00:53:00]

[00:53:30]

Many of these are upwind from schools, so they've been able to actually show that in school children who are downwind from these multiple applications—which are not regulated—that the kids' vibrance kind of fluctuate based on the indiscriminate, well maybe, let's just say the multiple use of these chemicals. Then you start saying does it mean that these kids all have acute toxicity? Of course, it doesn't. It means they have chronic toxicity—the kinds of things we're talking about here. They are much harder to diagnose that some people would say, "Oh, you're just making a story that really doesn't exist," but it does exist when you start actually looking at immune function, neurological function, and the interrelationship to environmental exposure.

Dr. Mark Hyman:

[00:54:00]

I think you're right, Jeff. The total load of environmental chemicals that we're exposed to are never looked at in total. An environmental working group did a study of newborns, and took their umbilical cord blood before they took their first breath, and they found, I think, 287 known toxins—217 of which are neurotoxic, flame retardants, phthalates, BPA, Teflon, and mercury, and lead, and pesticides. I mean, it was extraordinary what they found and this is from the mother getting delivered into the baby before they had any environmental exposures.

[00:54:30]

No wonder we have one in six children with a neurodevelopmental disorder, whether it's a learning disability, whether it's ADHD, or autism; these are all profoundly impacting our next generation. It's good that you brought that up. I want to close with some practical ideas of how this research and this changing paradigm should impact our choices if we want to have the ability to fix our broken brains, and also to have an optimal brain.

Dr. Jeffrey Bland:
[00:55:00]

I think, Mark—and you're a leader in this, so I'm saying the obvious—that you've been such a great champion of this, that the first thing is the enlightenment of our population that we have a lot more flexibility in how we function and we fully understand that our genes are waiting for information from the right environment to give the white light of good health. Whether it's our brain health, our heart health, our gut health that we have tremendous flexibility in how we function based upon how we send information through our lifestyle, our environment, our experiences, our diet to our genes. I

[00:55:30]

think that construct is so powerful in mobilizing people to say, "Hey, I'm actually the wizard in charge of my function. I just need to find the right people to help me. I've got universal knowledge already encoded for good health. I just need to unearth it, and allow it to be rated for it."

[00:56:00]

Then once you have that enlightenment, now, fortunately, you are prepared to say, "Okay, what things do I need to change based on who I am? What are the things that really are the most important drivers the actual things that for me make the biggest difference?" Now there's where the Functional Medicine provider comes to be of assistance because they're the kind of help on the detective story, right? To interrogate the right things to ask because not everything is of concern. Only certain things probably are really important for that individual, so what are the big things that make the biggest difference, and how do you action them in order to really create a positive outcome?

[00:56:30]

[00:57:00]

I think that these programs, like Dr. Bredesen's program for Alzheimer's, in which there are 33 or more different variables that he looks at in terms of personalizing approach towards that person to prevent or to treat Alzheimer's, is a good example of this model because he is saying not all 33 are equally important in every individual, so let's find the ones in that individual that are really the most important based upon their genes, their lifestyle, their epigenetics, and we're going to really work with that person to design a personalized approach. That is a paradigm shifting concept because now we're saying each person is treated as an individual. Each person is in one experiment of their life and we're going to help them to maximizing their capabilities by their own lifestyle and program.

BROKEN BRAIN

Dr. Mark Hyman:	So powerful, and it involves very simple things. Many things you don't even need a Functional Medicine doctor for. Changing your diet—we know the high-sugar, high-glycemic diets make an impact. The higher-fat diets now like ketogenic diets are being used. We know that exercise has a huge impact on our plasticity. It increases BDNF. It helps stimulate new growth brain cells, and new connections between brain cells. We know that sleep has a huge factor. You mentioned the glia in the brain. Well, the glia actually have a lymphatic system, which is through sleep is the way your brain cleans out like your body cleans out through your lymph system. If you don't sleep well that has a huge impact. The sort of stress reduction is required to help the brain function better. We know that stress shrinks your memory that are in the hippocampus, so there are really simple interventions.
[00:57:30]	

[00:58:00] Diet, exercise, sleep, stress reduction—it can all be done without a doctor and it will often care for 50 to 80% of the issues. Then, of course, there are going to be people who have heavy metals and who have chronic brain infections and who have other factors that need to be addressed. We can also do that through the role of Functional Medicine, so I think it's a very empowering message that we have neuroplasticity. That we can increase connections in our brain. That we can increase new brain cells at any age. I recall a study of cancer patients who were near death, and they gave them a targeted labeled ingredient that's made in new brain cells, and they found their brains lit up even at the moment of death with creating new brain cells, so we have this potential all the way through our life, and I think this is a very empowering message. Jeff, I'm really excited that you joined us for this documentary, and that you were able to enlighten us about this emerging research in science, and the trends that are happening. It's very powerful and exciting.

[00:58:30]

Dr. Jeffrey Bland: [00:59:00] Well Mark, I thank you. I think your leadership in this field is so extraordinarily important and I think we are witnessing a birthing of human potential through this concept that is really going to be transformative. It's going to be a transformative time when an individual recognizes that they have a lot more regulation and control than they ever believed and that by working together with teams of experts—not just a single person that knows all, but a team of experts—that can guide them and help them to assist in the development of their own personalized approach towards life leads us to maybe a century or more of good living, and compressing morbidity, and getting the most out of our genes. What an exciting time this is.

Dr. Mark Hyman: I'm down with that, a century of good living. All right, thank you, Jeff.

Dr. Jeffrey Bland: Thank you so much.

JENNIFER LOVE, MD | Amen Clinics

Dr. Jennifer Love: In undergrad, I studied biology and chemistry. I think that chemistry was one of the big foundations of exploring how things worked. Backing up even a little bit before that, I was a nursing major when I first started college. My nursing professors—I apparently used to drive them crazy. I was always asking questions about, "Well, why does this work? If we do something in this system, how does it affect this other system?" They would just throw their hands up in the air and say, "Go to medical school."

[00:00:30] I finally ended up down that path and going to medical school. After about nine years of medical training, I got my first job. All these questions that I had, there's so much information in medical school that you get, they say it's like drinking out of a fire hose. There's so much coming at you. But I realized when I was out in the day-to-day world that I was still stuck with the question of why. Why is this

[00:01:00] happening? So much of medicine is treading water. It's taking care of symptoms. I found myself trying to figure out how to get to the root of all of this. I've never really thought of myself as a functional psychiatrist. I just like getting in and coming up with something better than trying to calm down symptoms.

[00:01:30] With conventional psychiatry, it's largely driven by the pharmaceutical industry and managed care. Physicians are under time constraints to only spend a certain amount of time with patients. The reimbursements are for very short visits. It's difficult to be able to spend the time you need to really get at the heart of the issue. I think that's true not just in psychiatry, but in every discipline.

[00:02:00] I think some of the challenges with conventional psychiatry is that it's really based on symptom management. There's not a lot of research that isn't funded by pharmacological companies. It's really medication based and physicians are expected to prescribe medication, and then the insurance companies want therapy to be done by therapists because it's less expensive. You have this division of ... you have prescribers and then you have people who are coming in and trying to use therapy to get at the underlying issues. There's just a disconnect.

[00:02:30] My first job out of my fellowship training was with a big HMO company. If I said the name, you'd recognize them. I used to get in trouble for spending too much time with my patients. I would have patients who would come in and they were alcoholic or having a major depressive episode, and they'd never seen a physician to discuss it before. I was expected to do their entire evaluation and treatment

[00:03:00] in 20 minutes. It just didn't make sense to me that someone who is suffering from an alcohol use disorder ... My supervisor literally told me that I need to give them Prozac and Trazodone for sleep and then you're done and send them out. It just wasn't a good fit for me at all.

[00:03:30] When I fell into the practice and group that I'm with now, I think the biggest draw was the ability to take time with people to really get to know what's going on with them so we could look beyond treading water and trying to manage the symptoms of the moment, but get really at the heart of everything.

[00:04:00] The first question is: why is a person anxious? I think there are a lot of different reasons. I think every person who comes into my office has a different story. Some people have a very strong genetic predisposition to anxiety. Some people have been anxious since childhood. Some people come from very chaotic backgrounds. Some people have an onset in college and later. Finding out what is at the cause will then help me come up with a treatment plan that's individualized for them.

I think one of the big issues with anxiety for a lot of people is: if it's been going on since childhood, people may be really anxious and not even realize their level of anxiety because to them they're so used to it. They've always functioned that way. It's not really until you sit and listen to what their

[00:04:30] everyday existence is and talk to them about anxiety that they go, "Oh, wow. I actually really am anxious." One of the hallmarks with anxiety that I see is a total disconnect between the emotional part of the brain and the logical part of the brain. I would treat that very differently than someone who is having anxiety in a social situation or something.

[00:05:00] Someone who's had a traumatic event will have these emotional responses that are far out of proportion to what's going on around them. We need to have therapies that will center on connecting the parts of the brain that regulate emotions and logic so their emotional responses can be more in line with what's going on now. Someone with a panic disorder might respond to a different type of therapy, where we're looking at how they're thinking and what their thoughts are, and we want to [00:05:30] change those thoughts so they can change the way they feel. Some people, their fingers are so plugged into the electrical outlet that they need medication to calm them down so they can even participate in these non-medication therapies. It really depends on the person and what's going on with them physiologically so we can get started on the right treatment plan that's built for them.

[00:06:00] There are a lot of different types of therapy that can be just as effective as medication for treating mild to moderate anxiety disorders. For even more severe disorders, I think medications can be helpful to stabilize, but they won't really get at the heart of the issue. We probably have the most data for a type of therapy called cognitive behavioral therapy. The premise of it is simple: we feel the way we think; and, if we can change the way we think, we can change the way we feel. The premise is simple, but practicing it isn't always simple. It requires a well-trained therapist to walk that person through that. [00:06:30] It's really helpful for things like low self-esteem, social anxiety, certain phobias, even panic disorder it's really helpful for.

I've also sent a lot of patients for a type of therapy called EMDR. It wins first prize for the worst name of any therapy. It stands for Eye Movement Desensitization and Reprocessing. This is one of the best [00:07:00] therapies I've found in terms of really dealing with trauma, whether it's a post-traumatic stress disorder from a traumatic event, chronic emotional trauma, or childhood traumatic events. It's really good at helping connect the emotional and logical parts of the brain and helping people process efficiently so they're not constantly re-experiencing the past. That's the problem with a lot of anxiety disorders. People don't remember what's happened to them in the past. They're constantly re- [00:07:30] experiencing those emotions over and over again. EMDR is another great non-medication treatment. Then, of course, there's a lot of information on mindfulness and yoga and supplements that people can take and other non-medication treatments, too.

[00:08:00] Some people will come in and they'll tell me off-the-bat that they're anxious. They feel a racing heart. They feel like they have palpitations. They sweat. They have a feeling in their stomach. They have a very physiological response to stress that's very physical. Some people feel panic. Some people feel anxious or stressed. Some people, though, don't know how they feel. It's really trying to get at how they're functioning on a day-to-day basis. Are they really frazzled? Are they unable to pay attention and get things done because their mind is everywhere? Their thoughts are racing 100 miles an hour. They're always thinking about the same things over and over and over, and they can't focus in on what [00:08:30] they're doing. Those are a lot of the common signs.

I remember being in medical school, and one of the most ridiculous things I heard, and I was just a student, was that 50% of women will have a depressive episode at some time in their lives, and maybe only a third of men, but depression is nothing to do with hormones. I just wanted to laugh and say, "Have you ever met anyone in menopause? Have you ever had a female family friend, and monthly ... [00:09:00] there are these mood swings." That's not a depressive episode, but there are a lot of things that play a role in our level of mood on a day-to-day basis. Are we getting enough sleep? Are our hormones balanced? What is our stress like?

The big question is: when does it become a problem? It becomes a problem when it gets in the way of our everyday functioning; when you lose joy in life; when you're feeling sad most of the day, most days

[00:09:30] of the week. When things that have always been fun for you cease to bring enjoyment. When people around you notice a change. When you don't enjoy going to work, you don't enjoy seeing your friends, you don't enjoy hanging out with your family. When your work performance suffers. When there are functional issues that arise from it, then it's something that needs to be addressed.

[00:10:00] I got a phone call from a patient who had come to see me for depression. We had used medication for him because at some point he had been suicidal. He called me up. He was feeling much better on his medication. He said to me, "I think maybe I could have a little bit more." I said, "You're on a really decent dose. You just spent 20 minutes telling me that you're feeling better. Why do you think you need more?" He said, "If this amount works this much, then more could work more." I said to him, "What are you hoping to accomplish?" He said, "I'd really like more energy. I'd like to be more

[00:10:30] productive and get more done in the day." I asked him, "What are you eating?" He laughed and said, "Oh, don't even ask me that. I just eat junk all the time."

This was a guy who was so successful, by age 40 he had retired. He has a chef on call at his house and he was going and eating fast food all throughout the week. I had to say to him, "Look, if you go out and

[00:11:00] buy a high-end Mercedes, what are you going to put in your gas tank? You have to use a high-octane fuel. You can't throw sludge into that gas tank and then expect it to perform." I think that a lot of times we just are so busy and we're so programmed to buy whatever is in the grocery store and it's fine and we just stick it in our bodies, that we forget that our brains are much more of a high-performance vehicle than a high-end car, and that if it's important to have fuel in these high-end cars we need to have the right fuel in us as well.

[00:11:30] I always do a nutritional questionnaire when I'm meeting people and seeing what they're eating and seeing what their symptoms are. Are they having problems with concentration? Are they overly anxious? I may have different recommendations for different people. Probably everyone I meet needs to be eating more fresh foods, fresh vegetables and fruits, unprocessed foods. I think that most of my

[00:12:00] patients are stuck on processed foods, and I think that's a big problem. Getting a higher content of vegetables and fruits, fiber, and healthy proteins, and getting off the sugars and the unhealthy carbs is probably—across the board—my number one recommendation.

[00:12:30] I treat all of the chemical dependencies, from alcohol, cigarettes, heroin, drugs, to what we call behavioral addictions or process addictions, eating disorders, gambling, video games, the Internet— you can become addicted to almost anything. I deal with everything across the board. There's a lot of research that's going on in terms of what happens in the brain when we become addicted to a substance or addicted to a behavior. There's a lot that's written about dopamine and how a lot of addiction is trying to get dopamine boosted in the brain, whether it's speeding down the highway at

[00:13:00] 120 miles an hour, or someone who can't stop parachuting over and over and over again, or using cocaine, or someone with an eating disorder who goes on a huge binge.

The same part of the brain, called the ventral tegmental area, releases dopamine and it causes a huge dopamine rush in the brain. It doesn't matter if someone's taking an upper or a downer or they have a behavioral type of addiction. The same brain area is involved. A lot of the research that's going on right

[00:13:30] now is really centered around trying to regulate the dopamine system. But when I think about treating addictions, I really think of six different parameters, because it's not just as simple as are you using or not using? Do you do this behavior or don't? Because you can stop doing a certain behavior and be completely miserable and what's the point?

[00:14:00] When I'm looking at treating someone's addiction, I look at six different factors. I first look at what's going on biologically. That's a lot of what we do at our clinic, physiologically what's going on in the brain, in the body? Do I need to detox someone? Do I need to check their liver and thyroid status and all of that? What are the mechanisms going on in the brain that I think are contributing? Is someone really impulsive? Are they very anxious? Are they depressed and trying to self-medicate?

[00:14:30]

[00:15:00]

I also want to look at the emotional issues. What are the coping strategies that people have? When I think of emotions and the psychological factors, I think of, how do they manage stress, and what is the meaning of this substance to them? I had one patient tell me that giving up alcohol was the same as having a divorce. Another patient told me, "Marijuana raised me. I didn't have a mother who was around and I had marijuana." When people are that tied into a substance, the idea of sobriety is terrifying. You have to understand what that substance means to them psychologically and emotionally and what those coping strategies are.

[00:15:30]

I also look behaviorally. We all get into behavior patterns. I come in the house, I put my keys in the same place, I put my purse down some place. We have these life behaviors. People with addictions have the same thing; it's where they go; it's how they spend their time; it's who they're with, which gets into the social aspects, because you can't really treat an addiction unless you look at that. People who use heroin hang out with people who use heroin. I don't use heroin. I don't really have any friends who use heroin. We have to really look at how we reinvent someone socially and bring them into a community that is separate from their using community.

[00:16:00]

The final aspect I look at is spirituality. Some people see this as religion, but for me spiritually is reassessing, "Who am I? What is my place in this world? What kind of person do I want to be? What are the character traits I want to have? What is my level of integrity going to be?" That's really just as important in starting over when you're treating addictions than stopping alcohol or stopping the substance. If you continue to lie in sobriety, you still have these using behaviors, and you're not really going to have a transformative change.

[00:16:30]

[00:17:00]

I am fascinated by social media. We have the ability to create these online communities and just the fact that we call it social media, because in effect we're decreasing our in-person socialization. Yes, I can be social with my friends and catch up with everyone staring at a little computer in my hand on my couch in my PJs. I'm not actually seeing them. I'm not calling them on the phone. I'm not talking to them. I'm either texting them or just looking at their pictures, and suddenly that counts for community and connection. These Snapchats and Twitter and all of this, it's so interesting to see how communication has changed. But it's also important to look at what it's replacing at the same time.

[00:17:30]

[00:18:00]

I think that one of the reasons psychiatrists have been so put on the forefront in the last several years is this increase in rate of diagnosis of ADD. There's been a big push back from people saying, "Why is there suddenly more? We're over-diagnosing everything." My personal thought for years has just been the way that we live in real life when we go to school or we go to a job where you sit in a cubicle, you have to sit in a desk and not move, is so completely different to the speed at which information comes when we're not at work and kids aren't at school. They can get on the Internet, and everything's fast, and they play these video games that go really fast, and then they have to go and just sit and listen to someone speak. We're surprised that they can't pay attention.

It's an interesting question to look at, because why would we give all these people stimulants? Why would we give everyone medication to treat something that comes from overstimulation and change in environments?

[00:18:30]

One of the most difficult conversations I have to have with my patients is around technology because one of the number one complaints I have of people coming in my office is insomnia or difficulty getting to sleep. The reality is, people are watching TV, they're on the Internet, they're on their social media until late into the night. I have to look them in the eye and say, "I'm sorry, but you really do need to turn everything off a minimum of an hour before bedtime." It looks like I'm about to take their baby away. The look that I see on their faces, they're just terrified. It's a really difficult habit to break.

[00:19:00]

I have a young man I've been treating for over a year and his family brought him to me for a sleep disorder. The reality is, he's up on his computer until two or three in the morning, and then he wants to sleep all day and he's exhausted. They're telling me, "He's sleeping all day and we don't know what

[00:19:30] to do." I told them 100 times what to do. "You need to turn off the computer and go to bed at bedtime and actually sleep during the night." People don't want to do it. They're so enamored by what they're seeing, whether it's the video games that they get stuck on playing over and over and over, and they can't just shift and turn it off. It's very hard to turn off technology.

[00:20:00] There are a number of different types of relaxation training. There are some people who can do traditional relaxation and mindfulness very well. It's not difficult for them to quiet their minds. They are too busy to take the time to do it. There are other people who, as soon as they try to quiet down at the end of the day, they can't actually sit down and meditate because their thoughts are all over the place. That's where I'd have more of an approach of active meditation, because some people need guidance and practice in terms of getting their bodies to quiet down, because then the body gives the mind the feedback on how to quiet down.

[00:20:30] Active meditation is something similar to progressive relaxation, where you go piece by piece from head to toe and you tighten all the muscles and then you consciously relax them. You practice this going through the different muscle groups. It takes a body that's filled with a little bit of tension, you put more into it, and then you pull it out. People learn how to relax their bodies. Then, there's a direct message that's sent up to the anxiety centers of the brain telling them, "Relax down here. You can calm down." This is one of the reasons why it works so well.

[00:21:00] It's like getting a massage: you feel fabulous after you get a massage because you're pulling the tension out of all those muscles, so you're pulling the tension out of your brain. There's this total feedback between how we treat our bodies and how we feel in our minds. Even doing deep breathing techniques, where you really do good belly breathing, where you're not breathing in your chest but you're really letting that belly expand, helps keep your heart rate and blood pressure down. It helps with focus and concentration.

[00:21:30] A huge study came out a few years ago from UC Irvine. They were taking a look at the best ways to treat ADD. They looked at medications. Pharmacotherapy tends to work for about three years, and then you get the poop-out effect. The medications, the stimulants just don't work as well and people try to escalate the doses but they can't get the same response. They were trying to look at what has better long-term effects on focus and concentration than just relying on these medications.

[00:22:00] They actually found that mindfulness and relaxation had better effect. I wanted to call them up immediately and try to find who on earth was the person who was training these people with ADD how to do mindfulness, because I want his number, because all my patients need to see him. But, the reality is, it's one of the number one treatments not only for attention issues but for treating anxiety disorders and helping with mood too.

[00:22:30] I haven't looked at any of the studies of fMRI studies where you can see what's going on in real time as someone's doing it. We know that over time there are a number of physiological changes with relaxation techniques. What we think, from looking at SPECT imaging, is a big change that we can see when people implement these on a regular basis, is a decrease in the part of the brain that's called the basal ganglia. It's part of the movement center of the brain, but it's also part of the brain that we see [00:23:00] really overactive on SPECT imaging when people are very anxious; yoga, tai chi, or doing relaxation training, really calms down this part of the brain.

[00:23:30] I think if anybody has really big issues with a mood or anxiety disorder or an addiction, they need to give me a call. Putting it off isn't going to get you anywhere. We really need to sit down and come up with a comprehensive plan to help people move forward, to sit down and figure out, "What are your goals of treatment?" Not, "What are my goals for you?" What are your goals in your life and in your treatment, and then what are the steps we can take together to help you reach those goals so we can address any addictive tendencies, health concerns, nutritional things that are deficient, mood and anxiety components, sleep, or overall health, based on that person's goals, not mine?

JIM KWIK | Memory Coach, Host of KwikBrain.com Podcast

Jim Kwik: A lot of people don't know this, but when they see me on stage, I memorize a room full of people's names, like a hundred names, or a hundred numbers, or a hundred words, I'll do it forwards and backwards. I always tell people I don't do this to impress you. I do this to express to you what's really possible, because the truth is you could do it too; you just weren't taught how to do it because school is a great place to learn.

[00:00:30] What's learned? Math, History, Science, Spanish, but there are zero classes on how to learn, how to think, how to be creative, how to solve problems, how to listen, how to read faster, how to remember more. I always thought that it should have been the fourth R in school—reading, writing, arithmetic—but what about remembering? What about retention? What about recall? Socrates said there is no learning without remembering.

[00:01:00] I know this is possible for everybody because at the age of five, I had a very bad accident. I had head trauma, a brain injury. That left me with learning challenges all through school, all throughout elementary school, middle school, and high school. How did that manifest? I couldn't understand things like everybody else did. Teachers would have to repeat themselves four or five times. Then, I would just have to pretend I understood. I had no focus. I had a very horrible memory. Actually, it took me an extra three years to learn how to read. I grew up with these learning challenges.

I remember a few years after that, when I was about nine years old, I overheard one of my teachers talk to another adult, thinking I wasn't paying attention, pointing to me, saying, "That's the boy with the broken brain." When you're a child, that really leaves an impression. That was my identity growing up.

[00:01:30] Eventually, when I got to college, when I was a freshman, I wanted to start fresh. I wanted a new start. I wanted to make my family proud, show the world, show myself that I really did not have a broken brain. I took all these classes. I actually did worse. I was ready to quit school because I couldn't handle it anymore. A friend of mine was saying that, "Hey, going home for the weekend? Why don't you come [00:02:00] with me, get some perspective with my family before you tell your parents you're going to quit school because of your broken brain." I said, "Okay," and I go.

The family is pretty successful. The father is walking me around his property before dinner and asked me a very innocent question, which is the worst question you could ask me at the time. He says, "How's school?" I was like, "Oh my goodness." I just started breaking down. I tell him about my broken brain, how I don't learn like everybody else does, and there's something different there. He's like, "Well, why are you in school? What do you want to be? What do you want to do? What do you want to have? What do you want to share?"

[00:02:30] I noticed that questions really are the power of, questions in our lives, to be able to ask a new question to get a new answer. No one has ever asked me that question before. It took me a little while to answer. Then, when I go to answer him, he pauses. He takes out a journal out of his back pocket. He rips out a couple of sheets of paper, and he makes me write it down. I also noticed some of the most amazing minds out there—geniuses—they keep journals and they write things down. They don't know if it's because they're geniuses that they write things down or it's because they write things down in journals that they're geniuses. It's interesting.

[00:03:00] Anyway, I write down this list. It's like a bucket list. When I was done, I started folding up the sheets of paper to put into my pocket. He does something unexpected—he grabs the sheets out of my hand, and he starts reading my dreams. He starts reading my goals, my deep desires. I didn't realize that somebody else was going to look at it. I don't know how much time goes by, but when he's done, he's like, "Jim,

[00:03:30] you are this close to everything on that list." I'm thinking, "There's just no way." He spreads his index fingers about a foot apart. I'm like, "Give me 10 lifetimes. I'm not going to crack that list." He goes like this, like this to my brain, to my broken brain.

[00:04:00] He takes me to a room of his home I've never seen before. It is wall-to-wall, ceiling-to-floor covered in books. For me, growing up with learning challenges, never finishing a book cover-to-cover, I have a phobia of reading, it's equivalent to walking to a room full of snakes, for somebody who is afraid of snakes. What makes it worse is this person starts grabbing snakes, and starts handing them to me, all these books. I started looking at the titles. There are these incredible biographies of men and women in history, and some very early personal growth books.

He says, "Jim, I want you to read one of these books a week." I'm like, "Have you not been listening to our conversation? I have learning challenges. I have a broken brain." Then, he says, "Jim ..." I tell him about all my scores and I have a midterm. He looks at me and says, "Jim, don't let school get in the way of your education." I didn't realize at the time, it was a Mark Twain quote. I said, "That's very inspiring but I really can't commit to reading a book a week."

[00:04:30] Then—he's a very smart man—he reaches into his pocket. He takes out my bucket list. He starts reading each of my dreams out loud. Something about hearing another man who's, obviously doing well for himself, hearing my dreams being incanted out to the universe really shook with my mind, and my heart, and my soul something fierce. A lot of the things on that list were things I wanted to do for my family that they can never afford or would never do for themselves. With that extra leverage or motivation—and I talked about motivation as very key to be able to have a growing brain—to be able to

[00:05:00] fix your broken brain is having the motivation and drive to want to do that. With that extra motivation, I agreed to read one book a week.

Fast forward, I'm back at school. I have a pile of books I have to read for school, and a pile of books that I promised to read for my own improvement, and I can't keep up. I don't eat, I don't sleep, I don't workout, I don't spend time with family or friends—any of that. I just lived in the library, which is the worst recipe for fixing your broken brain. It's not very sustainable. I ended up passing out in the library. I fall down a flight of stairs. I hit my head again. I wake up two days later in the hospital.

[00:05:30] At this point, because I wasn't taking care of myself, I was down to 117 pounds. I literally was wasting away. I thought I died. When I woke up, another part of me woke up also. That part of me thinking, "What's going on? How do I fix this?" When I had that thought, the nurse came in with a mug of tea. On it, it had a picture of Albert Einstein, a genius. He was the opposite of what I thought I was. He's got an incredibly bright and better brain. It had this quote on the tea that said, "The same level of thinking

[00:06:00] that's created the problem won't solve the problem."

It made me ask a new question , "What's my problem?" My problem is I have a very slow, broken brain. How do I think differently about it? Maybe I could learn how to have a faster, better brain. I put all my studies aside, and I start studying this thing called my brain. I wanted to solve this riddle, how my brain worked, so I could work my brain. How my memory worked, so I could work my memory.

[00:06:30] I poured myself into adult learning theory, brain science, anything having to do with memory, or reading, focus, and concentration. After I started doing that, about 36 days in, it's like a light switch went on, and I started to understand things for the first time. I started to have better focus. I started to remember things better. I started to read faster. My grades improved. Then, my life improved dramatically after that.

[00:07:00] Now, the reason why I'm here still today—this is 25 years later—is I just couldn't help but wanting to help other people. I'm thinking it's so unfair that this wasn't taught and available to everybody because everyone is struggling and suffering more in this digital age than ever before with the information overload and overwhelm. All the villains are attacking our brain.

[00:07:30] I started tutoring this. One of my students, she was a freshman in college, she read 30 books in 30 days. 30 books in 30 days. Can you imagine what books she would read? She wasn't just reading. She was absorbing, and then retaining, and then understanding it. I wanted to find out, not how she did it, I know exactly how she did it, but I wanted to know why, going back to human motivation again. I found out her mother was dying of terminal cancer, and the books she was reading were books to save her mom's life, books on health and wellness from a lot of the experts that are in these series.

[00:08:00] I was blown away by that. I remember six months later, I get a call from this young lady, and she's crying, and she's crying, and crying. I can't get a word out of her. I find out they're tears of joy, and that her mother not only survived, but is really getting better. Doctors don't know how. They don't know why. They called it a miracle. Her mother attributes it 100% to the great advice she got from her daughter that she learned from all these books. That's where I realized that if knowledge is power, learning is our superpower.

[00:08:30] What is brain training and why is it important? What I believe is in this day and age, our wealth is not based anymore on our muscle power; it's based on our mind power. It's not our brute strength; it's our brain strength. What I'm interested in working with clients is, yes, mental intelligence. I want to get them to be able to remember facts, figures, formulas, and foreign languages. That's really important. Also, it's not just mental intelligence. We want mental fitness. Just as you're building your body, you're building your muscles. You want them to have energy. You want them to have strength, power, endurance, flexibility, agility, and speed.

[00:09:00] Your brain is like that also. Your brain can be trained for greater agility, speed, endurance, power, strength—all of that. That's really what correct brain training is going to help foster, where you're going to be able to remember things, have greater focus and greater retention. Being able to take this information because knowledge is not power; it's only potential power. It only becomes power when we implement it, to be able to take that information and apply it and turn it into action.

[00:09:30] My thing is this: we all can have better, brighter brains. What it takes, just as your physical muscles, you have mental muscles. The challenge here is we're not using our mental muscles to our greatest ability. What happens if you're not growing those mental muscles, then they're atrophying. If I put my arm in a sling for six months, it doesn't stay the same. It doesn't grow. It doesn't even stay the same; it grows weaker. A lot of our brain is what's happening there also.

[00:10:00] I talked about superpowers and superheroes a lot. I think everybody has these innate mental superpowers of focus, concentration, creativity, and so on. But I think there are three super villains that are attacking us on a regular basis that have never been here before. Number one: there's digital overload. They call it information fatigue syndrome, information anxiety. What's the result? We have higher blood pressure, a compression of leisure time, more stress than ever. Even if we have leisure time, we can't enjoy it because our minds are still multitasking thinking about all these other things.

[00:10:30] There's an epidemic of sleeplessness because of all this overload and overwhelm. There's so much information in this digital age. The amount of information is doubling at dizzying speeds. How many people feel like they go out there and buy books to help themselves, and they sit on the shelf? It becomes shelf-help instead of self-help. There's so much information, emails, social media, app notifications, text messages, newspapers, magazines, and so on. It feels like you're taking a sip of water out of a fire hose.

[00:11:00] If knowledge is power, then it's not only power; it's profit in this day and age. The faster you can learn, the faster you can earn. The amount of information is doubling at a dizzying speed that the president of Google says that the amount of information from the dawn of humanity to the year 2003, just a little over a decade ago, that amount of information now is created every two days online. People are drowning in information, but they're starving for practical wisdom. If the amount of information is doubling like this, the challenge is how we learn it, how we remember it, how we read it is pretty much consistent. That gap creates a lot of stress and anxiety. The number one villain is digital overload.

[00:11:30] The second challenge nowadays is digital distraction. Our brains are literally being rewired by our smart devices. One of the things I talked about—our morning routines—I think everybody has a to-do list. I really think equally important, it's important in today's modern day, is you have to have a not-to-do list. On the top of your not-to-do list, because the most successful people and the most productive high performers out there, they say no a lot. They say no to good, they say yes to great. One of the things you want to say no to is touching your phone the first hour of the day.

[00:12:00] When I say that, some people flip out because they're so addicted to their digital devices. I'll tell you two reasons why you don't want to touch your phone first thing in the morning. Number one: when you wake up first thing in the morning, you're in this alpha theta brainwave stage when you're most impressionable. When you're doing that, if the first thing you do is touch your phone, you're literally going through, and you're looking at getting your dopamine fixes on your likes, and your shares, and your comments, and tech notches. All those things give you a dopamine fix, and you're frying your brain. You're rewiring your brain for distraction.

I think a lot of people right now have troubling focusing. They'll read a page in a book, get to the end, and they'll forget what they just read. They'll go back, and reread it, and they can't concentrate. One of the reasons why is because of these digital distractions that we have.

[00:12:30] What's happening is there's something called decision fatigue. Decision fatigue is this research saying that we can only make a certain amount of good decisions in a day. After that, we can't. It could be the end of the day, we're at a restaurant, we're looking in the menu, and we can't decide what we want for dinner. It's that difficult. They found this research working with surgeons in terms of when they're making the most mistakes, and when's the best time for patient to get operated on, and so on. We all have this decision fatigue.

[00:13:00] That's why a lot of high performers—whether it's Mark Zuckerberg, or Tony Hsieh who runs Zappos— wear the same sweatshirt, they wear the same t-shirt every single day because they don't want to waste one of their decisions in deciding what they're going to wear that day. That's to the best of your ability for you to be able to manage and create routines in your life because, first, you create your habits. Then, your habits create you. One of the habits you don't want to do is touch your phone because it wires you for distraction.

[00:13:30] Besides that, the second reason you don't want to touch your phone is because it wires you to be reactive, because when you check your phone and you see your text messages, and your emails—and these are all things that people want something from you—you have fires that you need to fight. It's training you to be able to react to people as opposed to waking up in the morning, and having a clear plan for your day, and being proactive about it, and designing it.

[00:14:00] I talk about the difference between being a thermometer and thermostat. I think, the quality of our life, the quality of our brain comes down to whether we identify more with the thermometer or thermostat. Now, what does a thermometer do? A thermometer's main function is it reacts to the environment; it reacts to what the environment is giving it. The difference though is with the thermostat, a thermostat is different. A thermostat sets the standard. It sets a vision. It sets a goal. What happens to the environment, it raises to meet that standard. I feel like the happiest people out there, the ones that have better brains are this way because they have the locus of control coming from the inside.

One of the keys to fixing your broken brain so that it has more peace, positivity, and productivity, is to not touch your phone first thing in the morning, and to not indulge in digital distraction.

[00:14:30] The third super villain that is attacking our broken brain is this digital dementia. Number one is digital overload. Number two is digital distraction. Number three is digital dementia. What does that mean?

That means most of us are outsourcing our brains to our smart devices. It's keeping the names. It's keeping numbers. It's keeping our to-dos. It's doing simple math. If we talk about the brain being metaphorically like a muscle, it grows stronger with use, but it's use it or lose it.

[00:15:00]

Now, how many phone numbers, for example, did you know growing up? How many phone numbers growing up decades ago? You knew every single phone number. How many phone numbers can we remember right now? One, two, maybe three. Not that you want to be able to remember, and you have to study and remember hundreds of phone numbers, you don't want to be able to do that, but we've lost the ability to do that. What digital dementia is saying is we're outsourcing our brain to our smart devices, so our brains aren't getting the natural exercise. Our smart devices, in a way, are making us not so smart.

[00:15:30]

I think one of the big modern-day challenges people have as they feel like maybe they're suffering from a broken brain because senior moments are coming a little bit too early. They read a page in a book, and forget what they just read, or they feel absent-minded. They're in the shower, and they can't remember if they shampooed their hair, so they end up doing it twice, or they misplace things like their wallet, purse, or cellphone. Have you ever found yourself calling your own cellphone, hoping you kept it on, so it rings somewhere in your home, or you misplace things like your keys, or if not your keys, something

[00:16:00]

much larger like your car? You ever see the people outside of the mall parking lot using their car alarms trying to figure out where they placed their car?

These are challenges that are attacking us on a regular basis. One of the best ways to prevent brain aging, to keep your brain youthful and young, is by activating your brain. Here are two benefits that come out of it. By using your brain more often, you actually can live longer. There was a study that was on the cover of *Time Magazine* with these nuns—these super nuns. They're living well into their 80s, 90s, and above.

[00:16:30]

The researchers wanted to find out to what do they attribute that. Half of it had to do with their gratitude, their emotional gratitude, and their faith, but the other half had to with being lifelong learners. Throughout their entire life, they were mentally engaged in conversation, in games, and reading. By keeping mentally engaged and having dedicated themselves as lifelong learners, they added years to their life, but also life to their years.

[00:17:00]

What's really exciting is we've discovered more about the human brain in the past 20 years than the previous 2000 years combined. When you hear new science out there, like neurogenesis or neuroplasticity, basically saying that you could create new brain cells until the day you die, you could create new connections inside your brain until the day you die. What does it require? Probably just two things. It requires novelty and it requires nutrition. Novelty and nutrition.

[00:17:30]

It's like the human body. You go to a personal trainer, and they want to get your muscles, they want to introduce stimulus to it. They want to give it novelty or exercise. Then, they want to feed it with the proper nutrition, so it can grow and be healthy. Same thing with your neuro fitness, your mental fitness, if you will, by giving it new stimulus, either new thoughts or new body movements also because certain physical exercises you could do will actually build your brainpower.

[00:18:00]

There was a study in Oxford University that the act of juggling actually will create more white matter in your brain. We teach people how to not only juggle but to do other things like, for example, eating with the opposite hand or brushing your teeth with your opposite hand because we know that there's a mind-body connection. We know that one half of your brain controls the opposite side of your body. God forbid, if somebody had a stroke on the left side of their brain, if there's paralysis, it would manifest on the right side of their body and vice versa.

[00:18:30]

What we're realizing now is not just the brain-body connection. There's a body-brain connection, that using your body in certain ways could actually stimulate different parts of your brain. That's really exciting because, primarily, we have our brain that the primary function of a brain is actually to control our movement. As your body moves, your brain grooves.

One of the challenges in today's modern society, is we lead a very sedentary lifestyle. Most people are sitting at their desk all day eight to nine hours straight. They say sitting is the new smoking. What I advise people to do is to set their phone alarm every ... They call it The Pomodoro Technique. It's a time management technique saying that the average attention span is about 25 to 30 minutes. After that, there's a sharp decline.

[00:19:00]   Knowing that, if you want to maximize the return of your time and refocus your attention, set your alarm to go off every 30 minutes, maybe 45 minutes, and focus on one task. Then, when you're done, the alarm goes off, take three, four, or five minutes to do the things that are brain healthy. We're talking about movement. We're talking about deep breathing. We're talking about hydration because your brain is only 2% of your body mass, but it requires 20 to 25% of the nutrients, of the oxygen, of the water.

[00:19:30]   How do you improve your memory? First I would start with believing you can improve it. People talk about, "I'm too old," or "This runs in my family," and "I get these senior moments." What I find is, sometimes, you have to be careful of your self-talk because your brain is like a supercomputer, and your self-talk is the program it will run. If you tell yourself you don't have a good memory or you're not good with names, you will not remember the name of the next person you meet, because you programmed
[00:20:00]   your supercomputer not to, because the truth is only one-third of your memory potential is biological and genetic. Biologic and genetic, one-third. Two-thirds is completely in your control, and that's really great news.

If you want to improve your memory, I teach you to remember three things because if you ever forget something, where you put your keys, somebody's name, or anything, usually, one of these three things is missing. I want you to remember MOM, M-O-M. Let me ask you a question. Let's apply this towards
[00:20:30]   remembering names. Most people have trouble remembering names. Let's say that there was a suitcase here of $250,000 cash for you or your favorite charity if you just remember the name of the next stranger you meet. How many people are going to remember that person's name? Everybody. Everyone, all of a sudden, is a memory expert.

I want to point this out as your brain coach, it had nothing to do with your potential, and it had nothing to do with your capacity or capability. It had everything to do with whether or not you wanted to or not. The truth is you could remember things, you're just not motivated to remember because of the M in MOM stands for motivation. What is your motive for taking action?

[00:21:00]   I believe that there's a success formula. I call it H-cube. It goes from your head, to your heart, to your hands. That we could affirm things on our head. We could think things on our head. We could visualize things in our head, set goals in our head. If we're not acting with our hands, nothing changes. If we're not acting with our hands, usually, what's missing is a second H, which is your heart. The heart, which is the symbol of emotion, the energy emotion. It's the fuel that moves a car.

[00:21:30]   Tap into what they call your "why." Ask yourself, "why do I want to learn this? Why do I want to remember this person's name?" It's a very simple question. Maybe it's to show the person respect. Maybe it's to make a new friend. Maybe it's to practice these tools that we learned from the series because here's the thing, reasons reap results. Reasons reap results and rewards. Reasons come first. The M in MOM is motivation.

Now, what's the O in MOM? I want everybody who's reading this, I want to do this quick exercise. I want you to take your right hand, and just shake it out like this. Make a fist like this. Shake it out. Make a fist. Put it to your chin. Now, where's your chin, right? What happens is ... Everybody, I do this with an
[00:22:00]   audience of 10,000 people. 90% of them will go like this. They'll put it to their cheek, and not their chin.

The O in MOM stands for observation, observation. See, a lot of people, they'll blame all their memory issues to their retention. It has nothing to do with the retention. It has everything to do with their attention.

[00:22:30] One of the people who has an incredible memory is President Bill Clinton. I've had the opportunity to meet him a number of times. I remember the second time I met him. He remembered my name. He has an incredible memory. Everyone knows he's a great connector, great communicator, great charisma. He has an incredible memory.

I remember asking him, "How do you do that? I'm a memory coach. How do you remember these things?" He's like, "I don't use any memory techniques." He said, "Growing up, my grandfather in Arkansas would get the kids around and tell stories. Afterwards, he would ask questions to see if we're really listening, to see if we're really paying attention."

[00:23:00] I remember, we were at a fundraiser, and I was sat here, and I post this picture on Instagram. It's me, and then Forest Whitaker, Sir Richard Branson, Ashton Kutcher and his twin brother—I didn't know Ashton has a twin brother—and Bill Clinton sitting right next to me. When he's talking to me, I felt like there are a lot more important people at the table, certainly, in this room than I am, but when he's talking to me, he's completely paying attention to me.

[00:23:30] A lot of times, when you meet someone brand new, they're looking over your shoulder or they're talking to themselves. What I find, a lot of people aren't really listening. They're really just waiting for their turn to speak. They're thinking about how they're going to respond. If you want to have a better memory, you want to observe better. I really think that President Bill Clinton, his incredible memory, and his powerful presence with people comes from being powerfully present with people. That's something we could all do. We could all be present people in the now, and pay better attention.

[00:24:00] Finally, the last M in MOM stands for mechanics. I don't mean the person that fixes your car. I mean the strategy, the tool, the technique on how to learn another language, how to remember someone's name, how to read faster, how to give a speech without notes. I talk about motivation first because that's about caring, and observation, which is about being present. Then, you can put the mechanics on.

[00:24:30] I really think that a good memory training, there is no such thing as a good or bad memory. There's just a trained memory and an untrained memory. I think proper brain training and proper memory training really trains you to be a better person because when you're thinking about motivation, observation, and mechanics, in order to be ...

The art of memory is the art of attention. The art of memory is the art of caring. Being motivated to care about another human being because Maya Angelou said that people won't remember what you said, they won't remember what you did, they'll remember how you made them feel. Here's the thing: people don't care how much you know until they know how much you care. How are you going to show somebody you are going to care for their future, their family, their finances, their health, whatever it is you're offering them, if you don't just care enough just to remember them?

[00:25:00] I think the art of memory is the art of caring. The art of memory is the art of being present with people because that's what people really want. They want to be seen. They want to be heard. They want to seek first, to understand then to be understood. It's the art of observation. I think by going through a lot of these exercises what people are learning, it's just caring about somebody because here's the thing, nobody remembers everyone's name, but nobody forgets everyone's name either.

[00:25:30] I think genius leaves clues. You could role model yourself in saying, "Okay, I am the memory expert," meaning you, "and when do I remember things, and when do I forget things?" I tend to remember people I'm motivated to remember, someone I'm attracted to, somebody who could be good for my business, and so on because there's motivation there. You'll notice you remember people's names who are people you're really paying attention to as well.

One of the biggest challenges people tell me about is their memory. They say, "Jim, I want to have a better memory. I want people to say that I'm ..." I'm just hearing, "Well, I want to be better at sports." What sports specifically? Most people, their biggest challenge is remembering people's names. Have you ever met somebody, they gave you their name, and then seconds after the handshake breaks, the name just falls right to the floor?

[00:26:00]   Or it's not a short-term problem; it's a long-term problem. You're at the post office, you're at the grocery store, you're at the gym, and somebody taps you on your shoulder. You turn around, and you see someone you recognize, but for the life of you, you do not remember that person's name. What makes it worse is when that person has the nerve to remember your name. Or you're having a conversation, somebody's name you really should know, and somebody comes along, and you're in a position where you have to introduce those two people together. How do you get over it?

[00:26:30]   I want to teach you a really simple step on how to remember people's names. Really, seven steps. You can use any part of the seven. It will help you to remember names. I want you to remember to BE SUAVE. BE SUAVE. Next time you're at a networking function, you're at a conference, you're at a wedding, you're looking in the mirror, you're checking your makeup, you're checking your clothes, say to yourself, "I'm going to BE SUAVE."

The B stands for *believe*, because if you believe you can or believe you can't, either way you're right. You want to get rid of the automatic negative thoughts because those are self-programs that are going to self-destruct in your mind.

[00:27:00]   The E in BE SUAVE stands for *exercise*. I don't mean physical exercise, although one of the best brain acts is physical activity. These people who are more physically active would do better on mental acuity tests. They'll have their focus. They'll have a better memory, but I mean practice because practice makes progress. The bad news is it takes effort to improve your memory. The good news is it doesn't take as much as you think. That's the good news. I always tell people, I didn't say it was going to be easy, but I did tell you it's going to be worth it.

[00:27:30]   After that, the SUAVE. What do you do with SUAVE? The S is you meet someone for the first time, and then you *say* the name back to them. You say hello, using their name back to them. The U in SUAVE stands for *use* the name. Use the name in the conversation. You use it but you don't abuse it. You don't say, "Hi, Bob. It's nice to meet you. Bob, do you want to grab some lunch? Bob, do you want to eat blah, blah, blah." That would be an abuse. You want to use it three or four times in the context of the conversation.

[00:28:00]   After that, the A in SUAVE stands for *ask*. Ask. What's everyone's favorite subject? It's not travel, and it's not health, fitness. It's themselves. This is a really a great technique for people who have unusual names. Most times, you meet somebody, 80% of the time, it's a name you've heard before, but maybe 10% or 20% of the time, it's a new name. How do you memorize their name? Ask about it. What can you ask about a person's name? How do you spell it? Where is it from? Are you named after this person? What does it mean?

[00:28:30]   I remember, I was doing a training for the country's largest life insurance company. There were about a hundred or some people in the room. The training director's name was Nankita. Nankita. I was like, "Wow. That's a beautiful name. How do you spell it and where is it from?" I said, "What does it mean?"

She paused. I said, "What does it mean?" She looked at her coworkers, and she says, "It means graceful falling waters." I was like, "Wow."
Based on her coworkers' reaction, I was like, "Nankita, how long have you worked here?" She tells me. It's like, "With all these people?" She says, "Yeah. A lot of them are good friends. They were at my

wedding." I said, "Raise your hand if you knew that's what Nankita's name meant?" Out of a room of a hundred plus people, how many people raised their hand? Not one person.

[00:29:00] Here's the thing: the reason why you want to remember a person's name because a name is the sweetest sound to a person's ears. Think about the emotion that's connected to someone's name. Think about the first word that you learned how to write and how much love was associated, encouragement was associated with that. You want to ask about a person's name.

The V in SUAVE stands for *visualize*. Visualize. What do I mean by that? How many people are much better with faces than with names? You meet with somebody. You will say, "I remember your face but I forgot your name." You never go to someone and say the opposite, and you're saying, "Hey, I remember your name but I forgot your face." That wouldn't make a lot of sense.

[00:29:30]

What happens is we tend to remember more what we see than what we hear. There's a Chinese proverb that goes, "What I hear, I forget. What I see, I remember. What I do, I understand." What I hear, I forget. I heard the name, I forgot the name. What I see, I remember. I saw the face and I remember the face. When I do, going back to the practice and exercise, I understand. If you tend to remember what you see, then try seeing what you want to remember.

[00:30:00] This is more of an advanced technique than what most people do when they forget names. How many people do this, they go through the alphabet? Does it start with an A? Does it start with a B? Does it start with a C? They get really nervous and scared when they get to W, because there are not a lot of letters past that. Does it sometimes work? Yes. Sometimes, "Is it D? Oh, it's David."

Instead of that, what we're going to ask you to do is I want you to take the person's name and turn it into a picture. If a person's name is David, my picture of David is a slingshot. Why? David and Goliath. Imagine meeting David for the first time, and you imagine in the privacy of your own mind, without sharing this with David, you just hit him in the nose with a slingshot, and that represents David because what will happen is 30 minutes later when you're saying goodbye, you're like, "What happened to that guy? I shot him in the nose with a slingshot. What's his name? David."

[00:30:30]

If a person's name is Mark, imagine you're putting a little check mark on his forehead. A person's name is Mike, imagine they jumped on to the table and started singing karaoke on a microphone to remind you of Mike. You're like, "That's so childish, Jim," but who are the fastest learners on the planet? Children. How fast can a child learn a musical instrument compared to adult? How fast can a child learn another language compared to an adult? They use their imagination. They make fun of people's names. 80% of my friends got made fun of their names. That's how children learn through this source of imagination.

[00:31:00]

If a person's name is Mary, you can imagine getting married or imagine them holding lambs underneath her arms. Mary had a little lamb. When you say goodbye to Mary later on, you'll see those lambs. What's her name? It's Mary. If a person's name is John, you could picture whatever you picture. The V stands for visualize.

[00:31:30] The E, finally, in SUAVE stands for *end*. End. Because if you could walk into a room, and end saying goodbye to every single one of them by name, who are they all going to remember? They're all going to remember you, and that's unforgettable.

How do you fix your broken brain? The good news is one-third of your brain is predetermined by genetics and biology, one-third of your memory, and so on. That means two-thirds you control. I have found that there are 10 things you could do to really fix your broken brain. These are 10 things to have a quicker brain. I will give this to you, and then maybe we could also memorize also together as well.

[00:32:00] Number one is a good brain diet, a good brain diet because you are what you eat. Literally, what you eat becomes you. What's good for your brain? We know the foods that are good for your brain are things like avocados, blueberries, broccoli, coconut oil, salmon. You have green, leafy vegetables. You have all these things that are really good for your brain. You want to eat good foods. Good brain diet.

[00:32:30] Number two is getting rid of your negative thoughts. Getting rid of your negative thoughts. Dr. Daniel Amen, the brain doctor calls them ANTs (automatic negative thoughts). Number three is exercise. Exercise is good for your brain. Basically, anything good for your heart is going to be good for your head because it increases blood flow, and nutrients, and oxygen to your brain. Exercise is important for fixing your broken brain.

Number four are brain nutrients. Brain nutrients because when you're fast and on the go, maybe your food doesn't have all the nutrients it needs. Maybe you need to supplement with omega-3s. Maybe you need to supplement and get tested to see if you're low in B vitamins.

[00:33:00] Number five is a positive peer group. What we found—and I talk to Dr. Mark Hyman about this a lot—it's not just your biological networks or your neurological networks, it's your social networks. Who you spend time with is who you become. Are you around people who are zapping your energy? They're energy vampires. They're letting you go. They're not encouraging you. Or you're around people like a positive peer group, people that are teaching you things, that are challenging things to you, that are taking you to the next level.

[00:33:30] The number six key to fixing your broken brain is a clean environment. A clean environment, because we found through research that your external world is a reflection of your internal world. You know this anecdotally because how do you feel when you clean your home? How do you feel when you clean your desk? How do you feel when you organize your laptop or your desktop, if you will? Because that clarity goes from the outside-in as well. A clean environment is very important.

[00:34:00] Also, when I talk about clean environment, we're talking about clean water. We're talking about clean air. We're talking about a clean environment that has natural sunlight. We're talking about an environment that doesn't have toxins, pollutants, mold, and all the things that can affect your nervous system and lead to a broken brain.

Number seven, the seventh key to optimizing your brain, fixing your broken brain, is sleep. The lack of sleep is an epidemic right now. The problem is—because I came from an accelerator learning perspective—when you sleep, that's where you're consolidating short-term and long-term memory. When people suffer from insomnia, or sleep apnea, or any of these sleep issues, what happens to decision making the next day? What happens to our ability to make the decisions to solve problems?

[00:34:30] How focused do you feel on a bad night's sleep? How much energy do you have? How much brain fog do you have? You want to be able to fix and hack your sleep. There are so many things you could do. Anything from blackout curtains, to grounding devices, to getting rid of the blue light, not touching your phone at night, and so on.

After number seven, I would say key number eight to fixing your broken brain is simply this: brain protection. Growing up with learning challenges, I've had many head injuries, traumatic brain injuries,

[00:35:00] head traumas. How do you overcome that? How do you fix that? You wear a helmet. You avoid extreme sports because all those concussions ... Your brain is very resilient, but it's also very fragile. Brain protection. Protect your brain.

Number nine key to fixing your broken brain is new learnings. That's obvious for anyone who's joining us for these conversations because I feel like we're kindred spirits, because you have these growing brains already. New learning is where you create neurogenesis, neuroplasticity. The more you learn, the longer you're going to live, the more fulfilling it's going to be. Challenge your brain—that's how you create new connections.

[00:35:30] Finally, number 10 is stress management. The 10th key for fixing your broken brain is managing your stress. Most people don't realize all the anxiety, the depression, the challenges they have from this environment, because it's there all the time. It's like the fish never notice the water because when you're inside a jar, you can't see the label from inside the Jar. When you're living under this kind of stress, whether it's environmental stress, whether it's emotional stress, whether it's some kind of physical stress, relationship stress—whatever it is—work stress, we start getting accustomed to it.

[00:36:00] The problem with stress to your learning, to your brain, when you have cortisol, when you're producing adrenaline, it's good for fight-or-flight—something physical—but it's not good if you need to take a test. It's not good if you need to remember all these names. Not good if you need to give a presentation at work to a group of people because stress really shuts down part of your brain. You can't learn it really well. Those are my 10 keys for fixing your broken brain.

[00:36:30] Now, I want to give you what I call a quick recall technique for memorizing this list of 10 things to fix your broken brain. This is a 2500-year-old memory technique. It's a memory technique attributed to the ancient Greeks. The story goes: there was a Greek order named Simonides. He was giving a poetry reading. When he left the building, something really tragic happened. The building collapsed, and it killed everyone that was remaining. He had the responsibility of being the lone survivor to come back and help the family members identify their loved ones. He was able to do it though, based on where he remembered them sitting in the room.

[00:37:00] What we discovered through this, is that we remember where things are because as hunters and gatherers, we didn't need to memorize numbers, and words, and all those things. What was more important is we needed to remember where the good soil was, where the good food was, where the clean water was, where the enemy tribes were because that was our survival. What we're learning is that we store information in different locations unconsciously in our environment. Knowing that, what you want to do, a great memory technique for people who want to remember anything from a grocery list to giving a speech without notes.

[00:37:30] We get to train a lot of TED speakers to give those 18-minute talks. Have you ever wondered how people memorize the speeches, or how actors memorize their scripts, and so on? One of the ways they do it is through this technique. Let's say you have 10 key points you want to give on stage or at your next meeting, I think it's very important for people who are reading this series to learn with the intention of teaching it to someone else. One of the best accelerated learning principles there is, is to teach what you learned to somebody else because when you teach it, you get to learn it twice. When you're

[00:38:00] learning it with the intention of teaching it, you should pay better attention. You ask better questions. You take better notes. You make it personal to yourself to be able to express it to somebody else. I recommend everyone to do this for this exercise.

Now, we're going to take a location. Most people use their home because they're most familiar with their home, but because everybody who's here reading this, their home is different. I'm going to take a different location. I'm going to take your body because everyone's body is the same. We have similar parts. I'm going to take 10 places on your body, and we're going to name them together. When I'm

[00:38:30] done, I'm going to take the 10 keys to fixing your broken brain. A good diet, and getting rid of negative thoughts, and exercise, and we're going to put the first key in the first place, the second key in the second place, and the third key in the third place.

By the way, if you ever found yourself saying, "In the first place, this. In the second place, that. In the third place, that," like you're in an argument, that language came from this 2500-year-old memory technique. Now, that technique has almost disappeared. We're bringing it back, but that languaging is still there. Let's do this together. I want everyone to take a deep breath, and I'm going to name 10 places

[00:39:00] on your body. We're going to do it together. I want you to say it, I want you to touch it, and see it if you can.

[00:39:30] Number one is the top of your heads. Number one is top. Number two is your nose. Everyone say nose. Say nose out loud. Great. Nose. Three is your mouth. Three is your mouth. Everyone, remember three is mouth. We're just going down the body. Four are your ears. Five is your larynx, your throat. Six are your shoulders. Seven is your collar. Eight are your fingers. Where are your fingers? Nine is your belly. Ten is your seat.

Let's see if we can remember this. Number one is the top. Number two is what? Your nose. Number three is your mouth. Number four are your ears. Number five is your larynx. Six is your shoulders. Seven is your collar. Eight are your fingers. Nine is your belly. Finally, 10 is your seat. Those are your ten places.

[00:40:00] Now, if we wanted to remember, like let's say a grocery list, maybe you're in the shower or you're driving, and somebody calls you up, and say "Hey, we're having a party tonight." It's all about fixing your broken brain. "I want you to go to the health store and pick up these 10 things." You can't write it down because you're driving, or in the shower. I don't know why your phone is in the shower and people are calling you in the shower.

[00:40:30] What you could do is say, "Okay, avocados." Put avocados on the top of your head if you wanted to. Blueberries. I call them brain berries. They're coming out of your nose. Three is coconut oil coming out of your ears. You're like, "That's so childish." Who are the fastest learners? Children learn through imagination and play.

[00:41:00] Instead of doing that, I want to put the 10 keys for unlocking and fixing your broken brain. The first key was a good brain diet. I want you to imagine you're putting your good brain diet on the top of your head in the first place. Imagine the avocados there, the blueberries are there, the broccoli, the green leafy vegetables are there, the dark chocolate without the sugar, of course, is there also. Imagine that on the top of your head, and you could see it, feel it, imagine it.

I always think about what do I see and how does it make me feel. It may look a little silly because here's the thing when it comes to your memory, information combined with emotion becomes a long-term memory. You know this because the things in your life that you add emotion to, you remember better.

[00:41:30] Now, do we all have a song that will take us back for years because the emotion brings back the information? Maybe it's a scent, cologne, or a perfume. Maybe it's a smell, like of growing up, a childhood favorite food brings you back years or decades because information combined with emotion becomes a long-term memory. How do you make this emotional?

The second place is your nose. The second key for fixing your broken brain is this thing called killing ANTs, automatic negative thoughts. Get rid of those negative thoughts. How do you kill ANTs? Imagine ants coming out of your nose, and you're killing them. You never do that, but it's always impressionable. It's always unforgettable.

[00:42:00] The third place is your mouth. I want you to imagine using your mouth to exercise. Maybe you're doing pushups on your mouth. That's going to remind you exercise is good to fix your broken brain. Maybe you're doing lip exercises or something silly like that.

The fourth place are your ears. Your ears—I want you to remember brain nutrients. That's the fourth key for fixing your brain. You want to substitute with the essential nutrients that you need to fix your brain. What I would say is imagine coming out of your ears are these brain vitamins.

[00:42:30] Then, finally, as we get to the second half, number five is your larynx. That's your positive peer group, your happy friends. What are they doing? Maybe your positive peer group is coming here, and they're putting little happy faces on your larynx, like those yellow little smiling faces right there. You see them there, and you feel them. It's silly. It doesn't make sense, but that's what makes it memorable. We're halfway there.

[00:43:00] By the way, can you remember this? Number one is what? You go at the top of our head and there's a good brain diet. Number two, you go to your nose. What's going on with your nose? You're killing ANTs. Number three, you're going to your mouth. What's going on with your mouth? The exercising. Number four: what's coming out of four? Your brain nutrients. Number five is your happy friends.

Number six: here are your shoulders. When you remember six on the list was a clean environment. I just want you to imagine looking to your shoulders left and right, and somebody there is mopping, on the other side somebody is vacuuming, and that's what you remember. You look at your shoulders and you see that. That's number six.

[00:43:30] Number seven is your collar. I want you to remember for number seven, that is to remind you of sleep. I just want you to imagine on your collar, you have a necklace made up like a hammock. You have a hammock here, and you're taking a really nice rest here. You're sleeping in the hammock.

Number eight is your fingers. The eighth tip to fixing your broken brain is brain protection. I want you to imagine, look at your fingers, and you're wearing helmets. Maybe you have a helmet for each of your fingers. Maybe it's your favorite sports team. On your fingers, you see that. Right on your finger is brain protection.

[00:44:00] Number nine is your belly. I want you to remember nine is new learnings. What represents new learnings? A lot of people think of books. Imagine you have a whole bookshelf on your belly, a whole bookshelf with your favorite books on your belly.

Then, finally, number 10 is your seat. You want to remember stress management. How do you relieve stress? Maybe some people get a massage. Maybe they do yoga. Maybe they drink one glass of red wine or whatever it is. Just associate that with your seat. I don't want to know what your image is, but just imagine that as number 10.

[00:44:30] Now, you're on stage, or you're on camera, or you're talking to your friend, and you're like, "I watched this video. It's so awesome. Can I show you something? There are 10 keys for fixing your broken brain, and these are the 10 keys." Just literally go up your body, up your body and down your body. Number one is a good diet. Number two is killing ANTs. What's number three? Say it out loud. Number three is exercise. Number four, coming out of your ears is what? Brain nutrients, brain vitamins. Number five is your larynx. What do you have? Happy stickers, your happy friends.

[00:45:00] Number six, what's going on your shoulders? People are cleaning. That's your clean environment. Number seven, what's going on your collar? There's a big hammock there to remind you of sleep. Very good. Number eight is your fingers, what's on your fingers? Helmets, brain protection. Number nine, you have on your belly, a bookshelf to remind you of new learnings. Finally, number 10, you have stress management. Those are the 10 keys. That's how you memorize the 10 keys for unlocking and fixing your broken brain.

[00:45:30] One of the most important keys to fixing a broken brain, to have a better, brighter brain, is to control your routines, meaning control your habits because, first, you make your habits. Then, your habits make you. I think what's most important in your day is to really start your day off right, by jump-starting your brain. I have very specific morning rituals I do every single day that really jumpstart my brain, and also jumpstart my day. The reason why you want to focus on the first hour of your day is because if you can win the first hour of your day, you can win the entire day, because you kept positive momentum throughout the entire day.

[00:46:00] This is what I do every single morning. The first thing I do when I wake up, I go through a process of remembering my dreams. Remembering my dreams—this is the reason why a lot of people would want to do this, most of the time when you wake up, you had these dreams of inspiration, things that could really solve some of the problems you have, because when you're going throughout your entire day at

[00:46:30] work and through your life, you're solving problems. You're learning new things. When you go sleep, your mind doesn't stop. Your subconscious is still working on those problems. The challenge is when you wake up, you often forget what those answers are. Throughout history, our world is a reflection of a lot of the things we create in our world, actually, were birthed in someone's dreams.

[00:47:00] For example, art, literature, science. For example, Mary Shelley came up with *Frankenstein* in a dream. Paul McCartney came up with *Yesterday* in a dream. Elias Howe created the sewing machine in a dream. The scientific method, the periodic table, that framework was created in a chemist's dream. What are we thinking about? When I wake up in the morning, the first thing I do is go through a process of remembering my dreams. I just want you to remember this. Remember the acronym DREAMS. I use a lot of acronyms.

DREAMS, the D stands for - first - *decide*. Decide the night before that you're going to remember your dreams because decision is like incision. Incision means to cut. Decision means you're cutting off from the possibility that you're not going to, and you're going to. First, decide that's something you want.

[00:47:30] The R in DREAMS is *record*. Record. I mean keep a dream journal. Keep a dream journal by your bed. If you wake up in the middle of the night, have one of those little light pens, and write down your dream. Write your dream, so your recording will help you remember it.

The E in DREAMS stands for *eye*. What I mean by your eyes is keep your eyes shut. This is not in very specific order, but what you do is you train yourself when you first wake up to keep your eyes shut. Usually, the reason why a lot of people forget their dreams is they open their eyes, they get distracted, and they forget their dreams. Keep your eyes shut.

[00:48:00] The A in DREAMS stands for *affirmations*. Throughout the day—or even at night—what I say to myself is, "I'm going to have good dreams. I'm going to have peaceful dreams. I'm going to remember my dreams." Those affirmations are very powerful because your brain is like a supercomputer and your self-talk is a program that runs. When you say, "I'm going to remember my dreams," it's like have you ever had to wake up at a specific time for a very specific meeting early? You set your alarm for 5:30am and you wake up like two minutes before the alarm goes off. That's because you had the intention. You set

[00:48:30] that affirmation to do so. You could do that, also, that you're going to have positive dreams, and you will remember your dreams. That's your affirmation.

The M in DREAMS stands for *manage*. What are you managing? You're managing your sleep. We teach a number of brain hacks to be able to manage your sleep, but make sure that you have ... For example, you're in a room that's completely dark. You have blackout curtains because even the light on the alarm clock could keep you from getting a restful sleep. You want to keep it completely black to manage your sleep.

[00:49:00] Then, finally, the S in DREAMS stands for *share*. You want to share your dreams. You want to celebrate your dreams. You want to talk about your dreams to others throughout the day because if that's an intention point for you, you're going to start paying attention to it while you're dreaming.
The first thing I do when I wake for my morning routine, I remember my dreams. The second thing I do with my morning routines is I actually make my bed. You're like, "Jim, why do you make your bed? How is that good for a good brain?" I'll tell you a couple of reasons. First of all, you want to start your day with excellence, because I believe how you do anything is how you do everything in life. You want to

[00:49:30] take a couple of minutes, make your bed, make it perfect, and you start with the success because success breeds success and creates positive momentum.

The other reason why you want to be able to make your bed is because, again, how you do anything is how you do everything. You want to build some positive momentum, and carry that excellence on throughout your day. The other reason, also, is when you come back at the end of the day, you come back to success. You come back to a win. That's very important.

Expert Interviews – Jim Kwik

© 2017 Hyman Digital. All Rights Reserved.

229

[00:50:00]	Another thing I'll do first thing in the morning is I'll take a cold shower. We know that when you hit your knee, you put ice on it because it reduces the swelling. It reduces the inflammation. We know top athletes like Michael Phelps take ice baths because it reduces inflammation in your body that creates the disease, obesity, and all these big challenges. Taking a cold shower, not only wakes you up, but it helps to lower the inflammation in your body.
[00:50:30]	From there, I'll brush my teeth. You're like, "Jim, obviously, we brush our teeth." I would encourage you to actually practice brushing your teeth with your opposite hand. These are little exercises you could do that stimulate your brain because everything I'm talking about helps to wake up your brain and build on success. Using your opposite hand forces you to put your mind into your muscle. We find that the best exercises you could do to build your brain power are things like juggling, ballroom dance, martial arts, or music that requires you to use both hands and be dexterous. Brush your teeth with the opposite hand.
[00:51:00]	From there, I'll go into the kitchen and have a tall glass water. That's obvious, but when it comes to your brain, your brain is, again, 2% of your body weight, but it requires 20 to 25% of the nutrients. You use a lot of water when you're sleeping. You want to replenish that. That's when I take my probiotics because it's so important. Gut health is so important because your gut is your second brain, that microbiome. You're drinking lots of water. You're replenishing your probiotics there as well because you have a high concentration of nerves in that area.
[00:51:30]	After that, I meditate, I think it's important for everybody to have a mindful training or some mindfulness practice in your day because if you are suffering from digital distraction, your attention is everywhere, you need a time where it's just you in silence. You're focusing on your own breath. The reason why meditation is so important is, yes, it's nice to get all zen with yourself.
[00:52:00]	The other reason why is every time your tension goes somewhere, which it actually will, you bring it back. You're building your focus. Everything I'm talking about, you don't have creativity, you do creativity. You don't have focus, you do focus. You don't have memory, you do have memories. Everything that I teach in our coaching system is we take all these things, and we make them verbs, things that you could do, so they're process-oriented, step-by-step-by-step. What I'm saying here, you build your focus muscles because every time you bring your focus back to yourself or to your breathing, you build that fitness.
[00:52:30]	After I meditate, I'll make a tea. I like tea myself. I make either a turmeric tea, because turmeric along with pepper, it makes this golden milk with almond milk or something, and it reduces the inflammation in my body. Or I'll alternate between a turmeric tea, this golden tea, to what I call brain tea. I'll take aromatic herbs, ginkgo, gotu kola, or lion's mane, and make it into a tea, which are all good for your focus, memory, and attention. I'll add some honey. Some people like honey or some sweetener in there that's not sugar. Then, I'll add some fat in there also as well. That will be my brain tea.
[00:53:00] [00:53:30]	I'm drinking my brain tea while I'm doing my next activity, which is journaling. The reason why I'm journaling here is I'm writing down three things I'm grateful for because I think gratitude is the ultimate emotion. There are four keys for having an incredible mindset. An incredible mindset is the opposite of a broken brain. I'll give you those really quickly. Number one is a *growth* mindset. You always have to be growing because if you're not growing, you're dying. Nothing stays the same. Your brain has to always be learning; otherwise, it's slipping. You're green, you grow; you're brown, and you rot. You always want a growth mindset. The seminal work on it is called *Mindset* by Carol Dweck.
[00:54:00]	The other thing you want to build is your *grit*. The second chi is your grit. What I mean by that is your perseverance, your resilience. I remember, there was a big boxing, a match that was going on, and it was the largest one for the decade. I get a call from Sylvester Stallone saying, "Hey, do you want to watch the fight at my home?" I'm like, "Yeah. I totally wanna watch a boxing championship fight with Rocky." I have mixed feelings as I'm watching this fight. I'm sitting on his couch. It's me, Sylvester Stallone, and Arnold Schwarzenegger. I swear if somebody took a picture of that couch, people would be like, "Who

---

Photoshopped that Asian dude in that photo?"

[00:54:30]

We're watching this fight. I had mixed feelings because I'm all about brain protection. I've had traumatic brain injuries, and concussions and you have to protect your brain. Yet, I'm very curious about competition, and how it takes us to the next level. Afterwards, I remember asking Sly and Arnold. I was like, "What does it take to be a champion at that level? What's the difference between an amateur and a champion?" Arnold looks at me, and says, "Jim, the difference between an amateur and a champion is the champion could push through the pain period."

[00:55:00]

The champion could push through the pain period, meaning that if you're going to go work out, and you want to build a muscle, and you're doing ten reps or curls, the curls that you want to least do are probably 8, 9, and 10, the one you don't want to do. But if you use grit, going back to grit, and you push yourself through it, those are the same ones that are going to give you the most growth.

I believe in the maxim that if you do the easy things all your life, then your life is going to be very hard. If you do the hard things in your life, then your life is going to be easy. You want to build your grit. The other reason why I take cold showers is I don't like cold showers, I don't like ice baths, but I do it because—can I do another 30 seconds? As long as it's safe because I build by grit. It's growth. It's grit.

[00:55:30]

The third G, I would say, for the superhero mindset or really great mindset would be this thing called *giving*. Giving because we grow, so we have more to give. I think everything in the environment, everything grows or dies, or everything gives back to the environment, or it's eliminated, or it becomes extinct. We're here to be able to give, but we have to grow also. It's not murdering yourself. I always tell people self-love and self-care is not selfish. You have to grow, so you have more to give.

[00:56:00]

Finally, the fourth G, I would say, is *gratitude*. Gratitude because gratitude is the ultimate emotion. That's why when I'm writing down, going back to my journal, my morning routine, I'm writing three things that I'm most grateful for. Everybody talks about a vision board, and the things they want to be, do, have, and share. But I'm more passionate about my gratitude board, which are the things I'm most grateful for.

[00:56:30]

If people say, "I don't have a lot to be grateful for. I'm not wealthy or anything," I'd ask a different question. I would say, "For me, gratitude has nothing to do with financial wealth. I would ask yourself, how many things in your life do you have to be grateful for that money can't buy?" All the things that we have that money can't buy, that would go on to my journal. I start my day with three things I'm grateful for because I feel like I can't build on it unless I'm grateful for what I already have.

[00:57:00]

Then, I write three things that I want to accomplish that day professionally and three things personally. That's it, because everybody has a massive to-do list with dozens or hundreds of things on it every single day. I found that the high performers, the people really working their peak brain don't focus on all 200 things they need to do. They focus on the three things that are going to make the biggest difference in their life personally and professionally, they get those three things done, and they thrive.

After I do that, I do two to three minutes of intense movement. I do burpees, or I do pushups, or I do sit ups, or I do jumping jacks, just to get my heart ... That's not my exercise for the day, but it gets my heart pumping. It gets blood flow going into my body.

[00:57:30]

From there, I make a brain power smoothie. "Jim," it's like, "Wow, that's a lot of stuff." I'm saying you don't have to do everything, but as much of this as you can do, you really jumpstart your brain. We talked about great foods for your brain. We talked about avocados. We talked about blueberries. We talked about dark raw chocolate with no sugar in it. We're talking about green leafy vegetables. I'll put most of the green into a blender, and I'll just blend it up, and that's my brain smoothie. When I'm drinking my brain smoothie, I pick up a book to read. I think this is so important.

[00:58:00] I worked with a lot of actors, teaching to speed read scripts, memorize their lines. I remember I spent time with Will Smith right on set. Two things I got out of this. Number one: we're shooting from 6pm to 6am, which is insane. Imagine having to adjust your sleep schedule, and be ready, and everything else. I remember asking him this question. I was like, "How do you get ready at 3am, get prepared to go in front of all these cameras with hundreds and millions of dollars behind this movie? How do you show up like that and be prepared?" He's like, "Jim, I don't have to get ready." He's like, "I stay ready." I'm like, "Wow. That's a superhero mindset."

[00:58:30] Besides that, we were talking about how we keep ourselves fit. He's like, "Jim, I do two things every single day. I run and I read. I do something physical and I do something mental." When I say going back to your reading, I think it's important every day for someone to read 20-30 minutes a day because that's your mental exercise.

[00:59:00] Besides the fact, I teach speed reading; I teach the average person to read 300% faster, and understand more of it. Essentially, if we read something at 15 or 20 minutes, it normally takes an hour because leaders are readers, because if somebody takes ... In this series, we have these incredible experts. If someone has decades of experience, and they put it into a book, and you could read that book in a few days, you could download decades into days. That's incredible unto itself, because knowledge is not only power, knowledge is profit. I don't just mean financial profit, I mean all the treasures of our life, our health, our relationships, our career, and everything.

[00:59:30] I read, and I teach people how to read one book a week. I did a podcast on this episode on this. It's *How Do You Read a Book a Week*? An average person reads two books a year. That's it, two books a year. The average CEO reads about four or five a month. How do you do that? Really simple. I went to Amazon, and I was searching, what's the medium amount of words per book? I came out with a number like 64,000 words in a book.

[01:00:00] I was like, "Okay, the average person reads about 200 words per minute. I divide that together," and said, "Okay. That means the average book to finish is about 320 minutes." That's a lot of minutes, but I was like, "Well, if I divide that by seven, how many minutes is that really?" It comes out to about 45 minutes a day. That's very doable. 45 minutes a day to read one book a week. Leaders are readers. I read for 20-30 minutes while I'm drinking my superpower smoothie. From remembering my dreams, to making my bed, to making my superhero smoothies—that's how I start my day.

[01:00:30] Recently I was invited to the Cleveland Clinic Center for Brain Health. I was asked to do something very specific: to train the attendees, doctors, caregivers, some patients, and the local community how to improve their memory and their focus because their initiative is very powerful, they do all this incredible research on brain aging, dementia, and Alzheimer's, and they do a lot of caregiving to patients. What they're starting to incorporate more and more is the power of prevention and the power of lifestyle.

[01:01:00] When I went there and we filmed all these videos and—me presenting to this group of people—I addressed things that are most presenting for them. They wanted to talk about how to overcome absent-mindedness, how to improve people's focus, how to improve their day-to-day memory, like what they ate for breakfast that day. Sometimes, even when I'm working, this is a topic that is very near and dear to my heart because my grandmother was suffering from Alzheimer's when she passed, didn't recognize me, and didn't know my name. I was very young at the time.

[01:01:30] I wanted to fix her. Not only did I have my own suffering for my own brain injury at five, but a few years later, when I'd seen my grandmother, and when somebody is suffering in this way, and they don't recognize you ... I teach people on remembering facts, and figures, and foreign languages, and then the like. I think what's equally important is remember three things when it comes to your memory.

Number one: you want to remember your loved ones, like my grandmother. I want to remember those people that are closest to me. Besides loved ones, I want to remember my life, because I feel like that if

[01:02:00] your life is worth living, it's worth remembering. A lot of people, they don't even remember what they had for breakfast yesterday or today. You want to remember those magic moments in your life, your love, your life. Then, finally, your lessons.

[01:02:30] I have a friend named Marylou. We're talking about this definition of insanity that we've all heard. Insanity is doing the same thing over and over again expecting a different result. Marylou is like, "Jim, that's not insanity. That's just a poor memory." What that means is some people repeat mistakes in their life. They eat the same bad food or they get in the same bad relationship or they make the same bad investments or they hire same bad people because they don't remember the lessons in their life, the pain and the problems. I think that's one of the reasons why it's important to have a good memory.

[01:03:00] What I was doing, I remember even as I started training in this and learning these skills because I believe there's no such thing as a good or bad memory, there's just a trained and an untrained memory, and I would go spend time with seniors. I would teach them these methods. Even at the Cleveland Clinic, I was talking to patients. Sometimes, I would teach a technique, and talk about a lifestyle hack that's going to help them to remember more. Sometimes, I just got them to talk, and tell stories, and polish off those memories because I think one of the keys to immortality is, first, living a life worth remembering.

[01:03:30] What would my advice be to a parent who's watching this that wants to help their children? Maybe their children, they're struggling with learning, or they're struggling with their own broken brain, or they're struggling in school, like I was when I was a child. I would start with this, the question is not how smart your children are, it's how are they smart. I find that with children, having worked with a lot of children in this, and helping them with their focus, and their memory, and their reading abilities, and such, everybody has a preferred way of learning, first of all.

[01:04:00] It's nice to be able to honor that, that sometimes in our traditional school system, they only reinforce two kinds of education. It's like mathematical or verbal linguistic, like standardized tests. I'm saying that you are not your IQ—that IQ is actually being highly disputed, that your intelligence is not fixed like your shoe size. No matter where your children are, they could have growth. I come from that kind of belief.

[01:04:30] On top of that, I would say that it's not just honoring and valuing two kinds of intelligence. There are other kinds of ways that children are smart and adults ... It could be verbal, linguistic, and it could be mathematical, but also another form of intelligence or genius is visual and spatial. These are the great artists. These are the great architects. That's equally important as anything else. Somebody who's great with words and great in math.

[01:05:00] Another form of intelligence is interpersonal intelligence. Meaning, maybe that child is really great with other children. They have great connections and they're a great communicator, and such. Interpersonal. I would say another form of intelligence is intrapersonal. Where interpersonal is self to others, intrapersonal is self to self. I think an incredible superpower is self-awareness. I think you can only be happiest if you know who you are, and if you be who you are. Meaning, you have the curiosity to know yourself, and you have the courage to really be yourself. Intrapersonal intelligence is very important.

[01:05:30] On top of that—musical intelligence. Maybe your child is really ... Maybe they have trouble with learning math, or learning languages, or something like that, but they have a great musical gift. These are the future musicians, singers, songwriters, and so on. Maybe there's also kinesthetic intelligence. Some people might have challenges with math, or with music, but they have incredible intelligence in the human body. These are your athletes. These are your dancers. People that can move their body in ways that other people can't. I would say start working with the child—it's not how smart they are, it's how are they smart. Maybe they have other areas of intelligence.

[01:06:00] The other thing is, if I ask everybody to write down on a piece of paper your first and last name—and people could do this—they write their first and last name. Then, switch over to your opposite hand, and write your first and last name under it with your opposite non-dominant hand. I think, for the most part, that second time ... First time, it's faster, the quality is better, and it's more comfortable. The second time, it takes longer. It feels a little weird and uncomfortable, and the quality is not quite as good.

[01:06:30] Sometimes, what happens is when you're normally interested, or your children are normally interested in the topic, but they're not getting it; sometimes they're trying to learn it with the opposite hand. Meaning, it takes longer, the quality is not as good, and it feels uncomfortable for them because maybe the way the teacher prefers to teach is different than the way the student prefers to learn. It's like two ships passing in the night, and they don't even see each other, and there's no connection, and then there's no learning.

[01:07:00] I think as a parent working with the student, honor their difference because their difference is what makes them special. Honor their specific learning style. Some people love to learn by basing it on what they see. Other people like to learn by reading something. Other people prefer to have a discussion over it. Other people like to roll up their sleeves, they're kinesthetic learners, and they need to move around. Honor that individual. This is more like a whole self-learning where we're not treating everybody as an assembly line, a one-size-cookie-cutter-fits-all situation.

[01:07:30] The other thing I would say is really encourage them and the 10 things I'm talking about—lifestyle hacks. Meaning give them a good diet, optimize their brain, fix the hardware, fix that broken brain. Give them the right diet, help them with their negative thoughts, and make sure they're moving every single day because children now, they don't have their recess. A lot of that stuff is being taken out of schools around movement.

I want to create an initiative where classrooms are required to have standing desks, because they say that sitting is the new smoking, and being sedentary. You have to be able to move around. Make sure they're moving. Make sure they're around positive peers. Make sure they have a clean environment, all these things. Make sure they're getting sleep. Make sure they're not spending too much time on their digital devices because that's rewiring children's brains.

[01:08:00] You see these children out in restaurants or anything else—you can't take them off those iPads. They're really rewired. I would keep the negative influence, the EMFs, the toxicities ... Check your environment for environmental mold and all the toxins that could be affecting your children.

[01:08:30] For me, I like to do a lot of blood work and see food sensitivities. With Functional Medicine, to have a good Functional Medicine doctor, because you don't know if you're feeding your children foods that are irritating them, that they have allergies to, that's making them tired, that's distracting them, that's helping them to spread out their focus. All those things matter. Everyone always wants to know what the magic pill is. There is no magic pill, but there are magic processes. You have to do every single thing to be able to fix your broken brain.

JJ Virgin:

[00:00:30]

When my son was 16, he was crossing the street and was hit by a car. We estimate maybe 40 miles per hour, and no one saw it happen. He was literally left for dead in the street. The woman got out of her car, gassed it, and drove off. Thankfully, a neighbor pulled up, called 911 and he was airlifted to the local hospital. When we got there, the doctors told us that we needed to let him go. He had a torn aorta, which kills 90% of the people on the scene, and it had to be repaired. But the challenge was they couldn't repair it at that hospital because he had a severe traumatic brain injury. In order to fix it, they had to do it without a blood thinner. They had to airlift him to another hospital and the doctor said he would never survive another airlift.

[00:01:00]

Even if he did, he wouldn't survive the surgery. Even if he were managing to survive both those things, the chance he'd ever be normal was minuscule. My other 15-year-old son looked at that doctor and said, "So, maybe like a .25% chance he'd make it?" The doctor said, "That sounds about right." He goes, "We'll take those odds." He said to me, "Well you know, .25 is not 0. What do we have to lose?" Any parent reading this I think would say, "Hey, I'm going to fight, right? I'm going to fight for my son's life." We get to the next hospital. He survives the airlift. We have an amazing surgical team—five different surgical teams—working on him. He survives the surgery and then he is in a deep coma. The neurosurgical team says, "You know, we don't know if he'll ever wake up."

[00:01:30]

[00:02:00]

"We have no idea if he does, what his life will be like." I remember standing there hearing this and holding my son's hand and telling him ... There were like two fingers I could hold. Everything else was either bandaged or covered with road rash. He had 13 fractures. Bones literally sticking through his skin. I said, "Grant, this is going to be the best thing that ever happened to you," which is a ridiculous thing to say. I mean, this was looking so bleak, but I had to have hope. I said, " You're going to be 110%." From that point, I'm scared to death. I mean this was like the worst thing a parent could ever face, but I just went with this, how do I get my son to be 110%?

[00:02:30]

Now the doctors thought I was crazy, but it's interesting because when you start to lead with that rather than let's just get him to survive, I think everybody starts to treat it a little bit differently. Some of the doctors just kind of let me do some of the things I was doing. Immediately I put an SOS out to all my friends on Facebook and I had incredible help coming into the hospital early on. I had Dr. Hyla Cass come in right away, Dr. Daniel Amen. We were able to start to do some things that you wouldn't normally get to do and that the hospital actually wouldn't let us do, but we did sort of circuitously. These, I really believed, are the reasons that he's not only here today, but he's actually 110%.

[00:03:00]

[00:03:30]

Right away, the very first thing I did was I started taking things to help me with stress. I started doing some stuff to support myself, because I knew that in order to show up for my son in the hospital, I couldn't get sick. He was in the ICU and we had to go in there fully gowned, masked, and gloved. I made sure I put my self-care first. I think that's so important for every parent to hear because we tend to put ourselves last. I knew if I was making life or death decisions I had to be totally focused and game on. Then, one of the first things we were able to do was use essential oils and it wasn't something I was remotely familiar with. Someone came in and started using them with him and all I knew was that for the first time I started to see some response.

[00:04:00]

He wiggled his nose. He wiggled his fingers, which gave me some hope. We started using progesterone cream, which we were able to rub on him because it was a cream. There was some research out of Emory by Dr. Donald Stein showing that it helps reduce inflammation, which is the big thing that you have to do right now as your brain is so inflamed. He looked like the Incredible Hulk in the middle of the pediatric ICU. You'd walk in and he was so blown up from all the swelling from 13 fractures and all of the road rash. The next thing that I want to do—and this is where it became quite a challenge—was he'd been on five grams of fish oil prior to the accident.

[00:04:30]

[00:05:00]

I'm on a mission to get everybody on fish oil because I know that one of the reasons he's actually with us today was because his brain was protected going into this, because fish oil protects your brain from injury. You never know when you're going to hurt your brain. The chances we're going to hurt our brain is almost 100%. We all hit our heads. I knew I wanted to get him back on his fish oil and that's where the battle began, because he was bleeding and they were afraid that the fish oil was going to increase his bleed time and so they didn't want to do it. I got them to go to two grams, but I knew we needed to be much higher than that. The doses that they do in this situation is anywhere from 10 to 20 grams. I brought them all the research.

[00:05:30]

Dr. Barry Sears actually sent it to me. I had Dr. Michael Lewis, who wrote *When Brains Collide,* helping me with this, I had all the research and they go, "Nope. We won't do it. It's going to cause increased bleeding," even though there was nothing to show it would. When he spit out his feeding tube, which he did himself, we started doing it ourselves. First, I got him up to five grams, and we would always do it right around when they were going to test his bleeding time so I could check that. We never saw any change in his bleeding time. We got him up to 10 grams at the first hospital, and then when we went to the second hospital, we got him up to 20 grams.

[00:06:00]

[00:06:30]

When I went to the higher dose of fish oil, he went from barely speaking to speaking in sentences. It's very interesting, because when I went through all of this what I was told, when Grant was coming out of the coma, was that there was nothing you could do. That the brain has its own time schedule and now we wait. I'd already sent the SOS out to all of my friends in the medical community and I was so fortunate to get all of this information back. I knew that waiting was not the right thing to do and it just doesn't ever make sense. First of all, I'm not patient so I'm not going to wait. I said to this doctor, I said, "So there's nothing we can do?" She goes, "Nope. Not a thing." That's when I knew that I was just going to have to take responsibility.

[00:07:00]

I think that a key through-line for all of this, is that we have to take responsibility for our health and the health of our loved ones. No one's going to care as much as we do, and no one understands our own body and the people close to us like we do. I was able to communicate especially when we went to the second hospital where they were much more open. I got to the second hospital, Children's Hospital Los Angeles, and I said, "He's on 20 grams of fish oil," and they go, "Okay." They actually didn't check it, but by then he had massive files so it would have been a nightmare to look for it. They were like, "Okay. That's great." They put him on it. They were letting me do a lot more integrated approach.

[00:07:30]

I actually got into all the meetings with the entire team and talked about what I want to do from my side because here I am, I'm a mom, I'm a nutritionist. I've been working with my son and helping him with his bipolar disorder for years. As he was coming out of his coma, I knew best what to look for. I knew when he was going to get irritated when he needed to rest more than they would. We all worked together on it. I think the frustrating thing here is no one person is alike. No one brain injury is alike. To try to do one single protocol with the study, I don't even know how you would do it. The obvious thing to do is to look at the pathways and make the decisions. Here I looked at risk reward. There wasn't any risk for putting him on the high-dose fish oil.

[00:08:00]

[00:08:30]

Their perceived risk of an increasing bleed time was not real. The reward, the payoff was huge. There were already cases that had been out, the coal miner, Bobby Ghassemi, that had shown huge success, so why not try. When you look at this, and again this is the most extreme case, but that's where you really can learn. I've told my son, "Grant," I said, "You know honey, you're going to be a lab rat here." He goes "Okay." He's one who can really show us, because if it works in an extreme case, think what it can do for all of us. One of the things that we have to look at is our brains are ... they're easily injured. Kind of think of like having an egg in a hard head and we hit our head. We've got vibration injuries.

[00:09:00] We've got all sorts of toxic substances that we're breathing or drinking or ingesting, not that we're trying to, but they're in so many of the foods we eat and the air we breath. We're damaging our brain and it gets inflamed. One of the key things that fats can do is help put that fire out and help reduce that inflammation. The other thing they're key for is you can't communicate well without having good flow. They help with cell membrane fluidity. You have to have that in order to have your brain working well. This whole time I'm going through this with my son and it was four and half months in the hospital.

[00:09:30] That actually was easier than the four and a half years since then of helping someone come through a traumatic brain injury, but during that same time I'm the primary financial support for my family. I have two kids. I had a big book launching and then three more books. I'm running a company. I'm doing all of this. They were like, "How the heck are you doing this? I could never do that." I said, "You know what?

[00:10:00] Yes, you could and you would. We're never better than when we're challenged." When people are saying, "Well, how did you do that," I really realize that it all came down to mindset. So many people asked me what's the number one thing that's helped your son.

Well, the number one thing that helped my son was my younger son saying, "We'll take those odds." Us not going along with the first doctor who did a lot to keep my son alive, but looked at the situation and to him he didn't see that there was a miracle possible, right? My mindset said, "Hey, let's be open to

[00:10:30] possibility. He's not dead yet. We have to try." The big change for Grant was standing in that hospital and saying, "What do we need to do to help him be 110%?" It's a question that I've asked every single day since then, and this hasn't been an easy path. He's been suicidal multiple times, which 25% of people with brain injuries are suicidal. This is a major problem out there.

[00:11:00] We tend to think of it as something that happens to our soldiers or football players, but it happens because of domestic violence. It's the leading cause of death in children. It's 1.7 million people a year getting a traumatic brain injury. This is a major problem. Over 5 million people are disabled at any time in the US with it. You can turn it around and you can turn it around anytime. If you hurt your head five years ago, you can still massively improve it, but it's got to start with asking the right questions. For me,

[00:11:30] it was how do I get my son to be 110%. Then looking at every single thing that's out there that I could bring in to help him. I was looking at in preparing for this interview of like what did we do? It's this huge long list of things.

Now within that, I can tell you the things that were most successful for us, but that's us. It may be different for someone else, but it's asking that right question that made all the difference. My son, prior to this, early on had bipolar disorder. He still has bipolar disorder, but that led me down the path in the first place and ultimately probably saved his life because he was on a high dose of fish oil to start with

[00:12:00] that we've done for the bipolar disorder. Here's the thing: we've all got something. Everybody does; everybody's got something. I look at some of these things and I go, "What if his bipolar disorder is actually an advantage? What if ADD is actually an advantage? What if there are things about that that are going to be advantages and we can deal with the rest?"

[00:12:30] The first things I think we need to always start with, are cleaning up the diet, and helping the gut as much as possible, because there's so much we can do that makes a major difference. Even if it only made a 10 or 20% difference, hey, that matters. Whether you are a parent with a child with ADD, autism, or bipolar disorder, or whether everyone's totally what we'd call normal, which I don't know what normal is, you actually still want to do all the same things. Eat a diet that helps you maintain good

[00:13:00] blood sugar control and blood sugar balance. Eat good healthy fats to help nourish the brain and reduce the inflammation. Exercise, because if you look at the one thing that's probably the most key thing for having a healthy brain, exercise is so key for that.

In fact, there's a great study that UCLA did, where they showed that if rats don't exercise, their memory goes down, they slow down. The minute they're exercising, they have better executive function, they have better memory, their brain's working well. This is one of the key things we can do. Then really

[00:13:30] giving your child a sense of connection and purpose. It's the same things that we all need that are good for everybody. It's interesting. As Grant has gone through this process over the last five years, intuitively he's started doing so many things along with all the stuff I was doing. He started meditating. He started gardening and getting into the ground and earthing. He started doing high intensity interval training.

[00:14:00] He started doing the things that he needed to heal his brain too. It's like his body knew best. Dr. Hyman says the phrase I'm going to steal here, because I love it so much, that, "Sugar is our number one recreational drug of choice." It is the worst for your brain. It's going to create inflammation. That's what you want to have, not have an inflammation, but the other thing that it does is, eating a high sugar

[00:14:30] impact diet causes insulin resistance. That really causes problems in the brain, because in the brain you need insulin to come up to trigger all the communication, all the firing. Without that it's like your brain just got slow, old, inflamed and angry. Right? The other part that sugar does is it triggers the reward center in your brain.

[00:15:00] This is how we create this whole drug of choice situation is it triggers dopamine. You just keep coming back for more and more and more. In fact, they did this rat study where they gave the rat the choice between ... First, they gave him some kind of an opioid, I think it was morphine, and let him have as much as he wanted. Then he had Oreo cookies and he got to have those, and then he got to choose between them and he chose the Oreos for his reward; triggers the reward center in the brain and that's what they saw in that study. They both lit up the same reward center in the brain, but the other thing

[00:15:30] that it does, besides triggering that so you want to keep going to back for that dopamine hit, is that it will drive up serotonin and then deplete it.

Then it creates this really bad situation where you just keep needing more and needing more and needing more. You're creating inflammation in the brain and then you're creating insulin resistance, so now you don't have the insulin you need up in the brain for the communication, so again slowing you down, making you inflamed and making you angry—nothing you want your brain to be. The big

[00:16:00] challenge we have with sugar is that we've really been looking at it all wrong. I mean you just don't see that many people nowadays going out and getting a candy bar. We know better than that, but yet they'll get one of those energy bars and they're still loaded with sugar.

The ones that kill me are where it's hiding or disguised as something healthy like a lot of these smoothies or green drinks that are just a big sugar load. The big challenge there is that they're a fructose

[00:16:30] load. The worst sugar of all for the brain and for the body overall is fructose. It's used a lot because it's sweeter than glucose is, but the challenge is it makes you more insulin resistant. It actually can make your gut permeable so you're more sensitive to foods and you become food intolerant. It's more aging and it makes you fat. It goes straight to the liver and starts turning into fat.

[00:17:00] One of the key things, and I think back early on when Grant was a kid in school with bipolar disorder and ADD and all these things. Those are all titles. All I know is that if his blood sugar was balanced, everything was good and if it wasn't, things blew up. I still remember when he won some contest, and they gave him a pound bag of M&M's. They give this to a kid. I go, "You don't give a kid a pound bag of M&M's," and then he'd eaten them and they go, "He's climbing the walls. Come get him." I'm like, "I'm not getting him. He's all yours." As long as we keep things blood sugar balanced ... and that goes for all of us.

[00:17:30] In fact, one of the key things you can do to tell if you've eaten a hormonal winner for your meal is, how long can you go until you need to eat again. This idea that we need to snack every couple of hours is absolutely ridiculous. If you're eating a meal that's very balanced, and I'll talk about what that is, you should be able to go four to six hours before you need to eat again. What you want to really look at is the trifecta of protein, fat, and fiber because the protein and the fiber are going to slow down stomach emptying and help keep you fuller longer. Then the fat works to trigger the release of some chemicals in

[00:18:00] the brain to say, "Oh, we've eaten." That's why fructose is really problematic because it doesn't trigger that release.

[00:18:30] You're eating sugar, you're getting fat, and you're still hungry, which is a rotten way to be. It's actually really simple to do this. All you need to do is make sure you're getting some clean protein, and this is where we really want to think. There's such arguments right now over vegan, paleo, pegan, high-fat, and low-fat. It's like, here's the thing that we know: you could put all of us in a room and we'd all agree that you should under-process your diet. We should be eating real food, and that ideally you want to make sure you're getting a lot of non-starchy vegetables, right? That's key and important and we don't want to go get genetically modified food because that creates its own set of problems.

[00:19:00] Beyond that, we also need to make sure that we're eating animal sources of protein—if we're eating animal sources of protein—that have eaten the right foods too, while we're choosing the right foods, which is loads of non-starchy vegetables, a great rainbow of color, so we have these antioxidants that reduce inflammation and then will give us some fiber, some low-sugar-impact carbohydrates; things like squash, pumpkins, or wild rice, especially staying away from things like gluten that are toxic to the brain. Then make sure that the animal protein sources are wild, sustainable, or pastured so that not only is it that you are what you eat, it's you are what you eat, ate.

[00:19:30] If you're eating these factory cows and factory chickens—they're fed genetically modified corn and soy—now you have a problem too because this is getting into you. Remember, it's not just you are what you eat, it's you are what you eat, ate. You're getting the fiber from the non-starchy vegetables and the low-impact carbs. You're getting the clean protein from things like pastured pork and chicken and grass-fed beef and wild fish. Then you're getting healthy fats, some from that, and that's why that's key,
[00:20:00] because toxins are stored in fats. If you're eating animals fed toxic feed, you're getting toxins. It also changes the fatty acid profile to favor non-inflammatory fats.

Then in terms of healthy fats, I think avocado is one of the most miraculous foods on the planet, so is coconut oil. I know there's all this bashing right now of coconut oil, and actually people saying you should eat corn oil, which I was in a state of shock when I saw, because if you just look at the pathways and the science tells you everything, that's an inflammatory fat. It's one of the most genetically modified
[00:20:30] crops. That's a no-go. Nuts and seeds—especially if you could soak and dehydrate them or low-roast them—wild fish, olives, and olive oil. Healthy fats are key because they're going to help you feel fuller longer. It's going to help again keep your blood sugar stable with the protein and fiber, and then stretch that meal time out.

[00:21:00] The simplest thing that exercise does to help the brain is it gets a little blood flow to the brain. You want more blood flow to the brain. Even though you think, "Oh I'm out there exercising and it's making blood flow go to the working muscles." Yes, it does, but there's also a shunt of blood to the brain. You want more blood flow to the brain. That's key. Another key thing that it does, it's the single best happy drug out there because it will help raise endorphins so you'll feel better and lower stress hormones, which is the key component. You're raising up the good guys and lowering some stress hormones so you'll feel better.

[00:21:30] All the things that can happen when you have a brain injury where you get very fixed and you're not very flexible, and your cognition goes down and you can't remember things, exercise helps counteract all of that. Now the research for that is all done on aerobic exercise, but I like to do aerobic exercise in the form of high intensity interval training. I've seen some studies now showing that that actually just
[00:22:00] gets you those effects faster and more intensely, and that make sense to me because high intensity interval training gets all of the good from aerobic and training, and takes out the bad. When you do endurance-style training, you create more oxidative stress.

You're breathing heavier over an extended period of time and you create stress on your body, lowering your immune system. You can still get the benefits of what you would with aerobic training, which is all the blood flow and lowering blood pressure, and blood flow to the brain, with high intensity interval
[00:22:30] training, but you train your sympathetic nervous system to handle stress better because you go hard and then easy and hard and then easy. I'll contrast: endurance training would be going out for a 60-

minute jog, and high intensity interval training would be walk for a minute, sprint for a minute, walk for two minutes, sprint for a minute and do that to accumulate four to eight total minutes of sprints. You're going to do it in 10 to 20 minutes.

[00:23:00] When you do that, you actually raise growth and anabolic hormones. You don't have the oxidative stress that you had from the other exercise. You don't impact your immune system like you did with the other exercise. The key most important thing about it is that it doesn't take much time. I started out in this world as a personal trainer 30 years ago, and the number one reason people didn't exercise is because they didn't have time. Back then we used to tell them that you had to do it for at least 30 minutes or it didn't matter, which is ridiculous. The second reason was they didn't want to go the gym. This is

[00:23:30] something you can do anywhere and you don't need a gym. To me, the foundation for exercise is to do aerobic training in the form of high intensity interval training.

Again, because of the blood flow, because of the impact that it does to all of the great brain chemicals and because it also increases your brain volume. It increases your growth factors. It gets everything growing, moving and communicating in your brain. It was interesting, when Grant was in the hospital at Children's Hospital LA, they had such an amazing program. One of the first things they started to do with

[00:24:00] him was take him into this gym. Now I actually snuck in there with him and then I got in trouble because I was having him do push-ups on his knees, all sorts of stuff. They're like, "He's not ready." I go, "Yes, he is. He likes to be challenged." It's interesting.

He was still in a wheelchair at that time because he had a crushed heel and there were things that we found that we could do. You can use bands. You can use balls. I would say look for whatever you can do, if you can get the person in a pool. We got Grant out on furlough. We took him to the pool, put him in

[00:24:30] there, and he swam completely coordinated. It was amazing. Things he couldn't do yet on land, he could do in the pool. What I always say is, always look for the way and if there is no way to do that, then the next level would be to go to meditation. It's interesting. I have never been a meditator. I'm actually about to take my first class with Emily Fletcher. I do tapping instead.

[00:25:00] I'm a big fan of the Ortner's. Nick Ortner taught me tapping, so I do tapping. That's one of the things that got me through a bunch of this stress with Grant, but Grant found meditation and he started doing it himself. What was so interesting is, one of the things that happens as you come through a brain injury, is you lose your internal editor. You tend to be really into your amygdala and into fight-or-flight. He was easily triggered. It was really difficult to get him out into any kind of social situation, yet he needed that.

[00:25:30] Isolation was really damaging, it's damaging to everyone. There was a study that showed that social isolation is more damaging than smoking 15 cigarettes a day. He needed that connection but it would trigger him.

What meditation does for him is actually calm down that amygdala. Get him out of fight-or-flight. He now can tell when he's getting there and he goes into his room and meditates and it's incredible. That's

[00:26:00] what I see. I'm going to now learn how to do this, but for those of us that are anxious or start to get that fear up, this is one of the ways we can cool that down and get out of our fight-or-flight. As someone comes out of a brain injury, here's what I was told, "When he comes out of this brain injury, it's going to be ugly." Now I've never been around this. All I'd seen was television shows where people wake up and they go, "Oh, I love you. Hi."

[00:26:30] I thought Grant would wake up out of his coma, just open his eyes, look at me and say, "Hi, Mom." That's what I thought. I did not think that he would open his eyes, stare off into space and move his arm repeatedly for days on end. He didn't talk. He couldn't make any eye contact. Nothing. He came out of a coma over time. As he started to become more aware, he started to become super agitated. I would see this little thing coming up here. It was like the Incredible Hulk starting to turn green. When it did, we had

[00:27:00] to shoot him basically with tranquilizers to keep him from going berserk. When I first walked into the hospital when he was starting to get like this, he actually was in a straitjacket and that's when I knew.

[00:27:30] I was like, "Okay. We have to do something here. This is not how he is going to get better." One of the things that happens as someone comes out of a brain injury is they are in that fight-or-flight mode. That's the first thing that starts to wake up. It's happened to us now repeatedly, because we've been doing stem cell injections into his spine. When we do them, that's the first thing that comes back up online as that comes up more. It's like you lose your filter. You're going to say or do whatever you think. If you think someone's attacking you, you'll hit them. If you feel like you're scared, you'll yell. That doesn't work in society very well. What he's done to counteract that is meditation and learning how to control his brain.

[00:28:00] He's been doing neurofeedback and that's helped a lot too, because now he can recognize when it's coming and he knows what to do. You look at anything. I come from the weight loss world. While there's never one diet that's perfect for everybody. That's why I always look at this whole thing like the current fight over all this stuff I'm like, "Okay. There isn't one diet for everybody." When you have a brain injury, it's like, what's the extent of the brain injury? Was this the first brain injury? Was it a vibration brain injury? Was it a hard hit? What else was going on? With Grant as he was waking up, we knew that I had a son with bipolar disorder waking up. Bipolar brains are less stable brains to begin with.

[00:28:30]
[00:29:00] Brain injuries are unstable brains. I was like, "Who's going to wake up here?" We didn't really know. There were things specific that we needed to do there to really help stabilize his brain. CBD has been an amazing thing for him. When you look at it, there are still common factors for everybody that we can look at. Number one, you must reduce the inflammation, so what things are going to be key there. If I could pull out my key most favorite things, fish oil of course would be the number one, exercise, CBD. Besides helping with brain stability, it also helps with reducing inflammation. Then curcumin. Those were some of the key things that we started to do there. Then you've got to stabilize the brain. In fact, we've had him on medications to start with because that is so key.

[00:29:30]
[00:30:00] They can go into seizures, but a ketogenic diet has been a key player here to help and MCT oil. I always looked at, "Okay. What were the pathways? How do we get him off the medication as quickly as possible? What things could we do diet-wise there?" We have to do things to help stabilize the brain quickly. Ketogenic diets have been used for decades for seizures. That's another one, and MCT oil there to help. Then inflammation and stabilizing the brain and balancing your blood sugar is another key one. Then of course getting the blood flow to the brain. We were doing ginkgo, fish oil is going to help with cell membrane fluidity, exercise is key, recovery, and rest. When he first was coming out of the brain injury, it was like raising a really big baby.

[00:30:30] It reminded me of when he was six months old. He just was now 150 pounds and six feet tall. He needed to get stimulated and then rest and stimulated and then rest. He was sleeping about 18 hours out of the day. He would sleep throughout the night, and then throughout the day we would go and stress him, and then let him recover, and stress him, and recover. That's another key thing that you have to look at with the brain injury is really giving adequate rest and recovery. You do want to stress them so they can start to get better, right? Just like you have to stress the muscle, but then you have to give them adequate rest and recovery. Still, today he sleeps about 10 hours a night. He's still getting through it.

[00:31:00]
[00:31:30] That's another key thing is you hear, "Okay, it's whatever happens in the first six months or whatever happens in the first year," and that's not true. Yes, it's super important to get this in and start reducing the inflammation and help the healing as quickly as possible, but you can do these things to help heal your brain years later. It's never too late. You can always do these things. The most important thing that I've seen with Grant is that it's never too late and there's always something else you can do. When Grant was going through this process, there was a bit there where he was really suicidal and he was like, "I don't know why I'm here. I don't know what my point is." I said, "You know Grant, your purpose is to show people what's possible."

[00:32:00]   My son was basically dead on the street. The doctors told us to let him die. They didn't think he'd ever wake up. They didn't think he'd ever walk. They didn't think he'd ever hear. He's now better than he was before the accident, and he'll continue to get better. Now he knows that his purpose is to show people what's possible. The biggest limiter to what's possible is our mindset that tells us we can't do it, but if you flip that around and go, "Okay. What do I need to do to be 110%," and you open yourself up to possibility, anything is.

JOE PIZZORNO, ND | Author: *The Toxin Solution*

Dr. Joe Pizzorno: I've been involved in medicine now for about half a century, and over that period of time, I've watched quite a significant change in why people are sick. When I was first involved with patients back in the 70s, people were sick primarily because of nutritional deficiencies, nutritional excesses, lack of exercise, smoking, and the obvious choices people were making. Then starting around 1970, I

[00:00:30] saw a significant change in what was happening to people, and that is they're becoming sick because of what might be called the passive determinants of health. In other words, they're becoming sick not because of what they're choosing to do, but because of what was changed in the environment around them. Starting about 1970, we started using a lot more pesticides in our foods. We started using a lot more metals in our, you might say, manufacturing—and these things kind of leaked into the environment. We started using more and more water supplies that were less healthy, because as the

[00:01:00] population grew, some people had use water that had more levels of arsenic in it.

I started seeing more and more chronic disease. Not because of what people were doing, but because of what was in the environment that was poisoning them. As I started noticing more of my patients suffering from diseases because of toxins, I since started looking at, well, what percent of chronic disease is due to toxins? I hired a couple of really bright graduates of mine, and we spent a year looking at the research. I would now assert that the primary driver of chronic disease in the

[00:01:30] industrialized world is environmental toxins. I want to be real clear. I'm not saying that nutritional deficiencies are no longer a problem. I'm not saying that nutritional excesses are no longer a problem. What I'm saying is that we've actually added in an even bigger problem, and we're poisoning ourselves with metals and chemicals.

If you look at what happens to the brain when it's exposed to things like arsenic, cadmium, bisphenol A, or things of this nature ... What it does is it causes the neurons to become damaged. As neurons

[00:02:00] become damaged, they're no longer able to work as well. At the early stages, people don't really recognize that because we have a lot of extra functioning in our brains. As you start causing more and more damage, the first thing people will notice is, well, they don't remember that person's name quite as quickly. Or they'll start saying that they're talking and they had a word they know they want to use but have trouble finding the word. They may start noticing that things seem kind of fuzzy sometimes. It seems like maybe they're a little distant from the world. What's happening is the early

[00:02:30] stages of the brain not being able to function as effectively as it should. It's not dementia, it's not old age, but it's no longer quite as good as it was.

One of my big surprises in looking at the research was how calm environmental toxicity is. For example, most people don't realize that 10% of the water supplies in the US, they use the public water supplies, the ones where you expect the government would be paying attention to them. 10%

[00:03:00] of them have levels of arsenic known to induce disease in humans. Then, look at things like health and beauty aids. Like, did you put lotion on this morning? Did you put sunscreen on to protect yourself from the sun? Well, those things have what are called phthalates, and the phthalates are actually pretty toxic to the body. They do things like bind some receptor sites, so that you can't get sugars into the cells and, eventually, cause you to have diabetes. They also cause trouble in the brain, because they impair the function of the neurons as well. There are so many toxins I can talk about. Mercury,

[00:03:30] for example. If a person has so-called silver fillings, what they don't realize is that those silver fillings are actually 55% mercury. It leaks into the body and into the brain.

The CDC—the Centers for Disease Control—of the US government has put as their top five: arsenic, lead, cadmium, mercury, vinyl chloride, things of this nature. When I was looking at the research, I was looking at which toxins have the strongest disease correlations or causations. And I also agreed arsenic is number one, but then I looked at DDT. You might say, "Wait, DDT was banned 47 years

[00:04:00] ago?" But DDT is something called a persistent organic pollutant, which means that it's very difficult to break down in the environment. And once it gets into our body, it's very difficult to break down. The half-life and amount of time it takes for our body to get rid of one half of the DDT that we've been exposed to is between two and 10 years. What happens is DDT builds up in the body and the DDT is a neurotoxin. It causes oxidative stress in the neurons and your neurons degenerate more quickly. I

[00:04:30] would say mercury, arsenic, DDT, the organophosphate pesticides. They are very, very neurotoxic.

Oxidative stress is another way to talk about something called free radicals. What that means is that when certain molecules typically involved with oxygen in someway become imbalanced, they really

[00:05:00] then attach to anything that's around them. When they become imbalanced and they're near cell membranes, they attach to cell membranes and they cause the cell membranes to start to dissolve. If they're near DNA, for example, they connect to the DNA and it causes the DNA to become damaged. If they're near the mitochondria, for example—mitochondria are the little organelles in the cells that produce all our energy—they come in contact with the mitochondria. What happens when the mitochondria try to produce all these high energy electrons to produce this something called ATP,

[00:05:30] which is the energy coin in the body. If there's too much oxidative stress, it will actually damage the systems the body uses to get the energy from the high energy electrons.

Instead of producing ATP, we damage mitochondria. One reason why people, as they get older, have less energy and are more fatigued, because they have now burned out the mitochondria from the oxidative stress. Mad Hatter's disease was first discovered in people who made hats. The reason it was discovered is because these people making the hats were losing their brains. They're going crazy.

[00:06:00] They're getting totally out of control. When people were looking at what was going on, they realized that the hatters—the people making the hats—were using mercury compounds in the hats. By using mercury compounds, they were actually touching the mercury compounds with their hands and it was getting into their body. Basically, poisoned the brains.

There are questions to ask yourself to determine if you're likely to have toxins, and there's some ways you can measure the amount of damage being done to your body by toxins. Let's do the latter one

[00:06:30] first. There's this data laboratory test called GGTP—it's a liver enzyme. Normally, it's only measured when we're looking for people with hepatitis, because what happens when the liver gets inflammation from hepatitis, whether it's a virus or whatever else may be going on, the cells start leaking enzymes. They show up in the blood and now you know a person has hepatitis. It turns out that the body increases its production of GGT in the liver, in response to oxidative stress and to

[00:07:00] environmental toxins. The reason it does that is that GGT recycles glutathione in the body. It turns out, glutathione is one of the most important molecules to protect us from oxidative stress, and also to get toxins out of the body.

Our really smart bodies who were exposed to toxins, they increase GGT. The normal range for GGT is between 10 and 60. Anybody with a GGT above 20 actually has toxic load. Within the normal range, GGT goes up a portion of toxic load. For example, look at things like diabetes. Someone with the GGT

[00:07:30] between 30 and 50, well within the normal range, has an eight times higher risk of diabetes because they have so many toxins going on. There's another mark that can measure and that's in the urine, so GGT is measured in the blood. A marker called 8-OHdG can be measured in the urine. 8-OHdG is a measure of the amount of DNA damage that's going on in a person's body. The more toxins they're being exposed to, the more 8-OHdG that shows up in the urine.

[00:08:00] Then, if you want to look at, well, who is most likely toxic? Well, it's pretty straightforward. If you are eating conventionally grown foods, particularly eating foods that have been prepared and stored in plastic, you're getting tons of toxins into your body. Unfortunately, you're getting the pesticides like organic corn pesticides, organophosphate pesticides, from the foods that are being grown. If you store them in plastic, you'll get bisphenol A from the plastic. If you're eating soybeans that have been grown conventionally, you're getting cadmium. Unfortunately, one of the best predictors of how toxic a person is, are they eating conventionally grown foods or are they eating organically grown foods

[00:08:30]   that are stored in safe packaging?

Another way to determine how toxic a person is, do you use health and beauty aids? If you use standard health and beauty aids, they've got a lot of phthalate, and there's even lead still in some types of lipstick. It's a pretty significant source of toxins as used in standard health and beauty aids.

[00:09:00]   Another area to consider is, are you living in an area with high levels of arsenic in the water supply? 10% of the water supplies in the US have levels of arsenic known to induce disease. You have to look at how is the person living. Are they being consciously aware of toxins in the environment? Are they working to avoid those toxins? Because if you're not working to avoid the toxins, you've got toxins. BPA—we now know there are huge disease associations with BPA. People say, "Well, we'll use BPS and BPF instead."

[00:09:30]   If you look in the cells and at animal studies, they're just as toxic as BPA but because they're more recently being used, the human data for damage has not shown up yet. I'll guarantee you, 5 to 10 years from now, we'll find they're just as toxic as the bisphenol A. Let me be clear. I'm very, very aware of the huge problem with toxins, but I don't want to go live in a cave somewhere. I enjoy modern civilization. I like my computer. I like my motorcycle. What I want to say is, we need to put pressure on the manufacturers to produce these products in a way that they're not poisoning us. That's all possible and we can make choices. We make choices by only buying prepared foods that are

[00:10:00]   in glass, for example. Only buy food that's organically grown. Only buy health and beauty aids that have low toxins. Manufacturers ... It's not their intent to poison us. Their intent is to make a profit. Well, if you stop buying their products and start buying the products of the safe manufacturers, they'll get the message. We'll have safer products.

There's a huge variation in people's ability to protect themselves from toxins. First, there's genetics.

[00:10:30]   There's a thousand-fold variation in how well people make enzymes in the liver for breaking down toxins. Clearly, genetics has an effect but it's not determinative. We can do something about it. The most important thing we can do is to make sure our nutrition status is as optimal as possible. That's a problem, because if you look at conventionally grown foods and look at what's happened to the trace mineral content of those foods over the last 50 years, trace minerals have dropped between 25% to as much as 75% in the case of copper in vegetables. What's happening is, the conventionally grown

[00:11:00]   foods we were eating don't have the nutrients we need to make our enzymes work adequately to get rid of the toxins. It's not just toxin avoidance, it's also facilitating our ability to get rid of toxins.

Now, we're looking at getting rid of toxins. We want to make the liver work as effectively as possible with adequate nutrition, but we also want to make sure we're consuming as much fiber as possible.

[00:11:30]   As we evolve as a species and as we're developing our liver detox enzymes, the liver developed with the expectation of there being a lot of fiber in our diet. As we evolved as a species, we consumed between 100 and 150 grams of fiber a day. Now, we only consume 15 to 20 grams of fiber a day. When the liver goes through all this work to get rid of all this toxin dumped into the gut, if there's not enough fiber there, we re-absorb those toxins through something called enterohepatic recirculation. If you don't have enough fiber, even if you have a liver working reasonably well, it's even harder to

[00:12:00]   get rid of toxins from the body. I've actually seen a number of patients with remarkable results and if you look at my book, *The Toxin Solution*, I have about 25 case histories in that. I've had another 20 on my website, so lots of case histories.

I'll give you an example. 67-year-old woman, one of the wealthiest women in Canada, was at early

[00:12:30]   stages of dementia. She'd been having brain fog, her memory was spotty, her skin was dry, she was having trouble sleeping—all these problems going on. She was very worried. She thought she was basically losing her mind and her life was going away. She came to see me. I tested her. Super high levels of mercury. I put her on my mercury detox program. Now, the detox program I used with her and by the way, it's a slow protocol. You can do IV chelation therapy. It goes faster, but some people have side effects from the IVs, so I decided a safer, more natural approach. What I did with her, was I gave her a gentle drug called DMSA, only 250 mg every third night. Not very often. She wouldn't get a

[00:13:00] toxicity from the drug.

In addition, I gave her 2.5 grams of fiber a day. In this case, it was PGX. I gave her 2.5 grams of fiber twice a day to help improve the absorption of the toxins. Then, every day, I had her take N-acetyl cysteine (NAC), 500 milligrams. The reason I gave her the NAC is that it increases glutathione [00:13:30] production in the body and the glutathione is our most important antitoxin. Protects us from toxins, and for getting toxins out of the body. I gave her the fiber, so it'll absorb the toxins that are being dumped from the gut. I gave her the DMSA because it very effectively binds to mercury and to lead, and gets them out of the body. Both through the urine and through the gut.

What happened? Six months later, she said, "You know, I'm starting to feel better. My brain's starting to work better." One year later, she said, "Wow. I think I can get over this." A year and a half later, her [00:14:00] mercury went from 50, which is super high, to 3.5, which is very low. All her symptoms were gone but it took a year and a half. People need to realize that when they're being damaged by toxins, it takes time to clean up the mess. First off, you have to get the toxins out and it takes months to get the toxins out of the body. Then, all those enzymes that have been poisoned by the toxins, they have to be replaced. It takes months to replace and get new enzymes. Then, after that's all done, now the body has to repair the damage. It takes time.

[00:14:30] One of my strongest urges to people who are interested in detoxification, don't expect this to be a simple thing like, "Oh, I'll start detoxifying. I'm going to feel great tomorrow." No. It's going to take you time but the good news is that when you detoxify, you make a huge change in your health. Much, much healthier, much more vitality, and much lower disease risk. Glutathione is a fascinating molecule because we don't get it from our diet. Our body makes glutathione. In a way, I look at how [00:15:00] important is a molecule to the body is by looking at, well, what level does the body maintain? It turns out, we maintain the same levels of glutathione in our body as we maintain sugar, as we maintain potassium, and other very important molecules.

Glutathione is incredibly important to the body. Now, why is that? Glutathione does basically three things that are critically important. Number one, it's the most important antioxidant in our cells and in our mitochondria. If your glutathione levels were low, your cells would degenerate, your DNA would [00:15:30] degenerate, your mitochondria would degenerate more quickly. It turns out if you look at a species' ability to produce glutathione, it predicts how long a species lives. The longer-living species produces more glutathione than short-living species. The second thing glutathione does that's so important, is it plays a critical role in the liver for getting chemical toxins out of the body. There's something called phase-two liver detoxification. What happens there is you basically bind glutathione to chemical toxins, which makes them easier to get out through the bile and also through the kidneys.

[00:16:00] The third thing glutathione does, which is pretty interesting, it's responsible for pumping mercury out of the brain across the blood-brain barrier into the blood where the mercury can then be gotten rid of. It also helps get mercury out of the cells and also binds to the methylmercury we get from fish. It helps get it out of the body as well. Glutathione is an incredibly important molecule. There are basically three processes by which the body neutralizes toxins. It's called phase one, phase two, and [00:16:30] then excretion. Phase one is the way in which the body gets rid of a number of chemicals both very directly. For example, if you drink a cup of coffee that has high caffeine in it, well, we use phase one to break down and get rid of the caffeine. Phase one is very interesting and that is what's called an inducible enzyme.

The more we need it, the more we produce. There are about 60 of these phase-one enzymes in the [00:17:00] body, each responsible for different kinds of chemicals for detoxifying them. Now, many chemicals are too difficult to break down by phase one. What phase one then does is produce what's called activated intermediates, which converts the chemical into actually a more toxic form that's also more reactive and also easier for phase two to then neutralize. Phase one makes it an activated intermediate. Then, phase two binds the activated intermediate to another molecule, like glutathione, for example, which then neutralizes it and either makes it water soluble for excretion for the kidneys, or easier to get rid of through the bile.

[00:17:30] The final process is getting rid of toxins through the bile, so all three processes need to work properly. Big problems. Number one is, phase one is inducible, so you can produce more when you need it. Phase two is not inducible, which means that if you got a lot of toxins and phase one is producing more activated intermediates than phase two can deal with, you actually have a more toxic situation. Frankly, that's what happens with cigarette smoking. With cigarette smoking, we're actually pretty

[00:18:00] good at breaking down the carcinogens in cigarette smoke into the activated intermediates, but we actually produce more activated intermediates than phase two can get rid of. And that's why cigarette smoke is so carcinogenic. It's because you can't get rid of the toxins quickly enough.

In my early days of practice, I quickly became aware that food intolerance and food allergy is a huge problem. Now, notice I used both terms, food allergy and food intolerance. Food allergy means you developed an immunological reaction to the food, which means your body thinks the food is the same

[00:18:30] as invading bacteria. That's a problem. Then, we also have food intolerance, which is actually much, much more common. What that means is that for some reason, the chemical makeup of the food, or some chemicals in the food, are made of contaminates we can't detoxify properly, and they cause damage. Interestingly enough, by far the most common problematical food is wheat. Now, everybody knows about celiac disease but that only affects about 2% of the population. For them, they develop antibodies to wheat. And when they eat the wheat, it causes inflammation to the gut and you get

[00:19:00] inflammation throughout the body. You get all kinds of disease.

There's another problem with wheat and that is something called gliadin. And for susceptible people, when they consume gliadin, it comes in contact with the gut mucosa—with the cells of the gut. It tells the gut to become more permeable. When the gut becomes more permeable, not only does it let in more of the nutrients that we want, but also the gut is full of all kinds of toxins from the bacteria and such in the gut. It allows a lot of toxins from the gut to come in. It turns out that about 25% of the

[00:19:30] population should never eat wheat because every time they eat wheat, they have excess gut permeability for over three hours. You think about the average person, how often does the average person consume wheat? Many times per day. So the gut is always accessibly permeable, always allowing in these toxins.

Now, about half the population can eat wheat but not very often. Because for them, they get excess

[00:20:00] gut permeability for about one hour. As long as you're not doing it too often, that's not too big a problem. For about 25% of population, wheat is a great food because their genetics don't result in them getting excess gut permeability after eating wheat. I always decided if a patient was going to spend money to come to see me as a doctor, then I'm going to put them on my full aggressive protocol because we want to get things fixed. Here's how you do it the right way. Not everybody's willing to do that but I do talk about it in my book. What I do with patients, I say, "Okay, we don't know what foods you're reacting to. We can run some lab tests to see if you have antibodies to foods

[00:20:30] but it won't necessarily tell us what foods you're reacting to in non-antibody relating methods, chemically reacting to."

What I do with my patients is I put them on a four-day water fast. That's water. Nothing but water. I don't want them eating anything. No soups, no vitamins, no drugs. Nothing but water for four days. And then, every day, we introduce a new food. I start on the fifth day with a food which might be

[00:21:00] called the worst probable offender. I talk to my patients. I say, "Well, I think you may have some food intolerances." Almost always the patient will say, "Well, I know it's not X, because every time we eat X, I feel better." Okay, that's the worst food. I try X the very first day. I say to the patient, "Watch what happens after you eat the food, both during the day you're eating that food and the next morning." The reason I like doing this is because when you have avoided the food the person's reacting to for about four days—particularly for immunological reaction—they start becoming much, much more sensitive to that food.

[00:21:30] When they eat that food, they get a really strong reaction and now they have a psychological connection to, "Oh, I ate that food and look how bad I felt." That's kind of the things I've seen with people. For example, I had one fellow who was a psychological counselor, and he became a psychological counselor because he suffered from severe life-long depression. His depression was so bad that he actually was hospitalized, and had conditions and drugs and things of this nature. He came to see me—actually his wife dragged him in—which is pretty typical. Typically, the wife is

[00:22:00] bringing the husband in. He came to see me. I told him I thought he was allergic to wheat, and he was pretty desperate at this point because depression was a big problem for him. He came to see me. I put him on the water fast for four days. He ate wheat and said this is what happened. He ate the wheat and within 30 minutes, got so high, he was asked if he had just smoked a really strong marijuana cigarette.

[00:22:30] He was really high, feeling great for a few hours, and he crashed and burned and got so depressed, he couldn't get out of bed for a day. Okay. That was his reaction. It was disrupting his physiology; short term, oh it's okay, and then long term, devastation. What I do with patients, I say, "Four days of water. On the odd days afterwards, like day five, we'll give you food we think you're allergic to or intolerant to. Watch what happens that day and the next morning." Because sometimes when a person has a reaction, they don't notice a lot during the day. But then the next morning, they wake up all congested, all mucusy, wondering, "Why am I feeling so allergic? So mucusy?" Well, they're

[00:23:00] reacting to food, but sometimes the food reactions take a little while to manifest. Then, on the even days, I have them eat a new food that's low allergy, because I want to get some calories into them. I typically recommend avocados because I very rarely see people allergic to avocados. Almost always the first food I check is wheat because by far, it's the most common problem.

After wheat, I then go to dairy products, and then I go to peanuts, then soybeans, because in my
[00:23:30] experience it's also by far the worst. My experience has been that you don't have to find everything a person is intolerant to. If you just get rid of the worst ones—our bodies have remarkable adaptive and healing abilities—the body can deal with the lesser ones. It takes about two weeks, kind of alternating foods back and forth. When we've discovered a person reacting to foods, we say, "You can't eat that food at all for at least six months." Then, afterwards, we determine what foods are probably okay for them to eat. I actually then put them on what's called a four-day rotation diet. The reason for that is, when a person's been regularly eating a food that's damaging for them, that will cause a lot of gut
[00:24:00] permeability. If you give them a new food that's high in protein while you have a lot of excess gut permeability, they'll then become allergic to that food as well.

I want to apologize to all of my patients I didn't realize that with. It took me a while to figure it out because I'd take them off these foods that they're allergic to, have them stop eating those foods, eat the regular foods, they'd do fine for a while. Then, they start having problems again because they became allergic to the new foods that they're eating. Now, I do a four-day rotation diet. What that
[00:24:30] means is they don't eat any food, any more often than once every four days. By spacing foods for every four days, your body does not become allergic to it and your gut heals, and now you're not going to have a problem. After you've healed the gut and after the person's healthy, typically it takes about six months. Then, I'll have them try the foods that they were allergic to before to see if they can tolerate them. Not eat them real often but now we've got the digestion working properly, we've got their gut healed. Now sometimes, they can eat those foods and it's not a problem for them, but oftentimes they can't.

[00:25:00] Unfortunately, with wheat and dairy products, when people have been allergic to those, they usually can't get over it, but mostly everything else they can. Here are two pictures I want to show you. Here's a picture of my great grandfather, grandfather, father—and that little boy on the side—that grumpy little boy on the side, that's me. I got to see in my own family what happens when you go from a great grandfather who ate a Mediterranean type of diet, lived healthily, didn't involve himself to toxins, and lived before we entered all these toxins or put all these toxins into the environment. My
[00:25:30] great grandfather lived to age 95, never saw a doctor in his life, had no apparent disease, outlived his

wife by five years. I was the oldest of his 15 great grandchildren and we were at an annual family get together, he said, "You know, I've had a good life. Yeah, I think I'm done."

[00:26:00] He stopped eating and he was dead a week later. I think to myself, "You know, that's kind of the way to go." He was living independently, growing his own food, vitally active. I used to play strategy games with him as a precocious little boy. I'd play strategy games with him because I loved playing strategy games, because I'm really smart and I would beat all my friends playing these games. I hated luck games because I couldn't control it. I'd play strategy games with this old guy, he'd beat me all the time. I'm figuring, "What is going on here? What's going on? Maybe he must be smart, too." Not only was he smart, but he had all this experience, and his brain was working just fine. Then, we have my

[00:26:30] grandfather who was, I'd say, 75% the Mediterranean healthy lifestyle, about 25% the unhealthy American lifestyle. He also lived to age 95. He also outlived two wives, but he spent the last 22 years of his life in first a nursing home, and then assisted living, because his body broke down.

He didn't have near the vitality. He didn't have a lot of disease, but he didn't have much vitality by the end of his life. Then, there's my dad, whom I loved dearly and he was proud to be an American. He

[00:27:00] made sure not to teach his children Italian because he wanted to make sure we got into the culture, merged into the culture, assimilated, as they say. Standard American diet, smoked for a while, and then decided it was a bad idea, stopped smoking, didn't worry about chemical exposure. We had a garage, my dad liked working in the garage—solvents, you know, paint thinner—things like that. He didn't wear gloves, didn't worry about it. By the age 65, my dad could no longer drive safely at night. By age 70, we started seeing him deteriorating. By age 83, he had dementia. He was dead at age 88.

[00:27:30] When he died, he had had three heart surgeries, he had had osteopetrosis, osteoarthritis, hip replacement surgery—I mean, his body was just totally broken down.

When I was giving my lecture, I was shown this picture of all my forebears all standing together and I tried to find a picture of my dad when he was over the age of 70. None of my family, my siblings, none

[00:28:00] of us have any pictures of my dad after the age of 70. We were standing up, he was always sitting because he had such low vitality and so much disease burden. I say, "What's going on in my own family?" The genetics, you might say, "Well, maybe one had better genetics than the other." Maybe, but probably not. We all had pretty good genetics. Well, what's happening is, one group of genes was getting good nutrients and not many toxins, and the other genes were getting very poor levels of nutrients and lots of toxins. Now, here's a picture of me. In my late 60s, on a motorcycle. And what

[00:28:30] you don't see about that motorcycle is that, that's in Australia, with my wife on the back, motorcycling on the left side of the road. I was on the wrong side of the road.

Look at my level of function, I want to be like my great grandfather, not like my dad. I love my dad dearly but you know, we failed him. I'm really mad that we failed him so badly, and I want to thank conventional medicine for keeping him alive with all the disease. I want to throw rocks at conventional medicine and say, "I'm really mad at you because you didn't deal with the reasons why

[00:29:00] my dad was sick." That's why I became a naturopathic doctor, because I realize we have to deal with the reasons why people are healthy and why they're sick. Not simply try to use drugs and surgery and such to cover it up after everything's broken down. President Trump, would you please appoint me to the EPA? Let me be President of the EPA, because they have not been protecting us and it's really bad. We have all these toxins coming into our environment, through manufactured goods, through food, and through water, and things of this nature.

[00:29:30] What's going on? Why aren't you doing your job? If I had a blank check, I would much more deeply research the primary toxins that are causing the most disease—and that's very clearly arsenic, DDT, organochlorine pesticides, organophosphate pesticides. We have to deal with those things because they are killing us. I've been involved in medicine now for half a century. I think I know a couple of things. I've seen a lot of patients, and it's very clear to me that our bodies have a remarkable ability to heal if we just give them a chance. Now, what does "give them a chance" mean? It means getting into

[00:30:00] each person the nutrients that they need and getting out of each person the toxins they don't need. If you get the nutrients in, you get the toxins out, you'll have a dramatically better quality of life, less disease and much more longevity.

[00:30:30] The Mediterranean lifestyle is actually pretty variable. Some parts aren't as healthy as others, so I'll talk about the one that my forebears experienced. They lived in the foothills of the Alps and they did not have much meat available to them so they had a lot of vegetables they could grow. They had goat products, they grew chestnuts, they had nuts and seeds in the various types of plants they were growing. They had basically pretty much a vegetarian diet with small amounts of meat and occasional amounts of fish. They exercised vigorously. They were in the foothills of the Alps, so they're walking up and down hills all the time, and there was no manufacturing there, so they were not exposing themselves to chemicals.

[00:31:00] When they grew their food, they were using all-natural fertilizers—there was no toxins in them. They weren't spraying their foods because it turns out when foods have optimal nutrition, they're much more resilient to the bugs trying to eat them. Anyway, healthy Mediterranean-type lifestyle, real food, lots of vegetables, lots of nutrients, no toxins.

JOHN J. RATEY, MD | Clinical Associate Professor of Psychiatry and Author of *Spark: The Revolutionary New Science of Exercise and the Brain*

Dr. John J. Ratey:

[00:00:30]

I became interested in exercise as a treatment—a medical and psychiatric treatment—when I began my residency in Boston in the mid 70s, because that was the beginning of the burgeoning and blossoming of the Boston Marathon. Everybody was doing marathons, including many of my residents and co-residents in psychiatry. I began running, just like everybody, and realized this was a great way to treat depression. We had lots of anecdotal evidence of the effect of exercise on depression, from the past and the distant past. Hippocrates wrote about it in 300 BC in the first medical textbook, saying this is the way to treat depression. Get people walking, keep them walking. It relieves their depressive burden. I began to appreciate that and follow it all the way through.

[00:01:00]

[00:01:30]

[00:02:00]

As well, we saw a lot of people who had to stop marathoning, because Boston was full of these marathon people. When they stopped, they came up with interesting psychiatric problems. Certainly depression, anxiety. That's how I started my work in attention deficit disorder, because I saw a marathoner in 1981 who was a professor both at MIT and at Harvard and a MacArthur Fellow, and very, very prominent in his field and productive, unbelievable. However, he had to stop marathoning, and stop running because he had a bad knee. All of a sudden, got depressed. Then, after that, he developed the first case I'd ever seen. We documented the first case of adult-onset attention deficit disorder. That started my interest in ADHD. It was ADD back in those days. It led to many books and papers and lectures about attention deficit disorder.

[00:02:30]

[00:03:00]

He was a very productive guy who was always writing, always lecturing. He said, "Look, I get up and I can't figure out what to do till I turn on the screen." This is back when the computer was new. "Turn on the screen," and the screen would get him focused a bit. However, he couldn't get started, so he was procrastinating. He was forgetting things. He was unmotivated at times, which was never happening before. He was losing things, including his relationships. He was getting angry where he never got angry before. He was going to lose his girlfriend because he was just not on point. He wouldn't return phone calls. He did things that were very foreign to him.

[00:03:30]

This led to seeing it as an attention deficit disorder in adults. It wasn't even a big deal back then. People can't believe that, but it's true. In 1981, we didn't talk much about attention deficit disorder, even in kids. Then, for the next decade or so, we began to really expand the world of attention deficit disorder. My partner, who was my student, Ned Hallowell—Edward Hallowell—we both diagnosed each other with ADD, and many of our colleagues, many of our Harvard professor colleagues, as well as many, many patients. Then we wrote the book, *Driven to Distraction*, and it came out in 1993. That began to really change the world of attention deficit disorder.

[00:04:00]

[00:04:30]

Back then, it was thought to be something from the parents, or they weren't strict enough, or they were too strict, or just born a bad kid. Often confused with dyslexia. At that time, because we were interested in that and had been treating dyslexics for a while, eventually that changed. Our book was one of the reasons for that. We've sold about 2.5 million copies of *Driven to Distraction* up to this point.

[00:05:00]

When we exercise, we change our brains greatly. Our brains evolved—our human brains evolved to help us be the best movers possible. With that, our brains grew. Then, sometime when we began to get larger groups as hunter-gatherers—back 20, 30,000 years ago—we began to add language to our lives, and more complicated language, more complicated groups. Our big brains that evolved over 6-8 million years to make us the best movers, and the eventual evolutionary victors ... we use the same brain cells to think with, relate, to talk, so that our thinking brain is really our moving brain. The nerve

[00:05:30]   cells we added became used to talking and thinking and to do poetry and to do all the things we can do now as humans.

[00:06:00]   I'm fond of saying that physical movement—exercise, play, yoga, everything that we do movement-wise—is really a way to make our brains work and work better. A happy side effect is the positive effect on the body. We often recommend that people exercise before a big engagement or a test or a big meeting, because they'll be focused. They'll be on point. I start off my lectures usually with a round of Hindu squats or jumps, jump squats, with the audience, not just to relieve their stress and make them laugh a little bit and like me a little more, but it also turns their brain on. It makes them more attentive, less fidgety, and it makes for a better experience.

[00:06:30]

[00:07:00]   BDNF is brain-derived neurotrophic factor. It is an amazing little factor in our brain, a protein that we make when we use our brain cells. We have 100 billion of those brain cells when we're active, and you can't be any more active than you're moving. We use more brain cells when we move than in any other human activity. When they're active, they make this substance, BDNF. Early on, I called it Miracle Gro for the brain, because it's really brain fertilizer. It does everything that fertilizer does for plants and what we think of fertilizer. It keeps our brain cells growing, which is important, because if we're not growing, we're dying, we're eroding, we're losing. It makes our brain cells ready to be used.

[00:07:30]

[00:08:00]   The way the brain cells work is to grow and change, and that's how we learn anything, we understand things. Our brain has to grow in the information. We call that state of readiness to grow, neuroplasticity. We make our brains very, very plastic when we exercise, play, or move beforehand.

[00:08:30]   ADD or ADHD is definitely something we're seeing a lot of, and perhaps a lot more of these days. Our culture is ADD-genic, and has been. That's what we call it, meaning it produces people with short attention spans. That's because of our wonderful little gadgets that we are addicted to. From our cell phone to TV to video games to all the wonderful things that we have that make life very easy and make us into a situation where we're not training frustration tolerance in our kids, because all they have to do is start again in a video game, or start it over. This means they don't have to really pay attention for that long. We're now used to the six-second commercials and videos, and even TV and movies are quick to get us into a novel situation or a novel scene, because that's what holds people's attention.

[00:09:00]

[00:09:30]   It's such a tough call as to what to tell parents about technology, because it's so ever present. If the parents say to their kids, "You can't have a cell phone," or, "You can't use the iPad," yet they're constantly on it—which is the case most of the time—it falls on deaf ears. One has to be a family that says, "Okay. We're going to limit our screen time," which is now about nine hours a day, on average, for all of us. That means our kids are seeing this.

[00:10:00]   I have two grandchildren. One of the things that we've learned by getting them to do things like crawl forward rather than backwards—for my youngest, what was the object of excitement and interest that she crawled towards? It wasn't her teddy bear. It wasn't her little dolly at the age of one. What was it?

[00:10:30]   The cellphone. That was what she wanted, and that's what she crawled to. That's indicative of our society, because their parents are always texting and on it. My son-in-law is a social media guy, so he's really on it all the time. They begin to love it and cherish it and think it's great, even though they don't know how to use it.

[00:11:00]   When we go into schools and implement our program or implement a program of daily physical education or physical play, we see major changes in the school. The first thing we see is a drop in discipline problems. No matter what grade, no matter what area of the country, no matter suburbs or inner city, you see a drop in problems that are taken to the principal, or disciplinary referrals as they're called. For instance, we did this in Charleston, South Carolina, in a very troubled target school. In grades four to eight, about 130 kids every morning would come in, and instead of just hanging around, they did 35 minutes of vigorous play and exercise. The first semester, there was an 83% drop in

[00:11:30]

disciplinary referrals.

[00:12:00] What does that mean? That means that the teacher is no longer a policeman. That means that the kids are not disturbed as much by each other. That means they learn better, and they tested better, and all the things that we want for our kids happen. Then, we see the drop in absences, which is a big problem in our schools and has been for the past 15 years or so. Then, an improvement in grades and in test scores.

[00:12:30] We started a program when I was working with Reebok called Boks—B-O-K-S—which is now in 3,000 elementary schools in the United States, and we're rapidly expanding into Canada, Japan, and South Korea. There, it's a voluntary program. It starts that way. An hour before school, three to five days a week. The kids come in, and they've evolved in the past six years a very interesting curriculum to keep

[00:13:00] the kids moving all the time. The kids love it. The first 1,500 kids that we surveyed—this is grades K-5 when we surveyed these 1,800 kids, 1,500 kids or so—the very first time after a Boks semester, 96% of them wanted to do it again. What did that mean? That means they had to get up an hour early to get

[00:13:30] to school an hour earlier. They were losing sleep and all that, but they loved it, because it added such interest and enthusiasm in the kids. The teachers loved it, because the kids were much more well behaved, and especially those kids who have ADHD or dyslexia or other kinds of developmental problems.

[00:14:00] There's no particular exercise to treat depression, ADD, or anxiety. There may be some shades of one thing better than another, but all kinds of exercise are useful. Aerobic exercise is the center point, but

[00:14:30] yoga, weight training, strength training, Tai Chi—all those are great exercises. Some of the best are dance and martial arts, because with those two you get movement and focused attention, because you have to learn how to move and dance, how to make the move—unless you do a boomer dance, which is craziness. My daughters hate it when I dance because I just flail away. If you learn dance, you

[00:15:00] have to learn the moves correctly to the music with a partner or with a group. That's a huge demand on the brain. The same with martial arts. A good dojo or a good martial arts studio won't let you progress until you have mastered the moves and you practice, practice, practice. That really challenges your attention system early on. The kids don't even know they're training their attention.

[00:15:30] I wrote a new book, called *Go Wild*, where I talk about how we should be living according to our caveman genes, because we developed our genes over 8-10 million years when we were hunter-gatherers, and it's only been 10,000 years that we're not hunter-gatherers. Back then, we grew up and

[00:16:00] lived in the wilds. We lived outside. We moved a lot. We moved 10-14 miles a day. We ate up to 200 varieties of vegetables, and occasionally meat and nuts and berries. Our diet was varied. We also were outside as much as we could be, because we had to be.

[00:16:30] We have this need to be outside. It's called biophilia. It's something that we love nature. We love being in the wild. When we're not, we suffer. We constrict our lives. We know from studies that our brain, our immune system, everything gets better when we're outside and with the elements. It causes

[00:17:00] us to pay more attention – which is another big thing that we talk about in our book, *Go Wild* – about being mindful. Mindfulness training is meditation, of one form or another. When you're outside and moving, you have to be much more mindful than when you're in your secure environment. That's why we recommend that people, when they're exercising, be outside, rather than just on the treadmill or

[00:17:30] in the gym, because it presents different issues for you on different levels. You have to watch for stumps if you're running or walking, rather than on a treadmill, which is all predictable.

In *Go Wild*, I talk about rewilding our lives. That is, getting back to the way we should be. Which is moving all the time, getting out of the chair, changing our sedentary lifestyle, which is so pervasive,

[00:18:00] and exercising and playing, which is really important, especially for our kids and ourselves to continue to play.

Then, sleep is another big topic that we talk about in *Go Wild*, because sleep has so many benefits for

[00:18:30] us. One of the things I find traveling the world, no matter what country, everyone's sleep deprived. Everyone. The parents, the kids. Not just because of pressure, but because of toys, because of our digital world. We're constantly entertained in novelty with one form or another, so we cheat sleep. This is a big, big problem. You have to really work at it to get the necessary eight and one quarter hour in. It's hardly done by anybody.

[00:19:00] Diet. The more we have a varied diet, the better, because that's the way we evolved. Going from place to place, we had different vegetables and different fruits and different game at times, at different times of the year, in different environments. That was helpful to us, helpful to our immune system, helpful to making us who we are as humans. The big thing, of course, today is getting rid of glucose, sugar, starches, really paying attention to that, because it's even in whole grains. I know I step on

[00:19:30] people's holy writ, but whole grains are just longer packaged; it takes a little longer in our guts to break it down into pure glucose. It's not like pasta and rice, which immediately gets broken into sugar. This is a huge problem today with our obesity crisis, the diabetic crisis, and the metabolic syndrome

[00:20:00] crisis we are immersed in.

Also, the nature is to get outside, get moving, stay moving. Fall in love again with being out there, outdoors. Meditation or mindfulness, meditation training, gets you more mindful, keeps you more

[00:20:30] mindful. But it's really an attitude to pay attention to where you are, do things with purpose and with meaning so that you're much more present when you're doing them.

Then, the most important thing is community, being connected to one another. I'm working with a

[00:21:00] group that studies this kind of thing for the elderly. One of the big ways of keeping people well, keeping people from using Medicare B—we did this big study—is being more social and staying more social. It's even three times more important than if you exercise every day, which I think is one of the most important things you can do. Which is twice as important than, if you take medicine, taking it as your doctor prescribed.

[00:21:30] It all comes down to being connected. This is the biggest advice we have from *Go Wild*. Work together. Be involved with other people. Being in what we call a small tribe, because we, as hunter-gatherers, were in a group of about 40 or so people, maximum, and we knew everybody and we depended on

[00:22:00] everybody. You see this happening today in things like CrossFit—where that's a very interesting small tribe—or a Zumba group, or a running group, or a walking club, or just as people getting together now. We need to do that, because it gives so much to us in terms of health benefits.

[00:22:30] There's a lot we're learning. One of the things we learned about our diet is that we became fatphobic in the 60s, 70s, and 80s. We became low-fat people. That meant we became high-carb people, but we cheated ourselves on the good fats. One of the things that we've known in psychiatry since 1990 is that omega-3 fatty acids are perhaps as good a treatment for things like bipolar illness as are some of

[00:23:00] our bipolar drugs. With that came now a whole lot of research on looking at the omega-3s as a way to treat mood and anxiety, ADD, and autism. It has a positive effect on all of those pervasive problems. Plus, it's great for the heart. It's great for the skin. It's great for the bones. It's great for our

[00:23:30] connections in our body. It treats arthritis and the like.

We're learning more and more about all kinds of things that are good for us. Curcumin is a big deal

[00:24:00] these days. Another one that's coming is cannabidiol. It's a phytochemical in marijuana. It's not marijuana. It's not THC. It's CBD, which is a cofactor and a co-partner in the hemp plant and in marijuana itself. If you distill it down and get closer to pure CBD, it's amazing. It is a great anti-seizure

[00:24:30] medicine. It is an anti-anxiety agent. It's a helpful sleep med. But it's not a medicine. It's from our plants. It's very, very useful, and I think it's going to make an impact in the next three or four years. It's already there. It's one of the benefits of the marijuana culture.

[00:25:00] We really left the tribal idea behind a bit, because of our Western culture especially, we're on the move. We're not close to our families. We're not close to our extended families if we had them. We're

[00:25:30] moving around all the time. We're able to do that. It became a fashion to do that—to leave home after college or to go away from home to go to college. This became the norm. Then, we get to the point where we separate from others and we cocoon ourselves. Especially today with 24/7 news cycle, cycle

[00:26:00] of shows, of streaming, all the wonders of the Internet and the digital world we have at our fingertips, and we can entertain ourselves, and we can do that without anybody's assistance or help. We really don't have the kind of great connections that we need.

[00:26:30] When we look at the blue zones, which are areas of the world where people live to over 100 or so, what do we find? One, that their diet is pretty simple, focused on vegetarian and occasional meats; it can be in some areas really into protein with fish and meat. But, they're always moving. They're working, still. They're connected to the community they live in. It is quite remarkable, looking at the

[00:27:00] Caucasus, or in Okinawa where it started in Japan, and Italy. Small pockets of small towns where people were well over 90 and 100. They're still connected to everyone. Everybody around knows everybody else. That's so unusual today, when you can be living in a house and not know your neighbors for 20 years.

[00:27:30] One of the big points, I think, for people—certainly for when we talk to people with ADD—we tell them, never retire. Always be working, because that will keep the structure there. That's a good plan for everyone. Not to necessarily work at the same job, but to continue doing stuff on a daily basis, weekly basis—that enriches your life. You enrich your life by contacting others, being involved with

[00:28:00] others if you can. Not everybody has the idea of retirement being you just have a luxurious time, and you travel, and you play golf if that's your thing, or explore the world. Then, they end up sitting at home watching TV and being on Facebook all the time, or whatever. You need to really work at

[00:28:30] retirement if you don't have a directed goal or purpose, like work or a job or volunteering on a very regular basis.

City life is difficult, in terms of re-wilding, but it's there. One of the things that's happening in the US—and now in China, for instance—where there's really a problem in re-wilding, because there isn't any space that's green. But now, people, architects, city planners, are putting in green spaces, spaces that

[00:29:00] are natural for people to congregate in. There are a lot of parks and a lot of areas to go to to get outside, but it's difficult if you live in a high rise and you're surrounded by other high rises to get in touch with nature. You have to plan that. You take the weekends and you go out to the country, wherever that might be, to spend the time walking, enjoying, skiing, playing a game of tennis or golf or

[00:29:30] something, but you're outside.

The Department of Health and Human Services has said that every American should get 150 minutes a week of exercise. Most of that being moderate, some of that being intense or a high intensity, some of

[00:30:00] it being weight training, balance training, which is very important. All that. It's a good rule, because if you do 150 minutes a week, you will be in pretty good shape. Almost no one does that, except for people who are really into exercise. The idea—it would be somewhere near that—would be 30 minutes five days a week, at least. The best advice is to join a group that's doing this, whether it's a

[00:30:30] Zumba class, CrossFit, a spinning group, walking group, hiking group, or a skiing group. Those are the ideals. You really want to accomplish that because we need to move.

[00:31:00] A big thing these days is the standing desk. That's come to industry and schools. There are even treadmill desks, the tread desk. I had been talking about the tread desk for 10 years. And a few years ago, a fellow came to me and he said, "Well, I heard about your tread desk last year. I went online on Amazon. There are 100 different types of tread desks—a desk with a treadmill under it—100 that are available." That speaks to the ubiquity of it all. People are beginning to get the message.

[00:31:30] My biggest piece of advice to people that want to live a healthy life is to get connected and stay connected, because that is the spice of life. That is the meaning of life. That's what we should be doing. That's what we evolved to be connected to one another. It gets harder as we age to maintain

[00:32:00] that and not just think, "Oh, well, I'll just sit in my chair." You do that and you'll erode.

John Mekrut:	I spent 25 years in show business. Retrospectively, when I think about it, I was working with dysregulated brains for a really long time. I just didn't know exactly what I could do about it, other than try to manage their behaviors.
[00:00:30]	But that career sort of waned in its interest for me, and somewhere towards the end of it I had a daughter who was clearly a little different. She was our first child, and her interactions with the world were just a little behind—nothing that would sound an alarm, but as parents we observed there was something probably a little developmentally delayed. Let's put it that way.
	We got her into kindergarten, first grade, and all of a sudden the demands of life became much more apparent. Then, her interactions with the world became more obvious to us. Not so much when she was just hanging out with us at home.
[00:01:00] [00:01:30]	We went on a journey to find out what this was all about, and we had several different diagnoses. There was sensory processing disorder, attention deficit disorder. I think there was one more in there. I can't even remember what it was. But we finally ended up with an autism diagnosis, the subset of which was PDD NOS, which is very evocative of my daughter. Pervasively developmentally delayed, not otherwise specified. We don't know. And I was like, "Yeah, that sounds about right."
[00:02:00]	It set us on a journey trying to figure out what we could do to help this kid. She had behaviors that were really challenging. She'd scream and run out across the street through traffic. It was stuff that was really quite dangerous at times. In an effort to try and find out how we could help manage these, we visited the doctors, like you all do. What's wrong with my kid? We went to a developmental pediatrician, who sent us to UCLA, and we got this diagnosis. And we got into the system. The system is designed, by and large, to manage behaviors.
[00:02:30]	We entered the psycho-pharmacological arena. She must have done 15 or 20 major medications over a couple-year period. Anticonvulsants, antipsychotics, you get on the list. We tried just about everything to try to get some of these things to work for her, so that she could at least calm herself down to the point where she could have a meaningful interaction with the world. To an extent they worked. She wasn't as destructive. She wasn't as rageful. She wasn't a lot of things. She also she also wasn't my daughter.
[00:03:00]	It became very clear to us. We were at a holiday party at school and all the kids are singing. They had little hats on and were doing all this stuff. And my daughter was, oddly enough, right in the center, and was staring vacantly out into space, not singing—she could have been on the moon. It was unimportant where she was. She was not interacting with her world.
[00:03:30]	Her behaviors were managed, but at—for us—an enormous cost. So, we said okay. This is not going to happen. I can't live like this. I can't live with what I'm doing to this child. The guilt ... You saw me choke up a second ago. That's from my own guilt of what I did, with the best of intentions. I mean no disrespect to anybody we were involved with. Everybody is trying to find a solution for these kids and trying to find what we can put together that's going make them functional.
[00:04:00]	And I said, this road of pharmacology is clearly not happening for us. The side effects are too profound. Weight gains, lethargy, and excessive sleep—and you just can go down the list. Mostly, it was that vacantness that distressed me so much. That distressed my wife. A friend told us about this thing called neurofeedback. What's that? Oh, they put these things on your head. It trains the brain. Okay. Well, sure. We'll try it. We were trying anything. And I went to a couple of different

[00:04:30] practitioners. Joy Lunt, who is a veteran. She's been doing this for 30 years. Shout out to Joy. We did traditional neurofeedback, qEEG-guided neurofeedback. And we also, fortuitously, ran into another practitioner who did this different form of neurofeedback. This infra low-frequency training, which is how I ended up getting involved with it.

[00:05:00] But suffice it to say, all neurofeedback works. They work in their own way. There are five or six major types of neurofeedback to quantify it, but they all work. The brain is an amazing organ. It seeks information, homeostasis, to find calm. It needs to reduce fear and strategizes ways to manage its own behavior. Any information you give it, it will take it in and try to do something with it. But through this process of neurofeedback we got her to the point where we could get her off all her medications. If it did nothing other than that, I would have been thrilled. If we just got her off her meds, I would have been happy.

[00:05:30] We noticed an increase in her ability to interact with people. Her skill sets, these silly things—not silly in the sense if you're struggling with this. One of the symptoms we look for in clients coming to us, we ask them about their handwriting. People go, "Why are you asking me about my handwriting?" It is remarkable across ADD, autism spectrum disorder, and any number of conditions, handwriting is a

[00:06:00] huge marker. My daughter's handwriting was indecipherable. It had this really strange pattern, big letters, little letters. It was crazy. She now has the best handwriting in our family. It's almost calligraphic. It's so gorgeous.

The point is, she started to function over her body, over her emotions, over her socialization, her interactions with other, be it family or friends. That increase in her ability to interact with strangers,

[00:06:30] which was always a challenge in the spectrum disorder children, it all started to improve. We were like, "This is magical." And I agreed and said, "Yes, it is magical. And this is something I want to be a part of."

[00:07:00] That was sort of my transition, and I easily left show business behind. I said, "This is something I can do now for probably the rest of my life, as I can imagine it." It's an investigation into how the brain actually operates, and how it interacts with the body, and what's the whole system about. This is the cutting edge. In here are the answers to lots of our questions.

[00:07:30] I responded, personally, to infra low-frequency training because it deals in networks. There are several ways to look at what the brain does. Let's backup for a second. The brain's primary job is to detect patterns in the world, sights, sounds, whatever, and put them together into some kind of model that it understands and predicts the next second. It has to make a decision almost instantaneously—first of all, is this something dangerous? Is this something that's going to kill me?

[00:08:00] I think there's a common perception that our brain is there—our body is there, actually—to carry our brain around because that's its job. And I think it's entirely the opposite. The brain evolved over time to make sure your body stays alive. It's, in a weird way, almost subservient to the body. It makes decisions about what's dangerous and what's useful on a continuing basis to make sure that body stays alive and procreates. That's really kind of it. That's the job of life. Art, music, literature—those are all happy bonuses for our big giant cortex up here. The primary job is that we continue to function.

[00:08:30] Neurofeedback works—you can think of any system or any organism and they are all dependent on feedback. One-celled creatures have feedback. They reach out to something—it's either good or bad—and it makes its own way. It doesn't even have a brain. It makes a decision organically to move forward or to retreat. The higher animals like ourselves make much more complicated decisions about what's interesting, not interesting, fear making, what's appropriate response behavior in our system. We're always dealing with feedback. Feedback is the nature of life. We couldn't exist without

[00:09:00] it.

[00:09:30] There's biofeedback. Some of you are familiar, if you've ever had a mood ring—the first biofeedback device. It actually was measuring the skin temperature and would change the color of the stone in the mood ring. That's biofeedback. You're getting a witness of something that's actually going on internally. You're getting a visible manifestation of it. There's heart rate variability training. There's skin conductivity. There's measuring sweat glands. There are all kinds of biofeedback.

[00:10:00] Neurofeedback is a subset of biofeedback, in a sense, but we're using EEG signaling to present back as the feedback mechanism for understanding what's going on inside the brain. We're measuring amplitude. You put little tiny sensors on your head, very traditional stuff. It's been going on for 75, 80 years now. This is not anything that just happened yesterday. The amplitude of the signal is interesting because we want to find out what those variations are. What is the pattern that's being observed here by the brain, and how can it readjust to get a better pattern?

[00:10:30] It's seeking minimal energy expenditure. That's its basic goal. How can I get through this day, this minute, this hour using the least amount of energy as possible? The brain is a hawk. It uses 20% of whatever hamburgers and salads you want to put in your face. 20% of that is going right to your brain. It's very tiny. It's three pounds. Relative to your body mass, it's voracious. It's always strategizing to try and minimize that expenditure and do the best it can. It's seeking calmness. It's seeking homeostasis. It's seeking balance. That's one of its prime functions.

[00:11:00] So, by providing feedback in whatever manner you choose to provide it, you're giving information to that organ, the brain, so that it can make the best decision. How do I approach that? The brain is sitting in the dark. It's reading digital information coming from your ears, or your eyes, or whatever, so it isn't really interacting with reality as we perceive. It's processing information. What we do in neurofeedback is give it specific, in-the-moment, targeted information on its function. What are you doing right now? Is that useful information for you or not? If it's not useful information, stop doing it.

[00:11:30] What we mean by that is what we present to the client is a change of pattern on a video screen, let's say. It could be auditory. So, there'll be some flickering of the screen. The screen will appear bigger and smaller. It's very obvious to the person sitting the chair what's happening, but more importantly, it's obvious to the brain. "Oh my gosh. That's me," it recognizes over a period of time. That's why the training takes a while.

[00:12:00] It's not a therapy. It truly isn't. This is a training tool. This trains the brain in self-awareness and self-regulation. The second being derived from the first. It has to become aware of its own signal, and then it will organically strategize a way to regulate because that's its evolutionarily-designed outcome.

[00:12:30] We're presenting these variations in electrical signaling to the client sitting in the chair for their observation. Over the course of a few sessions, the brain finally recognizes, "Oh my goodness, that's me. The television isn't blowing up. That's actually my circuitry doing that. What do I need to do? What's the management I need to put in here so that will stop? Because I'm spending energy I don't want to every time. But it's a pattern. I have to discern it. I have to make a judgment about it. Tying into that is a dangerous concept."

[00:13:00]

[00:13:30] Your brain is always paying attention to every single change of pattern it witnesses, awake or asleep. You'll wake up at a random noise in your apartment. If there's a smell that's unfamiliar to you, it will bring you up out of a deep sleep. A sound in the other room, if you're intently focused on something, what's that sound? If you're driving down the street—the classic example—the thing you pay attention to is not the cars whizzing by, and the people walking in the street. Those are obvious. Your brain has already calculated those patterns in. That stupid Muffler shop thing, that will get your attention. The guy flipping the sign board for the telephone service, or whatever. Those are the things that are going to draw your brain's attention because they are out of pattern. The most vital element for the brain is pattern recognition. To find out what out there is out of pattern. Is it dangerous? It's a very fear-based mechanism. Apologies for that. It's why we're the most successful animals. We're very, very good at threat detection.

[00:14:00] That has obviously bad consequences, let's say, for people who are victims of trauma or PTSD—their threat detection is set way up here. So, they're constantly in perceived threat mode. It takes an enormous toll on their body because they're pumping out adrenaline, cortisol, and all the rest of it, to try to compensate for that state. What we're teaching the brain to do is recognize its own patterns, understand that it's its own, and then do your organic best to self-regulate.

[00:14:30] "Neurons that fire together, wire together," is a very common phrase known in neuroscience circles. And it's true. Your brain gets set into patterns that are comfortable. They may not be good for you, but they're known. Our job as neurofeedback trainers is to get the brain to recognize that those patterns are not useful, and to kind of unwire them. The good news is the brain is plastic. Neuroplasticity, great thing to know about.

[00:15:00] Probably about 15, 20 years ago, I think most neurologists would probably have concluded you're born with X, and that's sort of what you have until you die. Oh boy, is that not true. Your brain learns, takes in, and gathers new information, and learns new tasks and skills, until literally the moment you die. It's always ever-changing, always growing, always trying to take care of its best self. It's always in action. So, I know we'll talk, I'm sure, about things that you can do to promote that.

[00:15:30] But that neuroplasticity element is vital for what we're talking about here because the wiring patterns that one would have thought are immutable, are clearly not. That you can change. There's a tangential discussion to be had on placebo and all kinds of things. The willingness to change, the recognition that that's a possibility of change, I think, is vital to promoting good brain health, and bodily health, for that matter. If you're 300 pounds, and you're sitting on your couch eating French fries, if you have no conception that you can have a different life, it's going to be difficult. You have to

[00:16:00] be able to pretend, and say, " Yeah, I can eat healthy. I can eat better." A lot of it is the personal buy-in from the cognitive level of the understanding that things can change.

[00:16:30] Who is neurofeedback best suited for? Absolutely everyone. It's a training. You can train your body. People do all the time. People need to know they can train their brains. Your brain can have better function, always. SEAL Team Six uses neurofeedback, not because there's anything wrong with their brain. They know they can make their brain better. Trying to re-encapsulate what we do in the metaphor of peak performance.

[00:17:00] This is performance training. It's not about correcting deficits or something wrong with you, or something like that. If you have some symptoms expression, anxiety, depression, or lack of focus, ADD, whatever you want to name those things, this is just a matter of—I say that so casually— training your brain to move itself away from those dysfunctional patterns of behavior into more functional patterns, more performance-oriented patterns. It's not a difficult task, it just takes time and effort to do it, like anything else. A willingness to sit in my chair for endless sessions of watching dumb video products or whatever, and just exercising your brain to figure what it needs to do to strategize how to get to its best performance. It's not magic in any regard. I think people think of it

[00:17:30] sometimes, "Oh, this is like magic. I'm putting wires on my head, and I'm doing this." No, no, no, no. I'm revealing to you, the client sitting in the chair, your own brain.

[00:18:00] All healing is self-healing. Any doctor will tell you that. They set your bone. They're not fixing your leg, you're fixing your leg. They've just created a substrate. They've created the opportunity for your bone to heal. If they're giving you a medication for some condition, it's to allow your body to figure out how to marshal its own resources to fix your condition. The process is relatively obvious. We're doing the same thing in the brain. We're giving the brain the information it needs to make the course adjustments it needs to figure out how to best conduct itself in the world for best performance. It's seeking that anyway, but my goodness, why not give a targeted, specific, real-time information on

[00:18:30] how it's conducting itself right now, rather than having to guess about it? Changing your brain through learning is the reason we do this. Every piece of learning you can incorporate improves what you do.

[00:19:00] You get to ask the question, what are the best brain exercises? There are a gazillion of them. Certainly, get the apps. Sign up for Lumosity or Cognifit. They're great. Do Sudoku, do crossword puzzles. Learn how to dance. That's a great one. Highly recommended. What we're trying to do is engage ... Any brain exercise you want to do for improvement, try to find ones that engage the most of your brain that you can.

[00:19:30] If you're looking for the front of your brain, the frontal cortices, they're all about decision-making and action. The back of your brain is about sensory information. Try to find an activity: A) that you enjoy; and B) that can hopefully tie together as many of those as you can. That's why dance is so wonderful. It involves timing. It involves vision. It involves rhythm. It involves sensory data coming in, where is the position of your body in space and time? Decision about what you need to do. Where do I put my foot next? There are a lot of parts at play here. The more of those kinds of activities you can find that you enjoy, that engage those multiple parts of the brains, are going to be the most effective. Pick up whatever one that you want, though.

[00:20:00] The takeaway from this is, if you're looking to enhance the performance of your brain, find something you enjoy and go do it. Whether it's skiing, swimming, or whatever the case may be. Or chatting with friends. Human interaction is huge. There are lots of implications in there. Try to remember things. Try to actively seek out, last Thursday what did I do? You know, I'm speaking perhaps of somebody who has age-related cognitive decline, or something like that. Test yourself all the time. Make sure you're really paying attention to things. Don't sit passively and watch TMZ, sorry.

[00:20:30] My early experience with this training program was with my daughter, with her autism, but clearly, I discovered relatively quickly the broad implications that neurofeedback training can have for people. If I had to break it up in terms of my client load at this point, my anxiety is probably way up there. There seems to be an epidemic problem in our society. Anxiety, depression, bipolar disorder, migraine—go down the list. Neurofeedback has implications for all of these because the center point of it is this dysregulation in these networks.

[00:21:00] There are networks in your brain, which we really didn't know about until maybe 8 or 10 years ago. We knew clinically there was some reason that this low-frequency training was impactful, but we only knew it from a clinical or empirical point of view. So, fMRI research revealed there are networks in your brain, the default mode network being the primary target of our particular training. The default mode network is like the idle speed of your brain. If this setting is wrong, all of the higher [00:21:30] level functions are going to be out of whack because they rest on that basis. This network function, this network regulation is vital. It has implications for all kinds of things.

[00:22:00] Alzheimer's, people who have excessive default mode network activity produce voluminous amounts of energy, and therefore are producing more beta amyloids. Clearly, there's some connection here. I don't mean to say that any of this, by the way, is hard science. We're all puzzling our way through it. This is recent stuff that people are investigating, but the implications seem to be clear.

[00:22:30] Autism spectrum children have difficulties with their default mode network. It's not connected as well as with "normal folks." There are implications just for that alone. Anxiety, same thing. Depression, they're all ... There seems to be some connection to this default mode network. The target of the particular kind of neurofeedback that I do is to train that network, not exclusively, but as its main focus. Those networks operate at these very, very low frequencies (less than a tenth of a hertz, for anybody who's technically minded).

[00:23:00] Your normal functions that you would think about in the normal brain activity are in the multi-hertz range. Sleep or meditation is 10 hertz. Beta activity, conscious thought process, 15-30 hertz. Somewhere in there. This is one tenth of one hertz, and lower. So, it's a very unique brain space. Not sure exactly why. Probably to stay out of the way of all the other stuff. It's like submarines talking to each other in the ocean use long, slow waves to communicate. There's probably something similar going on in that regard.

[00:23:30] The default mode network interacts with other networks to create our function. The salience network decides what's important. The default mode network retreats, and the salience network hands it off to the executive control network to make a decision about what to do. These are all operating outside of your cognitive space. This is not anything you can think about, or willfully control in any regard. Our training attempts to tune the brain into those networks, and say pay attention down here. This is important. These variations that you're seeing on screen are variations in that network. Pay attention to that and try to regulate it—which oddly enough—it does.

[00:24:00] The connections between the gut biome and the brain are starting to be revealed. First of all, I have to give the nod out to the gut biome researchers, anybody who thought that what you eat might have an effect on your conduct. Going back 40 years ago, for goodness sake, you are what you eat. Yes. The health of your gut biome is vital to your function. There is a bi-directionality to that system.

[00:24:30] I'll use stress as an example because it's an easy one. When people are under stress, and what I mean by stress is not that you were hijacked, or you were kidnapped, or you were in a war. Stress is anything. Stress is just some change in your environment. You drive up and your parking space wasn't available. That's stress. Not really, but yes, it's stress. Now you have to make decisions, and you have to do stuff to reorganize your life because your parking space isn't available. Low-end stress, high-end stress. I'm not trying to compare the two. But stress is stress is stress. It provokes a cascade of things that happen, biologically, biochemically.

[00:25:00] For many years, we were only concerned about the biochemical side of things. I'll just digress on that for a second. There's a famous book called *The War of the Soups and the Sparks*, which I highly recommend, about the early 20th century dialogue between the people who were very much interested in pharmacology, about manipulating brain chemistry, versus the electrical people who

[00:25:30] were saying it's a co-equal venture. The brain is a bioelectric instrument. It has electricity, as one of its foundations. It also used chemicals, obviously neurotransmitters, etc., to help propel that function.

I'm not sure how an argument is easily made that the chemical part is the dominant one. It's clearly not. Otherwise, our chemical interventions with pharmacology would have worked far better than they do, and they would have had no side effects. So, clearly, that's like a blunderbuss approach to the brain. There's a wonderful TED Talk—I think it's David Anderson—on your brain is not a bag of

[00:26:00] chemicals, and where he talks about the implications of flooding our brains with SSRIs. To use as an example, where you're forcing open a channel of uptake in serotonin against the natural proclivity of the brain. Your problem is clearly a deficit in serotonin. I would argue, no, there's probably an electrical component to it as well, at the very least. Maybe there are some people who have a deficit in serotonin. I think that's unlikely.

[00:26:30] But you're forcing open those channels. What a surprise, there are side effects. You try to target a particular symptomatic structure by flooding an entire organism with a chemical. That doesn't seem wise, which is why I think we're seeing what we're seeing here in the lack of efficacy of a lot of the medications that have come out. Even the pharmaceutical companies are starting to give up on it because it's not a root that has born immense fruit, and the dangers are really, really high. The electrical side seems to be a much more interesting way to approach this.

[00:27:00] I'm circling back to, let's say, the anxiety person who comes in stressed. Anxiety is an expression of stress. Anxiety is not a thing, it's a symptom. Depression is a symptom. All of these things, I would argue that mental illness in its largest frame could easily be viewed as these are symptoms of something going on. This is an alert mechanism. You're depressed, not for some esoteric reason. Your

[00:27:30] body is telling you that there is something you need to do. You're anxious because your body and your brain together are telling you, you need to do something. This is intolerable. I make no judgment about the toleration level of somebody's anxiety.

So, by altering the brain's electrical capacities, by allowing it to witness that better self-regulation place, that better stasis point, that anxiety starts to diminish. How that connects to the gut-brain is

[00:28:00] when stress is reduced, which all of those chemicals that are being released start to abate, those chemicals ... you're anxious, what happens? Your stomach tightens up. Some people vomit. I mean there's clearly a body reaction to this that's being driven by a perception in the brain. So, it's all about the perception of the brain in many ways. It's a perception of the brain as to what's happening here that's out of whack.

[00:28:30] Why do people get hives? I mean you can go down the list of body expression. You sweat. All kinds of things can happen to you physically. That connection is clearly there. That perception on the part of the brain to drive a response in the body is clearly obvious. Just a little side bar note most people don't know—90% of your serotonin is produced in your stomach. I'm not sure why we're injecting it into our brains. It makes much more sense to solve the stomach problem, don't you think? That's my little shout out to the biome people.

[00:29:00] That bi-directionality, I think, is important to know. I think it's the next step. We're slowly putting this together. The gut biome people fixing gut dysbiosis is vital. You cannot function if you're consuming the wrong foods. If you have gut flora that don't make sense, have that tested. Check it out. Fix that. Take your probiotics. Do the things you're supposed to do to fix that.

[00:29:30] Additionally, I would suggest take care of the brain part. Make sure that your anxiety-stress levels are managed by your brain. There is evidence that increased stress and increased anxiety will give opportunity for bad flora to flourish. They're clearly, and we don't know exactly all the mechanisms yet, but we understand that they're there.

[00:30:00] Steven Porges has a polyvagal theory about the balance between the sympathetic and parasympathetic nervous systems, and how important that is. That nerve—it's the longest nerve, the longest neuron in the body—goes directly from the center of your brain all the way down through all your gut. What a surprise that it would be connected. We've lived through Descartes's nonsense long enough. The brain and the body are intimately connected. They're inextricable and each affects each other.

[00:30:30] Neurofeedback absolutely can change the connection between itself and the gut. There are those pathways. The vagus nerve is one. It's directly connected to all the organs in your body—your lungs, heart, liver, and spleen, and it's connected directly to the brain. Anything that affects the brain is going to affect those ultimately and finally. It's not just signals being sent upwards. It's also signals being sent downwards.

[00:31:00] There's some research done on irritable bowel syndrome, where if you did qEEG analysis of someone's brain and you can see the dysfunction, the dysregulation in their brain, you can almost predict, without knowing, that person probably has IBS. What a surprise.

Autism spectrum disorder children, three quarters of them probably have gut issues. Not surprising. The communication in their brain is not appropriate. They're not getting the right sensations to work with each other, so they're off. Not shocking. I can even extend it further to their food choices. A lot of parents struggle with limited food choice in spectrum children. I would hazard—I don't know this

[00:31:30]	for sure—but my guess is this is their defenses' way of saying I know these foods work okay for me. They're not going to upset me. It's your brain making that decision. It's by past historical analysis. So, I'm just going to stick with those four things. I'm going to stick with the tater tots, and the carrot sticks, and the whatever. And the chicken breast, or whatever the things are they might favor.
[00:32:00] [00:32:30]	The brain has figured out, it's always strategizing, "How can I minimize my upset? How can I remain stable? I'm not going to eat that kale because, nah, it doesn't look right." As many times as you say it's great, their brain is telling them something different. They haven't even ingested it. There's a decision made in the brain to refuse those particular foods. Yes, there is absolutely a bi-directional connection between the two. This is frontier stuff. This is not like 50 research projects have been done on this. But I think the indication seems to be, yes. And it would make sense. Of course, it's connected. Why wouldn't it be?
[00:33:00]	How we perceive who we are and how we are in the world affects all of our actions. It affects everything. It affects our choices. If you have a construction around your personage, that is, "I'm not worth anything," or, "I am valueless," you're going to make some bad choices. You can really damage yourself. I wanted to touch on this sort of spirituality part because I've been talking about the biomechanical part of neurofeedback, which is extremely valuable. That physiological restructuring your brain function.
[00:33:30]	There's another kind of neurofeedback I also use, which is called deep state training. It's about working in the alpha and theta ranges, which I would characterize as a more psychological form of neurofeedback. The alpha state is the meditation state. It ranges around 8-12 hertz, somewhere in there. It's a very easy place for most people to get to.
[00:34:00]	Theta is a state much deeper than that. It's right before you fall asleep. We're depriving ourselves of sleep, let me just say it that way, as a culture. We're setting up a culture right now where we're being dominated by push notifications and FOMO (fear of missing out). It's really ruling us. We're not taking the time ... Maybe it's because it's new. Maybe it's part of our biology that we're always on guard for the new thing. Maybe there are issues to be explored in there. But I think there's a psychological issue in it, too, that fear of missing out is leading us to overload our system with way too much information. Your phone has more computing power than the original computers that went to the moon. It's astonishing what that little device is. It's bad.
[00:34:30] [00:35:00]	People say, "Is technology good or bad for me?" Well, it depends on your perspective. It can be incredibly useful for you. There are wonderful apps and opportunities out there, and information to be had. There comes a time when you have to turn it off. Don't keep it at the dinner table. Don't keep it on your bedside table. There's a place and time for that kind of instantaneous connection with reality. There's a much more important place that is being neglected of time for self. Of time for just being quiet inside yourself and allowing yourself to resonate with your own inner being, whatever that may be. And finding some answers for yourself. The answers aren't out there, the answers are all in here. You can get information out there, and then you have to process it, internalize it, and make something of it, but the answer is always inside you.
[00:35:30]	So, the time for space, the time for distance, the time for reflection, are all vital. And I don't call it spirituality in a sense, but that deep state training we do in neurofeedback taps people into that separation from everything. You put an eye mask on. You're listening to tones that are telling your brain when you're in the right space. It's not like you have to learn a mantra or you have to figure it out or you have to go to a guru. No, this is you listening to yourself. Oh, that's the space, all right. And I'm getting a little tone, okay. And after a while, the loop starts to form of this is the space that I find desirable, and the effects on the people are so profound that they want to do it again and again because it's glorious.

[00:36:00] There's a psychological transference that happens in that state, which I find kind of fascinating. The meditative state, the easy enough one to get to, "I'm drifting. I'm feeling good," whatever. The theta state, that deep one, is really hard to find. I'm going to circle to that about the sleep quotient because in sleep that's where a lot of that happens. The theta space is where all that Jungian symbolical gets put down and memorized, but you don't know what it is. The space of alpha-theta allows the brain to

[00:36:30] process that, and turn it into a narrative that's understandable.

There are implications in this because we're so deficient in that theta space environment due to our sleep hygiene problems. We stay up until midnight. We have to get up at six, so we go alright. We used to go to bed when the sun went down and got up when the sun came up. That's the natural circadian rhythm of life. We forced it. And it's not just electric lights, it's a lot of things. It's a lot of

[00:37:00] technology. It's the phone, the television, it's all kinds of stuff. Work demands, etc., etc. We need to sleep more. We need to sleep deeper. We need to sleep uninterruptedly.

I tell people, "Put your phone in the other room." Don't use it as your alarm clock. Don't use an alarm clock, if you can get away with it. There's a wonderful alarm clock that wakes you up with smell. There's a natural progression to sleep, where you start to fall asleep and you drift down towards

[00:37:30] delta, which is the deep sleep pattern, but the transition point is that theta space. And then, there's a point in the middle of the night where you come up out of the deep delta space into a more theta experience. That's where memory formation happens. That's where short-term memory is turned into long-term memory. That's where the processing of some of that material, that even could be frightening, happens while you're asleep and there is no danger. Your brain gets to reorganize itself around some of this experience that it's had during the day.

[00:38:00] Sleep is also vital, by the way, just from a purely biological function, the lymphatic system ... Five years ago, the first major revelation of a new biological reality in the human body in probably 50 or 75 years, they discovered—we didn't know this existed—that the brain has waste materials and we never knew how it got rid of it. It just disappeared somehow. Well, there is an actual pressurized

[00:38:30] system in the brain that gets rid of your waste materials. And it happens when you sleep. It doesn't happen while you're awake. If you're not getting your sleep, you are literally damaging your brain.

Every time you short yourself on sleep. You might, "Oh, okay I'm going to do this for five and I'm going to catch up on the weekends." Every one of those five nights, you've damaged your brain. Permanently I don't know, but I'm not sure if I'm willing to take the risk. Get your sleep. Don't mess around. That's vital.

[00:39:00] It's implicated in Alzheimer's. The amount of beta amyloid that's produced during the day can't clean it out, where's it going to go? It's going to lay down like plaques in your brain. What a surprise. It has to go someplace. The implications are really, really high for sleep tied to good health of the brain and body. The recoupment of resources for the body spheres are pretty well known. But the brain, if it's, "Eh, it's just the brain, it'll be fine." No. It's not.

[00:39:30] Are we making ourselves sick with our thoughts? Sure. If you think of it from the perspective of brain wiring. Let's just use what I know best. Your thought patterns, if you continue to invest in them, will tightly wire together. Your perception of whatever that's fearful, that makes me angry, that makes me sad—whatever the thing might be—the longer and harder you hold on to those thoughts and ideas, the more robust they will remain.

[00:40:00] If you want to get rid of those thoughts, start thinking other thoughts. It's that replacement strategy. Those will then slowly dissolve. The circuits that fire together, wire together. The reverse is true. If they're not being used, the circuit is not being activated by your thoughts, it'll slowly disintegrate. The brain is an incredibly flexible place. It wants to use resources to the best of its ability, and if that's kind of useless, let's get rid of it. It can work either way.

[00:40:30] It's not like I'm proposing that we all just live in bliss. We all have problems. We all have things we have to worry about. We all have mortgages and car payments, and whatnot. I mean that's part of life. It's how much you obsess on them, and how much you value them, as the value you put on them as being disrupters of your life. This is not about eliminating stress. You're not going to eliminate it. Stress is a part of life and is actually a valuable component of life. It's an indicator to your system

[00:41:00] that, "Something needs attention. There's a stressor coming in, what do I need to do?" It's how you manage it. It's how you react to it that's important.

Managing your stress, putting it in the proper container. Is this the worst possible thing that could happen to me? Probably not. If you thought about it for a second. There's a—I can't quote it—

[00:41:30] Marcus Aurelius quote to that point. If you observe a thing you think is horrible, if you think about it for a second, "Oh, okay, it's not that bad," it's just not that bad.

I work in an integrative clinic, and we're on a path of putting together all of these things into a cohesive whole. Right now, it's largely organized around mental health issues. We're going to be bringing in the Functional Medicine aspects, and the gut health, and all the rest of it because it's important. Yes, I advise good diet.

[00:42:00] I personally do paleo as often as I can. For me, that's the most resident diet that I've come up with. I dearly miss pasta. I dearly miss bread, but it makes me feel better. Just in general terms, I'm not a dietitian. I can't give nutritional advice in that sense. I send them to the people I think they're going to get in value, and take their wisdom and experience as more gospel than they'll take it from me. But, yes, I absolutely encourage people. That's a vital part of this. To have your gut biome in order is

[00:42:30] fundamental. For me, it's the two parts. Get your gut in order, get your brain in order. Your life's going to be pretty okay.

There are many supplement manufacturers out there on the planet with, I'm sure, wonderful goods. I, again, do not have the science to pull apart which one is better than another. If somebody's feeling like they're not getting the proper nutrition from their regular diet, yes, sure go for it. I personally

[00:43:00] don't take a lot of supplements. I eat a really good diet, and I'm pretty comfortable with the way things operate. I could use a little more chondroitin probably for my hip, but it's not part of my regular regimen.

I don't necessarily tell people to take brain supplements, per se, unless there's something really sub-par going on. Especially in the age-related cognitive decline, I probably would get more behind it. I'm

[00:43:30] hoping if people eat good quality, organic foods that are locally sourced and they know where they're coming from, you're going to get most of the stuff you're going to need. If you're taking an SSRI, Zoloft, that particular article referenced, is changing the size of the hippocampus. You go, okay, and if it's going to solve your anxiety problem, perhaps there's a reason to do that. Unfortunately, Zoloft is prescribed for 10 different conditions, which may have nothing to do with the hippocampus.

[00:44:00] These medications are global in their impact on the structures of the brain. We don't know what they're doing. The longitudinal studies on the impacts of some of these drugs are woefully lacking. I am testament to that from the experiments that were done with my daughter, and I say that in a very non-pejorative sense. Most of the drugs she took were off-label use. Most of the drugs given to kids on the spectrum, or kids with ADD, for example, are not properly researched on dosage levels for 10-

[00:44:30] year-olds. They're just not. There's no data on it at all. It's complete guess work.

Wow. That's the one that kind of blew me away because we all assume these drugs are safe. No, they're really not. They're really not. I tell the story about aspirin, they just figured out about 10 years ago how aspirin works. We've been handing it out for 150 years. There are mechanisms that go on in here that we have no idea what the unintended consequences might be.

[00:45:00] If you need them desperately, take them for some short period. See how they're going to work for you to get you off that edge, that cliff, out of that funk, whatever that thing might be. Look for another answer because I don't think it's in pharmacology. I've met people who have 15, 20 years on benzodiazepines, and you sort of go, "What?" I can't fathom in my mind how that can actually happen to a person. Their brain is not deficient in benzodiazepine. That's not their problem. You're

[00:45:30] covering up a deeper problem with this particular person. I would suggest to their prescribing physician, let's look at a larger frame around this. And to the person themselves, you're not dealing with your situation. You're masking a symptom. Zoloft is just one. I could go down a list of medications that have profound effects of literally changing the structure of the brain. You are playing with fire if you are taking them.

[00:46:00] For parents of children with autism, specifically, do everything. Try everything. I tell parents who say, "Should we do this first, second, or third," it doesn't matter. Do them all at the same time, what's the difference. Your kid is not a science experiment. If neurofeedback is helpful, great. If occupational therapy is helpful, great. If sound therapy is helpful ... I'm a big fan of the listening program. It's a terrific program for people on the spectrum. It addresses sensory processing issues. If your kid likes any number of things, the list is quite long. We tried a lot, let's put it that way.

[00:46:30] We did Cogmed, short-term memory training. We did occupational therapy, speech and language therapy, physical therapy. We did martial arts, terrific one for kids on the spectrum. It teaches them body awareness. Teaches them control. Teaches them interaction with another figure—not a parent—interesting. Taking orders in a sense, memorizing their kata. There's a whole process of

[00:47:00] frontal cortex organization that has to be challenged in putting together the sequence of steps that they need to do to perform successfully their program. That's a great one.

I would try anything. ABA is very popular, especially with young children. If you have little ones who are really struggling to figure out how to put together the logical sequence of toileting, or how to hold a fork and eat from a plate, ABA's terrific for that. I would think over time, the older the child

[00:47:30] gets, it's probably not as useful. It's relatively, from my perspective, limited in terms of its impact because it's straight-up behavioral training. The more complicated a procedure gets, the more difficult it is to implement some of that stuff.

Neurofeedback, clearly, would be a go-to at the earliest opportunity. I've trained kids as young as two. People in my community have trained kids as young as six months. There's really no early time frame I can envision. They have to be willing and able to take in sensory information in some fashion.

[00:48:00] Ideally, visually, that'd be great. There are ways to do it just with a tactile buzzer, where they're getting a buzz. That gives them the same signal that their brain is producing, manifested in a buzzer device that rises and falls in volume depending on their brain function, of what's going on in their brain. There are ways to approach this. Sound is an easy one for kids who can't focus yet with their eyes—they can hear sounds.

[00:48:30] There are a lot of ways to get at the system at the earliest possible opportunity. My daughter was not diagnosed until she was nine. I came very late to this party. I don't mean to say it that way. Certainly, by no means is it a party. But I came late to this struggle on trying to get her function to increase. If you've had a diagnosis at two or three years old, just jump on it. There's no reason to wait.

[00:49:00] I would tell folks with autism spectrum children, though, it's a long road. It's a long, long road. My daughter still does neurofeedback and she's 20. Her brain is not yet there. She's 80% improved from where she was. I'm looking for that extra 20.

KIMBERLY CRESS, MD | Medical Director, TMS Serenity Center

Dr. Kimberly Cress:

[00:00:30]

I think my interest really first began in medical school. Interestingly enough, on my rotation in psychiatry was the first time I really was able to spend time with patients and get to know them. I had the great opportunity to work with a clinician who provided ECT, or electroconvulsive therapy, for an individual with Parkinson's disease. We were actually able to help this individual go from a wheelchair, and after ECT, he walked out of the hospital. It really showed me the biology behind treating his illness, in addition to looking at helping individuals from more of a biopsychosocial perspective. Meaning, helping individuals not only from the biological aspect, but also getting to know 'em from a psychological perspective so it really helped pull everything in.

[00:01:00]

I then continued my training, and had the great opportunity again of working with Dr. Lauren Marangell in the Mood Disorder Center at Baylor. And we had the opportunity to work in a whole host of different clinical trials that led to, for example, vagal nerve stimulation being FDA approved and various clinical trials. Again, really helping to see kind of the biology behind mental illness is where it kind of first began.

[00:01:30]

[00:02:00]

So TMS or transcranial magnetic stimulation is an MRI strength magnet—it's 1.5 tesla. It's equivalent to a magnet that's used in an MRI machine for helping with imaging for individuals. That strength of magnet is used in pulse on and off over a 20 to 40-minute period of time. It creates a magnetic field. That magnetic field then creates electrical current. As the magnetic field comes down, about three centimeters in depth within the brain, it then perpendicularly creates an electrical current. As you create electrical current, nerves fire. They release chemicals or neurotransmitters like serotonin, norepinephrine, and dopamine. Those are the neurotransmitters that we provide artificially through medications, and now we're able to facilitate their release utilizing the TMS. We're able to target where the magnet is treating and that's—in the treatment of depression—what's called the dorsolateral prefrontal cortex. It's basically the left front portion of the head. It's the area of the brain that's underactive as a result of the depression.

[00:02:30]

[00:03:00]

As the magnet pulses on and off, we're not only stimulating the release of those neurotransmitters, serotonin, norepinephrine, and dopamine, but we're also then facilitating the current, the circuits, to then fire that are involved in mood regulation. We know that within depression, not only do we have a dysfunction in these neurotransmitters, but we also have a malfunction in these circuits, so we're also able to come back and help facilitate the connectivity of the brain to help treat the illness of depression. We're able to do it in a manner that doesn't have the risk that come with medications. Oftentimes, individuals come in and part of the difficulty in effectively treating their illness is they can't tolerate medications. Common complaints will be they have sexual dysfunction, weight gain, tiredness, upset stomach, or other gastrointestinal-type symptoms. With TMS, we're facilitating the release of those neurotransmitters within the brain, so they're not going throughout the body and creating those physical symptoms, those side effects that can occur from medications.

[00:03:30]

[00:04:00]

It's a treatment that's extremely well tolerated. The most common complaint individuals might have is a little transient discomfort from the pulsing of the magnet as it's placed against the head. That pulsing, if you will, individuals quickly desensitize to it. They might have a little bit of a transient headache but it's nothing that an Advil or a Tylenol can't help alleviate. As they continue treatment, again—treatment lasts about 20 to 40 minutes—we're able to make these changes in the brain. Now, keep in mind with the TMS, it's a treatment that is done over multiple days. So, it's done five days a week for approximately six weeks in duration. Over that course of time, as we're facilitating changes in the brain, we're also helping neurons to regenerate. We know within the illness of depression, neurons can shrink, or what we call atrophy, and we can help facilitate the neurogenesis or regeneration of neurons, to help provide not only individual's mood getting better, but the longevity

[00:04:30] of the illness being under remission.

[00:05:00] TMS has been FDA cleared for individuals who have failed an antidepressant treatment. The reality is, more commonly individuals who come to my practice are individuals who have had not years but decades of depression. They've had multiple medication trials, and sometimes they're on multiple medications and still struggling. But the science tells us that individuals, when we treat them, and we treat them sooner within the illness and to the point of remission—meaning the depression is gone—those are the individuals that we can more effectively treat. Now, that doesn't mean we can't help individuals who have had long years of depression because that's who I am treating. I'm having great success with it. I mean, I've even had individuals who have failed ECT (electroconvulsive therapy) or even have vagal nerve stimulation (VNS) implanted in their chest and are still struggling with depression.

[00:05:30] Again, I want to emphasize the quicker we get them into a place of remission, not only can we help them get their lives back earlier, but oftentimes we can prevent the depression from recurring, because this is, unfortunately, a recurring illness.

[00:06:00] At this point, it's symptom based. As individuals are coming in, there are various scales, measures, that individuals can take, and it's just a questionnaire that individuals will fill out. For example, the Beck Depression Scale or the PHQ- 9, those are various grading scales that patients can fill out. So, we have them do them before the treatment, and of course along the course of the treatment, and then long term, because that really helps us get a measure of how individuals are doing acutely and long term. What we have found at the TMS Serenity Center is we've had individuals with a 72%

[00:06:30] remission rate. We are helping individuals and that's what I find clinically because a lot of the individuals I've treated are individuals I've treated for years.

I started a private practice in 2000, and I incorporated TMS in 2010. A lot of the individuals I was working with TMS, were those that I've treated for years that I was just not getting them to the point of remission or without depression despite their medications. Helping them to get their life back has been so exciting to see that transformation, if you will, and how they've been able to take charge of their life.

[00:07:00] Lisa actually came to see me for TMS back in June of 2010, now seven years ago. She is somebody who's struggled with depression since the age of 14, and through the years has had multiple episodes of major depression, requiring multiple medication trials. She's had multiple hospitalizations. She actually came to me on a variety of different medications including 60 milligrams of Paxil, 30
[00:07:30] milligrams of Remeron. She had Depakote at 750 milligrams twice a day and Geodon at 120 milligrams. Despite all that, she was still struggling with depression. She had seen a local news clip with regards to TMS and called and said, "I want help. I want to be at a place where I can start to live life again." She had been on disability for her illness and had worked as a teacher and was no longer
[00:08:00] able to work. We did TMS and she has done beautifully and is taking charge of her life. In fact, I saw her just yesterday and she said, "Thank God for TMS because it's given me my life back."

[00:08:30] As a result of getting her to the point of remission from the TMS, I've been able to simplify her medication regimen and so she's now only on 50 milligrams of Pristiq and two milligrams of Rexulti. With lessening the number of medications, that's enabled her to lose weight because a lot of the medications she had were facilitating weight gain, and she's sleeping better. I mean, she's just taking charge of her life in all different aspects.

[00:09:00] Treating depression is an art as well as a science. I see individuals throughout the day with depression and they're all unique. Everybody comes in and they have a different story in the sense that they have a different genetic makeup. They've had different environmental stressors in their life. Some have been abused. Some have had a neglectful childhood, and that has an impact on them and their brain functioning. As individuals come in, in trying to asses them and how to best treat them,

Expert Interviews – Kimberly Cress, MD

© 2017 Hyman Digital. All Rights Reserved.

268

you can't just create a standardized protocol for each individual. Quite frankly, that's even true with TMS. TMS has been FDA cleared for the treatment of major depression back in 2008, and there's a particular type of treatment protocol that we use.

[00:09:30] As individuals come in, they can have not only depression, but they might also have anxiety as well. As they're going through TMS treatment, sometimes we have to adapt their treatment protocols. For example, as this individual comes in and you see the heaviness of depression, and they're going through the TMS treatment, you start to see them improve and their mood lift. That underlying anxiety, which has always been there, might start to come out. Sometimes I have to change my treatment protocol with the TMS to adapt to where they are, because that's a reflection of their

[00:10:00] underlying illness. As a result, we adapt, we change the treatment protocol, and that's a way to best help treat those individuals and a part of helping them get to that point of remission. It's really analogous too, even with medications. Sometimes we have to add on or augment with other medications, because not one medication is going to take care of their illness. Even with TMS, we really specialize with regards to how we're treating.

[00:10:30] From a biological perspective, there can be a genetic makeup and each individual can be different, with regards to the genetics, which they can't control, of course, and that are part of their makeup. In addition to biological, the psychosocial perspective, and that environment they're raised in and the influence it has on them. For example, if somebody has been abused, that's going to have an impact on them and their resilience, and the plasticity of the brain is going to be impacted. That's part and

[00:11:00] so important in encompassing and taking care of the whole individual because again, when we take care of the whole individual, that's what's going to help them get to that point of remission. TMS is such an important treatment modality but as we help them function better with the help of TMS, we can then help them move forward and really get to some of their core issues because as I talk about abuse, those need to be addressed in a therapeutic setting.

[00:11:30] With psychotherapy and being able to get into self-esteem issues as well, that really helps in addressing and treating the whole individual because when there's that darkness of depression, it's hard to get into some of those core issues that are a part of them. With TMS, I've seen that we get them to that place, that they can now dig in and do the work that needs to be done. It helps them get to that place of peace.

[00:12:00] My goal is always to have individuals take charge of their life. I don't want their illness dictating what they can and cannot do, and I see that every day as a result of the dysfunction from depression. When they're at that point of remission, they can take charge and get their life back. The quality of the relationship with their spouse, family members, ability to make decisions about what they want to do with their career, or maybe going back to school or fulfilling their desires within their career development.

[00:12:30] Our science behind the genetic components of depression are still not there. That's one of the many areas of research and development that's currently going on. The reality, it's going to be multiple genes. We're never going to be able to target into just one. Stay tuned. My hope is one day—and I don't know if it'll be in my lifetime—that you can do a blood test and look at a person's genetic

[00:13:00] makeup and say, "Okay, you have this type of depression, and with this type of depression, then this is the treatment protocol that's going to work best for you." We're not there yet.

When individuals first come in, we have them fill out a variety of different questionnaires. We have them complete scales to look at in measuring the depression, the intensity of the depression, the anxiety, looking for other comorbidities that may be going on. For example, individuals with chronic pain that has an impact on their level of functioning as well. Diabetes, what's their blood sugar levels? There are so many different facets, and again, looking at the whole individual and what's a

[00:13:30] part of them, or have an impact in their ability to be able to function.

[00:14:00]

[00:14:30]

In addition to collecting that history, it's getting a story. Through the years, what have they been through? What have they tried from a treatment perspective? What's worked? What's not worked? To best assess, what's the best next step for that individual and helping them? Individuals who come in for a TMS evaluation, more commonly, they've had years of the illness, decades of the illness. They've had multiple medication trials that they've had maybe some response, but the depression has continued to come back. The question that I always raise, "Why would we try one more medication and expect a different response? Why would we think that this medication is going to give them point of remission when they've had a handful of medications that have already been tried?" We need to be thinking about TMS or transcranial magnetic stimulation sooner rather than adding another medication on and expecting a different result.

[00:15:00]

When we assess individuals, it's important to get a thorough history. Asking about their medical health should be a routine part of assessment. Had they seen their primary care provider? When was their last physical exam? When were labs last done? To assess and make sure that there are no medical conditions that may have an influence on their underlying mood disorder. Are they hypothyroid? Do they have anemia? There's a whole host of things that can be contributing factors to the overall sense of wellness. It's important to be comprehensive in looking at the whole individual.

[00:15:30]

[00:16:00]

Commonly, I see for individuals with depression, this sadness is pervasive. For some, especially men, it may be more irritability. It can come out in crying spells that come with feelings of hopelessness, worthlessness, or overwhelming guilt. Individuals can have an impact on their sleep. They may sleep too much or they may have disruptive sleep. They can find themselves having changes in their appetite. They eat too much. Sometimes individuals will use food to cope with emotions, where others are not hungry at all and will lose weight. They don't find joy in their lives. They have a tendency to isolate. Sometimes just getting out of bed is too much, or they feel like they have to force themselves to get out, and so their energy and their motivation to do things are impaired. Their ability to focus, concentrate, or make decisions is impacted as well. For some, they may go on to suicidality. It's not uncommon for me to have individuals who have thought life is not worth living feeling this way, feeling the heaviness and the darkness of depression.

[00:16:30]

[00:17:00]

Fortunately, more commonly, in the individuals that I'm seeing, that doesn't mean they have an active plan. It doesn't mean that they want to take their life. They don't want to commit suicide but it does reflect the heaviness. They will sometimes say, "Why is life worth living feeling this way? If I got cancer, I don't think I would care if I died." Looking at individuals and their struggles that they have, we always, certainly, want to first and foremost assess the risk and making sure that they're not acutely at risk of taking their life with suicide.

[00:17:30]

[00:18:00]

With regards to social media, there's a lot that comes to my mind when I think about mental illness. The first thing that comes to my mind is—over the years that I've been in practice—I'm amazed at the young age in which children, adolescents, will use the word "suicide." I think back to when I was growing up, you heard of suicide but it wasn't as common. And more commonly it seems like individuals will say, when they're frustrated or overwhelmed, "I just want to kill myself." I don't think individuals realize what they mean when they're saying that. We have to always be attuned to that, because that's a sign that an individual is struggling and we want to find out more. But I think, oftentimes, those are individuals that are just wanting to escape, if you will, that stressor that they're going on in life. It doesn't mean they want to take their life. My hope is that we can educate individuals to communicate and learn the coping skills to communicate that and to say, "I'm overwhelmed and I just need a time out."

[00:18:30]

Is that time out exercising? Is that time out a bubble bath? A drive? That can obviously vary for each individual. I think we need to really help individuals learn those skills to cope, rather than being at that place of just saying, "I want out." I think that can make a change for individuals at an early age. And we develop those skills, to give them skills to be able to cope and adapt as life continues on, and

[00:19:00] there are more responsibilities and demands of, especially, adolescence. There's so much that's put on them. When we talk about social media, it can be a forum for individuals to be able to communicate and talk about how they feel, which has some positives to it. But on the negative aspect of it, sometimes it can glorify how they're feeling. Are they using it as a media for attention

[00:19:30] and not really reflective of where they are? Sometimes, is it being taken to that extent of saying that I want to have attention and they can feed off of that? Having depression and suicide is not anything to be remiss about and we shouldn't be using these words flippantly.

[00:20:00] We need to help individuals think about how they're talking. And yet, on the other hand, I hope that it will help minimize the stigma of mental illness, and for individuals to get the help they need at such an early age. We're seeing younger individuals, children, adolescents, being placed on medications at an earlier age. If we can identify them and get them treatment at an early age, I think we can make such a difference in their life.

[00:20:30] If an individual is interested in TMS, my recommendation, there's probably a lot that you can Google and get on the Internet. The Clinical TMS Society is an organization of providers of TMS where you can get on the website and find a provider in your local community. I encourage you to do some research. As TMS is growing, there are more providers that are out there and so you have the

[00:21:00] opportunity to find somebody that may be very close to you. But then, do the research and find out how much experience they have. Are they up to date on education and involved in learning more about TMS?

For example, attending the Clinical TMS Society meetings. This is a new frontier. Neuromodulation is, I feel, the future of where psychiatry is going. There are more and more clinics out there that provide an opportunity to get the help in your local community.

[00:21:30] Neuromodulation is a general term with regards to how we can make changes in the brain. There are different treatment modalities. TMS, or transcranial magnetic stimulation, is one. Another one, for example, is TDCS. Direct current stimulation is another one. There are several others. TMS is the only one that has been FDA cleared at this point, but stay tuned. There's more to come.

MAGDOLNA SARINGER, MD | www.drsaringer.com

Dr. Magdolna Saringer:	My name is Dr. Magdolna Saringer. I'm a native of Hungary. I came to the US in my mid-20s to pursue my medical education and also to explore the world. After completing my child, adolescent, and adult psychiatric residency training program at the Albert Einstein College of Medicine and becoming board certified by the American Board of Psychiatry and Neurology, I was ready to start to apply all the modern tools that conventional psychiatry offers. Throughout my career, I had worked in children's hospitals, in day programs, emergency rooms, clinics, addiction clinics, so had a variety of different settings, and eventually I started my private practice.
[00:00:30]	
[00:01:00]	I treated a variety of mental conditions, mostly focusing on children. But in my private practice, I also work with adults. Among the mental conditions I treated were depression, anxiety, cognitive impairment, bipolar disorders, schizophrenia, basically everything that's diagnosed in psychiatry. It didn't take long that I became really disillusioned in what conventional psychiatry had to offer. Most of my patients were treatment resistant, they never regained a full function of their previous level, and many of them developed side effects from the medication.
[00:01:30]	
[00:02:00]	Then I worked in long-term facilities long enough, so I was able to see that what effect the ongoing medication management can have on a patient. After I got frustrated, I started to immerse myself to really look for something different; something more holistic and more humanistic. I immersed myself to look for and search the history of medicine. First of all, I was looking into my own culture, but also looked into the eastern culture to see that maybe there is something out there, what would be more helpful for the people who I came across in my offices.
[00:02:30]	
[00:03:00]	Fairly soon after, I learned about Ayurveda. As a matter of fact, I learned about Ayurveda at Canyon Ranch in the early 2000s when I was there, and that was the first time I heard about it. It really captivated my curiosity. It was so interesting to see. I really wanted to understand the interconnectedness between the individuals and the universe. I spent quite a bit of time to understand and really apply the principles on everyday life; but because of my background, my father is a scientist, my husband is a scientist, so I really had this need for reproducible data and really needed to see scientific evidence.
[00:03:30]	
[00:04:00]	During my study for the integrative medical board, I came across Functional Medicine. Then I knew that that's it, because Functional Medicine is the Western version basically of Ayurveda. Soon after, I joined the Institute for Functional Medicine and started the rigorous training to attain my certification. Since then, I'm really happy to have the opportunity to look for the root causes of my patient's symptoms and then provide them science-based and individualized treatment options for their well-being. That's why I got to Functional Medicine.
[00:04:30]	I would say that there are three categories, what I see are the major challenge areas. One is how we make the diagnosis. Diagnosis, patient come to the office and then the conventional psychiatrist immediately wants to put the patient in a box. The box is this man-made category of DSM-5, ever growing number. Then in their mind, it's constantly working on which category I can put this person in. During this time, they forget to really hear what the patient needs to say and where she is coming from. On the top of this, managed care and our limited time also does not allow for any deep and thorough assessment, and even time for listening to the patient. That's on the diagnostic end.
[00:05:00]	
[00:05:30]	There's also a problem that we identify patients with diagnoses. The patient is depressed, but we never looked into why; so why the person is depressed. From a conventional psychiatric point, the causation is that maybe they have a serotonin deficiency, or norepinephrine deficiency, or one of these neurotransmitters. This is such a simplistic answer and there is a disservice for the person, because one

[00:06:00]

person's depression is very different from somebody else. Maybe somebody has serotonin deficiency, but that person can have many other reasons why they became depressed. From a conventional point of view, that would be really important to look into at a deeper level why that person is depressed and what's causing it.

[00:06:30]

Then also, just going back to the diagnostic issues ... It's very simplistic and impressionistic, like what's my impression about what you are saying, but there's no objective. Regular conventional psychiatry rarely even sends the patient to do lab work to see if there are really hormonal abnormalities. Are there any vitamin deficiencies? Anything that can also cause the symptoms. Then, on the treatment end is very simplistic just to say that, "Okay, I'm giving you a medication and that's going to fix you," because medication is not the solution. In an acute situation, it can be helped for the patient. It can bring them out from a crisis situation, but keeping them on long-term medication is a disservice.

[00:07:00]

[00:07:30]

Then basically the studies—what conventional psychiatry is referring to are the six-week randomized double blind studies where the people they put in these studies are usually not the ones who work in the office. The ones who work in the office are usually the ones who are excluded from the studies because they have medical issues. They have substance abuse, and then they have many other things but not a criteria to participate in these six-week or even longer studies. The problem is in conventional medicine that we put somebody on medication.

[00:08:00]

[00:08:30]

I just had a patient the other day that at 16, she was put on Zoloft. She doesn't even remember why. Now she's 34, and has tried to get off many times by herself, but because she didn't do it properly; she's always failed over time. She's now here, and wants to know if she really needs this? Is there any way to stop taking medication? Then, on the treatment ... I worked quite extensively with really severely disturbed children. It's really very upsetting to see that these kids are put on medication at like four, five, six years old because they have behavior problems. Nobody even thinks about that maybe one day, it would be good to take these medications off before they develop millions of side effects. Then, I already do see that these kids are already obese. They already probably have non-insulin dependent diabetes, or something. They are already on the way to develop serious side effects.

[00:09:00]

[00:09:30]

On top of this, nobody looks at basics—what these kids are eating or what kind of physical activity they can do in in-patient units. In the United States psychiatric in-patient units, children have maybe an hour of physical activity; not even an hour, maybe less, and they are already obese, so they can go to their gym. They are just sitting on the bench. Then if they do a little bit of something, they get a reward of a lollipop or ... It's so many things, small and big; would be really good if the new generation of psychiatrists would think this way. Then they would be able to change it, and change the system, and change how they treat children.

[00:10:00]

[00:10:30]

What happened to this 30-year-old woman now, that's what she explained to me. Many times in her 20s, she just started to stop because first she thought that Zoloft is the same as taking Tylenol, so you can just stop from one day to the next. She really had serious side effects like she felt like she has a flu. Her joints were aching. Then the primary care physician immediately recommended her that maybe you are much better off if you go back. She did go back and felt better. What we did is that first of all, the taper is really important, the very slow taper.

[00:11:00]

What I suggested is that we do the workup to make sure her nutritional status is intact. I checked all of her hormones. Then also the microbiome, assessing the microbiomes to also make sure that I put the foundation down. We were going very slowly, almost like 5mg per week. She was on 100 mg, so she was not on the maximum dose. Then, she was able to get off, but it took about six months. Then, by the time her metabolic balance was in place, she didn't have any hormonal abnormality. We replaced the microbiome so she was able to tolerate this very slow taper. That patient I was working on about two years ago, and periodically she checks in because she's interested in the vitamins. They are the supplements. Then, she's doing good. Even my younger patients would benefit from this approach.

[00:11:30]

[00:12:00]

[00:12:30] I also have to say that I still have a lot of patients who come to my office and I give the speech about Functional Medicine, and lifestyle change, and then I'm very enthusiastic about it. I try to motivate them. At the end of my speech, they say, "You know Doc, I really want that prescription."

[00:13:00] Unfortunately this is for Adderall. Those are the kids who are in this competitive school systems. Then, the teachers, the parents are really pressuring them to study more than the time they have in the afternoon. They believe that they really need this extra amphetamine. I'm sure I would do great if I would start taking stimulants. That's very hard. That also takes a lot of psycho education, to educate

[00:13:30] the parents about the long-term effects of this medication. They are not just a quick fix. They have a lot of long-term effects.

[00:14:00] The mind, body, spirit approach, the first I was thinking about it. Then I really enjoy the teaching on this from Ayurveda, but also, of course, on Functional Medicine and then actually also on functional psychiatry. The way how I look at this is when a patient first comes to me, and that the patient first says that she has depression, or she's suffering, or she can't sleep, or she has depression, my first approach is that I would like to hear about her life. Then I would like to understand that why at this

[00:14:30] particular moment she has depression—what happened to her? What's happening at home, at work, and then also in her social life.

[00:15:00] Then, I look at depression as the end point, not the beginning; and then immediately I seek for the root cause. What causes? Why is it happening? Then when I do them, I spend an equal amount of time to look into the person's biochemistry and also the lifestyle changes. Then, also the psycho spiritual aspect of her life. Then what I've found, and I still have a great interest about the effect of trauma on people's life. When I'm talking about trauma, I'm not just saying that kids were sexually abused, or went through war, or horrible traumas but also minor traumas like relational trauma, like not being

[00:15:30] accepted, not being acknowledged, bullied, or humiliated even by parents. There are so many forms of insecure attachment, that's also in that psycho-spiritual area.

[00:16:00] The two really connect with each other. Maybe that person's biochemical individuality and there are many things she's doing great, but she's still depressed because of the psycho-spiritual stress, which she never addressed. Then, so trauma work and understanding and connecting, that's a good way also to treat psychiatric patients; not just depression, it applies to anxiety, PTSD, and so many things. That's

[00:16:30] one aspect of how the mind, body, and spirit are connected.

[00:17:00] There are a lot of people who come, and they don't talk too much about feeling depressed or anxious, but they have different kind of bodily sensations. They feel constantly bloated. The bowel movement is not normalized. They feel constantly anxious. It always comes with psychiatric problems. Then again, I try to understand their symptoms and their problems through this mind-body connection. Many of the treatment offers are basically targeting the autonomic nervous system.

[00:17:30] One of the areas I'm really interested in to offer and teach people is HeartMath—heart rate variability training. Some of them are really into it. That can really re-balance the sympathetic and parasympathetic nervous systems; so eventually they feel much calmer, and they are able to bring up

[00:18:00] the parasympathetic part of their autonomic nervous system so they feel more relaxed. That, of course, also comes with the connection between the nerves, the vagus nerve, you know that originates and goes up to the brain. The heart-brain connection is also significant. There are so many efferent pathways, which go from the heart to the emotional brain. If it's regulated and imbalanced, then the

[00:18:30] brain is receiving calming and positive feedback.

[00:19:00] For the MSQ, the Multiple Symptom Questionnaire, even if they just come for depression, or come for anxiety, or attentional problems, I always see scores of 30, 35 or up. It's really hard to bring down to below 20 or below 10, what would be normal because they have so many symptoms. The major one is really in the GI tract. The alteration of diarrhea, constipation, bloating. So many people have skin issues, skin rash, and many other things. Then also the sleeping problems, but the major one is

[00:19:30] digestion. That's how it manifests in many of the symptoms.

[00:20:00]	I had quite a few patients who came with digestive problems. The simplest thing can make such a huge difference. My experience lately is with people in their 40s, so in the mid-age patients who come. They complain that they have brain fog. They just can't understand and remember things as well as they did in the past. Then, I always do a very thorough nutritional assessment to see that what kind of food they
[00:20:30]	eat, because usually that's the first line what can cause problems. Then I always recommend them to stop gluten; so gluten is number one. This particular patient, we didn't do too much at the beginning. We're just sending out the labs; but I asked her to stop eating gluten. The month after when she came back for the lab review, she already said that suddenly the brain fog just lifted. Simple intervention can
[00:21:00]	make a huge difference.
[00:21:30]	If they are able to engage in more regular exercises, that also helped. Just going back to the GI, sometimes just for them to understand that it's not just their own genetics, but there are these millions and trillions of bacteria in different living organisms, living in our body. They also have their genetic messages and the products, what they make, re-establishing the flora. That can also make a significant
[00:22:00]	difference in psychiatric treatment management. Most studies out there are mostly for depression and anxiety, but I'm sure that as soon as science would be able to sequence these bacteria in everybody, that would also give a much more targeted probiotic recommendation, rather than just take one that
[00:22:30]	has everything in it. It would be much more precise based on what people have or don't have.
[00:23:00]	Ayurvedic medicine is so complex, but is also so simple. It's so interesting that's why it really captured my attention. The basic principle of Ayurveda; and Ayurveda, the translation of the word is wisdom of life. Then that really summarizes what it's about. Ayurveda is a medical metaphysical healing science. The basic premise is that they promote a human well-being. They promote health. They promote creative growth—everything that humankind needs. They also have a very organized system how they
[00:23:30]	recommend the individualized lifestyle plan.
[00:24:00]	What's interesting in Ayurveda is the concept of disease and the concept of how they look at health and disorders. What they say is that we all have health and disorder at the same time. It's just a balance and which one is taking over. Then they have this 5-point plan of what a person has to establish to have good health. Number one is the digestifier. They call it the Agni. Number two is the constitutional type. That's the Pitta and Kapha, it has to be in balance. That system is different for
[00:24:30]	everybody. The ratio of Pitta and Kapha is something that people are born with. The idea is just to balance it, keep it in balance. They have the same system for mental health, too. Their idea is that behaviors and morale are also somehow constitutional, but it's much more fluid; so people can learn
[00:25:00]	new ways through meditation, yoga, and nutrition.
[00:25:30]	Then their mental energies, that's how they call it, are the Sattva, Rajas, and Tamas. The Sattvic people, the ones who are very calm and doing good for the world, they are usually believing in a higher power. These are the optimal setups. The Rajas is the Rajic temperament, people who are more business focused, and they are more extroverted. They are not so into higher power. The third one is the Tamas. They categorize the behavior, what relates to this mental energy is laziness, no motivation, using others, something people don't really want. According to their principle, people should strive toward
[00:26:00]	achieving the Sattvic temperament. They have special recommendations for that.
[00:26:30]	Going back to the disease concept, the constitutional type, even the mental or the physical, was number two. Number three is making sure people are healthy and they avoid being diseased is that they have normal elimination, a regular elimination. That's imbalance. Then, the elimination is getting rid of the waste for that. That's very important in the system. The waste products are urine, feces, and sweat. Then number four is the senses; that all senses, hearing, tasting should work normally.
[00:27:00]	The last one is the mind-body and spirit connection. That should be in balance and should work as a whole rather than a fragmented piece. What they say is that if somebody's diseased because "dis"
[00:27:30]	means lack of something. "Ease" means comfort. The disease is lack of comfort. What they try to promote with these five elements or five basic elements is so everybody knows what they need to do

---

to stay at ease and not to go to disease.

[00:28:00] It's really fascinating to understand. They also have what I had trouble with. That's why I was looking for something more. The past diagnosis ... these Ayurvedic healers are really amazing. They can just put three fingers on your pulse and then make a diagnosis of what's going on inside your body; what kind of biochemical imbalances you have. I did see people who are able to do that. It probably requires a lot of practice.

[00:28:30] My approach with all of my patients is that I took a really thorough history of understanding of their life circumstances. I ask especially the anxiety, fear, trauma patients to fill out this questionnaire: the Adverse Childhood Assessment Questionnaire. That's a 10-item questionnaire. What's interesting is how many people score high, and then this is validated by the Kaiser Permanente Foundation in the
[00:29:00] 1990s. The lower the score, the better. Trauma patients usually get at least two or three on the broad-based population study of what the Kaiser Foundation did. The American population, at least ⅔, has one on the score.

[00:29:30] The patients we see, the people we see in our office, they usually have two or three. The reason why it's important is because I immediately assume that this patient has inflammation, because living in stress raises the cortisol level. Cortisol promotes inflammation. That's an important root cause, but I
[00:30:00] always look for the inflammation. The easiest way is I always do a very thorough diet history to see if eating the food would maintain the inflammation or not. Then I also do a GI and check the microbiome composition; so, I do like this kind of investigation. Then I also focus on trauma, like really see that from this ACE score; I have an idea already of what kind of traumatic events happened in their life.

[00:30:30] My first approach from a treatment perspective is, first of all, I make sure that they clean up their diet. For this population, I really promote physical exercise because there are so many studies out there that aerobic exercise specifically can help the brain with promoting the brain-derived neurotrophic factor
[00:31:00] production. Also, it helps to develop more synapses. I always do a HeartMath baseline assessment just to see where their autonomic nervous system is at this point. Sometimes, if they have sleeping problems and more complications of anxiety, I also like to see a cortisol diurnal variation.

[00:31:30] I already know if somebody is highly anxious, they probably have a high cortisol; but just to see that which part of the day is problematic. HeartMath gives me a baseline understanding, so then I teach them the technique. Then I really make sure. Now I'm working with IFM certified health coach. She's a great help for me. She's the one who is making sure that if the patient has questions even when they
[00:32:00] leave the office, they know what to do. Then, their practice can also be connected to my computer, my software. That's also helpful for many patients, not everybody, but some people like to be tracked.

[00:32:30] My coach helps to make sure of that, that's first. Then, from the medication point of view, when somebody is suffering from very severe panics, I had quite a few patients like that. I prescribe usually only short-term, but a low-dose of benzos like Valium, Xanax, or I prefer Klonopin because we already know why it works. We know that if they take it, they really feel much more relaxed. I make sure that medication management is just for the acute crisis, it's not for long.

[00:33:00] The health coach is a great help to the doctors and to any care provider. Especially working in hospitals, I know that people leave even when they're in-patient, and so they really had time to talk to the doctor
[00:33:30] and get the prescription straight. When people go home, everything is just gone. I am sure there are statistics of how many patients take the medication after they leave the hospital. From a private practice point of view, when I know my patient, I see which ones would really benefit from my coaching, and which ones would say, "No, I know it. I can do it." Then also self-motivated people can
[00:34:00] generate this internal coach, but most of my patients benefit from coaching.

I use apps so they don't feel so intimidated that somebody's calling on them. I use Twine, that app is pretty helpful. We set the goal on the session with the coach and then every week, they get a feedback,

[00:34:30] but they have to plug in the daily information. The most toxic foods on the brain is all over in the Functional Medicine field, but is still not out for the public, but it's absolutely sugar. The load of sugar, and then not just like fructose, like fruit sugar, but also these processed and synthetic lollipops and all the sweets, what we see. I know there are many studies done showing that the sugar is as or more

[00:35:00] addictive than cocaine. We're really kind of poisoning and making these kids addicted.

[00:35:30] I don't like to scare people, but some personalities need some scaring. I usually just tell them that we are starting the program. We clean out everything, what would be harmful for you. Number one is sugar. Then I would say gluten as well and dairy. Again, many of my patients really like dairy and especially kids. I want to make sure that it's grass-fed and organic, so the kids don't receive the

[00:36:00] additional hormones and what these poor animals were fed with. That's if they would like to.

[00:36:30] Then I usually do a genetic testing and that guides me further. Do they have a gluten sensitivity or lactose intolerance, especially older people? That's what I would like them to avoid. Then, at the same time, I always give everybody the information about the Environmental Protection Agency because they have the Clean-15 and the Dirty Dozen. I make sure everybody goes home with the sheet for the Dirty Dozen, so they get organic.

[00:37:00] For brain health, it's really the good quality fats. I've been doing this cognitive decline prevention program. I make sure that everybody is going toward the ketogenic state, because when the brain is on fat burning, that's the most beneficial. Some people have issues with ketogenics, some people can't. That is usually a gradual shift. I usually first introduce paleo because paleo is in the news. People know

[00:37:30] it's not scary. It's easier to do. I just ask them to do it for one month, so they don't feel like they can't have any good food anymore. Often, some people like to see numbers. In my office I have the ketometer. I tell them you don't need to go too high, you just make 0.4, 0.8, 1.2. That's not so difficult to achieve.

[00:38:00] If somebody has trouble, I also recommend the intermittent fasting. What's the best way actually to initiate this ketogenic state, because if they are able to stay fasting for I would say like 14 to 16 hours, from 6pm to 8am, or 6pm to 10pm, that's also a good way to get into this state of mind. Then,

[00:38:30] maintaining with good quality fish oil, and also good quality fat like avocados, nuts. I like ghee. Ghee for the variety of good quality fats and protein.

[00:39:00] What I recommend for people who are suffering from depression is to seek help, social connectedness, or feeling important. When somebody goes to see a therapist or a doctor, that immediately gives an importance that they are taken seriously. That's number one I would suggest. Also, if they come to me, I would definitely do the workup to see that if there are any underlying imbalances. If their condition is

[00:39:30] not so severe, I would also look into their diet and clean up and remove things that promote inflammation and gluten, for example. Start doing an exercise program. It can be a team sport. I'm great at recommending tennis or something that's interactive.

[00:40:00] If somebody has more severe depression, then the problem is they don't have much motivation to do all of these things. In this case, they need some intervention. Psychotherapy can be very beneficial, cognitive behavior therapy, or readjusting their nervous system with meditation. Also, just for them to

[00:40:30] know that depression is a stage, and it usually goes away. Of course, if it's severe and people are suicidal, then I don't say this. I say this, but then I'm more proactive of making sure that they are safe.

[00:41:00] Over the years, I also learned that, unfortunately, our society is not really tolerant of something out of the norm. Sometimes, when major issues happen in life like a trauma, somebody loses a job, and then they became depressed, that's not something that we immediately need to cover up. Social

[00:41:30] connectedness and leading them towards spirituality. I have so many patients who are even different kinds of affiliations like Judaism, Christianity, that can be also so comforting.

[00:42:00]

That reminds of my mother. After my grandmother died, she had a very severe bout of depression. That was the time when she reconnected to her faith. Then what she did, that was years ago, she enrolled to these orders, to be a societal member. She started to study the Bible, and then religion, and then she eventually became a teacher; a religion teacher for schools. I remembered that idea that she's connected, and then that really helped her to recover. She has never been on medication.

[00:42:30]

[00:43:00]

The future of psychiatry is—I went through my mind, and I planned it already. I planned a clinic in my mind especially if I was working with children ... what would be in that clinic; and what would be great for the future of mental health, especially brain health. Since I'm focusing more on brain health, I definitely would like everybody to look at the brain the same as their bodies, as their muscles. I mean you can go to the gym and build up your strength and your endurance, the same way you can do with the brain. I'm so into recommending people do brain gym time regularly; that's doing the brainHQ or one of these softwares, and they can do it online. It's fun. It's challenging. I think that should be a must. That should even be in schools to help people, rather than giving children ADHD medications.

[00:43:30]

[00:44:00]

Also making sure that everybody's educated on diet. They know what is harmful and what's good. Even in the clinic, there would be a kitchen where everybody can taste, and see, and go home with recipes; so, cooking together. The physical exercise part is not just aerobics but also strength training, which is also good for the brain. Then, also make sure that the people are connected, so organizing work. That's my next step I'm going to organize in my office, walks in Central Park.

[00:44:30]

You don't need to talk. We can talk if we want to, but it can be also just talking about nature and then discovering the beauty of the universe rather than thinking about the bad stuff. This kind of positive mindset, that's what I would really like to convey, to bring to the next generation of psychiatrists and also for psychiatric patients.

MAGGIE NEY, ND | Akasha Center For Integrative Medicine, Santa Monica, CA

Dr. Maggie Ney: I'm a naturopathic doctor and was always interested in health and wellness, and when I decided to pursue medicine, I spent a lot of time with doctors medical doctors in different clinics and hospitals and private practices. I realized medicine now is really just focused on diagnosing symptoms, diseases, and giving prescription medications, and it ignored what I found to be such a powerful part of health—diet and exercise and stress management. So, I wanted to become a doctor but have all that other

[00:00:30]   information as well. I think the biggest challenge conventional medicine has these days is the lack of time that we value in spending with individuals. We spend such a short amount of time and I think part of it's the insurance model that when we see someone with, for example, sinus infection, you could almost guess the treatment before even talking to the patient.

[00:01:00]   We need to—in order to give the best, most effective healthcare—look at the whole person. You can't do that in 5, 10, 15 minutes. You have to look at the complete physical, mental, emotional, and spiritual piece. All of that matters in making up someone and their health. Hormonal imbalances are when one or more hormones are being overproduced, underproduced, or not being officially metabolized out of the body. This can happen for a number of reasons. Poor diet. A diet that's high in sugar, processed foods, too much caffeine, too much alcohol, can all disrupt hormonal regulation. Lack of proper exercise can

[00:01:30]   contribute to hormone dysregulation. Too much stress can lead to hormonal dysregulation. Toxins in our environment can contribute it. We have endocrine-disrupting chemicals in the environment.

Things like parabens, BPA—they mimic estrogen in the body and disrupt our own natural hormonal rhythm. High stress is huge and contributes to hormonal imbalance, so there are a lot of variables. The

[00:02:00]   symptoms that can develop from hormonal imbalances for the brain: fatigue, depression, anxiety, brain fog, not feeling like yourself anymore. It's like you're looking through the world with different lenses. All of those really matter. When it comes to hormones and depression, you really need to look at all of them. Sometimes they're not easily measurable in the blood, depending on how old a woman is or where they are in their menstrual cycle. You have to look at all the symptoms, but estrogen, for example, is really a powerful hormone for depression.

[00:02:30]   Estrogen really helps awaken the serotonin receptors in the brain. When we're not exposed to healthy levels of estrogen, those receptors aren't being activated and we're not getting the benefits of serotonin, which is considered to be our happy hormone. Feeling good, being able to sleep, and less anxiety. Progesterone is another one. Progesterone is a hormone we're only exposed to from the time of ovulation to when we bleed to our periods. That level can fluctuate a lot in women. Certainly, in

[00:03:00]   perimenopause, when we're not ovulating regularly. We're not being exposed to progesterone and other times when women's estrogen/progesterone ratio isn't optimal. We can experience the effects of not having optimal progesterone levels. Progesterone helps activate GABA receptors in the brain, which calms and makes us feel relaxed.

If we're not having adequate progesterone, then the GABA, that important neurotransmitter, isn't being

[00:03:30]   efficiently used. Progesterone also affects dopamine levels. Low progesterone would contribute to low dopamine which is really important for the prefrontal cortex, which is our higher executive functioning, our mood, and behavior. There are a lot of different hormones that affect mood and depression. During perimenopause, one of the hallmarks or hormones is just going up and down, and not just being their normal rhythmic nature. And a woman's mood is absolutely feeling those effects. Eating a clean, whole

[00:04:00]   foods diet is very important. Increasing dark leafy green vegetables is key. Healthy sources of fat like coconut oil and avocado, good sources of protein throughout the day, keeping blood sugar stable,

[00:04:30] trying to avoid animal products that have been treated with exogenous hormone sources, because that also plays in a factor in our hormones. So, eating a really clean, whole foods diet; limiting sugar, processed food; being mindful of how much caffeine. A cup of coffee if you enjoy it, that's not a big deal. There are actually health benefits. It's when you need the coffee to function, when you need that glass of wine to wind down at the end of the night, that's when we're having an unhealthy relationship with these, with coffee and alcohol. Diet is huge. Exercise. There are studies that show that just 20 minutes of exercise a day helps increase brain neurotrophic factor, which helps to increase brain cells, and so that is huge getting women to start exercising at home.

[00:05:00] Stress reduction, and being mindful of stress reduction, and starting to realize that you don't have to do everything and say yes to everybody, and having boundaries. Recognizing chaos and drama and just saying no to it because that has an effect on our hormonal system. Eating too much sugar and foods that turn into sugar really easily like processed foods are pretty toxic to the brain. We get a rapid rise in

[00:05:30] glucose, which then plummets, which causes people to feel anxious and often depressed and crave more sugar. It also causes a rise in serotonin and then that plummets. Sugar causes a rise in dopamine and then that plummets. I think sugar is certainly the biggest factor in someone's diet.

Sugar is talked a lot about and we eat way too much of it. I think you can have a healthy relationship with it. There's not one health benefit to having sugar besides it tasting good, but you can still have sugar

[00:06:00] without sugar having you. The problem in our society is that people are just craving it and eating so much of it, and a meal doesn't feel like a meal until there's sugar at the end of it. When they're feeling down or tired, then they reach for that sugar. That's an unhealthy relationship and that's where we're seeing a lot of the toxic effects in the brain.

I think the most effective way, if someone's open and motivated, is to do a three-week strict elimination

[00:06:30] of sugar. I find that to be the most effective way because I do believe everything in moderation is just the healthy way to be in life. But it's hard to go from eating it every day to doing it twice a week and feeling really comfortable with that. It's much easier to eat in moderation—sugar or anything that's unhealthy— when you can do a strict three-week elimination diet. That's my number one way to help get people to be really aware of how much sugar they're eating and reset their palate. It's amazing what can happen if you can go just that three weeks without sugar or processed foods—how you can reset your palate and stop

[00:07:00] the craving. And then, when you reintroduce it, it doesn't even taste the same and you don't want it as much.

It's much easier to listen to your body and not overeat. I saw one today who's struggling with pretty significant PMS. I saw her for the first time about two months ago, and she came in presenting with depression and anxiety. She's a 28-year-old female working at a law firm, working long hours. Usually

[00:07:30] eating a bagel and cream cheese for breakfast, eating whatever they bring in. Sometimes it's a salad, and sometimes it's a sandwich. Snacking on sweets during the afternoon, living on coffee, and no time to exercise, not spending any time outside, drinking alcohol every night, going out after work late, having drinks. And she presented to me—she just couldn't understand, she used to feel great and now she's struggling with fatigue, depression, anxiety, and just really bad PMS, where all those symptoms are really

[00:08:00] exacerbated pre-menstrually.

She hadn't had a work-up in a while, so I did really comprehensive blood work. I did a micronutrient panel and I started her on a three-week cleanse. She was motivated and felt ready and wanted a change. I had her, for three weeks, eliminate all gluten, dairy, sugar, alcohol, coffee, but she was able to eat a lot of dark leafy greens, fruits, whole grains like rice and quinoa, millet, nuts and seeds, healthy sources of

[00:08:30] animal protein. Just getting rid of that sugar, the processed foods, the gluten, and the dairy. I also started her at that visit on a probiotic to help support the gut and the gut microbiome, and told her I'd see her in three weeks, see how she was feeling, and review all the blood work, and really make an individualized plan at that point.

[00:09:00] When I saw her, it was actually five weeks later, but she had gone through one full menstrual cycle and said her symptoms were so dramatically better just by the dietary changes alone. She also had cramps, and her cramps were significantly better. Her mood felt more stable. She was clear headed. She didn't have that brain fog anymore. That's very typical. In her particular situation, she was also low in magnesium and B6. We did a micronutrient panel on her. I started supplementing with those as well.

[00:09:30] When I saw her today, she reported even more energy, better mood, better sleep. It's really exciting work because they're working with their own bodies' natural ability to heal themselves.

[00:10:00] A woman's brain changes in relation to hormones that it's being exposed to. Let's just talk about some of the hormonal changes that can happen during a woman's life. Cortisol for example is a really key stress hormone. A little bit of stress is not bad for women. It's actually a little stress that can cause the cells of the hippocampus to grow and helps you remember better. It's the long-term chronic stress that actually plays a factor in a woman's brain and man's brain, too. Chronic exposure to cortisol with a woman who is under a lot of stress will actually cause those cells of the hippocampus to actually shrink. Estrogen is a key

[00:10:30] hormone for the brain and that also fluctuates a lot throughout a woman's cycle. During menopause and perimenopause when estrogen starts to drop, that has a huge effect on the brain as well.

People come to see me all the time for menopausal symptoms. It's not the hot flashes or night sweats that bring them into my office. It's the brain symptoms. It's the brain fog and not feeling like themselves and the depression and the anxiety. What we know about estrogen is that when it declines in

[00:11:00] menopause, it's not feeding their serotonin receptors so that can—for some women, overnight—switch their demeanor and behavior. Thyroid is another one. Women are more prone to getting thyroid disorders when they're in their 30s and 40s, and thyroid is a huge hormone that affects mood and depression. So, that's always important to make sure that women are monitoring those hormones as well. When we're born, hopefully we're born with healthy pattern of glucose and insulin. And that,

[00:11:30] actually, is partly dependent on how mom was during pregnancy that helps determine … But insulin levels, the more we're exposed to the sugars and the processed food as dietary changes, we have fluctuating levels of insulin.

When we eat a high-sugar, high-glucose meal, our insulin levels spike, and what that does is it causes the glucose to be absorbed into the blood. The more sugar we have throughout the day, throughout the

[00:12:00] chronic glucose exposure, then insulin keeps being produced in high levels. And our cells are basically, they've had enough. They stop listening. We're left with high insulin levels and high glucose levels leading to insulin resistance. And insulin resistance is now being shown to have a huge effect on the brain, actually causing a lot of neurodegeneration and neuroinflammation and contributing to Alzheimer's disease, which is now being considered type 3 diabetes. Insulin definitely has a big role in eating healthy throughout a woman's life, who can certainly keep that insulin level stable.

[00:12:30] Stress affects both men and women significantly and have long-term health consequences for both. I will say I think it's interesting—women and men both produce cortisol, the stress hormone, and adrenaline, epinephrine. They're stress hormones. Something different that women produce is a hormone called oxytocin, which is our feel-good hormone. It's what's produced during orgasms and breastfeeding, to help us feel good and bond. Men produce a little bit of that, but women much more. That's interesting. I

[00:13:00] think what we're seeing because of that, it helps explain how in times of high stress, women tend to be more looking out for others, connecting with others, taking care of others. I think that that explains some of the sex differences. I think an issue is, sometimes, women neglect themselves in those situations.

[00:13:30] I also think it helps explain why women are such good multitaskers. They can really handle a lot under times of stress. Vitamins and minerals are cofactors for every reaction in the body. For neurotransmitter production—neurotransmitters are the messages that are produced by the brain—you need vitamins and minerals to make them. If you have deficiency in any nutrient, then certain neurotransmitters aren't being produced efficiently. We know a lot right now about what happens in a woman's body when there is insulin resistance or nutrient deficiency. When a woman is pregnant and struggling with some of these deficiencies, it affects the baby, too. Everything when the baby is growing, they're getting it from mom.

[00:14:00] Yeah, there were some recent studies that are showing that optimal vitamin D levels during pregnancy helps to support the baby's language development later on. That's really exciting. That's really exciting news because vitamin D deficiency is epidemic these days. That's an easy nutrient to be tested for and treated with. There's more and more research showing that a woman's metabolic status during pregnancy affects the health of their newborn. We know that during times of obesity, there is usually

[00:14:30] insulin resistance. And that creates more neuroinflammation and neurodegeneration, and that's affecting the brain of the baby as well. What we're finding is that obesity in women who are pregnant contributes to more autism, asthma, ADHD, and more weight issues down the road in their offspring.

[00:15:00] For vitamin D, the normal range for a lab result is usually 30 to 100. I've seen some labs go down to 20, as the normal is 20 to 100. But the optimum range is really if you can get your vitamin D level to between 60 and 80, and that's where we're seeing a lot of the health benefits. Intermittent fasting is an eating program where you eat a certain amount of calories within a restricted time period, and the rest of the time is devoted to fasting. That can look like eating all your calories within a 12-hour window, and the

[00:15:30] rest of the hours devoted to fasting. What we're finding is that for certain people—particularly for people who are metabolically imbalanced, people with obesity, high blood pressure, high triglycerides—they respond really well to intermittent fasting.

[00:16:00] Men and women respond differently to intermittent fasting. Men, generally, are better candidates than women. Anyone who's had a history of not really being able to listen to their body and overeat or food restriction, they need to be encouraged to listen to their body and not a rule of when to eat and when not to eat. Anyone with any eating disorder, women who tend to be more thin or high stress, they don't do as well with intermittent fasting. Intermittent fasting, I would say, generally works better for men than women, although some women can respond and anyone who has these conditions of being just metabolically imbalanced.

[00:16:30] Eating a clean whole foods diet. I try to make it easy for people, too. There are so many books out there telling you what to eat, what not to eat. It's common sense. It's get back to nature and how we're supposed to eat. That's eating a lot of vegetables, some fruits, whole grains, nuts and seeds, healthy sources of animal protein, healthy oils, healthy fats. Getting as close back to nature. I always tell my patients, there's no bread tree or pasta bush. No cookie trees. We have to get back to nature and how

[00:17:00] we're supposed to eat. When we do that, it's really dramatic when we can cut out the sugar and processed foods—how you can wake up in the morning with a clear brain and more energy.

[00:17:30] Exercise is key. Moving your body, and if you can spend some time outside, that's key. Getting, again, back to nature and getting some exposure to nature. Sleep is essential. Trying to get at least seven to nine hours of sleep at night because that's when a lot of hormones and your immune system is rebalanced and our endocrine system is rebalanced. Stress reduction and being mindful of the stress in your life and taking tools to help reduce that stress, whatever that may be. Make sure to correct any nutrient deficiencies that you may have. Look at the gut and the gut health. If you have any symptoms—a

[00:18:00] GI imbalance, bloating, or gas, or burping—you really need to look at that because the gut microbiome and the brain health are so intimately connected, you really can't separate them.

[00:18:30] Getting your gut balanced is key. Hormonal. Again, if you're feeling like you're hormonally imbalanced, if your moods and your brain feel like they're fluctuating with your cycle, or you're entering menopause, looking at that a little bit more closely is really important. Sometimes that can be corrected just through the lifestyle modifications I've talked about. Sometimes you need a little extra support. For some women, they respond really well to the bioidentical hormones, which are hormones that have the same molecular structure as your body's own hormones. That can be helpful for some people. Then looking at the environment and cleaning up the environment. We're exposed to so many chemicals and toxins in our environment, and if we can just really start to be aware. It can be scary when we start to hear everything, but it can also be empowering. What I tell people is usually just get rid of plastic in the kitchen. Please try to switch to glass and stainless steel to store your food in. Get a glass water bottle.

[00:19:00]   The other thing is just being really mindful of your own genetics and your genome because some people metabolize toxins more efficiently than others. Some people are able to metabolize more hormones more efficiently than others, and when you learn about that, you can really make some key lifestyle choices that help optimize how genes are expressed.

MAGGIE WARD, MS, RN, LDN | The UltraWellness Center

Maggie Ward:	I got interested in nutrition very early on. I actually was thinking of medical school and I didn't really agree with how medicine was being practiced. Growing up as an athlete and a mother that cooked from scratch every day, she kind of got me into nutrition pretty early. I just felt like food is at the foundation of health, and I felt through food you can reach the most people. In improving what they eat, you're going to improve their outcome. So, I got interested really early on, and even when I knew I wanted to become a nutritionist, a dietician, I didn't really agree with how that was actually being taught, so I searched out different programs because I really wanted to learn about how to use food, how to cook food, and use food as medicine.
[00:00:30]	
[00:01:00]	I was very lucky to land into a program that really, at the core, is Functional Medicine. It's "try and figure out why people are ill," and a lot of that having to do with food and things they may not be eating, so I really got that training early on, and I was fortunate. I had a lot of culinary classes, which was really key to teaching people not only about nutrients, but how does that translate into really getting those nutrients, and how do you get it out of food and make it work for you? It started early on, and I kind of naturally fell into where I am now, which is perfect for what I want to do.
[00:01:30]	With mainstream nutrition, there's still not as much focus on quality. It's calories in, calories out. How do you figure out calories and just get that in? We know that calories aren't equal. You know, 100 calories in soda is not equal to 100 calories in broccoli. I think that is, unfortunately, missing in conventional medicine, or in conventional dietetics, I should say. It's still needed, because when people are acutely sick in the hospital, you need some of that training to help people survive, but I didn't want to practice nutrition in that way. I really wanted use food as medicine, and the quality makes all the difference. Our message here now in what we understand is that food is also information.
[00:02:00]	
[00:02:30]	You're not only providing nourishment, you're providing information to your body, which turns things on and off and communicates in a very specific way, of what you're trying to achieve, what outcome as far as health or trying to avoid disease. I think there's a disconnect, unfortunately, in a lot of conventional ways of learning nutrition, unfortunately. I think food and nutrition, whether it got someone sick or not, I think is always debatable. What I tell everyone that I work with, it's always part of the solution. For some people, that's 99% of what they need to do to get better, and I've seen that. Within weeks, people heal from their diabetes and joint pain, and things can turn around quickly.
[00:03:00]	For others, it's not as big of a piece of what they need to work on, but what I always tell them, "It's part of the puzzle piece," so you need to always be incorporating good quality nutrition to heal from whatever else might be going on for you. Nutrition, I think, can be challenging in a way that your health will sometimes dictate what you need to eat. When you're dealing with an infection or needing support around detoxification, your nutritional needs will change from that, so your need for protein might go up, and certain micronutrients go up. There's always that component, too. I think it's a really critical piece of healing, and that's why we incorporate it with every person that we see, in every treatment plan.
[00:03:30]	
[00:04:00]	Good quality nutrition, a good food plan, is the foundational piece of any treatment plan to heal. It kind of varies, I think, depending on how much of their food is going to make a difference for each person. The approach here at The UltraWellness Center with nutrition, I think, is very different than you'd see in any really conventional setting. I mean, one is time. We spend a lot of time with our patients. Unfortunately, in the conventional setting, even if you have a nutritionist work in the conventional setting, you don't have a very long period of time to work with people. In order to really make change happen, that can be challenging, especially around nutrition, because there's so much

detail involved in it, in helping figure out not only what to eat, but how are you going to do that and incorporate it into your day?

[00:04:30] I think the biggest difference is we spend a lot of time with our patients, so initially, when they come in, everyone that sees a physician then sees a nutritionist. Again, it's a really integral part of their treatment plan, and I think we have very good integrative care here. We work very closely with the physicians. We talk about cases. They make recommendations, and we support them and integrate it into making that work for that person. Nutrition is very much an art and a science, so even when patients might know what to do and are given the information, a lot of what the nutritionists do is figure out, "How are they going to do it?"

[00:05:00] We're supposed to eat more protein and do this, and this is what it looks like, but let's figure out, how does that work into your schedule, and your family's schedule, and your food preferences, and the foods that you maybe can't tolerate? I think we, as nutritionists here, are really trained in thinking from that functional approach of not just how much food, how many calories do you need, but are there certain foods that are not working for you? Are they making you sick? Are you not tolerating them? We have a lot of great lab data to guide us of what food that person is not doing well with. We have a lot of great nutritional labs to give us a better sense if certain nutrients are low, and how to improve that through their food, and sometimes some supplements.

[00:05:30]

[00:06:00] A lot of our work here is guided by the testing and the information we get through our testing, and that's not always available at a lot of other settings. We're trained a lot in mood and the emotional connections with food, which is, I think, really important. There are, for many people, emotional barriers to making changes, and that's always kind of first and foremost to get a sense of if that's there and helping people around that. Food is a very powerful thing, because we eat and drink for a lot of reasons. A lot of those reasons are good. We're emotionally connected to our food because otherwise we wouldn't be interested in eating.

[00:06:30] It's trying to find that balance of getting enjoyment out of your food, but not using it in ways that might have some negative impacts, around coping mechanisms and things like that. I think the nutritionists here, we're really trained in trying to identify barriers, not only the emotional standpoint, but the practical standpoint, and then trying to work that into making their food plan work for them. I don't think that's always really addressed in most other settings. A lot of it is because it takes time. We build a good rapport with our patients. Many of our patients stay connected with us and speak with us on regular time periods, and I think that makes a big difference to have that ongoing support.

[00:07:00]

When I'm working with someone developing a nutrition plan, often I'll request that they have some labs done with their physician. A lot of that can give some good information on which nutrients are low. Do they need some B12? Are they low in zinc, iodine, things like that? That can really help me fine-tune and determine what their deficiencies are, and put a plan together that's going to replete those deficiencies. We have a lot of testing we can do to help better determine if certain foods they might be reacting to are causing some inflammation, and therefore, some of their symptoms. We often know a lot of the foods that you usually have to take out to see if you feel better, but testing for reactivity to foods can be helpful.

[00:07:30]

[00:08:00] We do a lot of DNA testing now, too. We're still in the infancy around nutritional genomics, but it's rapidly expanding, and we're slowly getting more information of which way of eating might be best for this person. Do they do well with maybe more fat in their diet, or vice versa, can they do more carbohydrates? Are there certain genes they have that compromise their ability to detoxify? Are there certain genes that are indicating more of a need for certain nutritional support, to support various pathways in their body? I think this is a really exciting time in this area of nutritional genomics, to get a better sense of how is this person an individual with their genetics, and how do we influence those genes to present in a way that's really healthful for them?

[00:08:30]

[00:09:00] That's a rapidly expanding new area we've been incorporating into how we work with people. I think a lot of the foods that can confuse people around the health benefits are ... it probably goes back to false advertising. The food industry I always consider like a double-edged sword. I mean there are a lot of food products out there that are good, and they help people follow a certain way of eating and can be supportive, but then there's a lot of junk out there. And the advertising and the false claims can be very misguiding, especially for someone not very well versed in nutrition. When things say low-calorie, low-fat, sugar-free, or gluten-free, it doesn't mean it's healthy, and it can be misguiding and very confusing.

[00:09:30]

[00:10:00] I think that's where people get steered wrong so often. What I always tell people, too, is the foundation of a good way of eating is to eat food in its most natural form. If you're eating a sweet potato, you're getting a sweet potato. You're not going to go too far off course. I always try to steer people back to some basic principles around eating to help clear up some of that confusion. I think when you're eating whole, natural, unprocessed food in its most natural form, then you're going to be doing the best you can for your way of eating, and it takes out a lot of the confusion.

[00:10:30] I do think there are a lot of foods that can be damaging to the brain. I mean you think of our whole body as connected, so anything that's really going to do damage in the body is going to negatively impact the brain. I would say top of the list, if you put it in a bigger term, is processed food. I'm a big proponent of good quality fats in the diet, but there are a lot of fats that are very poor quality, and we're slowly learning that. Over the last decade, a lot of that information has come out, but very processed vegetable oils and hydrogenated oils—a lot of people are familiar with this term, trans fats—we've realized they've done so much damage to cardiovascular health.

[00:11:00] I think there are a lot of foods that can be damaging to the brain, and anything that's going to have a negative impact on your body, as a whole, is going to have a negative impact on the brain. I would definitely say the quality of the fat in the diet makes a big difference, so there are a lot of fats out there that are highly processed, a lot of these vegetable oils that we've been cooking with and hydrogenated oils. Any time a fat or an oil is superheated, you know, deep frying, things like that, it creates a type of fat that's very inflammatory to the body and damages the cardiovascular system. We saw that with the increase in heart disease that came with hydrogenating a lot of these oils. Your cardiovascular system is completely connected to your brain.

[00:11:30] I think the other major area of food that can be really harmful for the brain is the processed food in general, but a lot of the processed grains, the sugars, the added sugars, especially sugars that have been altered from their natural state, the corn syrups, the high fructose corn syrup. A lot of information is now coming out on artificial sweeteners and how damaging that is to the brain. I think that's a really big category of foods that we want to be careful with, and it's for a lot of reasons. I mean you could be eating a more whole wheat bread or whole grain bread, but still, once it's in that bread form, it's been stripped of a lot of its nutrients.

[00:12:00]

[00:12:30] You're getting food that's missing some of its really important nutrients, its fiber. And you're also getting food that your body is going to convert a little bit quicker into sugar. That's what we're realizing, is that the more glucose, the more the rapid rise of glucose in your blood and therefore also insulin, it has very damaging effects on the brain. I think a lot of the processed food, along with the artificial things that are added, the colorings, it's a whole separate category, the preservatives are chemicals and they definitely impact brain and cognition. Between that and the poor-quality fats in, unfortunately, a lot of diets, I think those are probably your two biggest areas of foods that are going to do damage to the brain.

[00:13:00] I think there is a long list of foods that are going to be good for the brain. If you want to put it into more simple categories, I mean good quality fat, just like there's poor quality fat. Good quality fat I'd put at the top of the list. I mean our brains are mostly fat, so to get the nourishment for your brain and for development, it's really, really critical. There are certain fats that are essential. There's a lot more information out about it, but your omega-3 fats, your omega-6 fats, they're essential because we don't make them, so we have to eat them. DHA, docosahexaenoic acid, which is one of the major fats you get from fish, we now know is one of the major fats in the brain, and that's why it's so important for developing brains. In utero and through early development, it's critical to get that DHA.

[00:13:30]   A lot of these fats are key for building proper brain or neurological systems. I think fats do other things too. There are many different types of fat in the diet, and I was talking before about the importance of keeping glucose down in the blood. When you have some good quality fat in each meal, fat does a wonderful job of slowing down the absorption of the sugar from the carbohydrates you eat. One of the ways to dampen that glucose and insulin response, is to have some good quality fat in your diet.
[00:14:00]   There are many sources of that. I mean, there are many different types of fat, and, honestly, I think we should be getting a combination of those fats, as long as they're in a whole food form.

The vegetarian/vegetable sources are your raw nuts and seeds. I mean those oils are very good for you when they're in the nut and seed and protected. Those are essential fats. It's a lot of the omega-6s and omega-3s. There are avocados and olives, which are monounsaturated fats. Monounsaturated fats are
[00:14:30]   now known for their cardiovascular benefits. If you have a healthy cardiovascular system, you're going to have a good, healthy brain, or cognitive system. All these vegetarian or vegetable-based fats I think are really critical, and even animal fat. A lot of that speaks to the quality of the animals you're eating, but good quality clean fish for those omega-3s are critical.

[00:15:00]   Healthy, pasture-raised animals, I think there's a place in the diet for many people. If you're eating an animal that is eating its natural diet, let's take the example of a cow that's eating grass and herbs and all of that, the fat quality is very different and I would say even inflammatory, in that animal, versus if it's a factory corn-fed animal that now has a lot more omega-6, certain omega-6s that can be more pro-inflammatory. Good quality animal protein, I think some of that fat is good for most of us. I would put fat at the top of the list, good quality fats for brain health, and then good plant food. The more
[00:15:30]   color in your diet, the better, such as dark green vegetables. The darker the pigment in a plant, the more we get these phytochemicals.

A lot of us now are familiar with this term antioxidants. Oxidative stress is a very natural process. We're all dealing with oxidative stress, but unfortunately, in this day and age with more psychological stress that we're all under, the more pollution that's out in the environment, we're under a lot more of
[00:16:00]   this oxidative stress that's being created in our body, and you want to counteract that with these antioxidants. Whenever you see a colorful fruit, vegetable, spice, herb, you know you're going to get a lot of these phytochemicals that are providing antioxidants to counteract that, and that's critical for the brain because we now realize the brain is really impacted by this oxidative stress that occurs, so getting a whole lot of color, a lot of plant food.

[00:16:30]   A lot of us are hearing half your plate should be leafy greens and reds and oranges and getting a lot of color. And spices and herbs, I think it's easy to overlook those. Cumin, curries, ginger, and cilantro—all of those are really rich sources of nutrients and antioxidants that we need, so we want to be really heavy-handed with our herbs and spices.

[00:17:00]   Five tips to make cooking easier... I mean there's a lot out there. What I tend to tell pretty much everyone I meet with is keep it easy. I think that's actually a big misconception about, if you're going to eat healthy, you have to cook from scratch. It's going to take a lot of time, a lot of effort and skill. But if you get a good vegetable, a pretty fresh vegetable, local, and then a good piece of protein, I just think there's very little you have to do to them to make them taste good and also be good for you. Have a good olive oil on hand, spices, herbs that will keep for a while. I think you just want to keep it pretty simple.

[00:17:30]   I think if you want to cook and get into sauces and dressings and all of that, that's fine, but that's going to be a little bit more time-intensive. You don't need to do that. I think planning ahead is so critical,

[00:18:00] too, especially the more busy your schedule is and the more mouths you're feeding. You need to take a little time each week. It's a little extra time out of your week, but you'll find ... my patients realize, "Wow, when I really think a few days through and plan the night before for the next day, everything kind of falls into place." Then it's just the way you eat. It's not that you're on a diet. It just becomes your lifestyle. So, I think a little bit of planning on the weekend.

[00:18:30] A lot of my patients decide to do a little batch cooking and do a little prep earlier in the week so that it carries them through the week. There are certain dishes, anything that's a little more liquid, water-based will freeze really well, so you can make a pot of stew, or chili, or soup, and freeze some of that. That can really kind of help people through the week or further down the line. So those, the planning ahead, the keeping things really simple, I think is important. I think it's important, too, to eat as a family. If there are multiple people in your family, everyone's got a little bit different nutritional needs. A lot of families I work with make separate meals for different people, and I don't think that's sustainable, nor is it really a good way to train especially younger people.

[00:19:00] Again, I mentioned my mother before. I mean, she cooked for nine people from scratch every day, and there were no extra meals made. What was provided was provided, and I learned to really enjoy and like and not be afraid of trying new things. I think within that, there's a balance. Everyone is a little bit different, so if there's some protein everyone can enjoy, everybody should be having a little bit of a vegetable, and then maybe there's a side dish that a younger person or someone who is growing and maybe needs a little bit more carbohydrate and more calories. You want to do that. I think preparing one meal is important.

[00:19:30] What I tell everyone I work with is part of that planning ahead is to make a little bit more the night before so that you either have a meal the next day, a breakfast, a lunch, something like that. You put the effort into making one meal, and it becomes two or three or more. It's also a money-saver, too, so I think that's important for most people.

[00:20:00] I think there are two main misconceptions about healthy eating, and I hear it all the time. It's a talk I have with pretty much everyone I meet. One, that it's time consuming. I always tell people I work full time. I'm pretty much a single parent. There's not a lot of time out there, but if you keep it simple and plan ahead, then it doesn't have to take much time. Also, that it's expensive. I think you want to do some additional planning and be mindful and keep an eye out for things that are cheaper. But if you plan properly, if you're eating mostly whole food, if you're turning one dish into several meals, it

[00:20:30] actually can be very cost effective. I know fast food is very cheap, but it does add up.

If you are cooking up a lot of legumes or a little bit of a whole grain and vegetables, you can make that last for a long time. It might look like an initial investment in the beginning, but when you break it down per meal, it becomes really inexpensive. I think that's why people think they can't eat healthy without breaking the bank, but I think most people can. Those are the two biggest misconceptions,

[00:21:00] and once people get a little more comfortable preparing food and plan ahead, finding what works for them, they realize it isn't difficult.

If you're trying to make a healthy way of eating work on a budget, it's just planning ahead, and there's going to be a little bit of prep and things like that involved. I encourage a lot of my patients to buy some frozen produce, frozen vegetables, because you can get organic and really good quality often

[00:21:30] very cheap. There's very little food waste around that because the frozen produce keeps for a very long time, so you don't have to worry about things spoiling. Doing that, you can buy things in bulk, whether it be produce or certain dry goods, whole grains and legumes, and some jarred goods that last for a long time. Keep an eye out. If you can, purchase a little bit more of that.

[00:22:00] Again, a lot of that can be made into soups and dishes that make several meals. That is a good way to make your dollar last longer. I encourage people not to drink ... don't spend money on drinks, even water. I think water should be pretty much the only thing most people are drinking. We do get fluids in our food too, but it amazes me how much money people spend on fluids, including water. You can get a little cheap filtering system if you're not comfortable with the water in your house and plan ahead and take that with you. That can save a lot of money, and obviously not buying fruit juices and things like that. That really adds up.

[00:22:30]

[00:23:00]

Again, batch cooking. Planning ahead and having food ready I think is helpful. If you make a dish and can freeze some of that, that's like having money in the bank and really can stretch the dollar. I do encourage people to buy good quality animal protein, and often you're going to spend a little bit more there, but a lot of it is about portion control. A little bit of animal protein goes a long way. Eggs are a good example. I tell people, get the best quality eggs because they're about 33 cents an egg. That's a really good nutrient-dense food for 33 cents. Even buying good quality eggs, that adds up to a lot of nutrition at a low cost. I think there are a lot of things people can do on even a really low budget to eat healthy.

[00:23:30]

If people don't like to cook, I think there are still ways around it. I often talk about assembling a meal. A lot of this, too, comes down to the time factor. I'll cut corners and buy things that are washed, chopped, ready to go, because that's where a lot of time goes. That sometimes will cost a little bit more money, but if someone can afford to do that, I think that's fine because a nice mix of greens, and if you can do a little good quality canned Alaskan salmon or you can even buy things that are already precooked, like a rotisserie chicken, and throw that on with just a little olive oil. I talk a lot about assembling meals for people that aren't comfortable cooking and putting a dish together.

[00:24:00]

Go to a good quality supermarket, and get meat that's already prepared. I think that's fine if it's good quality animal protein you're using. That's one way around it. There are some people that will spend a little more money and get some home delivery meals, and there are some of those out there that are good quality, so you can have that for backups. Every once in a while, people will bring in a cook to help them prepare a few meals over the week.

[00:24:30]

Even someone that's limited in their skills or doesn't enjoy cooking or has a very time-intensive schedule, I think there are still ways to put a meal together that's pretty easy. A lot of things can go in a blender and make a smoothie or a soup that way, too, without spending much time in the kitchen. It's just getting a few skills in place, getting people comfortable with handling their food, which I think is important for a lot of reasons. There doesn't have to be a lot of cooking involved.

[00:25:00]

[00:25:30]

For parents that have a child—I don't like to say picky—who is a limited eater. It's challenging. I think all children go through phases. Until I was a parent, I didn't really understand the whole dynamic that's involved, and again, how much of a role food plays for people, even in asserting their independence. I always encourage parents, and this is how I think a lot of us were raised way back when, but what's provided is provided. The parents decide what's going to be eaten and when it's going to be provided, and then you leave it up to the children to decide whether they're going to eat it. It's a little bit uncomfortable because none of us want our children to go hungry, but very few children will do that.

[00:26:00]

There are some cases where that can happen, but it's not very common, and I think people and parents, we need to know that it can take multiple tries to see a food. I really don't like the concept of sneaking food, either, into dishes because even if that child never tries cauliflower, it's been on the plate. It's been on the table. It does become part of their repertoire of what they have been exposed to and what they grew up with. I think it's important to model good behavior, to have those foods out there, and then leave it up to the children to decide what to eat. You can always play it safe and have a dish or a food there that you know they'll like, but not, again, make a whole other meal.

[00:26:30]

Learning to eat is such a life skill that I think a lot of our parents, unfortunately, either didn't learn it or they're just worried about whether their child is going to eat enough that they don't allow them to navigate and learn it on their own. I think it's really important to expose children to new foods, and let them try things, or not try things, and just get comfortable that it takes a little time for them to adapt to new foods or new ways of eating. A lot of it is good role modeling, and, "This is what we have," and then just not putting pressure on them to necessarily eat that food.

[00:27:00]   Most children come around to eventually eating some of them and getting more comfortable and then, I think, grow into adults that have better eating skills and cooking skills and all of that, too. It's challenging. I think for children who may be on the spectrum or have some cognitive issues, that's obviously another layer that can be challenging around food. Try to just choose your battles. Have the good stuff out there. Encourage them to eat the good food. This is where I think if it helps parents

[00:27:30]   follow a certain dietary plan, maybe that child needs to be off of wheat or something like that, if there is a good quality cracker out there that doesn't have the wheat in it, then I think some of that is fine, too.

A lot of what I do is help families to try to choose their battles and find what works best for them, and just keep exposing them to good quality food. For a child who is on the spectrum or dealing with some type of developmental delay, I think it's challenging, like everything else. Everyone is an individual, so

[00:28:00]   what that child might be dealing with might be very different from another child. I do think, from a nutritional standpoint, there are some concepts and guidelines that work for a lot of these children. We know sugar, processed food, artificial colors and flavorings, all of that, really needs to be removed. We've seen children, time and time again, really do better when you take the processed food, sugar, and coloring out.

[00:28:30]   I think that's a foundational piece that's really going to do good for all these children. We do find a lot of children have sensitivities to gluten as well as the casein and dairy, so that's a big part of our nutritional plans, and I've seen a lot of children really improve when you take those out. Taking out, say, the gluten, and sometimes you are removing, again, processed food that they weren't getting their nourishment and everything that they needed. Again, there's often a behavioral thing around food with a lot of the children on the spectrum, so it can become more difficult.

[00:29:00]   A lot of our families choose to make dietary changes together, so other siblings might become involved in the family, because it's really a supportive impact to that child, and they don't feel as isolated making some of these dietary changes. Again, it can be challenging with school activities and parties and all of that, but this is where there are a lot of products out there that we work with our patients to find some things that work for them, that they can put together to have them stay pretty

[00:29:30]   much low sugar and off of certain foods that might be bothering them. I really try to focus, too, on what to eat. For these children, it's critical. A lot of them need support with their detoxification system.

Getting in vegetables in any way we can, and into smoothies and juices, you know, green juices, things like that, can be really, really supportive for their detoxification system, and good quality fats. Pretty much all of our children get on a good quality fish oil. Very few of them are eating fish. We find their

[00:30:00]   omega-3 fatty acids to be very low. We were talking before about the developing brain. These children's brains are developing, and they need those building blocks. Getting a good quality fish oil and some of the oils that you get from some of the seeds and things are really important, too. That I would put at the top of the list as something to focus on, what to give your child who might be dealing with some of the cognitive issues.

[00:30:30]   I've had a few cases that have stood out over the years of successes with children that were on the spectrum. I had one child who was diagnosed with autism, and within about eight weeks had lost his diagnosis. His, a lot of it was dietary. Again, everyone is an individual, so depending on what's working against that person, it can take longer to heal as you're determining what's going on for that person. For this child, the casein in the dairy was a big issue, as was the gluten. There were a few nutritional deficiencies that we were able to determine pretty quickly and replete.

[00:31:00] This child also had quite a bit of lead in his system. Once we determined the source and started giving him a few things to help bring down the level of the lead in his system, in eight weeks, he was in a specialty pre-K, and he got promoted to a normal kindergarten. That happened very quickly. It usually will take a little bit more time. In general, what we see is language maybe coming back, better eye

[00:31:30] contact happening, and a lot of that is with the dietary things. Many of the folks that we see here, are very proactive. They've taken out certain foods they suspect to be an issue.

Once we really focus on, "Okay, you took out maybe some of the things that are problematic. Let's focus on what to put in. Let's get in some of the good fat. Let's try to expand on the vegetables a little bit more. Let's get creative in ways of getting more of these foods into them," that's where I think real healing starts. They're starting to replete, and I think that's critical. We focus so much in food on what

[00:32:00] to take away, and I think we need to focus just as much as what to put in. That's what is often missing for a lot of the people that come in, including the children on the spectrum.

We see a lot of children who may not be as typical a kid as we think, but their quality of life and their ability to interact and all that really, really improves significantly, and that's a lot of what our families are looking for.

MARK FILIDEI, DO | Amen Clinics

Dr. Mark Filidei: Functional Medicine is really getting to the core of all the problems, "Why do you have a certain condition?" It's actually unfortunate we have to call it Functional Medicine. We should just call it good medicine, but we still have to call it functional because we had to distinguish what's not functional. If you're diagnosed with rheumatoid arthritis for instance, here's your diagnosis and we are going to treat

[00:00:30] you at that level or going treat you with anti-everything drugs, but the next question is what's causing that. That's the next level down. That's Functional Medicine. It's really the core of your problem. We should all be doing this, it's getting there, but it's taking some time.

[00:01:00] I was actually into this when I was 12, really kind of precocious, taking vitamins when I was really young. Metabolism, health, nutrition was always on my mind from a really young age. This is just the extrapolation of that into my practice. It's proven to be the only way to fly really—with medicine.

[00:01:30] My practice was really similar to Mark Hyman's. I did the same thing Mark did. We're really on parallel tracks treating and diagnosing people with the same methodologies for regular medical conditions: diabetes, heart disease, and cancer. I came to the Amen Clinic about six years ago and then applied those principles to the brain, and that's been absolutely fascinating. Of all fields in medicine, mental health really needs this. Applying Functional Medicine to mental health has been spectacular for the patients and for myself, to figure out that this is just a giant hole in psychiatry, not knowing this stuff.

[00:02:00] Environmental toxins are actually a really big problem. In one aspect with technology, we're living healthier longer lives, but in the process, we're poisoning ourselves for the long run. This is having environmental consequences right now. You've all heard of phthalates and plastics. It's in the food we eat and they are one of the hundreds and thousands of chemicals now all of us contain.

[00:02:30] If you hear Dr. Pizzorno lecture, he's a specialist in this field, you want to run and hide in a corner. We're really toxic and eliminating those toxins, reducing that toxic burden can be difficult, but we really need to be vigilant and not get exposed. How do you not do that in your everyday life? Don't ever cook anything plastic or heat anything plastic in a microwave. Hot foods are not good in plastic. Try to always

[00:03:00] eat organic, fresh food not processed. Those are simple things you can do.

[00:03:30] The big knock against organic food: "We all know it's no healthier for you than regular," when it absolutely is. Even on a vitamin level, but certainly on a toxin level. Of the top foods you really want to avoid, farmed fish is probably the worst, GMO soy and everything made thereof. It turns out that commercially-grown dark leafy greens are grown with lots of pesticides.

There are certain things you can do. The environmental working group puts out a great little bulletin, *The Dirty Dozen and the Clean Fifteen.* You can use that in your everyday life when you shop. Certain things aren't that bad commercial. Other things you always want to buy organic. Those are again simple things you can do on a daily basis.

[00:04:00] Besides the pesticides, herbicides, etc., another thing you can do is don't spray for bugs in your home and find out what the landlord or the landscaping company is using around your house for pesticides. Mercury is a known neurotoxin, endocrine toxin. Most people have heard of the Mad Hatter. He's actually a real thing. These are people, back in old England, that used to make hats. They turned animal fur into felt with mercury salts and they literally went mad. It was a tremulous anxiety-ridden madness.

[00:04:30] You get the same thing with low levels of mercury, not quite so bad. Mercury toxicity manifests as anxiety, sleep disturbance, insomnia, and is a neuroendocrine toxin. It poisons all your endocrine glands so you have low hormones. It's an immunosuppressant so you can get sick and get cancer. From

[00:05:00] where do you get it? Fish and fillings. If you have those silver fillings in your mouth, they aren't silver. Those are 50% mercury. It's really ridiculous they're still putting these in people's mouths.

[00:05:30] When we do some special testing, they even have different reference ranges on the test if you have fillings or not. The levels are higher with fillings. You want to avoid that. The fish you want to avoid the most are the big ones that live a long time, so tuna, swordfish, shark. Fish don't make mercury, they eat smaller fish that have mercury in them and they accumulate it. When you eat it, you get it. Fillings and fish are two main sources, but then that's just one toxic metal. We have lead.

[00:06:00] A lot of this actually comes, believe it or not, in the air from China along with mercury. This gets into the vapor in the jet stream and drops over here. It's estimated that 20% of the pollution here in the LA basin is actually from China. Same thing with the northwest. It's a global problem, not just local.

[00:06:30] Arsenic is also a known toxin. People get poisoned with arsenic on purpose or accidentally. It's in the groundwater, in a lot of places. You're not likely to get lead or mercury in your water, but arsenic definitely can be there, especially if you're drinking well water, so you may want to check. We do a hair analysis test very frequently. It's a pretty good indicator of your metal burden. It's a good, quick, cheap, and easy way to start looking for metals. Arsenic shows up in hair pretty well. Sometimes on these TV shows, they'll dig up a body and see if they were poisoned with arsenic. They do hair sample testing.

[00:07:00] I was really awakened to the importance and widespread nature of Lyme disease, actually, when I came to the Amen Clinic. Looking back, I'm sure I missed dozens, if not hundreds, of cases before. I just wasn't aware. One of the first cases I saw here was a kid who was here for drug rehab and had started at 14 because he didn't feel good. He wasn't thinking straight, brain fog, some pain, some fatigue, couldn't do well in school and started using drugs just to feel better. One thing leads to another, you meet the wrong people. He ended up losing his entire high school time and college time to drugs.

[00:07:30] His mother is actually the one that figured out it was Lyme. Someone pointed her to a website that showed all the symptoms. He had everything on the list. She said, "Oh my God he's got Lyme." In fact, that's the case. He was out hunting a lot, got bitten, no one thought about it and no one checked until it was almost too late. That really opened my eyes to the whole issue. Since then, I've diagnosed hundreds, if not thousands, of people with Lyme from all across the country.

[00:08:00]
[00:08:30] We have six clinics. I see people from everywhere and Lyme is in every state. In California, it's not on the radar of any doctor, but it's here. More on the east coast, but it's absolutely here in California. Stanford did a study of 12 Bay Area parks in San Francisco and found that 6% of the ticks there had Lyme disease. Of that percentage, one was called miyamotoi, which doesn't show up in any Lyme tests. The most common type in California doesn't show up on a test.

[00:09:00] Lyme is called the great imitator for a reason. It can imitate virtually any psychiatric illness you can imagine, from attention deficit to depression to anxiety and insomnia. It can have profound effects on the brain. The spirochetes, which are the type of twisty bacteria they are, love neural tissue like your brain. You can have what's called neuroborreliosis, which is Lyme in the brain. We see this quite often especially in our patients from Lyme endemic areas. So, they may come in for depression or ADD and it turns out it's been Lyme disease the whole time.

[00:09:30]
[00:10:00] How do you treat it? It's variable. There's no one way to treat it. There are natural approaches that are largely herbal. There are antibiotic approaches and everything in between. Generally speaking, when you have chronic Lyme for years or decades even, the natural approach is usually preferable. If you catch Lyme right away, you take antibiotics, but that needs to be within weeks of your infection and then you can eradicate it. Years and decades later, it's a whole different animal literally. It's in three different forms. You have to use multiple antibiotics to treat it for a long time. You can get better absolutely.

[00:10:30] How do you diagnose Lyme? There's no great way. There is no great for-sure test. Largely, it's going to be a clinical diagnosis. Does it look and sound like Lyme historically? The testing is very problematic. Again, there's no great test. They all have their pros and cons. It's easy to miss chronic Lyme and there's also something called post-Lyme treatment failure syndrome, which maybe you had Lyme and you're treated and now you're still sick. Some people don't even believe that exists—the Lyme can't still be there.

[00:11:00] A lot of us Lyme-literate docs think it certainly can still be there. The treatment is always patient-based individual. It's really clinical and you can't rely on testing. We always do testing because if you find a smoking gun on a test, you're pretty assured you have something. Let me give you an example. You have a patient that's diagnosed with Lyme. They're very sick. There's a possibility this can be sexually transmitted. It's been documented, although it's kept under wraps.

[00:11:30] The first question is, "Should I have my husband or my wife tested?" We do. If they're positive, but they're totally asymptomatic, do we treat? No, I don't. You have no idea when to stop treating. In other words, you can have a positive Lyme test and not have any symptoms. It just shows that again it's a clinical diagnosis. If you're symptomatic and the picture fits, that's when you treat.

[00:12:00] How do you really get over it and why are some people sick and others not? Genetics play a big role. Your detoxification status and genetics play a role. If you're generally healthy, you might get the same infection someone else does and you're perfectly fine and yet the other person with some kind of issue is symptomatic. Lifestyle plays a huge role. Your general health plays a role. Genetics play a role. Toxins play a role. If you're exposed to mold in your house and you get Lyme disease, you're not going to get better until your mold is cleared.

[00:12:30] If you have a lot of heavy metal burden—mercury—you're still not going to get better because that's an immune suppressant. You have to get all your ducks lined up to treat all these chronic illnesses and that's what Functional Medicine is—looking at all those ducks and lining them up. What I tell all my patients is your body has to win this battle. The drugs aren't going to do it. Herbs aren't going to do it. Your body has to do it. How's it going to do it? It can't be suppressed with toxins, mercury, etc. You

[00:13:00] have to eat a good healthy diet. You have to sleep well. Iit's all the stuff our momma told us to do to be healthy. You really need that to get over any of these chronic illnesses.

[00:13:30] Mold is probably more of an issue than Lyme in this country. It's estimated about 50% of the buildings in this country are water-damaged buildings. It doesn't take much water to damage a building and cause mold. Mold and mycotoxins are all over the place and in certain individuals they can be very problematic. As with Lyme or any chronic illness, if you're susceptible and you have an exposure, you may get sick and stay sick for years even if you're out of the environment where the mold was for

[00:14:00] instance. Mycotoxins are similar to Lyme in that they're immunosuppressive. They can cause almost any psychiatric illness you can imagine. Stereotypically, mold cause brain fog, memory loss, attention deficit, anxiety, insomnia. Mycotoxins can do all of that and you can be exposed at work, at school, in your office, or at home.

[00:14:30] I'm actually going to be presenting on mycotoxins here in the near future. I just saw a patient that came to me with two complaints. One was getting sick all the time, multiple recurrent infections and brain fog, can't think straight. This is a fairly new onset. She's in her mid-40s, generally healthy, started shortly after moving into a new home that was a rental. I ask my patients very unique questions. What I

[00:15:00] ask everyone is, have you ever lived in a home that's had a water leak in it, a leaky roof or a leaky bathroom, or something where there's water? Yeah. Whenever I take a shower, water comes out the bottom of the stairs. I said that's not normal, there's probably a mold problem here.

[00:15:30] There was nothing obvious in the bathroom. However, there was a little discoloration on the wall and when the wall was opened up, complete black mold. When it was tested, it was the worst kind called stachybotrys—off-scale high. They couldn't even measure it. It was so high. She tested positive for mycotoxins in her body as well as other blood tests. With treatment, her brain fog is gone and mycotoxins are immunosuppressive. It could explain why she was getting infections all the time including the need for IV antibiotics for sacroiliac infections.

[00:16:00]   That was a case and there's many like that that people aren't thinking it's mold. You don't see it. This is not the stuff in the shower. This is the stuff that is behind the wall, in the attic, under the crawlspace and doesn't take a whole lot to get it started. Another case is one of our psychiatric patients in another clinic, at the Amen Clinic in New York, was referred to me for workup because their scan didn't look good.

[00:16:30]   This is a young guy, 30 years old, that had acute behavioral change, anxiety, insomnia, wasn't like himself. I spoke to him to rewind the story, which is always very important. When did things happen? Things changed when he moved back home from college. I said, "What happened? Was there any stress in the family?" "No, everything is great. No problems." "Where are you staying?" "I'm down in
[00:17:00]   the basement." "Okay. Were there ever any water leaks in the basement?" His mother was on the phone as well and she says, "Oh my God there was a water leak. It flooded two years ago. It floods almost every winter." I said, "Have you ever checked it for mold?" "Yeah there's mold growing behind the washing machine down there."

[00:17:30]   So once again, no one is thinking about this. The psychiatrist they saw before coming to our clinic was not thinking about this at all. It's an automatic knee-jerk-reaction—here is your problem. Here's your drug. Again, he tested positive for mycotoxins, treated, his anxiety got better. It was a really bad problem. They had to actually dig up the entire basement and surrounding part of the house. It was so covered with mold. In fact, I had many people on that block later call me for appointments because it was not just that house. It was the whole row that was having this problem.

[00:18:00]   Mold testing: don't do the home kits from Home Depot. Those aren't going to work. You need to get a good kit. You can get online kits that work well. It's called ERMI (Environmental Relative Moldiness Index). Those are government-approved tests really do work. You can check your house relatively cheaply to see if there's a problem. CIRS (Chronic Inflammatory Response Syndrome) is coined by Dr. Ritchie Shoemaker who's one of the mold gurus, certainly a pioneer in mycotoxin and mold toxin
[00:18:30]   problems. It's an immune-mediated inflammatory response to mold toxins but other things as well. Lyme can cause CIRS as well.

[00:19:00]   The main focus at least with Dr. Shoemaker's work is mold. It turns out if you have a certain genetic susceptibility, an HLA market (Human Leukocyte Antigen), you may be very susceptible to mold. What happens is your body doesn't recognize the antigen well and you can't get rid of it. You stay sick even if you were exposed years ago. It's an entire inflammatory response process that's rather intricate, but very helpful. That's usually based on lab work. He worked at a rather ingenious method for detecting this with blood tests.

[00:19:30]   There's this treatment protocol associated with specific steps. It's quite common to have this inflammatory response syndrome with multiple exposures including Lyme and mold. With mold, you really had to get a good picture of where it came from. This can be in the workplace, at home, or in a school. Schools have been shut down because of mold problems. This could be one contributing factor
[00:20:00]   to this rampant ADD we see nowadays. If you're toxic with mold, you're not going to think very well.

How do you know if you have CIRS? You don't, but that's why you have to have a high index of suspicion. As a practitioner, I always do. Most doctors are not thinking like that. That's why it's really important to go to a Functional Medicine physician because that's what we do. You have to be Sherlock Holmes and figure out what's going on.

[00:20:30]   The symptoms of mold exposure that are obvious are usually respiratory, so allergic-type responses. If your house is really bad, you're probably going to have some kind of respiratory response. Runny nose,

---

Expert Interviews – Mark Filidei, DO

[00:21:00] postnasal drip, cough, watery eyes, so kind of an allergy response. Especially, if it's only when in your house and you leave and you're better. That's a real big tip off. You may certainly be a candidate for investigating CIRS at that point.

[00:21:30] What's really critical and almost every case is when did things change and this is for CIRS and everything else. When and why did they change? That can be critical in determining what's really happening. If you were okay and then you moved into a new place when everything bad started, again big tipoff. You'd investigate that. Also of note, landlords are notorious for hiding mold problems. They don't want to find mold. It's very expensive to remediate and there are legal costs. Don't trust what people say.

[00:22:00] I had a case where a patient was obviously ill from mold. All the markers were positive. She responded to treatment. I said, "Have you had a problem in your apartment?" "Well the floors are warped from a water leak." "Okay, there's a problem." She had the landlord come and investigate and they hired someone to not find mold and they didn't find mold. She hired her own investigator who took her under the house and said, "Look up." and it was just barnacles of mold hanging off. It was obviously contaminated. Again, we have to have a high index of suspicion in any environment you're in, at work or at home.

[00:22:30] With complaints of brain fog and depression, I really treat it like anything that I see at the Amen Clinic. We do a lot of mental health-related stuff here. That's sort of our gig. It's really the same thing: what happened, when and why. Certain people are just born a certain way. You may have ADHD from the get go. That's different than at 10 you developed ADD, depression, or brain fog.

[00:23:00] For me, the number one question is, when did things change? If someone has brain fog, the first thing I'm going to ask is, "When did it start? When did you notice it?" "Well, it was 10 years ago." "Okay. Let's rewind the story and find out why." That's always critical to testing. I'm trying to figure out clues as to where to look. With Functional Medicine, we have many places we can look, lots of rocks we can
[00:23:30] turn over. We have to know which ones to turn over first and the history can really help you do that.

I'm an internal medicine physician. I do a lot of hormone therapy and Functional Medicine incorporates a lot of hormone treatments. I work with a lot of psychiatrists here at the clinic. I have a little running joke with them that we could probably eliminate 50% of all psych meds if people had their hormones balanced. That's maybe a bit of a stretch but there's some truth to that because hormones have a
[00:24:00] profound impact on your mental and physical health. Women going through menopause sometimes can't think straight. They can't sleep. Do you give them Prozac or do you give them progesterone?

I'd argue progesterone is the better choice, at least to start. Maybe, you have depression because your testosterone is gone. You can't sleep because your progesterone is gone. You have fatigue and memory loss because your thyroid is low. These aren't really addressed in almost any situation when you go to a
[00:24:30] mental health practitioner. They sometimes will look at thyroid but that's kind of it. Testosterone is profoundly important for mood, memory, motivation, libido; it's the mojo hormone. It's just really important.

[00:25:00] I've had very young men, 19 and 20, with low testosterone that have depression and low motivation. The question is always, why is it low if you're 20? It should be raging. It's environmental or infectious, so I've had multiple cases where low testosterone was due to Lyme disease or some kind of toxicity. You treat that and guess what? Their depression goes away, their memory gets better, their anxiety goes down. You wouldn't think about things like testosterone for anxiety but in fact if you have more
[00:25:30] mojo, you can handle anxiety situations better. With low testosterone, the key is age and it drops as you get older.

Men over 40, everyone over 40, their hormones drop. In those situations, you may need a replacement if something is not there anymore. Generally, under 40, you want to figure out why they're so low and

[00:26:00] try to treat that as naturally as possible. That can be done with exercise, diet and things like that, to a certain extent, but in some cases, you just need a little boost and there we use gonadotropin therapy. This is actually a prescription medication but it's increasing your own levels instead of taking testosterone mostly in men. In women, they have a fairly easy option. Sometimes just taking DHEA, orally over the counter, can increase their testosterone.

[00:26:30] There are many ways to look at and improve it. Really, it's kind of age based. What turns out to be the case in almost any illness you could imagine, physical or mental, is always going to be diet and lifestyle. You could take as many pills as you want but if you're not eating right, it isn't going to work in the long run. Diet and lifestyle are absolutely critical. That means exercise—physical and mental exercise. Cornerstone therapy. Everything else is secondary really. After that, then you want to be more vigilant about what you're eating as far as pesticides and toxins.

[00:27:00] Environmental awareness is very important. You could live a super healthy lifestyle and if you live next to a superfund site, you could be in trouble. You really have to be aware of what's going on at work and at home. Again, diet is absolutely cornerstone for almost every illness that I see.

[00:27:30] My diet recommendations are very basic and very similar no matter who I'm talking to. It's really about a low glycemic diet and organic as much as possible. There are two main food groups we want to reduce and that's fruit and grains. Some people freak out when you say low fruit, but fruit is all sugar technically. Avocado is technically a fruit that's all fat or good—there are exceptions like that. If you think about a fruit, it's all sugar. You really want to minimize that, but berries are awesome. There's a

[00:28:00] general consensus that purple foods are really good for your brain. That would be berries particularly.

Then low glycemic, so always low sugar index and fats are good. Fats are very important. These low-fat diets are disastrous for your brain so you really need good healthy fats. They've been given such a bad

[00:28:30] name. People still say, "I'm supposed to eat fats?" Yes, very important. Eggs are okay, too. I mean, unless you're going to be a fruitarian and just live on berries, it's hard to take too many. A handful of berries in a smoothie, you're fine. The limitations are when you eat good foods you're almost going to self-limit because they're filling. They're satiating, especially fats and you really want to try to get fats with every meal because of that satiety. If you get the right stuff, your body is not hungry.

[00:29:00] If you find yourself hungry after your meal, you probably didn't have a good meal. Now, we do use xylitol if someone has to have sweetness for some reason. Xylitol is a pretty good substitute. It's a natural sugar. It's actually medicinal and treats biofilms, which is a big problem with infectious

[00:29:30] etiologies like Lyme. It's used in nasal sprays to get rid of infections in your nose. It's used in gum not to get cavities. If you have to have something sweet, xylitol is an option.

Dr. Martha Herbert:

[00:00:30]

We label things with diagnostic labels, at least in the general medical community, not so much in the Functional Medicine world. Early on, in seeing patients with autism, I did that in a context of a neuropsychiatric clinical job. What I began to notice is that there are behaviors that are characteristic of autism, but that when I take a medical history of autism, or I take a medical history of obsessive-compulsive disorder of a patient with one of those things, there are many common features that I find in asking questions having to do with problems in general health.

[00:01:00]

[00:01:30]

The first thing I realized, and this was 20 years ago, was gut problems. Amazing how many people across these conditions had those problems. It wasn't diagnostic specific. What I've come to realize with autism is first of all, there are clusters of behavioral configurations. But underneath it all—just like 1/10th of an iceberg is above the water, and the rest of it is under the water—the parts that are below what we see behaviorally are a lot less distinctive one condition from another than the behavioral features. If you look at the kind of stresses that lead to these problems, they're pretty similar too.

[00:02:00]

As I came more and more to think of autism as a whole-body condition that arises from environmental, nutritional, and stress-related conditions, I realized that that's what's going on with everything else too so that it's better for us to look at it in the context of an epidemic of chronic illness more generally. Even in autism, there are so many medical conditions. It's not like they have these separate diagnoses. Here's the autism. Here's the epilepsy. Here's the irritable bowel syndrome. Here's the rashes. These are all emanations of some kind of underlying set of imbalances. That's true across the board.

[00:02:30]

[00:03:00]

Let's look at the underlying imbalances and where they come from and what we can do about it. When people talk about the brain in academia, on television, you get a picture of neurons in space. They're firing signals at each other. They're just suspended in space. Actually, in the brain the neurons are outnumbered by glial cells from four to one to ten to one in different parts of the brain. Glial cells do so much of the metabolic work that keeps the brain alive. Then there are fluids and flows and all kinds of things. The brain is a living, wet organ.

[00:03:30]

[00:04:00]

The brain emerged through evolution to help animals move around and organize themselves in space and to navigate gravity. What we're doing on the planet right now is we are messing with the fundamental parameters that govern the viability of life. We're messing with tissues. We're messing with the acidity of the ocean. We're messing with the carbon dioxide in the air. We're looking at coral reefs being gone within 25 years. Coral reefs are like, as a prominent microbiologist explained to me, a coral reef is like the biofilm of the gut. It's like the gut turned inside out. If we're looking at an ocean that won't support coral reefs within 25 years, how are we going to support the conditions that keep our fundamental interfaces with the world properly balanced? In our brains, we have a whole ecosystem of material things that keep the electrophysiological the way the brain generates brain waves, able to do that. We're messing with all those parameters.

[00:04:30]

I think we need to get this, the way we think about the brain grounded in the body. And the way we think about the body grounded in the world, in order to keep ourselves functioning well enough to think straight enough, to deal with what's generating our chronic illnesses and what's generating our ecological catastrophe that we're increasingly moving into.

[00:05:00]

There are a lot of overlaps between chronic diseases. There's a recent unpublished paper on *Research Gate* looking at the top diseases. If you look at the top diseases that have doubled, or more than doubled in the last generation, they all have in common certain fundamental metabolic optimalities like in nitric oxide. Peroxynitrite: it's a nasty thing to have. It messes you up.

[00:05:30]

I published a paper with my postdoc, Dr. Yau Wen. We took all of the genes that were available at the time, 667 genes related to autism and put them through some computer software to find pathways that they were in that were enriched with a lot of autism genes. Then we looked at things that were associated with these pathways. We had big overlaps with cell signaling, with cancer, with metabolic disease. Neurological actually wasn't as big of a deal as some of the other conditions. From that, we recently published a paper showing genetic overlap, specifically between autism and cancer.

[00:06:00]

[00:06:30]

Cancer is a mess-up of core metabolic and energy production mechanisms in our cells. You see these kinds of mess-ups across many chronic diseases. These mess-ups particularly manifest themselves in the brain in a subset of the many chronic diseases that are on the rise. I look at the problem as chronic disease. Then, the way it plays out in a particular person is based on their genetic weak spots or fault lines and whatever they've been exposed to.

[00:07:00]

[00:07:30]

There are number of things, which are common across many kinds of brain conditions, whether they be genetic, degenerative, traumatic, or psychiatric. You have neural inflammation. Neural inflammation is a stuckness in the brain's attempt to resolve stresses that it gets stuck in generating inflammation and continues to perpetuate it. It's hard for the brain to pull out of that. You see that in everything from Huntington's disease, to concussion, to autism, to schizophrenia, to depression, to other psychiatric conditions, to Alzheimer's, to Parkinson's. You also have energy problems. You have problems with mitochondria, the parts of our cells that make energy.

[00:08:00]

[00:08:30]

The brain uses 20% of the energy supply even though it only weighs three pounds, which is a lot less than 20% of the body's weight. The reason it does that, is it takes so much energy to fire synapses and connections. If you're having problems with your mitochondria, which is so easy to have, because of environmental insults as well as for genetic reasons, and most mitochondrial dysfunction is from environmental insults. There are tens of thousands of things, which can compromise mitochondria. If you have mitochondrial problems, the way that you generate brain waves is going to start getting imbalanced and disorganized. It may fall into different patterns depending on a lot of other things, but you have to go to the underlying generators in order to really solve the problem.

[00:09:00]

I see autism as what can be called an emergent property. Underneath the behaviors, and autism is defined purely behaviorally ... Underneath that, there are things that are going awry. What you see on the surface like the bubbles on top of the waves in the ocean are the behaviors. They are not things. They're the way the brain acts when it has certain kinds of stressors.

[00:09:30]

[00:10:00]

There are so many different underlying genes just in the ones which are associated with syndromes in autism, that are like well over 100 different genes and the mechanisms don't overlap. What I think of as the behaviors that emerge in autism or in other psychiatric conditions, are common pathways in the way the brain acts that you can get through many different genetic, molecular, and systems challenges. It feeds out through the brain waves and certain channels that create behaviors that a psychologist can classify. The way you get there is in many to a few relationships. Many different kinds of causal things to many fewer kinds of behaviors. That's why we can label it, but it doesn't help us to understand how it was caused or what we can do about reducing the severity or even if people can recover from some of these conditions. If you understand it this way, you understand that we can go in many places and help a little bit here, a little bit there, a little bit somewhere else. And that adds to something where the brain system gets some relief, and can organize itself with a fuller set of flexible options.

[00:10:30]

[00:11:00]

In our world of treating the underlying physiological, nutritional, toxicological infectious imbalances, we often see people do a lot better mentally, intelligently, emotionally. We can't necessarily explain that because we haven't fully integrated measurements and understanding of the brain into

[00:11:30]	Functional Medicine. I've run a research program called Transcend for over 10 years. That means Treatment Research and Neuroscience Evaluation of Neurodevelopmental Disorders. We thought a lot about how the measures that we can make ... I can measure glutathione or mitochondrial metabolites in the brain using magnetic resonance equipment. I can measure brain waves and how
[00:12:00]	their power, their energy and the way they are coherent and synchronized with each other change. These are different kinds of measures. Most researchers just look at one or another. We tried to put several of them together so we can say, "How is the physical part of the brain setting the stage for different kinds of activities? Then, how do the body biomarkers fit with that?"
[00:12:30]	What we've been doing in this world and Functional Medicine is looking at a lot of the body biomarkers, but not really integrating with the brain very well, so then when we say we're affecting ... Unless we can say that environmental metabolism causes autism or causes depression or other or anxiety, it doesn't really explain how that happens. It still doesn't change that, for the most part, we need to come at it by supporting the body. There are also top-down ways of supporting and helping the brain to reorganize and upgrade its organization. When you put that together, you're going to have a much more potent way of proceeding.
[00:13:00] [00:13:30] [00:14:00] [00:14:30]	Looking at autism for 20 years and seeing how much struggle there is with basic health, and then realizing that the basic health struggles we see in the body are also going on in the brain in ways that we can't see and that it's hard to measure. The brain has very exquisite chemical parameters for making certain signals. There are fluids all over the brain. If you have a nerve cell here sending neurotransmitters to the next cell over, those transmitters have to make it through the fluid. The acidity of that fluid or the alkalinity, the thickness, the stickiness, all these things are variables, not constants. The whole terrain of the brain influences the way the signals are going to be generated. How big of a network would it be possible to organize when you're trying to engage in activity. All of those parameters are up for grabs in terms of how much we upgrade the way ... These parameters operate in the whole body. In the brain, you have this amazing cellular, electromagnetic, energetic gel in which all the stuff is going on. It has a whole other level of importance.
[00:15:00] [00:15:30]	You can't just study neurons. You can't just study brain activity, the brain waves, or the parts of the brain that light up, which are a consequence of where those activities are going on. You can't just look at that. You have to look at everything that feeds them. We know that the electrical activity, and the places that it goes on, are different in neuropsychiatric conditions than they are in neurotypical people. We also know that there are problems with the energy, nutrition, metabolites, biochemistry, methylation cycles, and all kinds of things. All of biochemistry metabolism changes the way the brain waves operate. It's that universe, where things will start changing their shape and generate patterns and behavior, that we label.
[00:16:00] [00:16:30]	I recently gave a talk and indulged myself in collecting graphs of environmental factors that are going up with the same exponential curve as autism. Everybody comes to me and says, "Wow, look at this. It's going up the same way as autism. That must be the cause of autism." Well, there are dozens of things in the environment going up like this. There are dozens of conditions that are going up like this. Every time I take a medical history from someone, I find that there's a long history of clinical problems before a diagnosis emerges. We know that there are gut metabolism problems being discovered in people years before they get diagnosed with Parkinson's and other degenerative diseases. You need to look at all the things that contributed along the way and fixate on any one of them.
[00:17:00] [00:17:30]	It's comforting, psychologically to think that there's one thing but if we look at all of the things that we've changed from ancestral ways of doing things, not that ancestral ways were all right, but many of them were more grounded. We weren't processing food and taking nutrients out. We weren't putting chemical fertilizers and chemical pesticides, all of these things which are different, the list goes on and on and on. People didn't get oral antibiotics until the last few generations, knocking off their microbiome. There are a vast number of things, which are shifting very basic things in our body.

I think they all add up.

[00:18:00] By the way, I found the one graph by accident. I've been looking for these graphs. I found a graph that has patents and trademarks going up starting around the early 80s, right when the autism thing went up. What I think we've had is a vast economic deregulation, and the production of more and more things for the sake of keeping the economy going that have no necessary value, all the nanoparticles, all of these things, which if you actually think about, are really more about making money than anything else. I think that's the total load. I'm not saying that patents cause autism. I'm saying that it's all the stuff and that the whole economy is too big to fail. We just keep letting it do this.

[00:18:30]
[00:19:00]
[00:19:30] There are people who say that autism is not a disorder, it's a cultural variant. That has a lot of truth to it. I see people getting better from autism as opposed to having an identity that is autism. I don't see them losing things. I see them gaining options. It's an empirical question whether people who "recover" from autism or let's shall we say, "lose the diagnosis," are giving up some of their strengths. There are remarkable perceptual capacities in people with autism that exceed what neurotypical people can do. If they were to take the path of trying to heal their bodies, would they lose that? I don't know. I do know some people who have gone on that path and feel they're better off for having supported their nutrition. I feel really sad when I get reports from parents of people with autism, that they are viciously attacked on the Internet for depriving their child of the right to have an autism identity, by taking care of their nutrition and things like that.

[00:20:00] I like to see the work we do in helping people be healthier as a path to opening more options. When we have lack of nutrition or too many toxins, our system has a very hard time adapting. It has to do a whole lot of workarounds to get through the day. It's less stress on the system to not have those problems, to have a metabolism that doesn't work right. When you get into this evolution question ...

[00:20:30]
[00:21:00] I also think we're in real danger. One of the things I've been looking at is the decline of IQ. The IQ is going down. We are not nutritionally supporting our DNA-repair mechanisms. We're having many sources of many mutagens in the environment, many toxins, electromagnetic fields, and the nutrients we need to support our DNA repair are in short supply. Less vitamin D, less minerals like molybdenum and selenium that we need and less essential fatty acids. We are challenging our DNA and we're not supporting it. All these things are probably part of the rise in chronic disease that's in parallel with the ecological crisis.

[00:21:30] I'm concerned about devolution. I'm not really seeing advances in evolution right now. I'm really worried more about losses of evolutionary advances. We've lost so much biodiversity it's frightening. It just keeps going on.

[00:22:00]
[00:22:30] I see that food and supplements are complementary. I don't think you can get everything you need from supplements. I don't think you can get everything you need from diet. It's really hard to source optimally-grown or raised food, but I don't think there's any substitute for trying to do that. At the same time, between the soil having been depleted in so many places for so long, between organic being a label for not putting bad stuff in but not necessarily doing all the good things to raise it back, it's not a strong enough label for what we need. When you're environmentally stressed you often need far larger quantities of key nutrients to keep certain pathways going, both because of environmental stress and because of genetic weak points we are walking around with.

[00:23:00] I always insist with patients that we have to upgrade your diet as much as you can, and have as many nutrient-rich foods as you can. Then there are certain things we just can't get enough of. Vitamin C you can't get enough of in your diet. Certain minerals based on what we need, we need more than we're getting in our diet. Regionally, there are differences in soil. You don't know what soil it was grown in. The chemical fertilizers hardly replete minerals at all. We're all walking around

---

Expert Interviews – Martha Herbert, MD, PhD

with all kinds of mineral depletion. Magnesium, sulfur; very critical things that are not in good supply in our food, so it takes both, plus changing our agriculture and changing the way we're raising these foods. That's huge.

[00:23:30]

I grew up in the lower east side. Everything was ethnic. You could get every organ. You could get any kind of fish. You go to Whole Foods, you don't get organs. Every now and then they have chicken livers. It's really hard to get organ meats. You have to know where to go. Chicken feet are contraband. They're really good for broth. I think the industrial food production takes all these things and puts them into dog food or whatever they put them into. We don't get them. It's really hard to

[00:24:00]

navigate. People have to spend a lot of energy.

Also, another problem with food, is the same problem when people find that their child is sick or that they're sick. I never forget this privileged, middle-class family that came in some years ago. I diagnosed their child with autism. They said to me, "How could this be? We did everything we were

[00:24:30]

supposed to." There's this process of learning that what you were told you were supposed to do is really not about you; it was about marketing. You've got the process of reshaping your judgment to be your judgment again is a big journey for people. I wrote an op-ed 17 years ago in the Chicago Tribune about GMO. I said, "This is not an experiment. With experiments you have controls. This is

[00:25:00]

just messing around." In a real experiment, somebody plans it, they track it. None of that's going on. They're just doing it to make money. You promote low-fat milk and meanwhile you're selling the cream products over here, so you make up a story that the low-fat milk is good for you. They just make stuff up.

[00:25:30]

The behaviors that we call autism emerge from physiological dysfunction. The next question is, "Is autism something that develops through a cascade of physiological deteriorations, of health deteriorations in infancy that may even start before that?" I got funded by the Department of

[00:26:00]

Defense Autism Research Program. They actually fund research. They have a requirement for community participation and research evaluation that was set up separately from the NIH. I was funded to do a study of infants where we started sampling the mothers before the babies were born while they were pregnant. We got the placenta, the cord, cord blood, and kept measuring the mother while they were nursing, and took all kinds of things from babies two weeks, eight weeks,

[00:26:30]

four months, to 30 months when you could reliably diagnose autism.

We got brain waves, urine, stool, some blood spots, a whole bunch of neuro-functional tests. It's a huge amount of data; I could spend the rest of my life analyzing it. I'm working on getting the

[00:27:00]

resources to do that. We were hardly funded. It was a labor of love. We took EEGs. We have EEGs starting at two weeks. EEGs measure brain waves. Brain waves are measured in 1000th of a second. That's the time interval in which synapses occur. Now we are able to see a correlation between certain patterns in the brain waves at two weeks and the severity of outcome all the way out at 30

[00:27:30]

months. It's a very high statistical correlation. It maps with key behavioral areas that we see at 30 months.

[00:28:00]

It's looking to me like—and we're getting ready to submit this to publication now—the brain is irritable very, very early on. Perhaps because of stressors or exposures during pregnancy, or toxic body burden, or infection in the mother as well as whatever genetics. In most cases, people don't have the big autism genes. Then, you are more close to the edge of the cliff.

[00:28:30]

I also have data showing that if a family realizes, after their first child with autism, that they have to really change their act and improve lifestyle and nutrition, diet, reduce toxic exposure, the next child born is much less likely to have autism. When I say that we are seeing a high correlation between a

[00:29:00]

kind of irritability in the brain at two weeks, and how severe or not autism is at 30 months, I'm also saying that's not a closed deal but that choices that can be made, that are basically lifestyle, public health, common sense things. Once you get it, every choice needs to be a healthy choice. Once you

[00:29:30]

get that and you start doing high nutrient density, whole unprocessed, un-chemical food, you can radically lower the risk that this irritability will mature into a diagnosis. There may always be vulnerability and you may always have to be careful but, to avoid falling off a cliff, I feel something can be done.

[00:30:00]   I interviewed Anat Baniel while I was writing my book *The Autism Revolution: Whole Body Strategies for Making Life All It Can Be*. About 10 minutes into the interview, I realized that she was doing something of huge importance, that was very similar philosophically to work I had done years ago about the evolution and development of learning processes. She understood learning in terms of

[00:30:30]   when we're babies, the first way we learn is by moving our body and experiencing cause-and-effect in movement. The way we learn from movement provides a conceptual basis for further mental development. When a baby has brain damage, or brain inflammation, they either won't be able to

[00:31:00]   make certain moves or they'll make them but they won't assimilate the inflammation because the brain is too busy being inflamed to be absorbing and processing information.

What she figured out, was that when you go to teach the body, through giving it many of the learning processes in the body again, that it didn't complete it or it didn't work out. It's very flexible.

[00:31:30]   It's not a drill approach. You see a lot of upgrades in cognition. One of the things that's really interesting is that she's observed when she works with children who have a lot of gut problems and they're picky eaters, even if sometimes... Many of these children also doing diet and nutrition, but sometimes they're not. Even when they're not, they seem to get more settled and organized, and a

[00:32:00]   lot of the gut problems go way down without diet or nutrition. She still would recommend that they do that, but you implement these things when people are ready to implement them.

What we came up with was, that's a top-down approach where you are organizing the system so that the more organized it is, the less stressful it is to get through the day. Having a child with ADHD

[00:32:30]   who is all over the place, begining to feel who they are and where they are in space and allow them to focus and be there, they come down so much. A lot of the gut stuff goes away, probably through stress reduction and confidence. At the same time, it really helps to work from bottom-up. Really, working both ways ... There are things that are coming more and more into play now, supporting the

[00:33:00]   brain through light therapy, through LED light, through transcranial laser, which supports mitochondrial energy production. That's a top-down approach, also more physiologically oriented. These things can work together. All put together, you can upgrade the brain and the whole life.

[00:33:30]   The neural movement is the approach of helping the body have a more rich and complex map of itself in space. There are two ways of doing it for someone who could follow instructions. You can have a room full of people and they either sit in the chair or lie on a floor, and go through a series of movements that give you a sense of the full capacities of your biomechanical form in relation to gravity. Then your brain has more to compute with. Otherwise, you have these blank areas or

[00:34:00]   relatively blank areas. That's the neuro-movement. You can do this through instruction, or somebody can lie on a table and you can use your hands as a practitioner. With a baby, they're not going to follow instruction or with someone with a stroke they can't, so you have to move them.

[00:34:30]   I actually studied with her for five years, and I'm a certified practitioner now. I gave a talk at one of her conferences, actually her first conference, which wasn't a teaching conference. My talk was how neuro-movement helped me transcend and redeem my pediatric neurology training. It's so amazing for me. Pediatric neurology is a discipline where you're dealing with people who have brain challenges, often missing big pieces of their brains, strokes, malformations, the cells didn't grow right. What I'm watching with the neuro-movement is, children with these severe brain damage

[00:35:00]   situations coming out so much better than they ever would. We had a person in our training just now, who just finished recently, who had a stroke. She's a gorgeous 28-year-old. She was a model. She was a cheerleader for the Indiana Colts. She had a stroke. She came in after her discharge from rehab still unable to talk, spastic, drooling. Now she's walking around, she's a practitioner. She's a certified practitioner. It's amazing.

[00:35:30]

I feel like my job is to help systematize that. It gives so much ... I mean, I felt like as a pediatric neurologist, I'm looking at these things, I'm labeling them and referring them out to therapy. If there's this much more that can be done, it should become a standard of care. It's a very systems-oriented thing, the way that Functional Medicine is. It's based on fundamental properties of what I call "neuro-biomechanics." It's not just the mechanics of the body, but the way the brain is informed by that.

[00:36:00]

[00:36:30]

I'm the scientific director of the Documenting Hope Project and the principal investigator of the research arm. We see in the community people recovering from chronic disease. We see people getting over juvenile rheumatoid arthritis or idiopathic arthritis, asthma, depression, obesity, autism, ADHD. Kids get better. If this is possible, why are the methods by which people get their kids better not standards of care? Why do people have to run all over the place, putting it together? Why after 10 or 15 years of people recovering their kids, has there been no progressive documentation of how it's done?

[00:37:00]

We're taking 18 months for each kid, everybody's going to get the same testing so that we have clear benchmarks to compare. We're going to rigorously document what each person has at the diagnostic level. Then each person will get an individualized course of treatment. Everybody will get the diet upgrade, the environmental remediation in the home and so forth. The individual additional steps will be based on each person's results.

[00:37:30]

The things we do to get people better from these childhood chronic diseases are the same things that we need to do to regenerate a viable ecosystem. People need to know there are things we can do and when we help our health, we're basically voting with our feet to help our planet. We want to inspire people to go for the best they possibly can in themselves and their families. That's why we're doing the Documenting Hope Project.

[00:38:00]

[00:38:30]

Ever since I started hearing about people recovering, I thought, "This is extraordinary. We have to understand what are we transforming so somebody who's running around nonverbal can turn it to someone who's talking and functioning." I have a friend who has kids graduating college who were in special-ed. This was never supposed to happen according to what parents are told every day by professionals. We want the message to be, "Yes, yes you can." We can't promise a complete recovery, but there's so much you can upgrade. That's what we should be doing. We want to show it and document it scientifically and show the heart of it as well.

[00:39:00]

My colleagues and I started Transcend research in 2005-2006 to look at how treatments changed people, by looking at the different parts of the way we can measure the brain and body measures. We've done a lot of work. We've published papers. We haven't been able to really study the kinds of treatments that interest me the most, which are the whole body, health-promoting things.

[00:39:30]

[00:40:00]

I started an independent clinic called Higher Synthesis Health. Higher synthesis means to rise above and to integrate and that's what transcend means. This way I can have a place where people are actually undergoing multisystem improvement. I have there a research-grade EEG. I can do on-site EEGs. As we consolidate the Higher Synthesis Health project, we'll be able to add other kinds of brain investigations to show what changes over time. I really feel that this project needs to be grounded in real, complex treatment. In academia, you tend to pull out one treatment and do a clinical trial. I don't think people get better from one treatment at a time. They get better from a comprehensive strategy that evolves over time. Higher Synthesis Health is to embody a complex ongoing strategy for that person. The research measurement strategies are going on both in Transcend and in the Higher Synthesis Foundation, where we're working on collecting biomarkers for people to use in the community and data capture infrastructure.

[00:40:30]

Max Lugavere:

[00:00:30]

[00:01:00]

My background is as a TV presenter, producer, and journalist. I got my start in TV working for a network. My role in the to find a way to tell stories nobody else was telling in a way that was accessible and approachable to young people. The network was sort of like MTV meets CNN. My duties ranged from covering breaking news, to more heavy hitting journalism stories, to lighter topics that were peppered in. And ultimately, I was able to have free reign to cover stories that were important to me. Oftentimes my passions would steer me in the direction of health, and how technology is augmenting health, nutrition, things like that. I really got to cut my teeth journalistically with some of the top story tellers that were working in Hollywood when I had this gig. It also allowed me a really powerful calling card, because I was on TV, I had a verified check mark on Twitter. It allowed me to really access people that very few people get to do.

[00:01:30]

When I left that job with this background in journalism, I was exploring where I wanted to go with my career. I really wanted to go in a direction that was more honed and narrowed to the topics I was really passionate about, which have always been health and nutrition and things like that. Around that time, in my personal life, my mom started showing early signs of memory loss. I didn't have any prior family history of any kind of neurodegenerative disease. Dementia wasn't even in my vocabulary at that point. I didn't know what Parkinson's Disease was, I really didn't know what Alzheimer's disease was, other than this thing that old people get sometimes.

[00:02:00]

[00:02:30]

On the one hand, it was a traumatic experience. I went with my mom to some of the top neurology departments in the country, Johns Hopkins University, the Cleveland Clinic. And what I experienced there was what I've come to call diagnose and adios. Basically, you get these chemical band-aids prescribed, that when you do even a cursory dive into the research, you realize that the medications seldom work well and they have no disease modifying ability. What that means in English, is that all of the medications that are prescribed at this point to treat dementia have no effect on the progression of the disease. They don't slow it, they don't cure it, they basically just act like a chemical Band-Aid of sorts. And not a very good one at that.

[00:03:00]

[00:03:30]

That sort of compounded the trauma I was experiencing, coming to terms with the fact that my mom had some kind of neurodegenerative disease bubbling underneath the surface. And at that point, I was in between jobs. I had the time to really do a deep dive into the medical literature. I became obsessed with learning everything I possibly could about dementia, and specifically Alzheimer's disease. My mom wasn't diagnosed with Alzheimer's disease at the time, but I intuitively realized that Alzheimer's disease, being the most common form of dementia, might impart some insights that I might be able to use on one hand, and treat my mom with food and with lifestyle, exercise. Seeing if maybe improving her sleep might help. Reducing stress, things like that. Meditating. But then also, simultaneously, I became really obsessed, even more so probably with the notion of prevention, and trying to understand what I might do to prevent myself from ever developing dementia. Because, you know I'm a creative person and my intellect is my capital.

[00:04:00]

[00:04:30]

What I realized is that this is a very new area of research. Back when I first discovered this insight that changes begin in the brain decades before the first symptom, in my research I found that nobody was talking about it, despite the fact that the medical literature was filled with links and associations that were made between various risk factors and risk for neurodegenerative disease. I began putting all the pieces together and looking at research, both at the population level and more mechanistic research. Animal studies, randomized control trials, I put it all together. With research, you can't look at any one study in isolation. Research has to be viewed in the context of the larger body of work that exists. I realized if I really try to check all of the boxes, that I have a really strong chance in preventing this from ever happening to me. That was like a light bulb went off in my head. I became obsessed with the topic.

[00:05:00]   It helped me sort of diffuse the trauma that I experienced with my mom, and turn it into something really positive and proactive. I felt like I was really doing something to fight the disease at its core.

[00:05:30]   At a certain point, I realized that I have something that very few people have and that is access, media credentials. And I really wanted to use my skillset that I honed in Hollywood over six years as a storyteller to help spread this message of prevention. The way I conceived of doing that, at the time, was to create a documentary. I've never done a long-form documentary project, but it was an area that really interested me. I also realized that by doing a documentary, it would give me the excuse to reach

[00:06:00]   out to scientists all around the world. The top, top, top researchers in the field. Scientists tend to be very isolated. They tend to work behind closed doors and to be kind of camera shy. And what I found when talking about this topic, was that nobody was shy. Everybody wanted to be involved. I basically got "yes" from everybody.

[00:06:30]   I then did a Kickstarter campaign to raise initial funding for this project, and subsequently went around the world interviewing researchers and scientists and having conversations with them, becoming friends with them and then doing my own research and experimenting with my own biology. Getting my genes tested, changing my diet, going to get labs, tinkering with my diet, going to get new labs. It really became this passion of mine that I've been able to transition into a career. I have this documentary

[00:07:00]   coming out called *Bread Head*. It's the first ever documentary about preventing dementia aimed uniquely at a young adult audience, millennials. Changes begin in the brain decades before the first symptom.

[00:07:30]   And then in tandem with that, which I'm really excited about, I'm writing a book that's coming out very shortly called *Genius Foods*. If you consider *Bread Head* the prequel and my origin story, how a guy, who's not an MD or technically a scientist, was able to gather all this expertise on the topic, *Genius Foods* is everything I've learned. It's all of the hyper actionable, hyper accessible, approachable things that people can do to really optimize their cognitive function and make their brains work better, think more clearly, think faster. I really think it's a game changer so I'm super excited for that.

[00:08:00]   Scientists are not trained to interact with the public. We need scientists, we love scientists but they're very much focused on these really niche areas of research. And oftentimes, it causes them to, intentionally or not, lose sight of the forest for the trees. As somebody who had no prior training in medicine or science, it allowed me this ability to get a 30,000-foot view on the science, and connect dots

[00:08:30]   that I think is very rare for clinicians and scientists alike to connect. When I came at them with this idea that this is a topic I was going to make relevant to young people, they thought it was a project that really needed to see the light of day, and found it to be really important.

[00:09:00]   The other thing is that it takes, on average, 17 years for what's discovered in science to be put into day-today clinical practice. There's a huge lag between what we discover in research, and what your average primary care physician knows about and puts into practice in the clinical setting. I really wanted to be a catalyst because I felt like 17 years is not time we have to lose where our brain health is concerned. I

[00:09:30]   think my passion, personal story, dedication to responsibly communicating science, which is evident in all of the content I create, really made me a trustworthy character for these researchers to feel comfortable to open up and communicate their science. Also that their research wasn't going to get mangled.

[00:10:00]   I have one foot in science and one foot in media, and so I can speak for media and tell you that media—more often than not—mangles science. That was evident with the recent *USA Today* headline that went viral that was an interpretation of this American Heart Association statement that we should all avoid saturated fat. Media does a terrible job of covering science. There's no question about that. They want clicks more than they want anything, and that was very evident in the *USA Today* headline that said that

[00:10:30]   coconut oil isn't and has never been healthy.

[00:11:00] My passion is not to drive clicks to my website, it's to really get the truth out there. I think that researchers saw that and they're aware that media generally does a very poor job of communicating science. Poor at best, irresponsible at worst. My passion really is about communicating these ideas responsibly, more than anything else.

[00:11:30] So, a lot of people consider millennials the care givers on deck, and that is why millennials should be interested in this topic. I see millennials as patients on deck because I know, based on my research, that changes begin in the brain decades before the first symptoms of memory loss, 20-30 years by some estimates, and even longer by others. This is what will ultimately manifest as the clinical presentation of Alzheimer's disease and dementia, and is a lifelong cascade of events that build up in the brain. It's something that young people really should be conscious of their whole lives, the same way we want to do certain things so that we look better come summer time and we're at the beach in our bathing suits.

[00:12:00] Our brains really are who we are. Our brains make our minds the same way that our joints produce movement. There's no question that if there are steps we can take to make our brains work better, to make us think better, to make us be less depressed and less anxious ... I mean, the world is already an anxiety-producing place. We don't need to be made more anxious by our diets. This is something that is relevant to every single person, if that person has a brain. I have no doubt that roping in young people is going to be something my projects do. I've already been able to see that a lot of my followers are young people, which is surprising because I do talk quite a bit about dementia and aging.

[00:12:30]

[00:13:00] I was never an athlete but I became interested in weight training and physical performance because I really enjoyed going to the gym. I saw profound mental benefits from exercise from a very young age. It was just a bonus that it also made me look more athletic, even though I was always terrible at sports. Since I started going on this journey to really figure out the optimal diet for brain health, I've really lowered my consumption of carbohydrates, both in the form of overt sugar but also in the form of grains. I used to believe that the more grains we ate, the healthier we would be. I would avoid white rice like the plague but if you put a huge bowl of brown rice in front of me, I would eat every grain of rice in that bowl. I thought, more brown rice, more health. The same thing for bread. I would eat lots of whole wheat bread. I would eat copious amounts of bread if it were whole grain. But if it were white, I wouldn't touch it.

[00:13:30]

[00:14:00] In reality, the impact these foods have on your blood sugar is very similar. When I started doing the research into how sugar affects the brain, my consumption of these kinds of foods really dwindled, to the point where I rarely eat grains, if at all. I don't avoid them completely, but my consumption of them has dramatically lessened. What's interesting is that by adopting a brain-healthy diet, not only do I feel like my brain, memory, and energy levels are better than they've ever been, but so is my body composition. As a side bonus, I'm actually leaner and stronger than I've ever been. And that's not my focus. My focus is brain health.

[00:14:30] There are really interesting associations made between blood sugar and brain health. Depending on the marker of brain health we use, there have been associations made between even slight elevations of blood sugar, both fasting blood sugar and a marker called the A1c. The hemoglobin A1c, which is basically a three-month average of your blood sugar. And brain shrinkage. The higher your blood sugar, the smaller your brain. What hasn't really been known up until, I think recently, is the direction of causality. Do we have smaller brains and that causes us to reach out for more sugary foods? Do more sugary foods actually shrink our brains? There is a lot of research, a lot of science tying various dietary patterns that are higher in fat to better brain health. The Mediterranean diet, for one, is the dietary pattern that's inherently higher in fat. It's rich in extra virgin olive oil and fatty cuts of meat, fatty fish, things like that. And they tend to have a significantly reduced risk for developing Alzheimer's disease, dementia, and also cardiovascular disease.

[00:15:00]

[00:15:30]

[00:16:00] There have been randomized control trials, which is hard data, showing that when you consume more fat in the form of nuts or extra virgin olive oil, it actually leads to improved brain health outcomes in

---

[00:16:30] terms of cognitive function. Cognitive function is improved and things like that. Going back to what I was originally talking about, trying to figure out this direction of causality, there have been very large trials showing that by improving metabolic health, we can actually significantly delay cognitive decline. When we talk about improving metabolic health, this is a really complex topic. The best way you can improve your metabolic health is, without question, avoiding sugar and avoiding processed carbohydrates.

[00:17:00] It's not just sugar and carbs. We need to sleep better. All of us need to get better sleep—even a healthy person. If you have one night of poor sleep, the very next day you're essentially pre-diabetic. Your insulin sensitivity is handicapped and that's not something that persists. Sleep is incredibly important for making sure our hormones are working properly. Insulin, one of our body's chief metabolic hormones, which is sort of the gatekeeper to allow cells to process sugar, is highly affected by sleep. Stress is another one of those things that's really important for metabolic health. And exercise. A study was just

[00:17:30] published showing that young people today are as sedentary as 60-year-olds. Leisure time and physical activity is at an all-time low. Exercise is an incredible way of bolstering metabolic health, especially to build muscle, which is something I really focus on in my workouts.

[00:18:00] One of the big buzzwords in the wellness community are superfoods. And "superfoods" is not a very scientific term, but it's basically a term given to foods that are pretty healthy. What I've done with my work is, I've isolated foods that I call genius foods. These are the foods that really have a strong body of evidence to suggest that they're very good for cognitive function and brain health. Just to name a few of them, I consider eggs to be a genius food. For decades eggs were demonized. The yolks are rich in cholesterol, and for that reason we were told to avoid them because we were told that by eating cholesterol, the cholesterol in our blood would go up, which is actually completely inaccurate for the

[00:18:30] vast majority of people. I am a huge fan of eggs and I consider egg yolks to contain everything required for the development of a healthy brain.

[00:19:00] This makes sense when you consider that one of the first structures to develop in an embryo is the nervous system, which includes the brain. An egg yolk is literally designed by nature to have everything needed to grow a healthy brain. Eggs are definitely a genius food. I also consider dark chocolate a genius food. Chocolate that has above 85% cacao content is rich in a plant compound called polyphenols. Specifically in chocolate, these polyphenols in a form called flavanols. They are really beneficial to the brain and have been shown to improve the functioning of the hippocampus, which is the brain's memory center. It's a very vulnerable structure in the brain. It helps our brains process memories. And

[00:19:30] it's one of the first structures to be damaged in Alzheimer's disease. So, chocolate actually makes your hippocampus work better.

[00:20:00] Again, it has to be dark chocolate because the darker the chocolate, the less sugar. Even better, I like to snack on cacao nibs, which are basically pure cacao. Eggs, chocolate, and I mentioned extra virgin olive oil. Extra virgin olive oil is profoundly good for the brain. Again, it's rich in polyphenols that reduce inflammation. Extra virgin olive oil can reduce inflammation on par with low-dose ibuprofen, without any of the negative side effects. There is lots of research now connecting ibuprofen, which is a very common pain relieving drug, it's an anti-inflammatory drug. But it's not without its side effects. There's a lot of research now connecting ibuprofen use to cardiovascular events. Extra virgin olive oil actually

[00:20:30] makes your heart health better and it makes your brain function better, so definitely very healthy.

I think it's no secret at this point that fatty fish is very beneficial to the brain. Fatty fish like wild salmon - and sardines are rich in the building blocks the brain uses to create new brain cells. I try to eat a good portion of fatty fish two to three times per week at least.

[00:21:00] The question is, "Does the diet need to be high in fat to be good for the brain, or does the diet need to be low in carbs?" My perspective is that the diet really needs to be generally low in carbohydrates. By necessity, you're going to end up eating more fat, because when you reduce carbs you're going to end up eating more fat. The real benefit in that sort of diet is the reduction in circulating insulin. It's not that we need to eat more fat to produce more ketones, it's really that fat doesn't raise levels of insulin.

[00:21:30] Insulin interferes with a lot of the body's processes.

[00:22:00] That being said, when we do replace carbs with fat, there are some fats that are healthier than others. As I mentioned, we really want to consume more extra virgin olive oil. A lot of people now talk about coconut oil. Coconut oil is definitely good for you in moderation, but the evidence surrounding fats and oils really is in favor of extra virgin olive oil as the oil we should be using the majority of the time in our kitchens. I think coconut oil is great to cook with. It's a saturated fat so it's very heat stable at higher temperatures. It also has a kind of fat in it called medium-chain triglyceride. The medium-chain triglycerides in coconut oil, there's a lot of really exciting research surrounding them and how they might

[00:22:30] potentially benefit the brain by supplying an alternate fuel source to ailing brain cells.

In that capacity, I think coconut oil, and specifically MCT oil, could be very beneficial to the broken brain. Again, in terms of the weight of the evidence and the oil that I use mostly in my kitchen, it's really mostly extra virgin olive oil. I think that if you want to prevent dementia, you should cut out the added sugar

[00:23:00] and the sources of refined carbohydrates in your diet. That's step one. That's like the bottom of the broken brain food pyramid is cut out added sugar. No sugar sweetened beverages and that includes fruit juice. Definitely eliminate processed carbs from your diet. You basically want to avoid the aisles in the supermarket and avoid food-like products and stick to whole foods. Vegetables, dark leafy greens, meat,

[00:23:30] fish, eggs, nuts. Those are the foods that you want to concentrate on.

When it comes to grains, I think the vast majority of people consume too many of them. I would say definitely cut down or eliminate grains from your diet and see how you feel. Some people do better with more carbs than others. If you're insulin sensitive, which is the minority of the population, sadly in the

[00:24:00] United States, then you can reintegrate carbohydrates into your diet post workout, maybe once or twice a week. I think carbs are not evil, they're just over consumed. We misuse them today. I think in the post workout window, carbs from a sweet potato could actually be beneficial because they help your muscles store sugar, which could be used for the next workout.

[00:24:30] Unfortunately, 75% of the population in the United States is either diabetic or prediabetic. Therefore, for that population, that's essentially a carbohydrate-intolerant population. I think recommending grains is irresponsible. I think they should actually cut out grains, which are generally very energy dense and nutrient poor.

[00:25:00] When you go one step up on the broken brain food pyramid, I think eliminate grains if you're having metabolic problems, as most people are today. Eat more healthy fats. Add fat back to the diet. Don't be afraid of grass-fed butter. Don't be afraid of coconut oil, especially when we're talking about cooking with it; it's a very safe fat to cook with. Unlike the industrial seed-ingrained oils we've traded saturated fats in for, which are very unsafe as they're very prone to oxidation. Drop the soybean oil, vegetable oil, canola oil, and corn oil. Bring back grass-fed butter, coconut oil, and extra virgin olive oil. Consume

[00:25:30] copious amounts of extra virgin olive oil. We want lots of it. That's what the research shows really benefits our brain health. You can consume a liter of it a week and it seems to really improve cognitive function.

Obtaining an optimal brain is not just about diet either. It's about making sure you're sleeping well. I'm not just talking about getting more sleep. I'm talking about higher quality sleep. We really want to cut down our use of smartphones and technology at night. The blue light from those devices, whether we perceive blue light or not, tells our brains that it's daytime. Our brains are operating on operating

[00:26:00] system 1.0 and when we're looking at bright light, whether it's from our TV screens, smart phones, or laptops, that sends a signal to our brains that it's daytime. Our brains don't want to wind down when it's daytime. Our brains want to forage for food and procure a safer environment for our tribe. Making sure

[00:26:30] we're sleeping better, I think, is really important because many of the brain's custodial efforts occur while we're sleeping.

[00:27:00] Exercise is one of those things. The body of evidence right now is so strong that your average neurologist really should write exercise on a prescription pad before he writes anything else. Exercise is unlike any drug that's on the market. Exercise actually has a disease-modifying ability. It can slow the progression of many of these neurodegenerative diseases we're talking about. I like to incorporate movement into nearly everything I'm doing. In general, I like to keep my workouts either low and slow or hard and fast. None of this middle ground stuff, which doesn't really accomplish anything very well, in my opinion. I like to move more and do aerobic exercise throughout the day—whether it's taking the stairs instead of using the elevator, biking to work, or just walking around more. Just walking was shown

[00:27:30] recently in a randomized control trial to improve cognitive function and vascular risk factors in people with vascular dementia. Walking is truly medicine. And it's very simple. It's something that we can all do.

[00:28:00] At the other end of the spectrum, I'm obsessed with high intensity interval training—exercise that really pushes your body to the limits. That limit is going to be different for me than it is for you. Everybody has a different threshold of what constitutes high intensity. Whatever that means for you, you really want to make sure you're pushing your body to that threshold. When you work out at that level of intensity where you can really only sustain 20, 30, maybe 40 seconds of exercise, you're literally sending a text

[00:28:30] message to your genome to cause yourself to adapt and grow stronger. That's not something we get with lower intensity exercise. That adaptation, that stress response, occurs both in our muscles and in our brains. High intensity exercise is profoundly important.

Neuroplasticity is the ability of the brain to change throughout life. It was once believed that the human

[00:29:00] adult brain reached its peak level of performance at around age 25, only to begin a slow decline until death. If you were a person that developed dementia or had a learning disability, there's not a whole lot you could to do improve the way your brain worked. As of the early 90s, if I recall correctly, we now know that the human brain is able to grow new brain cells in the memory center of the brain throughout life. This is something that was previously considered impossible. We're able to make new connections,

[00:29:30] and "rewire the brain" under certain circumstances.

This is something I think is profoundly empowering that our brains are actually plastic. Neuroplasticity, really what that implies is that the brain, rather than being this sort of static thing carved out of stone

[00:30:00] that we inherited and couldn't do much to change, is actually more like plastic. It's malleable. And the way we can change the way it functions and manipulate it is through our diets and our lifestyles. Eating a brain healthy diet really promotes the neuroplasticity of your brain. Neuroplasticity tends to decline with age, but it's not necessarily inevitable. We can really have a positive impact on our brain health and our neuroplasticity at any age. The research really shows this now.

[00:30:30] Again, it's a profoundly important idea and I think at the end of the day, in real human terms, what that means is that we're no longer helpless. We no longer have to settle for the brain that we think we have. We can transform our brains at any age into our biological best. Whatever that means for you, whatever that means for me. It's different for everybody. But at least at this point we don't have to sit on our hands.

[00:31:00] If you're like me and you have a parent that has dementia, I think what I've learned is that you really have to be vigilant in your own self education. Learn what you can about the ways in which diet and lifestyle can modulate brain health, and do your best to lead your parent to a healthier lifestyle; a lifestyle that includes more exercise, better sleep, less stress. Maybe sign them up for a meditation

[00:31:30] course. Go through their kitchen with them. Tell them, explain to them why certain foods are bad for their brains and why others are really good for their brains.

At the end of the day—and this might seem counterintuitive—at a certain point you have to detach. Stressing yourself out over what your parent is doing can compromise your own brain health. Stress is the enemy of the hippocampus, which is the vulnerable memory processing center of the brain. To use a

[00:32:00] line that everybody knows, you can lead a horse to water but you can't make it drink. Ultimately, everybody is going to live the life they want to live, whether or not they have dementia. I think it's really important to do your best to get your parent on a track that promotes brain health, no matter what age. Also realize that if for whatever reason they don't listen to you, or they don't take as much of a proactive approach as you, you have to separate yourself.

[00:32:30]

What I've found is that it can be really stressful to the caregiver. Again, stress is very damaging and I'm all about that prevention. I think we have to do as much as we can to inform our loved ones, but then there's a certain level at which we have to detach. Know that we've done our best, we've given the information, we've been teachers to those that matter in our lives, but at the end of the day, people live

[00:33:00]

the way they want to live.

So, *Bread Head* is my documentary. It is basically the world's first ever millennial-focused film about preventing dementia. My goal in the film is not to pick out bread as the sole smoking gun when it comes to Alzheimer's disease, because that would be inaccurate. That's not my goal. My goal, though, is to

[00:33:30]

expose the relationship between hyper-processed foods and our risk for developing dementia and Alzheimer's disease. What I think might surprise some people is that I consider bread a processed food. It's humanity's oldest processed food, but it's a processed food nonetheless.

When you walk down the street, you don't see people eating stocks of wheat. They're eating sandwiches. Wheat has to be processed into the form of bread. Bread, your average slice of whole

[00:34:00]

wheat bread elevates your blood sugar quicker than table sugar. It's very energy dense in a time when we are less active than ever. It is rich in carbohydrates, which we know we need to be eating less of. It contains gluten, which presents a problem for many people because it happens to be everywhere. And eating more bread is just adding insult to injury. I consider bread to be a processed food. The film really looks at the role of sugar and the advice we've gotten over the years to consume 7 to 11 servings of

[00:34:30]

grains per day, and how that affects the health of our brains. I'm super excited to debut that.

It also goes deep into the notion of Alzheimer's disease as type 3 diabetes, as many researchers are now referring to it. This is no longer a niche idea. The medical literature is packed with references to

[00:35:00]

metabolic dysfunction in the brain as playing a role in the worsening and maybe even the development of Alzheimer's disease. This is a very compelling idea to me. The type 3 diabetes hypothesis is really compelling and when you look at the research now that's coming up by the day, showing the link between our diets and our lifestyles and our brain health, it seems to be a really strong hypothesis.

[00:35:30]

In trials where patients are put on plans that help improve their metabolic health, cognitive function also seems to improve. Whereas, Alzheimer's drug research, when drugs have reduced amyloid plaque in the brain, have turned up nothing but failures. It really strengthens this notion that amyloid is sort of

[00:36:00]

like a bystander in a more fundamental problem in the brain. The latest research really seems to show that the problem that begins more than any other problem in the Alzheimer's brain is metabolic despair. If that's true, I think eating a diet that preserves the metabolism of the body, and thus the brain, is really the way to go.

MONA KARIMPOUR, DO | Amen Clinics

Dr. Mona Karimpour: [00:00:30]	Since an undergrad, I was very interested in psychiatry, actually more in the brain. I did a lot of research on Parkinson's disease and then that got me interested in doing more research, so I did some research after medical school on schizophrenia. And then, throughout medical school, I actually did a rotation at the Amen Clinics and that's how I got interested more in Spect Scan Imaging and Functional Medicine pertaining to mental health and mental illness. When I finished residency, my first job was at the Amen Clinics and I've been here since 2011.
[00:01:00] [00:01:30]	At the Amen Clinics, our approach is a little bit different, because we look at everything holistically, and we have a lot of different providers. First of all, we do Spect Scan Imaging, so we look at blood flow to different areas of the brain, then we also have supplements we can offer and provide. We also have TMS here, we offer IV Ketamine, neurofeedback, and we have a PHE who does biofeedback, neurofeedback, and qEEGs. We are a very comprehensive clinic and I think that's what allows us also to be very holistic because we get that information from the other providers that are specialists in that field. We have our DOC meetings and so we are all constantly communicating and looking more towards cutting edge approaches so we can be comprehensive and better help our patients.
[00:02:00] [00:02:30]	Relationships and community—this is basically a big part of what mental health is. As a psychiatrist, we're looking at things from a biocycle, social, and spiritual approach. Biologically, we're looking at genetics. A majority of patients who have depression or anxiety in their family lineage, you'll see that the parents are probably struggling with the same thing, or people who have bipolar or schizophrenia. That's the biological perspective and that also integrates with the relationships and communities. As individuals, we're growing up in different bubbles in our communities and so being raised by a parent who is bipolar or is schizophrenic or depressed, you are then learning from modeling and the social interactions you have with them. And then, let's say for example, if they're depressed, if they're isolating themselves, you are growing up in an isolated community to some extent, minus the school system that you're in as a child. And so that can have an effect.
[00:03:00]	Also, in our current day society, we're dealing with a lot of social media and little kids now are playing video games instead of back in the day where they used to go out and play football and be interactive. Again, there's a lot more of that isolation and that whatever channel, whatever video game they're on, that's also affecting their relationships and their mental health.
[00:03:30] [00:04:00]	I mentioned social media, but social media can go both positive and negative. For example, if someone is a bipolar parent or concerned maybe their child will develop bipolar, they have that opportunity to actually seek out support groups online. They could look to see if there's maybe a local group, maybe there are educational resources out there. Luckily, going online isn't as expensive as it used to be. If someone is concerned, they can go online, read about new resources, get educated, and further seek help instead of ... You know sometimes people can actually suit themselves with, instead of proper medications, they try to suit themselves with substances and that could actually go down to a worse path.
[00:04:30] [00:05:00]	I'm not sure if social media is training our kids and adults to have ADHD per se, but I am aware ... I was watching CNN the other day and a lot of the apps they're creating, it creates an addictive type of drive, especially a lot of the video games. Even with the way we text and incentives they provide, the emojicons all of that—it creates this where we're getting used to the stimulation of the TV, of the iPad, of our iPhone, and it's a reward kind of rewarding system. It does create a lot of, depending on what apps kids are looking at, mental health issues such as, it can create anxiety, some addiction, ADHD, and things like that.

[00:05:30]

[00:06:00]

How do I prevent that from happening? I think it needs to happen from a young age. You need to limit your kids from playing video games, you need to be aware of what video games exactly they're playing and monitor them. I think monitoring is a huge effort of being aware of what your children are doing because that's what's going to create good habits or poor habits. Instead of having your child have an iPad in front of them for five hours so you don't have to worry about calming them down and get them hooked on to that game, could you limit it to something where it's more educational and have them be there for half an hour, learn something, and then bring them to the dinner table without the iPad and say, "Okay, let's have a family dinner, let's communicate where we have the emotional warmth instead of this cold iPad in front of us?"

[00:06:30]

I see adolescents 13 and up. With the use of social media, I've seen an increase in depression and anxiety more towards our adolescent and the young adults because the lifestyle changes you're dealing with, the developmental stages you're dealing with, you're dealing with high school which in general, high school there's a lot of peer to peer competition, there's been a lot more bullying. And with the use of Facebook, Instagram, social media, they're able to Snapchat a picture of someone they are bullying and it can just go viral. With that, I've seen a lot of, especially in that age group, even college, it goes pretty viral with the use of social media, misuse of social media, and it can cause a lot more depression and anxiety.

[00:07:00]

[00:07:30]

When we're talking about shameful feelings of inadequacy, low self-esteem, usually that goes down the path of people feeling depressed and then spiraling into anxiety. How to prevent it? A lot of that just has to do with again that biocycle social approach. What kind of community are they raised in? How are their parents monitoring them? What support systems do they have? Who are their friends? And going back again to social media, I mean, if they're looking at Instagram shots of someone who has made their shape or their face look like something it really isn't, then that person could feel a lot more inadequate. I think also with educating that you know whatever people put on Facebook, that isn't reality. I mean some people are just picking their happy days and putting it on there. And so, if someone's thinking, "Okay, how come my life isn't as great, and doing that comparison?" That's going to create even more feelings of inadequacy.

[00:08:00]

[00:08:30]

I think with educating, with making people more aware that what you're seeing on social media, what you're seeing or what little piece of insight someone might be providing you doesn't necessarily mean that's what is truthfully going on in their lives. I think that's where it's really important to help people and make them aware that people tend to share just what they want you to see. You know, you're not alone if you're feeling sad, there are a lot of people out there feeling sad. If you're feeling nervous and anxious, there are millions of people out there. I think that's the key point of educating and forming and letting people know they're really not alone.

[00:09:00]

[00:09:30]

With social anxiety, things they can do are: one is actually coming up with a powerful positive mantra, something that makes you happy you can resonate with. The other thing is practicing that, kind of like a meditation, maybe 10 minutes in the morning, 10 minutes in the evening, practicing that positive image you have. Doing it in front of the mirror for example if you're nervous about going out. Another practical thing is, it's what I call finding your happy place. Use your five senses to think about something that calms you down, soothes you, and makes you happy. Maybe you can see yourself sitting by the ocean, hearing the waves, smelling the salty water, the sun on you. Using your five senses and taking 10 minutes in the morning and just thinking about that, your happy place, 10 minutes in the evening, doing the same thing. Basically, the more and more you practice that, like a marathon runner, then when you do go into a social area where you're nervous, you can just kind of excuse yourself, go to the bathroom, get up, walk around and just think back to your happy place and soothe yourself.

[00:10:00]

The same practical tools for anxiety can help with depression, also. There are different modalities, you can go to Amazon and purchase. The *Feeling Good Handbook* uses the techniques of Cognitive Behavioral Therapy. You write down the negative thoughts you have, then the negative feelings

[00:10:30] associated with that negative thought, and then what negative behaviors do you do associate with that? It's kind of like in the old days when you say journal. Well, this is more of a structured approach and you would basically journal it down and then you would come up with, okay what's the opposite positive thought? What's the opposite positive feeling I have and what are the behaviors I do?

[00:11:00]

[00:11:30] When you actually put something like that down on paper and you look and see, "Okay, I'm looking at things from a negative standpoint when in reality if I look at it from a positive standpoint, I can actually start feeling better and doing more positive things. When I look at it from a negative standpoint, it's a negative self-fulfilling prophecy so I'm kind of shooting myself in the foot." And so that's a technique at home. If you need the workbook to do, you can just purchase it online and basically that would be another way that would help with depression. Also, a lot of support groups. There are a lot of different support groups for someone who is battling with cancer, and that's what has made them feel depressed. Finding a support group, a cancer support group maybe at your local hospital, something like that is also very useful.

[00:12:00] With traumatic brain injury, actually that's where we use Spect Scan Imaging. We've done a lot of research and with our retired NFL players, it's also very useful because with our other set of scans, it's a very helpful diagnostic tool. Also, we have at the Amen Clinics a protocol where we've done hyperbaric oxygen treatments, we've enhanced supplements, we've educated our patients about certain areas that have been affected that can overlap with certain areas that can cause depression. With optimizing everything, looking at blood work and then following them on our protocol, we actually can help sometimes either halt the worsening depression and/or dementia or kind of brain injury, or actually sometimes we've even been able to reverse it. That's one of the things we do at the Amen Clinics that is very useful and helpful.

[00:12:30]

[00:13:00] With a lot of sports, a lot of contact sports, there definitely needs to be lot more precautions, awareness, and education about not just with traumatic brain injuries but also what subsequent problems can occur from it. I have a lot of patients who will come in and say, "I'm a football player. This is my passion. I love it." Or skiing or surfing ... and the very first thing I'm going to say is, "Well, use safety precautions, wear a helmet." And I will educate them because if not, this is what can happen, you can have damaging consequences.

[00:13:30] So am I going to take away a thriving football player's passion or am I going to look at the entire risk and look at their benefits and educate them and tell them let's look at prevention? Prevention is to wear a helmet, try not to get tackled or slaughtered on the field, and then let's reassess if something does happen, let's reassess, and see how bad was your brain injury. Did you have a concussion? I also like to look at everything from a holistic standpoint. If someone is very happy and passionate about playing football, I'm not going to take it away and say no—you know—and get their parents and everyone onboard, don't play football because you enjoy it. You always have to look at things from a risk benefit ratio and then I think educate and inform your patients and then keep reassessing and going step-by-step based on their lifestyle and what makes them happy and also what are some things we can do to prevent traumatic brain injuries.

[00:14:00]

[00:14:30] Holistic doesn't just mean that I'm going to tell people, "Okay, you know what, do half an hour of cardio daily, take supplements, meditate and do yoga." In my book, I don't see that as holistic. Holistic, I look at people from every single angle. Are they in an abusive relationship? Are they taking care of themselves? And then of course, depending on the severity of their illness, do they need supplements or are they going to benefit from medications. When I speak of holistically, I'm looking at the person as a whole within their society, not just supplements being the holistic treatment versus medications. In

[00:15:00] more mild to moderate cases, I would be thinking, "Okay, let's look and see, especially if we look at what is going on psychologically and socially, can supplements help?" If not, if things are more moderate to severe, then, definitely, I would say, I don't think supplements are going to help right now. Let's start with medications and then go from there and see how you're doing.

[00:15:30]   For someone who is in pain right now, I definitely will recommend to reach out to a local support group and find someone who is a psychiatrist, psychologist, is educated in this field. You can call the Amen Clinics and reach out and set an appointment with someone who's educated and can help in the field of mental health.

Dr. Nancy O'Hara:	I started my career as a teacher and taught children with autism. I was a really lousy teacher, so I decided to take the easier road and go to medical school. And it really was the easier road, but I was a typical, traditional pediatrician and seeing a lot of kids on the autism spectrum, a lot of families. It was
[00:00:30]	one child in particular, a four-year-old, with severe allergies, asthma and autism who was only eating a white diet, that typical dairy, pasta, bread, and nothing else. I was trying for a year to get him off that diet because I thought it would affect his allergies and his asthma but his mom couldn't do it. They went away on vacation and he got a diarrheal illness. They called our office. The nurse at the office said, "Take him off dairy. It'll make his diarrhea better." She took him off dairy and he started talking for the first time, a four-year-old.
[00:01:00]	She called me and she said, "I'm working with him full time. I took time off from work." I said, "That's got to be it. Keep doing what you're doing." She kept doing what she was doing. She came back from vacation and he got over his diarrheal illness. She put him back on milk, he stopped talking. She called me. I said, "Well, it's got to be the transition, the flight. Keep doing what you're doing. It'll get better." Thank God, she didn't listen to me. She took him off milk again, he started talking. She put him back on, he stopped. Three or four times, she did this.
[00:01:30]	She found my mentor, Dr. Sidney Baker. She came to me and said, "You have to go meet this guy." I thought, "Well, this is crazy. Diet can't affect autism. It's ridiculous," but I was going through five years of infertility and I thought I'll go as a patient and that changed my life. I got pregnant and about 20 years ago, started an integrative consultative practice for kids with neurodevelopmental problems. That little boy is now in college.
[00:02:00]	Sid is an amazing soul and probably one of the most brilliant men I've ever met. When I went to see him as a patient, he found that I was very yeasty, had a lot of toxicities, silver fillings. I detoxified myself, changed my diet, went casein and gluten free and felt amazing. I said to him, "I'd like to do what you do." Every day off I had—one day a week—I would basically sit at his feet and work with him for two
[00:02:30]	years until he finally convinced me to try to do it on my own. I tried to do it within a general practice for a while but the week before I quit, they told me I wasn't giving enough vaccines and was spending too much time with patients. I thought I have to do something different. That's when I started the Center for Integrative Health and Sid and I still work together today and it's a great experience.
[00:03:00]	PANDAS is an acronym for Pediatric Autoimmune Neuropsychiatric Disorders Associated with Strep. That means that any child who has an acute onset of OCD, tics, anxiety—it's associated with a strep infection—may well have PANDAS and that treating them for that strep infection with the antibiotics
[00:03:30]	may help them get over their OCD and tics. This was first discovered and named in the 90s by Sue Swedo who's a director of the National Institute of Mental Health. It's been a very controversial diagnosis for many reasons. It's hard to identify. Sometimes, the association with strep isn't very clear. People don't want to think that an infection could cause anxiety, tics, or OCD.
[00:04:00]	In 2012, 30 physicians got together, tried to make it less controversial, and tried to rename it PANS, Pediatric Acute-onset Neuropsychiatric Syndrome, which included other infections like mycoplasma and viruses and other things that could lead to OCD and tics, like exposure to anesthesia or exposure to pesticides. In general, the only overriding factor is an acute-onset. You talk to parents. They'll say, "On
[00:04:30]	July 12th, my kid was fine. On July 13th, they started ticking like nobody's business." That's the history that tells us this could be part of the problem.

[00:05:00] When you find a child with PANDAS or PANS, you first have to make the diagnosis. It's a clinical diagnosis. There's no test you can do that makes you sure that this is PANS or PANDAS. The test results could be positive, meaning you could have high strep titers or they could be negative. It's really the history: when I see a child that has that kind of an acute-onset of those symptoms—anxiety, aggression, tics, OCD, behavioral regression, an 11-year-old that all of a sudden wants to play with a four-year old, those sort of things—then I will do a trial of antibiotics or an antimicrobial herb and see if they get better.

[00:05:30] If they get better within a week to two weeks from something that may have been going on for months, that's my diagnosis. I then may go on to do more testing or more support of their immune system, but it's really about looking first could this be part of the problem and then using an antibiotic or an antimicrobial herb to start treating it. They should first try to go to their pediatrician. If their pediatrician isn't knowledgeable about it, there are great parent associations. New England PANS, the PANDAS [00:06:00] Network, and there's also a Physician PANDAS Network, PPN. You can find physicians that are literate in this type of diagnosis you could go to.

Lyme disease, like PANS and PANDAS, is a clinical diagnosis. There's no test you can do that definitely proves you have Lyme. Lyme is a multisystem diagnosis too, meaning that it's not just about the germ, [00:06:30] the spirochete that you get from a deer or a field mouse or whatever that causes the disease. It's the way the body reacts; it's the metabolic changes, the immunologic changes, the nutrition deficiencies and that then affects the body and the brain because the brain is downstream of everything. With Lyme disease, you can get symptoms like rash or joint aches like we typically hear about but you can also get brain effects. You can get anxiety, depression, chronic fatigue, or autism. Lots of different diagnoses at [00:07:00] the core could be secondary to Lyme.

[00:07:30] There's one young woman who was very near and dear to my heart. She was a 13-year-old who was a tremendous athlete, straight-A student, doing wonderfully and all of a sudden, developed severe anxiety and OCD, and couldn't leave her home. She became more and more restrictive until she couldn't move from one small piece of her family room to even get to the bathroom. She became disheveled. She couldn't eat. She couldn't interact with anybody. She was scared of everything. She was admitted to the hospital. Doctors went to put her on multiple psychiatric medications. When we looked at her history, [00:08:00] she had been treated for Lyme twice, the year before and about six years before but only treated for a very short period of time.

[00:08:30] When we did our testing, her Lyme testing was markedly positive. When we started treating her for Lyme with antibiotics, immune support, metabolic support, her symptoms slowly but surely turned around, and now she's doing great. I would say that the lesson she taught me was that we can't just look at brain illnesses, mental illnesses, or psychiatric illnesses as the brain. We have to look at other things that may be going on in the system that could be affecting behavior.

[00:09:00] With autism, I think we look at it as a neurologic or a brain disorder. For me, autism is a brain disorder that happens downstream from several other medical problems. Kids with autism often have immune problems—gut problems, metabolic problems—and those are missed because we say this child has autism, but if we look at the underlying mineral deficiencies, dietary problems, or gut problems, we can actually help them to be not just more available for their therapy but possibly recover.

[00:09:30] There's a great saying: genetics load the gun but environment pulls the trigger. I'm sure you may have heard that before but autism is a genetic susceptibility but we have to look at all the environmental factors that may be affecting the child's development and act on those. I think all brain disorders, whether it be anxiety, depression, possibly even schizophrenia, are due also to immune disorders. In the [00:10:00] womb, the neurological system and the immune system are very closely linked. When we have an immune disorder, inflammation, an autoimmune disease, an immune dysregulation, we can also have neurological dysregulation. We see that with all kinds of brain disorders. If we treat the body, we can help the brain to get better.

[00:10:30] We have an integrative practice that tries to integrate all the therapists to treat autism. I started my career as a teacher, so I'm very invested in behavioral therapy and other therapies for kids with autism. We have to look at what's going on for them medically, so first and foremost: diet. The gut is not the second brain; I think it's the first brain. If we're not giving our kids a good, anti-inflammatory, whole foods, non-processed diet, we're not doing the right thing by them.

[00:11:00] Then, we look at what supplements, minerals, and vitamins they may be needing and we do that. Then, we look at other illnesses like Alzheimer's, Parkinson's, NMDA encephalitis, and see what we can learn from those diseases and what medications or supplements help those people that may also help our kids with autism. Then, we also look at homeopathy, intuitive therapy, and other therapies that may help them in general. One of those may be hyperbaric oxygen. We don't use it in every kid but in

[00:11:30] children with inflammation, Lyme disease, cerebral palsy, or traumatic brain injury and concussions, it may be an adjunct to the other therapies we use.

[00:12:00] Hyperbaric oxygen is where you give oxygen at a higher percentage. What we're breathing is 21% oxygen. Depending on the unit, you can give anywhere from concentrated oxygen—which is like 28 to 35%—to up to 100% oxygen. More importantly, you give it at an increased pressure. You help that oxygen get into the cells and decrease the inflammation, and also improve the mitochondrial function because that's something else that's affected in a lot of our kids. The mitochondria are the energy cells of all of our body. When our energy cells are not working, our energy is dysregulated. That doesn't mean we may be lethargic. We may have chronic fatigue but we may also be revved like we see in our kids

[00:12:30] with autism. It's sort of like that car idling where the engine revs without us pressing on the gas. That's what our kids with autism are like and HBOT can also help that.

[00:13:00] OCD is obsessive compulsive disorder. OCD can come from many different factors. One of them is PANDAS or PANS. If you have an infection with strep, mycoplasma, viruses, or even with Lyme, you can have a new onset, an acute onset of OCD. That's one thing we look at, to see if that could play a role. The other thing is many kids with OCD have very low serotonin levels and serotonin is what we all need to be calm and chill out. Melatonin is what we need for sleep sometimes, or to get over jet lag effects. Often, our kids have very low serotonin or dopamine levels. We need to give a supplement or

[00:13:30] sometimes a medication to help increase and regulate those serotonin and dopamine levels.

[00:14:00] Sometimes it's affected by diet. A lot of our diets are high in inflammation and high in glutamates. Glutamates are not just MSG (monosodium glutamates). Glutamates are in a lot of our foods, a lot of our cytotoxins. Decreasing that with supplements such as GABA or taurine may also be helpful in decreasing OCD. I think all of our children, no matter their diagnosis, should be on probiotics. All of us have depleted our ecosystems of the plethora of germs we need. We need a lot of probiotics. The best way to get it is in our diet—fermented cabbage, sauerkraut, kombuchas, and kefirs—but if we can't,

[00:14:30] then take a good probiotic supplement. That's not a probiotic in a yogurt, but it's really taking a good supplement that may be 10 billion, 50 billion, 150 billion units of probiotics.

[00:15:00] That's one of my favorites. My other favorite is essential fatty acids. They're essential and it's what we should all eat but in our American diets, we're very bereft of those. It's why the Mediterranean diet is considered to be a much healthier diet. These are good oils like olive oil, coconut oil, flaxseed oil, macadamia nut oil, but we don't get enough of that. The lighter the oil, the less the essential fatty acid. We may get it in fish like some of our fattier fish like mackerel, anchovies, salmon, but again, we don't eat enough of that. A good essential fatty acid supplement can be very helpful.

[00:15:30] There are some great studies out of Harvard and Oxford in England looking at essential fatty acids in treating mental illness and in treating ADD and ADHD. 80% of our children with autism are bereft of vitamin D. We're not getting enough sun exposure. We're living inside more without vitamin D exposure so they need vitamin D. Another one that's really important is folinic acid. Many children in the autism spectrum have a defect in folate regulation and so they can't folate from their foods, which you get from green leafy vegetables, by the way. Not many of our kids are eating that anyway, but folinic acid is very

[00:16:00]   helpful in, again, calming and regulating the hyperactivity that many of our kids have.

[00:16:30]   I'd say another one of my favorites is something called PharmaNac, which is N-acetylcysteine. It's a nice way of getting glutathione in. Glutathione is something all of us need. It's what we all use to detoxify our bodies. I think you'll hear more and more about it when you listen about heart disease or cancer, but what we know from research from Jill James and Dick Deth and others is that 71 to 72% of our kids with autism have a decrease in good glutathione.

[00:17:00]   Glutathione is meant to stick to the things we're supposed to get out of our body—the toxins, the chemicals, the metals—these sort of things. Our kids with autism have, instead, glutathione where the sticky parts are stuck together. If your sticky parts are stuck together, they can't effectively stick to and detoxify your system. I'm a big proponent of anything that can increase glutathione. That's broccoli, broccoli sprouts, sulforaphane, N-acetylcysteine, B12, the folinic acid I was mentioning, and anything that can help support our natural detoxification in this very toxic world.

[00:17:30]   The cell danger response is something we all have. Let's say you're exposed to a virus. What your body does is put out this response called the cell danger response. It's where our cells release cytokines and mitokines to fight inflammation and fight the virus. When the virus is treated and goes away, then the cell danger response retreats, but in kids with autism, their cell danger response never turns off. It's a persistent cell danger response.

[00:18:00]   I always use the analogy to an army. If you have an enemy army attacking you, you send out your sentries. Those are the cytokines, the mitokines, the inflammation response and your sentries are looking to try to fight off that enemy. But when that enemy goes away and retreats, your sentries go back and everybody in the army rests and re-nourishes themselves and all of that. If your cell danger response is always on and you're always putting out those cytokines, you're always in a state of
[00:18:30]   heightened alert in your body, always in a state of inflammation. What do you see when you're in a state of inflammation? Hyperactivity—that deer-in-the-headlights look that our children with autism have, that hypersensitivity.

[00:19:00]   What do you do when you're at war? You close down your borders. You close down your cell to cell communication. That persistent cell danger response also leads to a lack of communication, lack of social interaction. This research is coming from UC San Diego and a group of researchers led by Dr. Bob Naviaux who's another brilliant man. He has been doing research on a medication that has been used for decades for African sleeping sickness, some medication called suramin, and his first study of this was
[00:19:30]   released and showed that this antipurinergic medication can turn off that persistent cell danger response. It can cause an awakening of a sort in children with autism.

[00:20:00]   I highly recommend looking at the research by Bob Naviaux. The most recent article was in the *Annals of Clinical and Translational Neurology* just released in May and more research will be done looking at that. I think it may be a key to unlocking some of the problems we see in autism. Suramin is not yet available; it's just available in research. I was just in Africa lecturing and mentoring some physicians and even though it's used there for African sleeping sickness, it's not something they even have easily available. The next phase of studies is about to be done but there hasn't been any other antipurinergic medication that comes close yet. I think the closest we can come to is by helping our children to detoxify, as I was
[00:20:30]   saying earlier, with glutathione.

[00:21:00]   I think the other thing that will help and what I have used is something that repletes our ecosystems. All of us have depleted ecosystems. It's from wearing shoes, using toilets, living indoors, more C-sections, less breastfeeding. We all have depleted our biomes of the germs that we need, and so one of the things that may reset this abnormal cell danger response and this autoimmune, immune dysregulation is something called HDCs. This is something William Parker at Duke is studying and that my mentor, Dr. Sidney Baker, is harvesting in his own clean lab. These are grain beetle worm eggs.

[00:21:30] Sounds disgusting, I know. Back hundreds of years ago when we used to eat grains that were dried in vats, we used to eat grain beetles and grain beetle worm eggs. This is something that resets that immune system response. When I was talking about those cytokines and their persistent cell danger response, one of those cytokines is tumor necrosis factor alpha and these grain beetle worm eggs

[00:22:00] decrease that inflammation and help to reset that persistent cell danger response. That is one thing I've used and seen work quite well in some of our kids.

I had a young man with autism, a teenager with a severe onset of perseverations (repeating the same thing over and over again), anxiety, sleep problems. He was literally climbing the walls. His parents

[00:22:30] weren't sleeping. He wasn't sleeping. He had been admitted to the hospital. He had tried lots of psychiatric medications, lots of other supplements and medications. I tried these HDCs, the grain beetle worm eggs. Within a very short period of time, he was sitting next to me, talking to me, conversing,

[00:23:00] being calm, sleeping at night. That has continued as long as he continues on these HDCs. There are a lot of kids like that. It's not just one story but that one definitely stands out.

There's lots of research going on right now in the areas of autism. I think we can't just focus on the genetics, although there is a genetic susceptibility. We need to look at the environment and how the environment is affecting our kids. I think the most exciting research right now is coming out of UC San

[00:23:30] Diego on the cell danger response and the use of antipurinergic medications. Other exciting research is coming out of Duke and Dr. William Parker and the use of HDCs and other immune modulating effects to decrease the inflammation in the autoimmune reactions in our kids. I think autism is an autoimmune disease. It's not only neurologic dysregulation, it's immune dysregulation. Any research we do that looks

[00:24:00] at the immune system, as well as the neurologic system can be very helpful in these kids.

I think we often use the analogy of an onion and onions just make me cry but if we look at our children as a gift, and when they have autism, they may re-wrap in many layers of wrapping paper. What we do as integrative physicians is try to unwrap those many layers of wrapping paper to get to the true gift

[00:24:30] inside but whether we get to that true gift or they have several layers of wrapping paper, seeing that child as a gift can help them to see themselves as a gift. That's number one.

The second thing is to look for somebody else that's been through this. There's a great group of parents, TACA (Talk About Curing Autism) and they have many mentors who can be very helpful to parents.

[00:25:00] Looking at others, SPED-NET groups, NAA, finding other parents who have been through this, they can help lead you down the right path. I think look at your child's total body. I always say kids crave that which they're most sensitive to. If your child's craving a certain food like milk, for instance, take it out 100% for three weeks and see what happens. You may see a different child at the end of those three

[00:25:30] weeks. If you don't, then pig out on it and see if you see any regression, but just start with one thing. Find one thing that may make a difference for your child and try that, and don't give up.

NORMAN DOIDGE, MD | Author: *The Brain's Way of Healing*

Dr. Mark Hyman:	Dr. Doidge, your career's been focused on something called neuroplasticity. How would you define that and what is neuroplasticity?'
Dr. Norman Doidge: [00:00:30] [00:01:00]	Neuroplasticity is a property of the brain that allows it to change its structure and its function in response to mental experience and activity. It's not, as some people sometimes say, just brain change. If you think about it, think of Alzheimer's. That brain is changing, it's degenerating. It's actually losing its plasticity, so it's important to keep in mind that neuroplasticity, in some ways, involves mental experience and activity. Sometimes, in the lab, people forget that because you can take chemicals or electrically stimulate a brain and see it change and say that's plasticity. But that's highly artificial, and they're working with networks that evolved to process mental experience and activity. The reason I emphasize that so much is because we're not just going in there and trying to use chemicals or electricity or magnetism or something like that to arbitrarily change brain structure. We're always, in some way or other, also using mental activity so that we can actually sculpt our brains in meaningful ways, ways that we evolved to do.
Dr. Mark Hyman:	It's like if you want to build your muscles you have to work your muscles, right? If you want to build your brain ...
Dr. Norman Doidge: [00:01:30]	Right. Towards a particular end.
Dr. Mark Hyman:	Right. Yes, if you want to be a swimmer, or a weightlifter, or a basketball player, or a dancer, it's all different. In the same way, your sort of work has explicated the fact that by having different brain activities, by different brain exercises, if you will, you can do brain lifting instead of weightlifting, and that actually has a huge impact in restructuring the brain and reorganizing its function.
Dr. Norman Doidge: [00:02:00]	Yes. Something like an exercise, a highly repeated mental activity, is one way to develop brain structure. There are also other ways and we can sometimes do it in concert with many kinds of activities sometimes, which are not repetitive. Sometimes brain change comes very, very quickly.
Dr. Mark Hyman: [00:02:30]	Yes, I would see that. We were just chatting about the ways in which you can see very quick change in patients. I had a patient with ADD who had all sorts of inflammatory issues, gut issues, environmental toxic issues, lead, and we corrected those things in two months. He went from having illegible handwriting to having perfect penmanship, without any other input. But you're saying for really more damaged brains you need more focused inputs, whether they're music or magnetic stimulation or different brain exercises or different kinds of activities, that actually will help rewire the structure and function of the brain.
Dr. Norman Doidge:	Right.
Dr. Mark Hyman: [00:03:00]	In your career you've been focused on brain healing. You wrote a book about brain healing, and the question I have is, "What are the advances in thinking and practice around brain healing that can help people recover their brain function?"
Dr. Norman Doidge: [00:03:30]	Sure. The first one is that it's okay for you to say brain healing, because for about 400 years the words "brain" and "healing" really weren't used in the same sentence, and that's because neuroscientists, going all the way back to Descartes, always conceived of the brain as some kind of complex machine. He saw it as a hydraulic machine. The discovery of electricity lead people to start talking about the brain as though it was hardwired, a hardwired machine with circuits. We still talk about circuits, and the development of the computer has led people to talk about the brain as though it's a computer and

it's a form of computer hardware. The problem with this machine metaphor is people forget it's a metaphor. Machines do many glorious things, but they don't grow new parts, they don't change or reorganize themselves, they don't heal.

[00:04:00]

Dr. Mark Hyman: I wish my computer healed when it wasn't working.

Dr. Norman Doidge: Yeah, there you go. This metaphor basically gave rise to what I call the Doctrine of the Unchanging Brain, and clinically it gave rise to a neurological nihilism; a belief that when something's broken, there's nothing that can be done. I can't emphasize how powerful that's been, even though we've discovered that the brain is neuroplastic. Now, in everyday mainstream clinical practice, people still

[00:04:30] frequently behave as though it's a machine. First of all, just attacking, undermining, exposing the impoverished nature of that metaphor, has led us to be able to stand back and try new things. What have we learned about the brain? Well, as we said before, literally thousands of experiments that it's a use-it-or-lose-it brain. The circuitry has to be developed and maintained to some degree. We've

[00:05:00] learned that plasticity within the brain is competitive, meaning that if you develop a certain area for a particular mental function and then you don't use it for a long period of time, other mental functions will start taking over that cortical real estate, if you will, in using it.

We've learned that if you don't develop certain brain maps in childhood, like maybe kids with learning

[00:05:30] disorders don't do, if you have very focused, appropriate, targeted, incremental brain exercises, you can develop processors they didn't have. I wrote about that in my first book, *The Brain That Changes Itself*, and the Arrowsmith School was one example of that. We've learned that if you have a stroke and a certain brain area dies, with appropriate stimulation and activity by people who know what they're doing, areas adjacent to that lesion can take over those functions, or areas in the mirror hemisphere

[00:06:00] can take over those functions. There are many, many things we've learned, but in *The Brain's Way of Healing*, my latest book, what I tried to do was, instead of talking about neuroplasticity or this idea of neuroplastic healing in a low-resolution way, I tried to break it down. I've now spent almost 20 years studying this and been to five continents looking over different kinds of mechanisms, and there are

[00:06:30] many different ways to skin a cat. There are many different ways that neuroplastic interventions work. What I found was that there are five sorts of key types, or stages, of healing that the brain can go through that often get blocked when a person is injured or has damage, and different people need different stages addressed.

[00:07:00] We're beginning to refine that. These five stages are the first time someone has proposed stages. I'm not locked into there being five. There may be more, but they're all different, and it allows us to sort of find where different interventions fit.

Dr. Mark Hyman: Take us through those five stages of healing, because what you're saying is really revolutionary. I don't want to step over how dramatic this shift in our paradigm is. It's about what the brain is capable of,

[00:07:30] and how we can then intervene in medicine to fix the problem, and these five stages seem like a culmination of your work around how to heal the brain.

Dr. Norman Doidge: Sure. I'm going to do that, but let me tell you one thing before I tell you the five stages, which is why I thought they were necessary. We've gone from a state where mainstream medicine has, really for decades, said to people who have a traumatic brain injury that, you know, if you have a concussion or

[00:08:00] a mild traumatic brain injury, wait a number of weeks and 80% of you will get better. But 20% don't, and for those that don't get better, what we said they should do was just rest, or rest and restore, or rest and pray that they restore.

Dr. Mark Hyman: Rest and pray. That's a good medical prescription.

Dr. Norman Doidge: The patients that got better were fine, but there are many, many patients out there who haven't
[00:08:30] gotten better. In fact, traumatic brain injury is the number one cause of combined death and disability if you put them both together. It often affects young people too. As I was traveling around and

| | studying and researching these things, I've now come across twelve different interventions. Thirteen actually, for traumatic brain injury alone, and people who have traumatic brain injury don't have a lot of money to spend on just anything, and I was trying to figure out, which ones do we use for which person? It's a work in progress. That's why I had to say, "Well, what is blocked in this patient?" |

[00:09:00] studying and researching these things, I've now come across twelve different interventions. Thirteen actually, for traumatic brain injury alone, and people who have traumatic brain injury don't have a lot of money to spend on just anything, and I was trying to figure out, which ones do we use for which person? It's a work in progress. That's why I had to say, "Well, what is blocked in this patient?"

The first stage of neuroplastic healing, the one that I think I preferentially attend to in any patient, is attending to any problems in cellular health, brain cellular health. That's neuronal health, glial health, because most of the cells inside your brain are called glial cells. We thought they were support cells for the neurons, but in fact the glial cells also have communicative capacities.

Dr. Mark Hyman: And they're also your brain's immune system.
[00:09:30]

Dr. Norman Doidge: Yes, so I always attend to that first. If you were to think of something like traumatic brain injury, I describe light therapies. They affect cells, the mitochondria, hyperbaric oxygen, there's fantastic work now, out of Israel, showing that hyperbaric oxygen indeed is helpful for certain people with traumatic brain injuries, so that would be a cellular intervention. The interventions for autistic kids that deal with inflammation are people who've had toxic exposures, which are a lot of people in America as you are
[00:10:00] all directed at cellular health. The reason I go there first is, one: you can have some spontaneous recovery because once the cells are functioning, life experience is enough to stimulate those circuits to sort of play catch up. Two, why would I want to put a person through various kinds of brain stimulation or exercise if their cells aren't healthy? So that's the first phase.

[00:10:30]
Dr. Mark Hyman: So cellular health, you're talking about light therapy, you're talking about hyperbaric oxygen therapy?

Dr. Norman Doidge: Yep. All the detoxification therapies, all the things that address dietary causes of food sensitivities and allergies. A lot of the things that Functional Medicine does.

Dr. Mark Hyman: Detoxification?

Dr. Norman Doidge: Detoxification, yes. Many of the things that Functional Medicine is leading the way in.

Dr. Mark Hyman: Adjusting all the triggers in environmental toxins, you've got microbio, triggers of inflammation like dietary allergens or sensitivities.
[00:11:00]
Dr. Norman Doidge: Yes. These, obviously we know they're important in many, many brain problems. I mean, clearly, at least a subset of depressed patients are showing a subset of inflammation, as you well know.

Dr. Mark Hyman: Yes.

Dr. Norman Doidge: Many of the childhood learning disorders, the autistic spectrum, are involved in this. Multiple sclerosis, and probably a lot of other brain problems, and then there's, of course, all the cellular things that are going on that are predisposing people to things like strokes and vascular dementia.
[00:11:30]
Dr. Mark Hyman: Cellular health is a huge concept that has many, many interventions.

Dr. Norman Doidge: Huge. Yes, and we all probably could benefit from attention to that. The next thing that happens is because it's so powerfully a use-it-or-lose-it brain, when the brain isn't working properly, circuits tend to go dormant or shut down. They're there, they're memory based circuits, they contain memories of circuits and so on and so forth, but they go into a kind of turned off state. In my book, I explain how I
[00:12:00] know this to be the case, but in brief, if you can find a circuit that's dormant and give it just a little bit of stimulation, it comes online very quickly, especially if you've addressed this underlying cellular problem. We know it's already there, it's just dormancy in biology is a kind of last ditch defense of an organism when it's failing to function or achieve homeostasis. It says, "Okay, we're going to shut down
[00:12:30] now. Maybe things will change environmentally and we'll be able to work," but until then there's

something called learned non-use.

Dr. Mark Hyman: I can remember all the Chinese I learned in college and forgot?

Dr. Norman Doidge:
[00:13:00]

It probably could be evoked and brought back much more quickly than you think if you immersed yourself. One of the reasons we know that circuits shut down is based on the work of Edward Taub. Basically, he did some spectacular animal experiments, which lead to the most important treatments we now have, I believe, for stroke, for people who lose the use of an arm or a leg. And, basically, what

[00:13:30]

he discovered was, let's say, when a person has a stroke, for about six weeks to several months, there's a period where there's kind of chemical chaos in the brain. There's blood that has to be reabsorbed. There's inflammation. Cells die and release all sorts of toxic problems and so on. We've known about that crisis for, well, over a hundred years now. It's called dialysis. A person might have a stroke in a

[00:14:00]

small part of the brain, let's say right here, and try to use his left hand, but because of dialysis, because of this very global chemical chaos in the brain, it doesn't work.

Because people were locked in this idea that the brain was like a machine with these different modules, they assumed that what rehab should be was, during the dialysis period, basically just keep

[00:14:30]

giving them a little bit of exercise to kind of prime the pump. And by the end of the six weeks, dialysis is over, you'll see what's left. And if they can just do this, that's the end of rehab. Because rehab wasn't about building new circuitry. It was just about priming the pump. Here's what Taub found out; Taub found out through these fantastic interventions, that one of the reasons the arm stops working is because, during dialysis, you're trying to use the arm and you learn that it's not working, so the circuit

[00:15:00]

shuts down completely. Now, the circuit may be damaged, but it may be less damaged than we think. He called this learned non-use, so what he would do for a treatment is he would take a person who lost the use of this arm, say, and they would be tempted to want to use this arm to make up for it. He put this arm in a sling or a cast so they couldn't.

Dr. Mark Hyman: Immobilized the good arm.

Dr. Norman Doidge:
[00:15:30]

Yes, and then incrementally trained this arm. He would find that he could restore a lot of lost function, and when he did brain scans on this, he found that the areas that were now being used were very close to the original lesion, just around it, or in the opposite hemisphere. I mean, he also did extraordinary experiments with animals where, for instance, he would disconnect nerves, let's say the nerve for this arm, and he would put the arm in a cast immediately after he disconnected the nerves so

[00:16:00]

that it couldn't try to use the arm and learn that it wouldn't work. Then he'd take off the cast, and within a few training sessions the arm could work.

Dr. Mark Hyman: Even with the cut nerves.

Dr. Norman Doidge: It's actually spectacular. And these things have been replicated, and it tells us there are many things we don't understand about how the nervous system works, but yes, even with cut nerves.

Dr. Mark Hyman: That's extraordinary.

Dr. Norman Doidge:
[00:16:30]

Another time, he cut nerves in both arms, put casts on both arms so that they wouldn't learn they couldn't use them, took off the casts, and they could use them. I have these things on film.

Dr. Mark Hyman: Extraordinary.

Dr. Norman Doidge: Yeah. The nervous system doesn't work in a simple point-to-point way. Where, for instance, that's what Mike Merzenich and others have shown, that if, for instance, most people think that if you touch this area there's a nerve that goes straight up into this part of the brain and it's a one-to-one correspondence between this and this, but that's actually not how it works.

Dr. Mark Hyman: [00:17:00]	Unbelievable.
Dr. Norman Doidge: [00:17:30] [00:18:00]	It has to do with the timing of the input. I mean, Merzenich was able to do things like take a nerve, cut it, twist it, and wait six weeks or so and then stimulate the finger, and the brain map was completely normal. You would think it would be all mixed up, like let's say you had a nerve bundle that carried these two fingers and you cut the nerve and twisted it. You'd think it wouldn't work, but over time it has to do all with the timing of the input. All of this is to say that there's this phenomenon that was first discovered in stroke, or first demonstrated in stroke, called learned non-use. But what I started to find in my clinical work, and Ed Taub started to find in his clinical work, is that learned non-use applies not just to stroke, but to most brain problems, because it applies to cerebral palsy of course, which is similar to stroke, but it applies to some degree to MS and other problems. I realized that learned non-use, whenever a function isn't working, there's a tendency to try to use it, it fails, and it goes dormant. If you can find ways to stimulate the dormant circuitry, we have the second stage of neuroplastic healing, neurostimulation.
Dr. Mark Hyman: [00:18:30]	Yes. What do you use to stimulate it?
Dr. Norman Doidge: [00:19:00]	Well, the easiest way to stimulate is to get the person to try to do what the circuitry was for, so what Taub would do for neurostimulation is very simple. He would do very, very simple physiotherapy exercises for the arm, but whatever the circuit requires. Taub's work can also work for language, so therefore you use words and the other way you can do it is you can, I'll get to this in a minute, but you can put lots of spikes into a circuit just to reawaken it in general, and then get the person to do a mental activity while the spikes are coming through the circuit.
Dr. Mark Hyman:	We've talked about cellular health and neurostimulation, but there are three more. The next one is neuromodulation. Tell us about that.
Dr. Norman Doidge: [00:19:30] [00:20:00]	One of the things I was taught in medical school, and I bet you were too, was that let's say someone had a stroke and they couldn't move their right arm, and they lost 90% of the function of the right arm. We were told just look at the CT scan, look at some kind of scan, you'll see 90% of the brain area governing that function is dead. As I started to see people getting better from neuroplastic intervention, I realized that just couldn't be possible and that there was a lot of sloppy work actually going into that correlation of 90 to 90. In fact, studies of lesions and loss of function show that there's very little correlation. It's stunning. There's far less correlation between the location of the lesion, there is some, but far less than most people think in the loss of function, and the size of the lesion in the loss of function. What I started to realize by studying a lot of EEG work and quantitative EEGs of different conditions, is something like this is happening.
[00:20:30] [00:21:00]	A person loses 90% of the function. Some of the cells are dead, that's true. Some of the cells, though, are metabolically compromised along the damaged area. At the simplest level, some of them are sick cells that are near the dead cells, and sick cells don't necessarily fall silent. They fire at irregular rates. In general, we talk about neurons as though they're on or off, but really, neurons, the only time they're really off is when they're dead. What happens is a neuron has a firing rate, which is usually a fast rate that signals that it's on, and then a slower firing rate that means that it's off. Sometimes that's reversed, but when a neuron is sick in some way or other, it doesn't necessarily fall silent. It often will fire at a slower rate or some kind of irregular rate. These neurons, these sick neurons, are giving off junk data, and healthy cells near them are receiving junk data. Then there are some healthy cells that are functioning just fine.
[00:21:30]	A person could have lost 90% of the function, but only a small number of the cells are actually dead. You could figure this out, for instance, if you were to take something like an MRI and a SPECT scan and map them together, and you would see the difference between the dead tissue and the areas that are somehow or other compromised. This is happening in many, many conditions, and it gives rise to what I call the noisy brain, which is a poorly modulated brain, where the cells are sending out a lot of junk

[00:22:00] data to healthy cells. Sick cells are sending that to healthy cells, and so those cells aren't working and then they can go into learning non-use. The trick here is to resynchronize the brain, and you can do this by all sorts of mechanisms. We're just beginning to show some of them. One of them is neurofeedback, which is, again, a mental experience kind of intervention to modify the brain waves, which is the electrical activity of millions of feedbacks.

[00:22:30]
Dr. Mark Hyman: Neurofeedback is essentially where you use your brain to control its function by thinking differently and experiencing differently, and you do it by basically playing video games with your brain.

Dr. Norman Doidge: Yes. You basically will put some leads or sensors on the brain, and in very sophisticated versions you can put a lot of sensors on the brain, and when, let's say the brain is firing very slow waves when a
[00:23:00]   person should be wide awake and concentrating. They're firing the waves that are closer to sleep. That person might have a version of ADD or a traumatic brain injury, something like that. You can set up a game where in the very few times that their brain fires faster, more appropriate waves, they do well in a video game and they get rewarded. And every time they have lots and lots of slow waves when they shouldn't, they don't do as well in the video game. You could set up a race between three boats. You
[00:23:30]   just tell them something like the middle boat should move ahead. That's all they know. They don't have to know how their brain is working or anything like that, and the brain's pattern recognition will just be firing constantly and gradually, it'll train down the slow waves and up the more appropriate waves. That's one mode of neuromodulation.

Dr. Mark Hyman: I've done it. It's pretty wild you can actually control a game with your thoughts.

Dr. Norman Doidge: Yes.

Dr. Mark Hyman: And your brain waves.
[00:24:00]
Dr. Norman Doidge: Again, neurofeedback. I'm not interested in any individual intervention. I'm interested in families of intervention. That's one. I describe another intervention, which I'll be talking about at the IFM tomorrow probably, where you basically do very, very mild electrical intervention on the tongue.

Dr. Mark Hyman: Sounds fun.

Dr. Norman Doidge: Yes. You're not shocking the tongue, Mark, and you're not shocking the brain. What you're doing is you
[00:24:30]   have very, very mild stimulation. It feels like champagne bubbles going off on your tongue at a particular wave. Now, why the tongue? The tongue is the royal road to the deepest part of the brain. You don't have to crack open the skull. You don't have to use medication to get to the deepest part of your plastic brain. There are at least as many nerve pathways from the tongue to the brainstem, which is this kind of master control center, as there are from the ear into the brain. You think about how much information you can get through your ear from music and speech and so on. By modulating the
[00:25:00]   waves on the tongue, it goes through the cranial nerves into the brainstem. I'm going to describe how you can get the entire system to reset in cases of things like traumatic brain injury and Parkinson's, multiple sclerosis, and so on, from the bottom up.

Dr. Mark Hyman: What you just said was basically heresy, that you can reset the brain in Parkinson's, Alzheimer's, strokes, I mean this is just groundbreaking.
[00:25:30]
Dr. Norman Doidge: If you believe that the brain is an inanimate machine, it's heresy. If you don't, if you understand that it's plastic, if you believe that the brain is something that's, as we often hear, in your head, then it's heresy. At some level of course in anatomy textbooks, the brain is in your head, but of course the brain
[00:26:00]   is seamlessly connected to the cranial nerves, the sense organs, and the body. The body did not, as some people often say, evolve as infrastructure for your brain. Neuroscientists often do this, but we say it all the time. You are your brain. We speak about human beings, as though this from the neck down is an appendage support system infrastructure for the brain. Ray Kurzweil and some people

---

[00:26:30] would like to just take all the ideas and export it into a computer and make a human being. This idea that somehow the body evolved from the brain is just crazy. I mean, brains evolved millions of years after bodies did, and they didn't evolve to be the master of the body. They co-evolved with the body to work together with the body. The emphasis in the work I do is always on non-invasive ways of changing the brain.

[00:27:00] The easiest way to get into the brain is through the same windows the brain uses to receive information from the world. Your sense organs, your eyes, your ears, all of your sense organs, are what are called in engineering terms and in biological terms, transducers. All the transducers do is they transform energy patterns from one form of energy into patterns of energy in another form of energy.

[00:27:30] Microphones take sound energy and put it into electrical energy, speakers take electrical energy, put it into sound, it goes into your ears, which converts the sound back into electrical and so on and so forth. Transduction, transduction, transduction. It's happening all the time, but we can use these transducers, these evolutionarily-derived or God-given or however you want to think about them

[00:28:00] transducers, if we know what we're doing, to influence using patterns of using to influence and sculpt aspects of the plastic brain.

Dr. Mark Hyman: What are the techniques of neuromodulation?

Dr. Norman Doidge: For instance, let's say that tongue one, years and years of working on the proper waves found out how to basically override noisy brain firing in the brain stem by just giving sensory input on the tongue at a

[00:28:30] particular rate with a particular wave form. For instance, take autistic kids. A lot of people think that the essence of autism is the inability to model other minds. There's a lot of literature on that, and a lot of autistic children have that problem for sure; but it can't possibly be the essence of autism. I know that because I've seen interventions that help autistic kids.

Dr. Mark Hyman:
[00:29:00] Yesah, you talk about reversal of autism in your book.

Dr. Norman Doidge: In rare cases it happens. In many cases, symptoms, if you follow the different stages of neuroplastic healing, can be ameliorated. There are many kids with autism who've made improvements. I know there are many scientists who talk about it as though it's completely genetic and that it's irreversible. There's not scientific data, as Martha Herbert points out, there is no scientific data for those claims, and we're finding more and more cases of kids who, with various kinds of interventions, can make some improvements.

[00:29:30] One of the things about autism is most autistic kids are hypersensitive to sounds, and they'll cover their ears. We used to think, well, that's just one of the many symptoms in that autistic package. Well, it turns out to be an absolutely crucial symptom for those kids, and here's why. When you walk into a room, let's say it's a party, a gala, first you hear booming, buzzing, confusion, and then over a while

[00:30:00] your ears will, because they have the equivalent of a zoom lens in them, an auditory zoom, hone in on the frequencies of human speech. Well, autistic speech can't do that.

Dr. Mark Hyman: Can't filter out the noise.

Dr. Norman Doidge: No. Their auditory zoom is very frequently not working, which is why certain sounds, particularly machine-like sounds, just drive them crazy. Now, why should a machine sound drive you crazy? Well,

[00:30:30] here one has to speculate, but I rely on the work of Stephen Porges to some degree, who's a master of the human nervous system. If you look at different species in the course of evolution, species communicate with each other in particular frequencies, so we're communicating in a frequency of human speech. We often evolve to communicate with each other in frequencies that our predators can't hear. Our predators have certain frequencies, which often scare the living daylights out of us. If

[00:31:00] you think about *Jaws* or a movie about aliens, there'll always be some low boom, boom, boom threatening sound, and the filmmakers put that in because they want to stimulate the fight-or-flight response in the audience.

Dr. Mark Hyman:	It works.
Dr. Norman Doidge: [00:31:30] [00:32:00]	It works. But imagine you're an autistic child and you don't have an auditory zoom, and you're hearing things like that all the time. You go into fight-or-flight. When you're in fight-or-flight, there's another evolved system in mammals. That is the social engagement system, and that's how we relate to each other. It's interesting how much of the social engagement system is governed by cranial nerves. You're looking at me, and your eye position is cranial nerves. You're focusing on human speech. You can do that, you have a functioning auditory zoom, cranial nerve-related, and your facial expression is cranial nerve-related and so on and so forth. In the sound based interventions we've used, there's a lot of great work done in Toronto on that. You basically train that auditory zoom by using modified sound to gradually teach the child to differentiate human speech, and that's a kind of neurodifferentiation, the final stage and modulation of the fight-or-flight system.
[00:32:30] [00:33:00]	Once that auditory zoom is working, and sometimes it can start working in two or three days, kids who didn't look at their parents will go over and hug them for the first time. That's pretty remarkable, because if the essence of autism is the inability to relate and model other minds, that shouldn't be happening without any kind of training, you know what I mean? What happens is you turn off the fight-or-flight system by correcting the auditory zoom, and their social engagement system, eye contact, longing for warmth, reaching out, is turned on immediately. I'm not saying this listening-based therapy is the only intervention I'd use for autistic kids. Of course, I would address those earlier stages of cellular health.
Dr. Mark Hyman:	Well, you bring up a very important point, which is almost an anathema to conventional medicine, which is multimodal interventions. Which means that traditional medicine is a single intervention, a drug or treatment for a single outcome. You give this drug, you give this therapy, it works for autism. That's failed miserably. For everything, for Alzheimer's.
Dr. Norman Doidge: [00:33:30]	For many reasons, yes.
Dr. Mark Hyman:	You're talking about multiple interventions working on different aspects of brain dysfunction. Whether it's diet, exercise, sleep, light, sound, taste, movement, all these things are ways of accessing the brain that have really been neglected and almost ignored in conventional medicine.
Dr. Norman Doidge: [00:34:00]	Well, I think it's fair to say "ignored" would be a polite way to talk about it, the kinds of dismissals, because it doesn't fit with certain models. One is a machine.
Dr. Mark Hyman:	Or randomized controlled trials don't work for it.
Dr. Norman Doidge: [00:34:30]	The issue here is this: much of modern medicine is taught as though these problems are all linear, like one billiard ball hits another, which hits another, which hits another, which hits another, which hits another. But these systems are not linear systems. They're constantly reciprocally interacting and there are emergent orders and so on and so forth. The other thing is we have our genetic variation, but neuroplasticity shows us that our brains all wire up slightly differently, so we're all very different and the idea, you say you have a brain, but of course you could easily say in your skull are 150 different organs. I mean, that would be a more reasonable way of talking about the brain because there're so many different functional sort of parts, and they can all link up and de-link.
Dr. Mark Hyman:	It's a network.
Dr. Norman Doidge: [00:35:00]	Yes, but it's the most dynamic network that we know about, because it can constantly reformulate itself. That's another very important point for all of medicine, but particularly if you're dealing with something as sophisticated as the brain. These linear models are not the appropriate model. You need complexity theory to address these things and you need to understand that every brain injury is different. Two brain injuries have as much in common, for instance, as two bombed out sites do from

[00:35:30]	30,000 feet. In one city, they took out the electrical grid and the harbor, and the other city, they took out the residential areas and the financial district. Up close, brain injuries are different.

Dr. Mark Hyman: Yes.

Dr. Norman Doidge: The idea of, let's say we wanted to study an intervention for a brain injury. Not only is the damage different, in other words two different people in two car accidents are hit in different parts of the head. Neuroplastically they're wired up, so they perform functions in different parts. One person was
[00:36:00] an alcoholic, does lots of drugs, hasn't exercised for 25 years, has a low IQ, and never completes anything, and the other person has none of those things. The same intervention, to put those different people, to put together apples and oranges, figs, rotten figs, pomegranates together and to just say, "Well, they all had brain injury and we're going to do one thing for all these people," that's just a fiction. That's not science.

Dr. Mark Hyman: You're talking about a personalized approach to brain health that's customized for each individual.

Dr. Norman Doidge: Brain health and disease. Sure.
[00:36:30]
Dr. Mark Hyman: We only have a few minutes left and there are two other aspects of brain healing you talk about. You talked about cellular health, neurostimulation, neuromodulation. What are the other two?

Dr. Norman Doidge: The next one I've called neurorelaxation. It's the most tentative of the phases, but I felt I had to put it down because in a number of these interventions, let's take the sound intervention for kids who are
[00:37:00] autistic, or people with traumatic brain injury. I just observed something that had never been recorded in the literature, which is often these people would sleep something like 16 hours a day for five, six, seven days. I called it a neurorelaxation phase. It seemed, you might say, well, they were just catching up on their sleep. Everyone with a traumatic brain injury has sleep problems, or most of them do. Maybe they're just catching up on their sleep, but it seemed like the brain was moving into some kind
[00:37:30] of huge stage where it was just regrouping and preparing for new learning. We know, for instance, that when you sleep, certain channels in the brain open up that allow glymphatic channels, which are recently discovered, which allow it to drain out the buildup of toxins. But sleep is very, very important for neuroplastic consolidation. The reason I highlighted that stage, is because I wanted patients who were going through these interventions to anticipate it could happen to them and clinicians not to
[00:38:00] interrupt that profound, unusual amount of sleep that some of them experience, because it tends to be self-limiting. It's not as though they're completely desynchronized.

[00:38:30] Then the final stage is neurodifferentiation. We map the world and when a baby is born, everything we know from work on animals and brain scan kinds of work, a baby might be born with a very diffuse map of its fist and gradually differentiate its fingers. All of your brain maps work that way. They start off with low amounts of distinctions or information in them, sort of like Columbus' outline of America, and then they become highly differentiated. Let's say the circuit goes dormant, as so often happens
[00:39:00] with learned non-use. Those maps get either de-differentiated, they kind of regress and become simpler, or they become chaotic. One of the things we do is we teach very fine distinctions in the final phase. The brain is now, cellular health has been addressed as much as we can, it's been stimulated, modulated, it's had its relaxation. Now it's ready to learn, and we are redefining the brain maps, and we do that with kids with learning disorders. We do that with all sorts of things, and that's basically
[00:39:30] making very fine distinctions. Brain exercises can also teach you to do that.

Dr. Mark Hyman: How do you intervene in that stage?

Dr. Norman Doidge: An example would be, let's see a very easy example. Not all brain exercises are alike. Some brain exercises, and I have no financial relationship with BrainHQ, but that is the one that was developed by Mike Merzenich and his team, and there are 150 studies showing they are effective for many different
[00:40:00] things. All these meta-analyses that merged together brain exercises that were not carefully developed

[00:40:30]	with brain teasers and things that are just rebranded as brain exercises, those are not valid meta-analyses. Again, it's apples and oranges all being mixed together. These are really fine brain exercises that can help people, who as they age, I'm not talking about Alzheimer's, as they age, one of the things that happens to all of us or most of us as we hit our 40s and 50s and 60s, is we're replaying a lot of already mastered skills.
[00:41:00]	When you're young and you go to school and you study for a French test or something like that, you are really taxing your brain and turning on a part of your brain called the nucleus basalis, which helps you consolidate connections. Many people, as they get older, may have been in the same job for 20 years, they may have lived in the same house, the same city, the same spouse and stuff maybe, and so the engagement of the brain at that high level of learning has not gone on often for 20 years. The parts of the brain that allow you to learn and maintain fine distinction of the brain maps haven't been adequately exercised.
Dr. Mark Hyman:	So, learn French when you're 50.
Dr. Norman Doidge: [00:41:30]	That's a very good thing to do. Exactly. Just as a person who wants to maintain their physical health will do some interval training, they'll challenge themselves. You have to do that to maintain your cognitive health. One of the ways you'll do it, for instance, is when I'm speaking to you, you're registering all the distinctions between the sounds that I'm making. Many people, when they're 40 and 50, they go to a party and they're introduced to two people and they say, "I'm going to remember this name," and they don't remember the name. Part of the problem is that their auditory processing maps haven't been taxed enough in the last 20 years, so the name doesn't stick.
[00:42:00] Dr. Mark Hyman:	So, use it or lose it.
Dr. Norman Doidge: [00:42:30]	It's a use it or lose it thing. These brain exercises would teach you to make very, very subtle distinctions. When people do these brain exercises, what they find is suddenly they can remember things at parties and things like that, but they can do much more than that. These brain exercises have helped people who've had radiation, or people who have chemotherapy often get a kind of mental fog. These brain exercises can reverse that. Appropriately applied, they can help certain people who've had traumatic brain injuries. They shouldn't be used on everybody, but for some people they're helpful. That's a kind of neurodifferentiation.
Dr. Mark Hyman:	That's great. This is a powerful new model of thinking about how to resurrect a brain that's poorly functioning. Your work is just extraordinary, because it's opening a new world, the possibility of brain recovery, which has heretofore been thought impossible. I really appreciate your work. Thank you for it. Thanks for joining us today.
Dr. Norman Doidge:	Thank you.

OMID NAIM, MD | Hope Integrative Psychiatry and La Maida Institute

Dr. Omid Naim:	The impulse to create what is now Hope Psychiatry came about as I started out in community psychiatry, working with high-risk youth, working with the most sick and most at-risk youth in the county up in the Bay Area, in a particular program that was a wraparound program. There were intensive services, and seeing the value of a community approach. What I was seeing is that we were providing these services when people were at their worst. What we were actually doing is recreating a natural environment in which families, parents, the youth themselves, people are being supported by multiple caregivers. It seemed really clear that what was working really was community, and the feeling that we should be offering that at the outset of treatment, rather than waiting for people to get so sick.
[00:00:30]	
[00:01:00] [00:01:30] [00:02:00]	During that time, I also learned about body-oriented psychotherapy approaches. Learning about trauma, being something that's from a more ecological holistic lens, rather than a psychoanalytic or behavioral issue. What we call mental illness is really the consequence of us being disconnected from what our natural environment is like, and that most depression, anxiety, PTSD, excluding things like schizophrenia, they're actually, I think, mostly normal reactions to an abnormal environment in modern life and we should be designing a clinic, imagining what a clinic should look like based on that. We should actually be trying to support people in reestablishing their own innate capacity to heal, their own innate resilience, and to bring community together as the primary resource.
[00:02:30]	If you come to our clinic, what's different is that the questionnaires will go through all aspects of your life: how you're eating, the kind of work you do, how close are you to friends/family, what are your relationship patterns, as well as what a conventional psychiatrist would do, which is mostly ask a symptom checklist. Conventional psychiatry right now diagnoses based on symptoms, and the paradigm really is that those symptoms are the disease. If you're depressed, what that means is that you are excessively sad, excessively tired, lack of motivation, lack of drive, isolating.
[00:03:00]	In our model, in our concept, in our belief system, that is actually the end result of the problem. And so, one of the first things I do is when we gather up all this information, we look at how all aspects of the person's life are manifesting these symptoms, and try to really change the perspective of the person. Most people are coming in with a perspective received by our culture that if I'm depressed, I have some faulty gene, or something traumatic happened when I was young, and I'm damaged from that. There's a broken mentality people come in with. What we try and do is reorient the conversation, and one of the most important things to say is that the symptoms are actually the results of the problem. They're not the source of the problem, and so our focus is really to tend to the root cause.
[00:03:30] [00:04:00]	The starting point of thinking about that is we're primarily biologically still tribal in our nature. If you look at most mammals, most primates, they live in groups. They live in tightly interdependent groups and the mammalian way of life is like deep interdependence. What that means is that our biological systems, our nervous systems, really if you look at evolution, there's the reptilian evolution, the next thing being mammalian. What that really means is a lot of the wiring in our nervous system is designed towards connection and reading each other's motivation, so we can work in what's called a flow state. We're not having to think about what we're doing, that we're actually reading each other, responding to each other, so that we can act together, fast.
[00:04:30]	If anybody's watched a National Geographic show, the horse, the zebra that's caught alone, or the seal that's caught alone, is in massive terror because if you're a mammal and you're alone, you've lost most of your advantage in terms of survival. We're still carrying that same wiring, and so we are belonging, feeling part of something, feeling part of a group, feeling deep relationships that with a sense of interdependence, that nurtures our nervous systems. That provides our nervous systems something

[00:05:00] essential, like a plant needs water and sun. These are essential components to our being in balance.

[00:05:30] One of the ways we talk about in our clinic is to reorient the conversation about why something happened, and really step back and look, what is it like to go through the things we go through and have very little community? I came through residency learning to really focus on how did early childhood affect a child? And really, that often meant how did the mother or the father fail the child in some way? What I like to do is change that perspective for clients, and say let's really step back and look multi-generational, and let's ask where was the extended family? Where are all the other people? I think that the idea that the nuclear family should do everything and be able to provide everything is a real false, actually design, in terms of our innate nature.

[00:06:00]
[00:06:30] So, belonging is, I think, essential to our nervous systems. Another side of that is that our ability to be there for other people is what triggers a lot of our core resilient traits. When you look at who gets ill and who doesn't, there's a chemical imbalance theory that's been going around for the last 30, 40 years, and that, I think, is a real false paradigm. If you look at the general population, there are high rates of those genes and high rates of those biological traits in people that don't get depressed and don't have anxiety. The real difference is what we call resilience factors. And so being in deeply interdependent relationships triggers in us courage, bravery, patience, and compassion. These are resilient traits that we can move through difficulty, hardship, pain, and suffering, and not allow our predispositions towards depression or anxiety to overtake us.

[00:07:00]
[00:07:30] We are mostly living completely outside of our norm. The idea is that we've societally moved on; but biologically, we're still primates that lived out in the wild, deeply interdependent communities, whole foods, bursts of intense challenging activity on a regular basis, as well as long periods of time of rest, play, good sleep. And so, if you look first at it in terms of physically, our bodies are having to manage a lot of technological stimulus and it's not getting a lot of natural stimulus. Unless you're living really out in the open, the rhythms that trigger our nervous system are very different, living in modern life versus a natural life.

[00:08:00] If you look at time and nature, if you look at challenging activity, if you look at food ... our food system is completely different in modern life, and especially whether it's whole foods versus refined foods or whether it's the soil being depleted of essential nutrients because of the way we're over-farming. And so, these things all deplete our nervous system's ability to be flexible, resilient, and respond to things well.

[00:08:30] The main problem, in terms of community, is that we no longer need each other. Because of progress, we can, for the first time in history, a person can go through their entire adult life without ever actually relying on anybody. You can survive that isolated, but what does that do in terms of your needs for connection?

[00:09:00]
[00:09:30] I think that we undervalue community because the culture has kind of moved forward with this individual mentality, especially in America. I think America is just an extreme of a Western mentality, but in America especially, we value the pioneer. We value the frontiers and we value the singular hero. And yet, at the same time, if you do a survey of people, if you ask at a dinner table around your friends, and bring up these kind of conversations, how many of us feel like that we're doing too much and that we can't complain? How many people are feeling overwhelmed, being so alone? I think we're subject to a culture that really promotes individualism, and there's a lot of pluses to that. There's a lot of value in that, but at the same time, I think there's a diminishment of community. I think in my generation, nobody would question, "Is it right for me to take the best job and move across the country and leave certain people behind?" In terms of biologically, I'm wired to feel dependent on and obligated to.

[00:10:00]

[00:10:30] I just got off the phone, actually on the way here, with a colleague of mine who's struggling with his mom. He is moving forward in his life and his mom is feeling very anxious about him not being around anymore. He shared with me that this is something that's going multiple generations in his family.

Expert Interviews — Omid Naim, MD

People spread out across the country, and he's saying I'm seeing that it's time for me to cut my ties with my mom because she's so bitter, and her bitterness comes from how her mom expected too much of her.

[00:11:00] I was really urging him to actually step back and think about this in a different way. To think about it, he's now an adult. He is now an elder in his family. He's now an elder in his community, and did it help his mom to be resentful and blame and move on from her mother? Even if it's easy right now for him to just cut her off, is this really going to help him versus if he goes back, works through his anger and finds his compassion, his care, his patience, his willingness to be generous with his mom right now and take care of her because she's not well. What will that actualize in him? And that's what I believe love

[00:11:30] is, is that process. Not a cathartic experience, but love being that willingness to grow and expand ourselves for each other, wherein in that process, we then grow and sacrifice for each other. Those are our most innate capacities, and that's a beautiful and transcendental thought, you can say, but at the same time, it's basic mammalian behavior. Love is what binds us together.

[00:12:00] I think that willpower is necessary. Spiritually, we have to all go through that point of real confrontation with what do we believe in? What do we care about, left all one? To make changes to our health and to make changes to our lives, if we're thinking about the larger population and how we are going to manage health care, that kind of change. It's very hard for each person to be able to do

[00:12:30] that on their own. I think that friend power is natural power. It's how we function. It's actually to support each other and also to hold each other accountable. We can't hide in groups. We can't hide places in which we're not really living up to our best. Again, as mammals, we're so wired for group

[00:13:00] behavior, and so the power of that.

What I want to say on this subject is that I don't think we can really solve our healthcare problems if we don't start thinking that way, because we've done amazingly in health care in terms of acute conditions, heart attack, end stage diseases like cancer. What's really breaking our system are chronic conditions like mental illness, diabetes, GI issues. These are all chronic conditions that are lifestyle-related and they're all preventable.

[00:13:30] If you look at what resources we need, we need coaching. We need supportive programs for people to change their behavior. What we're really talking about is that we need community. What I often say is that the solutions are simple but difficult. They're actually not that complicated.

[00:14:00] It's like doing yoga. It's taken me two years of trying to touch my toes without bending my knees. It's quite simple but it's very hard. It's very hard for me to do that over the last two years. If I'm all alone doing yoga, it's different. Anybody who's done anything like yoga, if you've done it in a class, the energy in a group is so powerful, and that motivates us. There's something I think that's also intangible. I think I'm describing it in terms of mammalian behavior and why we're driven to be in groups. But if

[00:14:30] you've ever been in a group, if you're in a yoga class, and there's an energy you feel, and that's, I think, something that's intangible that we can study and understand better. But it's something real. There's a potency, the feeling that you're a part of something.

There's a lot of research on this, in terms of amount of use, and people who spend X number of hours a day on Facebook, that it does lead to lower self-esteem, and it correlates with depression. I think that in terms of the research on whether there's a link, I think that's not a question really, at this point. I

[00:15:00] think that at the same time, we're not going to get away from technology, and I think balance is somehow really important.

The question you asked was, "Why?" I think that, again, it goes back to how much we are group animals and how much we are reading each other's behavior, and what's going on also, in terms of American culture. I have a friend from France, who often says Americans are known as being very

[00:15:30] optimistic. I think we can be very positive, very optimistic, that pioneering spirit, but I think there's a need for more balance. I think a lot of the problem in social media is that we're really presenting only

[00:16:00] the best side of ourselves, and so connection is becoming entertainment. We're replacing feelings of interdependence, feelings of connection, by stimulation and socializing is not the same thing as friendship. I think that's what's getting really confused.

[00:16:30] Socializing, I would consider as more entertainment. It's play, which is also really necessary. As animals, we need play. For entertainment, we need play, because we're here to enjoy our lives, but it's very different than friendship. And so, the terms of friendship, I think are being defined on social media, and the terms of friendship are that you have to be positive, you have to be interesting, you have to entertain. There's this celebrity kind of energy that's taking over.

[00:17:00] There was a study done in the 1950s of people exiting high school and how many of them wanted to be famous, under 15%. Most recently, a similar study, over 80% felt that being famous was a number one goal for them. You can look at that in a positive way in the sense that the self-esteem movement was the last 20, 30 years. Telling our kids that they can do anything, there's a lot of positivity to that, but that can also create a lot of pressure because that means I have to hide the parts of myself that are human, my frailty, my fragility. That's what makes us human and that's what gives us the most meaning in life. You can't have meaning without struggle, and so a lot of people, I think, struggle with emptiness because of this.

[00:17:30] If you go down to the level of the nervous system, and what I've been talking about so far around being disconnected. What that means at the level of the nervous system, is we've become very disembodied. What that term "disembodied" means is that we're not connecting with our emotions as part of our human experience. In the West, especially, we're a culture defined by, "I think, therefore I am." My thoughts, my conscious mind, that's me.

[00:18:00] Belief in our own thoughts serves us when it's connected to what's happening in the moment. Our nervous system has many components to it that read and sense the environment, and guide us on how to respond. Like my stomach letting me know I'm hungry, pain lets me know that there's some force on my body that's causing trauma. Anxiety's primary purpose is to let me know there's something dangerous, there's something concerning in my environment. So, our emotions are bodily experiences. They're sensations in our body that inform us, and then we have this capacity for thought. We have [00:18:30] this capacity for reflection, to reflect and be able to choose. To be able to decide how to handle the situation.

[00:19:00] What's happened as we progress more and more in modern life, we're more and more disconnected from our sensations. We're more and more disconnected from reading the environment and a very common experience in modern man is feeling stuck in his head. We can become disconnected, or what we call disembodied. There's a word, embodied cognition. In the West, we're a culture that starts with the Cartesian idea of, "I think, therefore I am," very top-down.

[00:19:30] When we really look at the neuroscience and, I think, the human experience, we're actually very much bottom-up, in the sense that our senses, my heart, there's a lot of research now on how the heart has its own nervous system that stores information about relationships. The gut stores a lot of information about safety, and so we're informed a lot but we're now very disconnected in modern life, and we can create ideas in our minds, stories in our mind that become hindrances to really reading the environment and what's really happening. I think that's what we call the human condition. It's the human condition being this sense of somehow not quite being in the world anymore. I think that phenomenon is neurologically being stuck in our heads and no longer being as connected. I think that's related to how we manage depression and anxiety. We view these sensations, panic, sadness, or [00:20:00] heaviness. Rather than listening to those senses as information, we experience those as one more way that my body is betraying me, and we apply our own stories to it. I am weak ... ideas around what we need and what we don't need.

[00:20:30]   How do our thoughts impact chronic disease? I think the most important aspect of how our thoughts need to shift about chronic disease is our relationship with the sensations, our experiences. Reconnect with what our body is trying to tell us. Experiencing sadness, anxiety and concern, experiencing pain, again this is my body telling me what I need. This is my body telling me there is something out of balance.

[00:21:00]
[00:21:30]   When you're looking at chronic conditions, most chronic conditions are actually acute conditions that have become chronic, and I think that step of acute becoming chronic has a lot to do with the story we tell when we experience something. I think that mental health as an industry has created this problem a lot. We started out telling the story of faulty parenting and then faulty genes and chemical imbalances, and so our beliefs govern how we respond to some stress or pain or discomfort. If we have learned that there's something going wrong, that means that something is out of your control, your genes or something out of your control from your childhood is governing what's happening, you respond very differently than if you respond with resilience, with consciousness, that my emotions, my pain, that's my body telling me what I need, and alerting me to how to get in balance.

[00:22:00]
[00:22:30]
[00:23:00]   The first thing is reframing the story, so really truly listening to somebody's story, and then looking for places where there are set beliefs on why things happen. And then, asking us to take a step back and really reframe that and looking at where there are patterns as to how we perceive what's happening to us, and really asking us to question that. We don't come into this world with set beliefs. We come into this world very pure, just responding to our environment. Part of adapting, part of growing up, is learning how the world works, and we need to develop beliefs, because we can't decide at every moment, basing on all decisions, but sometimes we can get organized around core beliefs that I'm too much or I'm not enough, how I should be as a woman, how I should be as a man. Our culture can impose on us really narrow definitions of who we can be, and that can limit our ability to respond resiliently to stress and pain and hardship. We act based on what we think we should be doing versus really listening to what we need.

[00:23:30]   When you look at programs that help people transform their lives, when you look at healthcare programs or mental health programs that are resilient-based programs where it's really about transforming how I respond to the stress, there's a lot of research done on this. There are several key factors, one being the ability to change some daily practice, whether it's eating differently, meditating, or yoga. Another one being that you do it within a group, knowing that you're part of a whole group that's all committing to some change.

[00:24:00]
[00:24:30]   The most powerful one is meaningfulness. People who are able to go through some transformational change successfully, most often they have been able to connect that with something meaningful in their lives. Really, what does meaningful mean? Meaningful means that there's something that is beyond just my survival. This is actually not just about me. And so, I think the key is to start to really think about where do we derive purpose and meaning in our lives. Most people, eventually it comes to others or comes to the world as a whole, it comes to the Earth. Whether it's the climate or a sibling who needs something, or it's a coworker who needs something. I think it's really about shifting and realizing that the opportunities are all there. We may be able to go it alone in terms of survival, but feeling a part of something important, that's what it is to feel like you belong. There's a sense of a shared mission.

[00:25:00]   Neuroplasticity is a term that describes how the brain learns. We've known that if you exercise a certain muscle, the muscle grows. What you do over and over again, it strengthens. We know that in terms of the body. The brain, for a long time, was thought to be fixed. Once you go through adolescence and the frontal lobe grows, you're stuck with the brain you have, and we now know that's no longer true. Even into our 80s and 90s, if we decide to commit to doing something differently, regularly, it actually changes the architecture of the brain. It's based on a protein called myelin.

[00:25:30]	Our brains are really electric conduction systems, and just like if you insulate a wall, the heat doesn't leak, and that means you can preserve energy. When we do something repeatedly, patterns that get laid down in the brain, that happens to a protein called myelin that insulates the neurons, and so you get these reliable patterns. Just like your muscle can grow if you bikeride, if you decide to go for a bike ride, your brain also lays down a pattern of how to ride a bike and how it does that is this protein, myelin.

[00:26:00]

[00:26:30] Myelin breaks down every 21 days. I think that's why there are a lot of 21-day challenges, because it's really built around this idea of the half-life of myelin, the protein. What this means is that it really speaks to what I think a lot of people do know, that character matters, that routines matter. While I may have inherited a predisposition to depression or anxiety, I can also develop new habits at any point in my life that promote resilience and my ability to respond to sadness or to fear more robustly and more reliably.

[00:27:00] I think what it really means, which to me is the excitement of the paradigm shift we're in right now, is that we have this neuroscience that I can teach people about their own nervous systems, about their own body. I can tell people, "You know what? If you do this for 21 days, it's going to be really hard at first but by 21 days, your body is going to now have this mechanism where it becomes reliable, and that's when it becomes a habit." The negative cycle you get in, is really only there because it became a habit because you keep doing it. While that first week or two is hardest, committing to change can make a huge difference. It becomes a new habit and habits become your character.

[00:27:30] With genetics and the biological revolution at the end of the 20th century, there was so much we've gained in terms of understanding the relationship between our genes and our behavior; but I think that there was a false translation that happened that everything is, like, you have a gene for black hair, you have black hair. I have a gene for depression, I have depression, and if you're really looking at the epidemiological data, that's just not true.

[00:28:00] I think the difference is, I think, what's really coming back that the neuroscience is showing is that choices really matter. Routines really matter. Habits really matter and building character really matters. And so, I'm excited because we can be non-reductionistic about this, or I can look and say— what is a genetic predisposition bringing to your story? What does your early childhood and family structure bring to this story? What does your lifestyle bring to this story? What does the food system that you're subject to bring to this story, as well as character? How can you construct a character? How

[00:28:30] can you imagine the kind of person you want to be, and how can we together build a plan where you can actually get there? That's a much more exciting story. That's a much more inspiring story. The problem with many of the biological theories is they remove you from the experience. They remove your story from the experience. You're just subject to things that are outside your control, and I think neuroplasticity is a really valuable thing for us to know and to be able to teach people.

[00:29:00] The problem with refined foods is that we get these bursts of sugar. We get bursts of glucose into our system and our bodies are not designed for that. Sugar and carbohydrates, they trigger endorphin release. They also trigger serotonin release. That's that good, cozy, warm feeling we get when we overeat. That kind of numbing feeling, that's an endorphin high, but that's not the ideal way of getting

[00:29:30] sugar. I kind of equate that to getting money from a loan shark. He's ready to give you a burst of what you need but you're going to be in more debt, because if we are seeking out these bursts of serotonin and bursts of endorphins for feeling good, whatever goes up fast, comes down fast, and that's the problem. So, if we're seeking it out because we're needing comfort, then we are going to need to go back for more comfort. And that's why I've come to think actually sugar is the gateway drug in terms of creating that spike and depression, spike and depression. Where you get a burst of energy and then

[00:30:00] you're kind of feeling low and moody, I think that actually sets a lot of people up for other substance abuses.

[00:30:30] The key here is, like, serotonin is comfort and then dopamine. So, most antidepressants are either designed to boost serotonin or dopamine. Dopamine is the challenge neurotransmitter. We really are mostly designed actually to forget the food and then build comfort. And so really, it's comfort. What are all the other wonderful ways that can nurture us with comfort? Number one is actually physical contact.

[00:31:00] I come from a culture where physical contact is a lot more normal. We hug, we kiss, and what's lovely is to kind of see how much science is showing how touch is very essential to our nervous system. But then, if you also step back from a basic sense, look at all of the primates and mammals, touch is how we know that we are safe. The most basic part of comfort is knowing that I'm safe and knowing that I have others around me, and there's no better way than actual physical touch. It makes sense that, really, we're designed to actually seek serotonin through the comfort of safety. That's the most common thing when I work with people who struggle with addictive behavior, is helping them through meditation, mindfulness, and slowing down, and starting to become their own monitor, asking

[00:31:30] themselves with compassion and curiosity, "What is it I'm really seeking right now?" Let me get the food or the drug as a solution and let's get away from a judgmental stance on that and actually say you are seeking something. You need something. You're not getting something, but let's name what it is you really need and then give you a chance to explore ways you can get it that feel more nurturing to you, and that are more sustainable.

PEDRAM SHOJAI, OMD | Author: *The Urban Monk & The Art of Stopping Time*

Pedram Shojai: I was pre-med at UCLA. I had figured out sometime around high school that the easiest way to keep your parents off your back is to get good grades. I just started getting straight As and I was very good at school. As the son of immigrants who came to America, you're either going to be a doctor, lawyer, or engineer at that time.

[00:00:30] I went straight to UCLA. I was going to be a doctor. I was on that track. Then I started to become exposed to the medical system as a young man at UCLA. Interned with a couple of prominent doctors, I was shocked at what I saw compared to what I thought the profession was at the time. It's a big challenge when you come from a motivation that's Vitalistic to then get into a mechanistic framework where everything was about drugs and interventions that were pretty aggressive.

[00:01:00] At the same time I met a Tai Chi teacher on campus at UCLA. All of a sudden, I'm in this place where I'm feeling energy and I'm feeling better and I'm out in the sun doing all sorts of interesting exercises. I'm having all this life coursing through me while walking down these stale hospital corridors, handling patients that don't have much hope and dealing with doctors that have probably just as little for what they're able to do for them.

[00:01:30] I snapped. Now I look back, and I realize that the attending doctor I was working with was an angel because he put me on a different path in my life. I found a Kung Fu master I was studying with. I started to escalate my training with him. It turns out, he was a lineage holder under a temple training tradition that was unbroken from China, which is hard to say because most of those people were killed in the Cultural Revolution.

[00:02:00] My grandmaster made it out and I became the senior student of this person. All of a sudden, I'm doing this very different type of training. Then Chinese medicine became self-evident. It was the healing part of the same traditions I was learning. I never looked back. It was fascinating to me. It was interesting. I jumped in.

[00:02:30] My parents weren't too happy about it at the time. Their kid goes to UCLA and then goes off to become a witch doctor, right? I said, "Look, you know I'm always going to land on my feet. I'll be fine. Trust me, there's something here." It led me down a very interesting path.

The thing that really attracted me to Chinese medicine, Oriental medicine in general, is this notion of vitalism. When given a chance, the body can fight and be resilient and really build up its immunity, its strength, its resilience. It was part of a system where almost all of the ancient medical traditions were Vitalistic.

[00:03:00] Then, only after about World War II did this mechanistic, allopathic vision of medicine really take hold and become the way we operate. It's replaceable parts and mostly it's steroids and antibiotics and surgery. Now we're in a heyday, we're in a renaissance where all sorts of interesting things are happening. When I was studying this stuff, the options were limited.

[00:03:30] Chinese medicine to me really looks at the body as a whole, it looks at the person as a whole, and as compared to the Western framework where if it's a mind thing you go see a psychologist, if it's a spirit thing you go see your priest or your rabbi. The doctors have different specialties.

In Chinese medicine, this one individual looks at you and your entirety and addresses your concerns, whether they be your marital issues or the food you're eating. All is part of a holistic gestalt in your treatment. For me, that was very interesting. It seemed to speak to a lot of the problems modern humans seem to be having.

[00:04:00] Depression is an interesting subject because there's such a huge spectrum. Is it years of frustration that have now collapsed in on themselves to become depression? Is it food intolerance that's led to years of drain of the Vitalistic energy that keeps the body going so you just don't have enough juice to be happy
[00:04:30] and be there? Is it situational? Is it circumstantial? There are a lot of reasons someone would be depressed.

When you're looking at a holistic framework you look at the body in its entirety and say, "Okay, well, listen. Your systems are down. You're not sleeping well. Let's adjust your digestive capacity to bring out more energy from the food you're taking. Let's get you moving, let's get the energy in your body flowing, let's get some sunshine."

[00:05:00] All these things become part of a prescription for someone who, say, has depression. The depression isn't a deficiency in an SSRI. It becomes a worldview that has been shifted based on some sort of internal locus of control that's been lost or compromised. It's not always easy. Looking at the whole person, looking at the situation, and then coming up with solutions that are dealing not just with the biochemistry and the neurochemistry, but the socioeconomic status. Maybe you're depressed because you're broke all the time.

[00:05:30] There are a lot of reasons these negative items stack. As we know, people that have depression end up stacking more and more depressive items until eventually there's this feeling where you can't get out from under it.

As a Doctor of Oriental Medicine, we look at this and say, "Okay, well, what parts of your life can I start to lighten? What parts of your metabolism can we start working with? How can I give you little wins every single day and bring up a little bit of energy so we can then reinvest that in moving forward?"

[00:06:00] Asking a person who is depressed and down and out to put more time and energy into things is very challenging. It's like asking someone whose pockets are empty for cash. I have to find where I can loosen up some energy and enthusiasm and then work with that to move forward. I think Chinese medicine is very well-suited for that.

[00:06:30] I had an episode when I was running multiple medical groups in my twenties. I got over my skies. This thing grew and then the insurance coverage started to change. Money started to dry up. I didn't adjust and let go of people and all sorts of things that trained managers would do fast enough. It created a lot of financial stress.

I metabolized it as best I could. It helps to know Tai Chi, it helps to know Qigong, and meditation and all that. There's an old saying in the martial arts. It's, "I don't care how good you are. If you stand in the
[00:07:00] ring, eventually you're getting punched in the face." For me, it became this real understanding of how to shift the nature of a circumstance instead of stand there and get punched in the face with stress.

I can metabolize a lot of things. I'm a martial artist. I'm a yogi. I have all these things I can learn to offset
[00:07:30] the pain. Why stand there in the first place? I learned the hard way and lost some hair in the process. I really found my way around navigating life, boundaries, and circumstances better so you can resolve some of these problems and not stand there and have to have your systems deal with them.

When we're in our rest-and-digest physiology, it's when our body is doing what it's supposed to be
[00:08:00] doing, it's healing, it's clearing out toxins, it's digesting food. All of these parasympathetic functions are where we're supposed to be 99% of the time. This sympathetic nervous system is amazing to get us in and out of a crisis. It's designed for that.

[00:08:30] What's happened in the modern world is that these stressors, the sound of a screeching car tire, the sound of a helicopter, a text message that might be bringing something stressful, these are all starting to elicit calls to this emergency system that's not supposed to be used to the extent that it's being used and that we are so far over in the overuse and abuse of this sympathetic nervous system, that we're starting to become more and more wired for stress.

[00:09:00] It's starting to break our brains. It's starting to collapse our adrenal function, which means store more fat, have much worse temper, and not be able to be present because when you're here, when you're present, there is that parasympathetic feeling. Most of us have this low-grade anxiety because the stress is overwhelming and it's usually just bubbling up.

[00:09:30] That has a lot to do with the modern world, if you will, but also our interpretation of events, our ability to have better boundaries, and allow for certain things to come into our life. A lot of it, I've found is also just counter-management, time management, being able to say no to things when you already have too much on your plate. I think a lot of us have become people pleasers and oftentimes, take on more than we should and our bodies can account for. Then we're in time compression. That puts us into sympathetic overdrive again. It becomes a very vicious cycle.

[00:10:00] The gentleman who coined the term stress, Hans Selye back in the 50s, talked about distress, which is the negative type, and then eustress, which is the positive type. Stress has only a negative connotation within our culture. We know this in peak performance, we know this in all of the modern sciences coming out, which show that positive stressors that don't break you down and keep you on that razor's edge make you better.

[00:10:30] There are lots of good reasons to have stress. If it weren't for stress we wouldn't get out of bed. You get stressed when you don't have food and you have to go get it. Life brings on stress but then the ability to match that stress with what you need to do to deliver, render, show up, and learn and grow from that event oftentimes—if it's a razor's edge sometimes you fall over and it becomes detrimental and sometimes it helps you grow.

[00:11:00] I think the modern human needs to learn to find that line of stress and stay right under where it's overwhelming so that it becomes a growth tool in life. You can use stress to continue to grow and then you understand how stress works so that when you unplug, I call it drinking from infinity. You stop time.

You go hard, you work hard, and then you unplug and you relax fully and deeply so when you come back up you have the reserves and the resilience to grow again through stress as a tool.

[00:11:30] One of the most important things to do for managing stress is I always advocate with patients to look at their phones or their calendars and show me where they've built in times for rest and relaxation. You'll book an appointment for a hairdresser, you'll book an appointment for calls at work, and all these things that line up on the calendar. Then we say to ourselves, "Hey, I want to have quality time with my kids." "I want to spend more time with my wife." "I want to rest. I want to do yoga." Then, when I look at someone's phone I don't see any of those things in there.

[00:12:00] Making appointments with yourself and learning to leave that space and hold that space for yourself creates a bit of that work/life balance so that then we can decompress. It's like, "What am I supposed to be doing right now? I'm so freaked out. I feel guilty. Someone is watching. I'm not doing my homework." We have this anxiety that's always there instead of learning to unplug and be like, "No, no, no. This is my break right now. During my break I don't want to talk about work. I'm actually going to lie on the floor and take a nap or whatever I need." Giving yourself permission to relax I think is the first stop on that journey.

[00:12:30] Meditation, we've known for thousands of years, is a wonderful tool for self-discovery and relaxation and all these wonderful things have passed down from the Himalayas. It's like, "Okay, great. It's old. It must be true." Now you look at the data that's coming through and everyone is so excited about what it does to the brain and builds the resilience and all sorts of things that help us with neuroplasticity.

[00:13:00] You know, I didn't need that data back when I was a monk in the 90s because when you see a seasoned meditator, you see it immediately in their face. They're glowing. There's this feedback loop that's already there because you notice that this is a calm, beautiful person.

[00:13:30] What it's doing are multiple things. One, it's basically pulling our energy out of the limbic system, that fight-or-flight animal brain that's just like, "Get food. Survive. Get a mate. This is stressful." It brings us up into our higher centers. The prefrontal cortex in particular, is interesting because that is where negation of impulses happens.

When we want to separate ourselves from the monkeys it's our ability to say, "Monkey, no," to an impulse that really gets us into our higher human functions, morality, ethics, all these wonderful things that have helped us build society. Stress pulls us out of that.

[00:14:00] When you're meditating you start to build this part of the brain. That's the part that says, "No, you know what? I don't think you want to have that cheesecake. I know it sounds like a good idea right now but no cheesecake. That's not on your diet." It's that moment where that voice can come in and stop us from making terrible decisions, whether it's in our marital life, business life, or just our everyday diet.

[00:14:30] That comes from empowering the part of the brain that runs that show. Meditation clearly shows that that's what it can enhance. If all I had for negation of impulses, meditation would be the best drug in town. It does way more than just that.

[00:15:00] There is no one right way to meditate. I think that meditation has actually been taught incorrectly in the West in many ways because it's basically been relegated to a funky, Himalayan form of a Quaalude, right? Which is, "I'm going to get really stressed out and then I'm going to do my thing and try to come down again." I put it to you that I see meditation as an operating system.

It's something that should be running in the background at all times. Basically, having you become aware of how you feel, thoughts that come up, and say, "Hey, listen, you're starting to get agitated. What is that?" If you had 15 open windows on your desktop and you're supposed to be working on a document and then your Skype and your IM and all these things are going off, you can't focus on anything. That's how our mind works.

[00:15:30] Meditation would be cruising through that mental desktop just closing those windows and keeping you focused on what it is you're doing here and now. There's breath work meditation, there's mantra, there's yantra. You can work with sound, light, visualizations, prayer as coupled with meditation. There are lots of ways to climb the mountain. I tend to tell students that you need to go with where your disposition is. If you're an artist and you're visually inclined maybe you want to use visuals for your meditation. That's your way in.

[00:16:00] I think one of the core disciplines in meditation that should be learned by all and then practiced to whatever extent makes sense is slowing and monitoring the breath because that is anchoring the attention on something that's real. You can't go very long without breathing. It ties you in with the core physiological need of your body and it brings you into focusing in on something that's happening here [00:16:30] and now. That in breath and out breath you have, some wonderful space to navigate internally that you become aware of once you slow down enough to perceive it.

There are a lot of neurotoxic elements inside of our foods. There are a lot of heavy metals. There's a lot of toxicity in general in our culture now. First stop: just eat real food, eat organic food. Try to grow your own food. Mitigate the damage because there's a lot that is coming at us at all times that would compromise our health.

[00:17:00] A lot of these things lodge in the brain, a lot of these things can be causing things like Alzheimer's and dementia and really damaging our ability to process because the brain is an electric signal generator and it's got a lot of electrical conductivity that runs through it. Anything that gets in the way of that, especially if you're talking heavy metals, becomes a very big issue. This is probably one of the core issues of our time.

[00:17:30] Now meditation helps build up higher cortical function. I've looked at some studies that show increased density in those parts of the brain. It's really about training the brain to rewire the circuitry towards parts that are those higher functioning centers. It becomes an incredible discipline in mind/body awareness that I feel when coupled with movement practice where you're using eyes, mind, body, and
[00:18:00] breath to coordinate the sensory motor strip on top of the cortex, that's when people start to become fully integrated.

I've seen lots of interesting work with kids with ADD and attention deficit issues becoming more embodied and using mind/body practices to really bring balance to the brain. The mind/body practices on one end are wonderful but you have to stop the bleeding. You can't be chewing on lead pellets and
[00:18:30] doing meditation and getting away with it. It has to be a lifestyle hygiene issue coupled with a practice.

I look at meditation like flossing for the mind. You do it because it's the right thing to do and moves you forward. If you have four hours to sit and cultivate enlightenment practice, great, good for you. You have more time than most. At least it will help offset and keep you away from the walls caving in if
[00:19:00] you're just in a busier phase of life right now and you need something to help you that is healthy and holistic.

I like all movement because we do so little of it. I'm a martial artist, I'm a Kung Fu guy. Tai Chi and Qigong are very specifically designed to help influence movement with brain and body and breath and all these wonderful things that are built into their architecture. What are we talking about?

[00:19:30] We're talking about moving the right hemisphere, coordinating it with the left, moving the upper and the lower body, and challenging the brain in a basic cross crawl. If you look at a baby going from creeping to crawling, that type of neurological development is an incredibly important part of our human development. If you look at how we have stopped moving, the inability of the body to move across hemispheres and up and down has created blockages in the circuitry of the brain.

[00:20:00] We're just as optimized as we could be because we're not moving. I want three-dimensional, multi-dimensional, multi-plane movement and a lot of that comes through the core and then uses the whole body in moving so you can move in an intelligent way using your physics in the right way.

The world we live in is nuts. If you're lucky you get eight hours a night to sleep, which is wonderful
[00:20:30] because you're lying down and recovering and all that. The average American is spending over an hour a day getting to and from work. When they're at work, they're spending about eight hours sitting at a desk doing whatever they're doing.

We're talking about very few hours in the day where we're moving. Our ancestors were hunting and gathering, they were moving around all the time. When they were sitting they were sitting on the floor
[00:21:00] where their body weight had to be supported by their postural muscles and their hips would open up. There weren't all these unnatural positions that were compromising the biomechanics of the body.

Couple that with nutrient deficient food that's calorically-enhanced and calorically-rich just to fill you up and store calories. What we're doing is we've skewed the entire math. What we need is energy to burn, move, and fuel the movement of this incredible, incredible machine that can jump off cliffs and do 15 tumbles and dive into the water and all sorts of things we see on YouTube. We're capable of that. What
[00:21:30] have we done to support our ability to move? What have we done today to do that?

[00:22:00] I'm a big fan of environmentally hacking everything: a standing desk at work, having a timer that goes off every 25 minutes to do five minutes of exercise/stretching/breathing/whatever it is that you need to check in with your body. What that has shown to do is bring up the active metabolic rate so that then your resting metabolic rate is higher so you're burning more calories at rest, you're using your postural muscles, you're moving around, you're not shutting down the circulation, and in doing so you're keeping the body much more resilient and healthy.

[00:22:30] Couple that with getting outside, getting some sunshine, moving around, getting all your social interactions back instead of being stuck on a phone. We have a bit of a homecoming where humanity can come back to being vibrantly alive instead of becoming these drone automatons that we see in cubicles everywhere. It's the wrong direction.

Everyone talks about the healthcare crisis being a healthcare debate. It's a healthcare finance debate. The healthcare debate is what we do every day, how we eat every day, and how we live. It's a lifestyle issue. The medicine and all the interventions that come that are super expensive, once we've broken it, that's because we are not living correctly. The front end is everything. It starts with movement.

[00:23:00] It doesn't take a neurologist to tell you that lack of sleep makes you crazy. Sleep is incredibly important for the remapping of neurons, of consolidation, trimming, of thoughts and emotions and processes that happened all day. It's like you eat a meal, you have to digest it. You have an experience. Your mind has to digest it. That's what happens during sleep.

[00:23:30] Psychologically, it's incredibly important to just give your brain that down time to start processing the events of the day, that are coupled with emotions, anxieties, and all things that come with having a human experience to rectify and bring things into balance. That's an important part.

[00:24:00] There's also an important part with growth hormone where we're actually helping heal the body's tissues, grow, and do the things we need to do to substantiate using this body the way it needs to be used. One of the major immunomodulators is melatonin. When we go down, it's when we shut down the amusement park to clean things up, to test everything out, to pressure test the rides, and make sure tomorrow is going to be another good day.

[00:24:30] If we don't get that, we start to have issues carrying forth in the next day. Look at the kind of behavioral fallout. I didn't get enough sleep last night because my baby was up. This morning I had to have that third cup of coffee because, Lord knows, I've still got to show up and still be who I need to be at work.

By 10am, my blood sugar has crashed. I'm snacking on things I would otherwise not be snacking on, going back for some more coffee, and now I've thrown off my blood sugar, I've thrown off my adrenals, I'm at this place where I'm wired and tired and by the end of the night I'm not really as friendly as I should be to my children.

[00:25:00] You see this incredible fallout that carries forward into life, that comes from a poor night's sleep, that then becomes behavioral, becomes marital problems, all these sorts of things that we see. It all starts from starting to slow down.

One of the things I tell my patients and students all the time is three hours before bedtime, no more artificial lights. We like to have candles on in the evening. Think about it. Hundreds of thousands of years, our species sat by fires and had torches and candles and that's what light was. That red light does not drive our physiology into imbalance. It doesn't keep us up. It doesn't keep us cranking the way [00:25:30] society would have us do.

Once you start learning to decelerate in the evenings, to value sleep, and give yourself that sacred, empty space to go down, recover, and heal, that's when you start to see the benefits ripple out across your health, relationships, waistline, everything.

[00:26:00]   You want to have a healthy brain. You need to move your body, you need to breathe deeply. You need to couple whatever you're doing with exercise and understand your relationship with food. Your brain likes fat. Good, healthy fats. Avocados, olive oil, all you want. Feed your brain so your brain feeds you. Then you are in a matrix of better decisions. You're in a matrix of having more energy.

[00:26:30]   What happens when you have more energy in life? When you have energy and clarity you have the power, the personal power, to make better decisions, to move your career ahead, to spend that extra time with your kids. All of the things we miss out on when we're not present and we're checked out are a function of not having enough energy to our brains.

[00:27:00]   Once you start to feel this and you start to move with it, investing a little bit of that energy into furthering this trajectory, your brain starts getting more resilient and healthy and charged with more energy, there's no turning back. It's like a light bulb goes off and that light then becomes the guiding light of your life. You will have a much better, fulfilling life because of it.

DR. RANGAN CHATTERJEE | Author: *The Four Pillar Plan*

Dr. Mark Hyman:	Dr. Chatterjee, you run an extraordinary mission in the UK, and you created a show called *Doctor In The House*, a BBC show where you go into people's homes and help them transform their lives using Functional Medicine. Tell us why you're doing this, and what do you expect to get out of this?
Dr. Rangan Chatterjee: [00:00:30] [00:01:00]	This show, *Doctor In The House* is a series of documentaries that's gone out on BBC Television. I think what my aim with this show is, is to demonstrate to people that no matter what condition you have, there are things that you can do with your lifestyle every single day that are going to improve it. Now, look, sometimes, you can reverse disease. You can absolutely prevent disease, but even if you don't have a label or a disease, actually making changes to your nutrition, making changes to your lifestyle can actually improve the way you feel, whether that's just your mood, your energy level, fatigue, all these things. I don't think people really realize that, so I've been very lucky to actually have this opportunity. Whether it's Type 2 diabetes, which I helped a lady reverse in 30 days, which two years on, she still does not have Type 2 diabetes, or whether it's fibromyalgia. Fibromyalgia pains, one in six weeks or anxiety attacks went down by 80% in six weeks. I used a different approach. You know, Mark, Functional Medicine, I used that framework to help me look at these problems in a different way.
Dr. Mark Hyman: [00:01:30]	It's really extraordinary. I think about the show. It's called *Doctor In The House*. You literally go into people's homes. You stay with them. You watch them. You explore their house. You understand the patterns that are going on there. What exactly do you do? You go into the house and just hang out and look in their fridge or cook with them? Tell us about how this all works.
Dr. Rangan Chatterjee: [00:02:00] [00:02:30]	Yes, well, it really depends on what that family's complaint is. The first thing to understand is - I don't know when I knock on the door for the first time. I don't actually really know what's going on there, okay? I'm not involved with choosing who that patient is and what their problem is. My job is, like it is with every patient in my clinic, is to do the best that I can for them. In this last series, it was quite a pretty complex case. It's actually much more complex in the first series, but when you strip these things back and you look at what are the factors in that person's life that is contributing to the way they feel, you can always do something, always. Look, what do I do? Well, in the lady who had Type 2 diabetes, what's amazing about going into someone's house is that you start to see things that you would never see in your clinic.
[00:03:00]	In clinic, we ask patients questions. They give us answers, but the thing is, is that often, they won't tell us the truth. That's not because they want to lie to us. It's because they will filter the information that they think you need to hear. What was happening in that house, I was seeing breakfast, lunch, dinner, nighttime snack, what is in their fridge? What are they really eating, rather than what they tell me they're eating? On a personal level...
Dr. Mark Hyman:	You do a fridge biopsy?
Dr. Rangan Chatterjee:	I did a fridge biopsy. Yes, absolutely, but not in every case. Not in every single case, but there were a few cases where I had to go in and actually really re-educate them on what should be in their kitchen.
Dr. Mark Hyman: [00:03:30]	When you went in there, what were you finding? Often us doctors, don't get that window, but it's extraordinary to actually see how people are living, their stress levels. Are they exercising? How they manage their lives, what they're buying, what's in their cupboards? You know how they're

cooking, when they eat. You get to see an extraordinary amount of information that tells you something, so what were the things that you found?

Dr. Rangan Chatterjee:
[00:04:00]
Yes, well, it's the things ... We know well, Mark, the things we talk about all the time that it always comes down to the same things in people's kitchens. There are too many refined and processed carbohydrates, breakfast cereals, refined breads that have sugars as an ingredient.

Dr. Mark Hyman:
Like a double whammy, flour and sugar.

Dr. Rangan Chatterjee:
Yes, ready meals.

Dr. Mark Hyman:
It's like bread that doubles as cake.

Dr. Rangan Chatterjee:

[00:04:30]
Yes, exactly. Then, you open the cupboards, and you see all the soft drinks, the carbonated drinks, even the diet drinks. There's so much in there that, I think sometimes, we in the health world, we talk about these things. We assume that the message is getting out there, but you go out there in the real world...people still don't know how toxic these foods are for the way that their bodies feel but also how their brains feel. Food is a big thing. It never ceases to amaze me how simple changes to someone's diet within days can impact the way they feel.

Dr. Mark Hyman:
Days, right?

Dr. Rangan Chatterjee:
Within days.

Dr. Mark Hyman:
As a doctor practicing medicine, we prescribe drugs.

Dr. Rangan Chatterjee:
Yes.

[00:05:00]
Dr. Mark Hyman:
We rarely see drugs have that big an impact in such a short time.

Dr. Rangan Chatterjee:
Yes.

Dr. Mark Hyman:
Even in a long time.

Dr. Rangan Chatterjee:

[00:05:30]
I am on a mission in the UK. I'm on a mission to help transform the way that the public views health because I think we see the brain as separate from the body. I think we see the heart as separate from the liver, as separate from the gut. What we're realizing now is that the body is this interconnected being. Your hormones influence your brain. You gut microbiome influences your brain. Everything interacts with each other.

Dr. Mark Hyman:
You're talking about going into people's homes and noticing things that cause brain damage. What were the things you found that were most affecting people's brains and cognition and be able to focus and be present?

Dr. Rangan Chatterjee:
[00:06:00]

[00:06:30]

[00:07:00]
I think there's four key things that I saw in people's houses that were affecting their brain. They're the four things that I think affect our health, in general, and the four things that I think we've all got control over - what we're eating, how we're moving, the quality of our sleep, and our stress levels. The top two for me that I saw would be food and stress. I think stress is something that people often don't think about with their brain health. I think it's a big problem these days. We're living in a society where we're overworked. We're under-slept. We've got a constant stream of emails, tweets, Facebook. We're never switching off. For me, I find my email inbox stressful. We know that this psychosocial stress raises levels of our stress hormone cortisol. Cortisol damages our brain. If cortisol is too high for too long, it can damage the cells in our hippocampus, which is

where we lay down our memory. I think if people really understood that, and we can help people understand that, that actually, the stress in our lives is impacting our brain function.

[00:07:30] I always talk to people. "Get 10 to 15 minutes of me time every day. Switch devices off. Just sit there. Read a book. Meditate. Do some yoga. Something, but just focus on that one task." I see that having profound impact all the time. I make it simple, Mark, for people. I have made deals with my patients before. They say to me, "Oh, doctor. Meditation, I've heard about that, but I don't have time to meditate." I said, "Okay. Can you commit to two minutes a day?" That's short, because they think I'm going to say they have to do 20 minutes a day. I remember on the first series of *Doctor In The House*, I had a lady with menopausal symptoms. Her daughter wanted to prescribe hormones for her. She didn't want that. Again, in four weeks, we got her menopausal [00:08:00] symptoms down from 15 out of 17 on the British Menopause Society questionnaire down to two out of 17. A critical component of that was this 15-minute relaxation in the evening.

I made a deal with her. I said, "Look, you have four minutes to brush your teeth every day, right?" She goes, "Yes." I said, "Why is that?" She said to me, "Well, because it's been prioritized since I've been a child. That's just my normal habit." I said, "Let's make that meditation your normal [00:08:30] habit, but let's start with two minutes a day. If you could start with two minutes, that becomes five minutes. That becomes 10," but if I start with 15, 20 minutes, they do it for two days. They don't manage to do it the third day, and they give up.

Dr. Mark Hyman: Yes. That's powerful. Yes, that's very powerful, this meditation. People don't realize. They think it's just a way of relaxing, but it actually reprograms your biology. It increases stem cell production. It decreases inflammation. It boosts your immune system. It helps regulate your [00:09:00] hormones. It improves your blood sugar control. I mean it's got massive effects, and I think one thing people don't realize about stress is that it causes a leaky brain. We talk about leaky gut, but there's a barrier in the brain that protects the brain. When they're stressed, that barrier breaks down, and a lot of that outside influence is going to harm the brain. This is quite extraordinary. Tell me more about this gut issue, because I know that you focus a lot on the gut. You were sharing a story about an obese kid who had gut issues, allowed him to fix those and ended up helping him lose a lot of weight. How do you approach the gut from a point of view of Functional Medicine within these patients?

Dr. Rangan Chatterjee: Yes. Look, I think this is something I didn't learn at medical school, but this has been part of the
[00:09:30] training with the Institute for Functional Medicine and all the additional education that I now do. I've learned that the health of the gut is critical, yes, for the health of the brain, but also plays a critical role in things like obesity, mood problems, all kinds of things. How do I approach it?

[00:10:00] Well, first of all, I want to understand what that patient is eating, okay, because we know that the biggest and the fastest way to change the health and the composition of your gut bugs is by changing your diet. There are so many tests you can do. I sometimes run stool tests to have a look at what is the combination of bugs inside us? I think a lot of people still don't understand that we've got trillions of bugs that live inside us. Actually, it's the combination of those bugs and the [00:10:30] community that is probably more important than actually the individual components. One of the biggest measures I look for now is the diversity. How diverse is your gut?

Depending on what I find, that will also dictate what I then do with the patient. This 11-year-old boy you mentioned who was obese. He was extremely obese, and he was struggling with his weight. His fasting insulin was 33. Now, depending which doctor you ask, we want to see a fasting insulin under four, certainly under six, so 33...

Dr. Mark Hyman: ...was off the chart.
[00:11:00]

Dr. Rangan Chatterjee:

[00:11:30]

Off the charts. In six weeks, we got it to nine and a half from 33, but we did that with two measures. Yes, we cut out refined and processed carbohydrates. Things like your refined breads, your cereals, the sweet drinks, the muffins, the doughnuts... We increased healthy natural fats, a lot of avocados, a lot of nuts, a lot of good quality meat and fatty fish, but also, we put a rainbow chart on this little boy's fridge. All the colors of the rainbow were there. I said, "You have to tick off every color every single day, okay?" He did it.

Dr. Mark Hyman:

Not by eating Skittles though?

Dr. Rangan Chatterjee:
[00:12:00]

[00:12:30]

Not by eating Skittles. You know, you've got the lycopene in tomatoes, or as you guys say, tomatoes. You've got the blue-purple pigment in blueberries. What people don't realize, I think, is that there is communication between our gut and our brain. When our gut makes chemicals, and those chemicals, via the vagus nerve, actually are attached to receptors in our brain. That can change the way our brain operates. It's very, very powerful to understand that by changing what you eat, changing the health of your gut, you change the health of your brain. Fiber, I think, is very, very key. I'm not talking about All-Bran. I'm talking about the fiber from plant foods like if you eat every color of the rainbow every single day, you're going to get lots of different sources of fiber.

[00:13:00]

The fiber comes down. Your gut bugs feed on that fiber, and they make short-chain fatty acids. These are chemicals, really, that are anti-inflammatory. They help our immune system. Some studies are showing they're anti-cancer. It's really incredible. Just by increasing plant-based fiber in your diets, not only are you getting all these polyphenols, not only are getting all these lovely phytonutrients, but you're also making compounds in your gut that influence your brain. It's remarkable.

Dr. Mark Hyman:

[00:13:30]

Yes. It's interesting you mention the short-chain fatty acids. Most people don't know what those are, but they're basically the fuel that the bacteria make to feed your colon cells. It's really a very symbiotic relationship. We know that for example, like you said, all these fibers help one of the most important compounds called butyrate, but when you eat wheat flour, which I don't mean whole wheat or regular wheat, flour is treated with a compound called calcium propionate, which is another short-chain fat that's very toxic. It can cause ADD, behavior problems, autism, inflammation. In fact, in animal models, it induces autistic behavior when you inject it into the animals. While you're eating all these bran and processed foods, not only are we getting the sugar, but we're getting some of these really adverse compounds.

[00:14:00]

A lot of people suggest that this approach, Functional Medicine, is expensive. It's difficult. It's hard to do. If you don't have resources, how do you get it done? The testing, the supplements... but the truth is, you and I know that it actually isn't that hard with basic principles like you mentioned - food, sleep, exercise, stress reduction that are either free or food you have to buy anyway. Just change what you buy. It can actually have an enormous impact on your health. How do you do this if you don't have resources?

Dr. Rangan Chatterjee:
[00:14:30]

[00:15:00]

Yes, Mark, that's a great question. It's something that people always say. Even when I went around the country in the UK filming *Doctor In The House*, I would stay with families from all different sections of economic backgrounds. Cost would sometimes come up, but what I've realized like you've already mentioned, is that 80%, I would say, is free. 80% of what we need to do with our lifestyle for most people is freely available to us. If we talk about these four pillars: food, sleep, movement and relaxation, okay, what can people do in their diet? Very simple, if you reduce refined and processed carbohydrates, breads, muffins, pastas, the ones that are highly-processed, and you increase healthy natural fats like avocados, nuts, fatty fish, that's something you can do immediately with your food that's going to have an impact on your health.

Dr. Mark Hyman:

That's true.

Dr. Rangan Chatterjee: [00:15:30]	Movement. Whatever someone is currently doing with their movement, they can self-assess and go, "Am I moving enough?" If not, maybe something simple like just putting an alarm on your phone once every hour to remind you to get up and walk around the block. A tip I say is drink more water because if you drink more water, then, you have to get up regularly to go and pee, but it gets you up.
Dr. Mark Hyman:	If that's really an exercise, go to the bathroom, I think you're in trouble.
Dr. Rangan Chatterjee:	I agree.
Dr. Mark Hyman:	Better than nothing.
Dr. Rangan Chatterjee: [00:16:00] [00:16:30] [00:17:00]	Look, it's about meeting people where they're at. It's all very well for me to say, "You need to do X amount of exercise every day." That will work for some people, but I like to break it down and make it simple. Whatever somebody is currently doing, if they move more, that's going to have an impact on their physical health, on their brain health. I like the 10,000-step that you target. I think it's a really good easily measurable target for people. I've seen it with patients. They can get to the evening. They've already done six and a half thousand steps, and they're like, "You know what? I'm going to go for a quick walk before dinner." It's something measurable for people, but the other thing with movement is I think we've really neglected muscle and strength training. I always talk to my patients, whether they're 20-year-old patients who want to get fitter and stronger or whether it's a 75-year-old patient. I go through, and I'm there in the consultation room with them, showing them exercises because what I've realized, Mark, is that you can refer to various specialists, but there's something powerful in that interaction with that patient. If I then take my jacket off and say, "Hey, look. What about this? Can you do this?" I will do that in the consultation room with them to inspire them because our job, I believe, is to inspire a patient when they walk out to make them feel, "I can do this."
Dr. Mark Hyman:	You drop down, do 50 push-ups in the exam room?
Dr. Rangan Chatterjee: [00:17:30] [00:18:00]	I had done that, but no. Sometimes, I've got patients like a 72-year-old lady I had in-clinic a couple of weeks ago. She was nervous. I said, "Okay. Well, look, I've got this thing that I call a five-minute kitchen workout, that I teach people to do in their kitchen." I try and remove the obstacle of paying for a gym membership, getting a personal trainer. I love the gym. People like having a personal trainer. That's great, but I'm saying you can do a five-minute strength workout in your kitchen every single day. A recent couple I treated...they were in their early 60s. They hadn't done any form of strength training for maybe 20, 30 years. They were concerned about their brain health. They said, "Doctor, what can I do?" I explained to them how strength training is very important for their bodies and how exercise in general, but strength training also increases levels of BDNF, brain-derived neurotrophic factor, which is like...
Dr. Mark Hyman:	... Miracle-Gro for your brain.
Dr. Rangan Chatterjee: [00:18:30] [00:19:00]	Exactly, Miracle-Gro for your brain. Who doesn't want Miracle-Gro for your brain. They were nervous. I showed them what they could do in their kitchen. Just five simple exercises, a wall press-up, a kitchen worktop dip. I showed them. I talked them through it. When they came back a few weeks later, they said, "Doc, we were scared, but we started doing it in the kitchen." Within two weeks, they were doing it seven days a week in their landing upstairs while their evening bath was running. This is a couple in their 60s, no strength training at all, but by showing them that it is free, it is simple and it is doable, they felt great. They started doing it every day. I think every single patient has the ability to do that.

BROKEN BRAIN

Dr. Mark Hyman: [00:19:30]	It's true. I mean I often do what I call the seven-minute workout, so two minutes longer. All you need is a chair and your own body, and it's powerful. It's a high-intensity workout. It's strength training. It's portable. You can do it anywhere. It's extraordinary, the power of that. I hadn't done a ton of integral training, and I do this bicycle loop. I do it in about, usually 55 minutes. All winter, I didn't ride my bike, and I did this seven-minute training. When I started riding my bike in the spring, I was riding five minutes faster day one, which was striking to me that my body responded that easily and quickly. It's very powerful.
Dr. Rangan Chatterjee: [00:20:00]	I was going to say, Mark, sleep is something that I don't think people realize how important sleep is. We talk about brain health. We talk about the beta-amyloid protein, this protein which accumulates in our brain in conditions like Alzheimer's disease. We know that when we sleep deeply and we sleep for long enough, actually, our body processes a lot of this waste that builds up, including beta-amyloid protein and clears it out.
Dr. Mark Hyman:	I think your brain only detoxifies at night.
Dr. Rangan Chatterjee: [00:20:30] [00:21:00]	Exactly, and what I think is so powerful about that is if you explain that to a patient, you give them the science that they need to understand how important that sleep is. It's not just about, "Hey, you need to sleep more," because everyone knows that, but how are we going to help our patients sleep better? The first thing is we have to explain to them why it's important for them. If we'd done that, then often, all someone needs to do is prioritize their sleep. For many people, that's all they have to do because in the world that we're living in today, if we're not prioritizing sleep, sleep tends to fall by the wayside. There's too many temptations with Netflix or whatever. I'm as guilty as anyone of being tempted.
[00:21:30]	Sometimes, all people have to do, and I say it to them. I say, "Look, what about the next seven days? All you do is you go to bed half an hour a night earlier. Tell me how you feel in seven days." I'm telling you, more often than not, people feel better. They make better food choices the next day because they've slept better. They've got more energy. They feel sharp in their brain. That brain fog has gone down. These are simple free interventions that people can do. It doesn't cost money.
Dr. Mark Hyman:	No, no, no.
Dr. Rangan Chatterjee:	It doesn't cost anything.
Dr. Mark Hyman: [00:22:00]	The food thing is interesting because well, yes, I think that eating well is expensive. You don't have to get the most expensive cut of meat or the most expensive rare vegetables, but eating just real food doesn't have to be that much more. In fact, I went to this family as part of The Doctor Oz show that I was on where we went in Florida. They lived in a very small little house, family of six, very poor. We got them eating real food. I went to their house and visited them. I saw coconut oil and almonds and avocados. I said, "Wow, isn't this expensive for you?" They're like, "No, it's actually cheaper than what we're eating before because we bought a case of soda for each of our family every week."
[00:22:30]	You start cutting out all this stuff that they're buying, the processed food, which is actually pretty expensive when you think of pennies per nutrient. When you actually look at how nutrient poor it is, you're getting that very much for your money. You're getting a lot of calories, but not a lot of nutrients. They actually felt better. They lost, I think, 300 pounds as a family, and they loved it. They started spreading to their relatives. It was done on a budget, and I think there's a big myth about how it's expensive to eat real foods. It's really not.
Dr. Rangan Chatterjee: [00:23:00]	Yes. The first family I ever went to, first part of my documentary series, *Doctor In The House*, I remember really clearly the very first day. I met the family. I had not diagnosed Type 2 diabetes at

[00:23:30]	that point because I hadn't run bloods. I hadn't done anything yet. They didn't know what was going on with their health. That's why I came in. That evening, the father of that family said, "Hey, doc. Come on, let's go. I'll tell you what we normally eat." I went in the car with him, and we drove 15 minutes out of town to a fast food restaurant. We went through the drive through, and he ordered four meals, but each family member, so there's four people in the family, had two meals each. This cost 48 pounds. We're talking about $65, something like that. That's just for one evening meal. They were doing this about five nights a week.
[00:24:00] Dr. Mark Hyman:	That's right. People don't realize.
Dr. Rangan Chatterjee:	Yes. It was amazing because what was interesting about that, that what he said, "Doc, I feel a bit embarrassed that you're going to see all these." I said, "Hey, don't. Look, I just want to observe. The more I know about what you're currently doing, the more I can help you." What was interesting is that A, that's a lot of money, and when I moved them over to eating real fresh whole food, they were saving money.
Dr. Mark Hyman:	Saving money, right.
Dr. Rangan Chatterjee: [00:24:30]	The other things was he felt bad in front of me that he was eating this. Actually, one level intuitively as a family, they knew that actually, what they were eating wasn't particularly good for them. I think a lot of people around the country, around the world know that fast food and junk food is probably not good for them. The question is, why are they not changing?
Dr. Mark Hyman:	Because they don't know what to do.
Dr. Rangan Chatterjee:	Exactly. That's the key. That's what we need to help them see...what else they can do.
Dr. Mark Hyman: [00:25:00]	Yes, that's powerful. I think that's true. I observed the same thing. I mean they actually don't know what to do. They know what not to do. They try not to do it, but if you take a rotisserie, I mean a chicken, a couple of chickens, whole chickens, throw them in the oven. Make a salad, some roasted sweet potatoes, that's much less expensive to feed a family of four than going to a fast food and spending $60.
Dr. Rangan Chatterjee:	Yes, absolutely. I agree. I think it's really important that message gets out.
Dr. Mark Hyman:	By the time he gets there and comes back, it's about the same amount of time spent, actually.
Dr. Rangan Chatterjee: [00:25:30] [00:26:00]	Yes, so that's him. Then, there's the gas cost of driving 15 minutes there and back. That's half an hour driving, and a $65 meal. That's a lot of money if you're doing that five nights a week. It's really remarkable. I think a lot of time, in the wellness community, we often don't think that we don't have that realization that there's actually a lot of communities out there who don't know this and need help and understanding. I'll tell you something I feel incredibly passionate about. I don't know what it's like in the US, but in the UK, a lot of doctors will say, "Ah, you know, patients don't listen. They don't listen to what we tell them." I've got a problem with that because I genuinely believe that people don't want to be unwell. If we can explain it to that patient in a language that they understand, that it means something to them. I find, by and large, people want to make that change.
Dr. Mark Hyman:	They do.
Dr. Rangan Chatterjee: [00:26:30]	If we do this right, if you've got 10 minutes with a patient or 15 minutes or 20 minutes, and you say to someone with Type 2 diabetes, which we know can also affect your brain, your blood sugar...if you talk to them about medication, about what you need to do and what drugs you're

[00:27:00]	going to need to be on and right at the end, you say, "Yes, but also, if you can just change your diet, lose some weight, that's going to help you." That's very different from starting off and saying, "Hey, you've got this condition. Yes, we've got some drugs, but look, there's plenty you can do with your lifestyle. I'm going to teach you. I'm going to show you what you can do. Are you interested?" I tell you, people say yes. I think it's the way that we don't prioritize as a profession, we assume patients won't do it.
Dr. Mark Hyman:	Yes. It's when we say, "Well, I told them to lose weight and eat better and exercise. They didn't do it." I'm like, "How helpful is that? Eat better, exercise. I'll see you in three months. If that doesn't work, we'll use drugs." Well, that is not good medicine.
Dr. Rangan Chatterjee: [00:27:30]	Exactly, so I think we can make a difference. We can change people's health, and people want to get healthier. People want their brains to function. Who wants to wake up with brain fog? Nobody wants that because it impacts not only their health, but it impacts their relationships with their spouses, with their children, with their work colleagues. That then causes more stress. Stress releases cortisol. Cortisol starts to damage your brain, and you're in this vicious cycle. What we need to find is the lever to turn for that patient to start. Instead of a negative cycle, let's start a positive cycle that helps feeding more and more health.
Dr. Mark Hyman: [00:28:00]	Dr. Chatterjee, how do you keep your brain healthy? What do you do every day to maintain your health? I mean you work hard. You travel. You're on a TV show. You have a clinic. I mean it's not easy.
Dr. Rangan Chatterjee:	It's not easy.
Dr. Mark Hyman:	You have a family, two kids.
Dr. Rangan Chatterjee: [00:28:30]	Yes, you're right, Mark. It's not easy particularly when traveling because when you're in your own environment and you've got everything surrounded by you that actually helps you stay healthy, it's okay but obviously, I'm traveling at the moment, traveling out here to see you and do our filming. It is incredibly difficult. What do I do? Okay, first of all, I'm prepared. I remember you saying a few years back about not getting yourself in a food emergency. I think you're spot on because if you're not prepared, you're going to find yourself hungry, tired, craving something. If you're in an airport, often, there's nothing but sugar or processed foods. Like I said, how do I keep myself healthy, because I do live and breathe this myself.
[00:29:00]	Again, I talk about food, movement, sleep, relaxation. Food, I will eat whole real food pretty much every day even when I'm traveling. Did I do that six, seven years ago? No, okay? It was a slow process. Was it hard at first? Yes. It had its challenges, but now, it's normal for me.
Dr. Mark Hyman:	It's automatic.
Dr. Rangan Chatterjee: [00:29:30] [00:30:00]	It's automatic. I'm not even tempted anymore. My taste buds have shifted. I've re-tuned them in to what whole natural food is, so I will eat that every day. I'll take tins of wild salmon with me when I'm on the road. It will be in my backpack just in case I'm hungry. I can peel it open and have something. I will make sure that I work out every day, even if it means, from my bed, if I just hit the deck and do push-ups and tricep dips and squats. Sometimes, that's all I'll do, but it all helps. It doesn't have to be a one-hour gym workout. Little bits can really help. I will prioritize sleep. That is something that changed me maybe two or three years ago.
Dr. Mark Hyman:	As doctors, we're trained, "Who needs sleep? We stay up all night. Be on-call."
Dr. Rangan Chatterjee:	Yes, but I will genuinely switch off at home. I will switch off maybe at 8:30. That's my cut-off. I will put my computer off. I won't answer emails. I often won't take calls after that time. I will get to

[00:30:30]	bed early, because I find when I do that, everything else gets easier, but my weak spot, the one area I struggle with is the stress piece because, you know, running around, trying to do multiple things. I find it tricky, but I tell you. When my son was three years old, sorry, when he was a bit younger, I remember, he wouldn't sleep very well. He would be up several times a night, but I disciplined myself to get up early and do just five minutes of meditation every morning. I tell you, I felt like a different person.

Dr. Mark Hyman: Totally.

Dr. Rangan Chatterjee:
[00:31:00]

My energy went up. I was less reactive in the day. Recently, that's fallen off again, and that's the one area I struggle with. It's trying to discipline myself to do that. For me, if I do it when I get up, it happens. If I don't, it doesn't happen. Simple as that.

Dr. Mark Hyman:

[00:31:30]

[00:32:00]

That's powerful. People say, "Well, I'm too busy to meditate." I find I'm too busy not to meditate, that just taking that time in the morning. I can do it in the car, on a plane. I can do it in the subway. Even at the end of the day, I'll always try to do it 20 minutes twice a day. I think, "Well, 40 minutes. Who has 40 minutes in a day?" It's made everything else so much better. It made me more focused, more ability to think, have more energy, better sleep, less anxious, less reactive, better able to be present for what I'm doing. It's magic. I never would have imagined it was that powerful. I think people underestimate the importance of hitting the pause button and stopping the stress response, which happens automatically, but the profound relaxation and healing that comes with meditation or some similar practice is just not something that happens automatically. It actually has to be an active process.

Dr. Rangan Chatterjee: Yes, I agree, Mark. I think one thing we have to do as a community is demystify meditation because I think lots of people have lots of hang-ups about it. Is it religious? Is it deeply spiritual? Do I need to sit and chant? They've got all these misconceptions.

Dr. Mark Hyman: It's like exercise for your brain.

Dr. Rangan Chatterjee:
[00:32:30]

[00:33:00]

Yes, exactly, but it can be ... Let me give you an example. My wife, she cannot stand the thought of plugging into an app and having someone guide her through her meditation, because she can switch off naturally. She doesn't like that. Me, for example, I struggle a bit with that. I like the act of plugging into my app and pressing play and someone talking me through it. Two different ways of doing it, but they suit different people. I think there are many ways that people can meditate or be mindful. As you say, it's simply about pressing that pause button. It doesn't matter how you do it. Actually, some patients, I say, "You know what? Maybe for you, it's as simple as finding your favorite bit of music, putting it on and immersing yourself in it, but don't be scrolling your phone at the same time. Put the lights off. Close your eyes and just listen intently to that music." That is a form of meditation.

Dr. Mark Hyman: Sure, sure.

[00:33:30]

Dr. Rangan Chatterjee: It's about finding the right one for that patient, I think.

Dr. Mark Hyman: All right. Thank you, Dr. Chatterjee, for joining us today, appreciate it.

Dr. Rangan Chatterjee: Thanks, Mark. My pleasure.

BROKEN
BRAIN

RAPHAEL KELLMAN, MD | Microbiome Medicine Pioneer & Author:
The Microbiome Diet, The Whole Brain

Dr. Raphael Kellman:	We've been taught by science and colleges, universities, medical schools, that bacteria are bad. They're disease-causing, they're virulent, they're pathogenic, they're something we just have to obliterate and get rid of. It was the big enemy.
[00:00:30]	With the discovery of the incredible, staggering numbers of bacteria in us, in the microbiome, it was the greatest turnaround in medicine, in science in 150 years. From bacteria being disease-oriented, virulent, pathogenic, now, all of a sudden, they're our greatest allies. In fact, that's what the research is showing, that bacteria on Earth, and within us, have one primary goal: to promote healing and to promote life outside of us and the world at large and within us. That's bacteria.
[00:01:00] [00:01:30]	But for 150 years, we've been taught the opposite, and that's because that's the way medicine was evolving. The beginning of technology and the development of antibiotics was the real big first tremendous growth in medicine and therapeutics and drug interventions. And with it came a very, very powerful feeling that we now can control what was thought to be the enemy. It was the enemy to us in those days because we saw when someone had a disease, an infection, maybe meningitis, perhaps, and they were possibly going to die, we gave them an antibiotic, and they survived.
[00:02:00]	The enemy was the bacteria. The hero was the antibiotics. The same thing with tuberculosis, but that was just a small clip, a small part of a big picture that now we're privy to see. We're seeing the big picture, that yes, there was a small battle that we won then, but when we look at the totality, in fact, bacteria have won the great war against antibiotics.
[00:02:30]	For all these years, because we believed in the power of antibiotics, fueled by the pharmaceutical industry, that we believe these are our modern-day heroes. That's why, for so many years, we've literally fallen in love and we're enamored with antibiotics. But now a revolution is happening, and it's not that antibiotics will have no role. But the whole idea, the whole approach, the whole paradigm to the treatment of disease in general—especially the brain, but even infectious diseases—is beginning to change.
[00:03:00]	The question I always hear, "Are we overprescribing antibiotics?" Well, the answer is yes, for sure we are, but we forget that most of the antibiotics we humans consume come from eating poultry. The poor chickens and animals are being fed antibiotics constantly for various reasons, and we are the victims. They're the victims, but we're the victims as well, because most of the antibiotics, 80% that end up in us don't come from the doctor—they come from the chickens we're eating.
[00:03:30]	That being said, nevertheless, antibiotics in the doctor's office are definitely overprescribed. Doctors tend to give antibiotics for upper respiratory infections. Why? Because patients want a treatment. They want something.
[00:04:00]	Luckily, for us who are involved in more holistic or Functional Medicine, we have many, many things to offer patients other than antibiotics. But for some doctors who don't prescribe the antibiotic, the patient leaves disappointed, so there's a pressure upon doctors to prescribe, and yet frequently, they're not needed. Studies show that they're really not needed at all for upper respiratory, even for bronchitis. Even in children, it's so questionable about ear infections, how to treat.
[00:04:30]	But we now realize that we're overprescribing. I think as time goes on, we're going to realize that there's really a very limited role for antibiotics. A very important role, but as we learn more and more

---

[00:05:00] about the power of bacteria to heal and the power of a healthy microbiome to heal, that will be the main treatment. Not only for treating the brain, inflammation, autoimmune diseases, helping with depression and anxiety, but also for the treatment of infectious disease. We're going to now turn to our greatest ally, the microbiome, to help heal our patients, people who are sometimes gravely ill from an infection.

[00:05:30] The microbiome is so critical for brain health. When I think of the brain, I automatically think of the microbiome. To me, the microbiome and the brain are really part of one whole. They're really inseparable. In fact, I believe that the whole brain is not just what we find from our neck up, but it's also what's in our gut, and they're part of one system. To separate them is arbitrary. I like to think of them as one unit, as one whole, and I'll give you some reasons why I believe that to be true.

[00:06:00] Number one: embryologically, the gut and the brain start out at the same point. One goes up, and one goes down. But when two cells start from the same place, they always retain a memory for each other. That's why I love studying embryology because you could learn about how different systems are interconnected so deeply even though they're so far apart. Embryologically, they were one when we were first developing. That's the same thing with the gut, with the microbiome, and the brain. They really were one at our origin.

[00:06:30]
[00:07:00] The microbiome and the gut. The gut, the gastrointestinal system, is the housing for the microbiome, the trillions of bacteria, the friendly bacteria. They have direct communication to the brain. There's a bi-directional highway. They're constantly speaking to each other in so many different ways, in many different "languages," and they're communicating messages to each other. These messages are part of a communication system that really outshines any type of communication system we know of today without modern technology. It's really staggering. This communication actually mostly originates from the microbiome up to the brain and is 400 times the amount of messages coming from the microbiome to the brain than from the brain to the body.

[00:07:30]
[00:08:00] This is where the origin of communication starts, and the microbiome speaks to the brain and determines, "Should the brain be in a state of inflammation? Should the brain reduce its inflammation? What types of messenger molecules should the brain start producing?" And on and on and on, so therefore, the microbiome has such a strong and intimate relationship with the brain, from the beginning, from the get-go, and it continues on and on until the moment that we die. We now have the ability to significantly bolster, enhance, and improve that flow of communication; both improving the gut in the microbiome, and most importantly, improving the brain.

The problem today is that we're experiencing such a devastating effect on the microbiome. People always ask me, "Why do we get sick? Why are so many people sick?" That's a really good question because if we go and reckon with that question, we're not going to really understand why our patients got sick in the first place. Where does it come from?

[00:08:30]
[00:09:00] Genetics plays a very, very small role. Very small role. The origins, mostly, are in the outer environment, in outer ecology, from toxicity in the outer ecology in the world, and toxicity in the inner ecology in the microbiome. The amount of bacteria in the outside world is just inexplicable, so too with the amount of bacteria within us. They outnumber us, possibly 10 to one. Some people say we're 50% bacteria, but either way, the numbers are staggering. We are really a huge ecology—but this ecology is very vulnerable to being disrupted.

[00:09:30] It's very easy for it to lose its integrity and how robust it ought to be. Toxins in the environment like pesticides, chemicals, various toxins that we're exposed to on a day-to-day basis, the overuse of antibiotics—there are so many reasons why the microbiome is becoming weaker and weaker, and with it, diseases, chronic disease, and diseases of the brain are rapidly growing, reaching epidemic proportions.

[00:10:00] The overuse of antibiotics, and antibiotics in poultry, the insecticides and pesticides that are found in abundance in the foods we're eating, nonsteroidal anti-inflammatory drugs—these are medicines that have been used to such a great extent. I see so many patients who were put on a drug like Protonix, or Pepcid, or Prilosec, because for a few months they had burning in the esophagus or in the stomach or an ulcer. The doctor put them on Prilosec, but they never took them off of it, so years later, they're still on it. What I'm finding is that may be a greater problem, a more significant disruptor of the

[00:10:30] microbiome than even antibiotics.

I see so many patients with unexplained chronic gastrointestinal symptoms and brain symptoms like cognitive decline, and people in their 50s with brain fog, difficulty concentrating, brain fatigue,

[00:11:00] depression, and anxiety, with concomitant gastrointestinal symptoms that really have been alluding gastroenterologist. They have no answer, so they're suffering with the gut problem together with the brain problem, and neither could the gastroenterologist help them, and neither could the psychiatrist help them. This represents a whole new field of how to treat these two conditions, which are really one condition. This is the interrelationship between the microbiome and the brain.

[00:11:30] All these different chemicals and medications affect this delicate balance of the microbiome, but also stress disrupts the microbiome. A poor diet—not just the typical unhealthy diet of our day—refined carbohydrates and junk foods … Even people who eat a pretty good diet, not taking into account what our bacteria want to eat is an unhealthy diet for our microbiome.

[00:12:00] In my book, *The Microbiome Diet*, I describe the types of foods that all microbiome like to eat. When we sit down to eat, we also have to think about our wonderful neighbors that live within us. What they want to eat—but in the end, what they want to eat and what we want to eat are really one and the same. Once we start adopting the diet that is what we're really meant to be eating, it not only heals our bacteria, our microbiome, but ultimately, it will heal us as well.

[00:12:30] What's amazing is that the microbiome bacteria produce some of the same chemicals—the neurochemicals, the neurotransmitters—that the brain produces, which is quite amazing in the sense that bacteria are so similar to neurons. They're really, like I was saying before, opposite sides of the same coin. Neurons and bacteria are almost like brothers. Maybe they're really one and the same to some degree.

[00:13:00] They both, as I said before, start out embryologically at the same point. They produce some of the same neurotransmitters. For example, we all know the brain produces serotonin. We know the brain produces dopamine. We know the brain produces GABA, melatonin, and all kinds of neurotransmitters. Many of the psychiatric medications were designed to increase the levels of these

[00:13:30] various neurotransmitters like serotonin—like the SSRIs, Paxil, and Prozac, etc.—they raise the serotonin. But what's incredible is that our bacteria in the microbiome produce Prozac, too. They don't produce Prozac, but they produce what Prozac wants to do, which is to increase serotonin.

[00:14:00] Our bacteria in the microbiome are producing dopamine, serotonin, norepinephrine, and GABA, and these messages are going to the brain, sending signals to the brain and part of this incredible communication system in the brain. They're part of the conversation. These messenger molecules are also sending messages to our stress system, what we call the HPA (hypothalamic-pituitary-adrenal) axis. The microbiome, the bacteria are also sending signals to the gut cells.

[00:14:30] We're talking about an interconnection of bacteria and brain cells, and it's so complex and such an incredible web. You really can't separate bacteria from neurons in the brain.

It is well-known now that inflammation is a precursor and a cause of so many diseases. Various brain diseases, whether we're talking about depression, anxiety, or neurodegenerative diseases like dementia, Alzheimer's, Parkinson's disease, multiple sclerosis, ALS—you name it—or everything in

[00:15:00] between. People have all kinds of brain symptoms and people complain of broken brains that defy elite diagnoses.

[00:15:30] The root of this invariably is inflammation. The immune system is in a slightly overactive state. It's sending signals, we need to be in an alarm state. We can't just go on with regular living in peace and equanimity. We have to be alarmed. We have to be in a state of vigilance, hypervigilance. Where is that message coming from?

[00:16:00] By and large, it's coming from the immune system in the gastrointestinal tract. It's well-known now that 70%, or perhaps 80%, of our immune system is found within the gut. And interfacing with that bulk of the immune system is the microbiome. If the microbiome—the incredible ally of trillions upon trillions of cells—if in any way they lose their power, they become less integrated. They lose their ability to really maintain a very healthy control center. Then immediately what happens is, so many of

[00:16:30] their vital functions begin to falter.

For example, one of the most important roles of the microbiome is to tame the immune system, to keep it in check, to keep it in control, to organize it, to send the signals to the immune system what to do. In fact, the microbiome educates the immune system. It teaches it what is a friend, what should

[00:17:00] you send inflammatory processes against and what you shouldn't, who's part of our oneness, our ecology and who's not, what's a foreign compound and what's not.

That education, the teacher of our immune system is the microbiome. If the immune system is not balanced and it's in a hyper-excitable state, you automatically should make the deduction that there's

[00:17:30] something off with the microbiome. That inflammation instantaneously creates inflammation in the brain. And when you have inflammation in the brain, it sets the stage for all the different diseases and all the different types of dysfunction that this whole series is discussing. The root cause is inflammation, and the root cause of inflammation is an unhealthy microbiome.

[00:18:00] I find it interesting that in between the microbiome and the brain is the thyroid. It may be a coincidence of billions of years of evolution, or maybe there's something to it. I like to think of the thyroid as sort of a relay station, showing that it plays such an important role in brain health.

[00:18:30] It's probably—other than the microbiome—is one of the most important variables I want to look into when someone has any type of brain issue. It doesn't matter what it is. Whether it's depression or brain fog, whether it's MS, Parkinson's, dementia, Alzheimer's, or everything in between. Confusion, difficulty concentrating, focusing, a little anxiety in the morning and depression in the afternoon, not being able to recall names like you were able to do five years before ... All of these, I have to consider the possibility of a low thyroid.

[00:19:00] Why is that the case? Like I said before, what are the origins of disease? It's ecological problems. Sure enough, there's a whole category of chemicals in the environment called endocrine disruptors. These endocrine disruptors don't have to be at high levels in the environment to really create havoc in our endocrine system. The endocrine system is a hormonal communication between systems.

[00:19:30] The reason why it's so vulnerable to these endocrine disruptors—like phthalates and BPA and dioxin, etc.,—is because the endocrine system relies on receptors like antennas where the messages are picked up. These antennas are very vulnerable to damage. Even a small amount of a toxin could damage this whole relay station—and there are so many points along the incredible web of

[00:20:00] communication—that is so easy for the system to become damaged and scrambled. Messages can easily be scrambled.

What system is most vulnerable? Which gland is most vulnerable to endocrine disruptors? The thyroid, clearly. The problem is, though, while it's well-documented that endocrine disruptors are causing disease in the animal kingdom with fish and reptiles, but also in humans, doctors are not picking it up

[00:20:30] sufficiently in the clinical setting, in the doctor's office. The question is, why?

[00:21:00] First of all, doctors have gotten used to only doing a very limited type of test, like just TSH and T4, or free T4, while there are many more things to test. There's something called total T4 and total T3, and free T4 and free T3, and thyroid antibodies, and reverse T3. But even if all of that is done, we have made assumptions in medicine and premises that have really never been proven to be true.

We've all been taught that if there's a problem, you could pick it up in the blood. For example, if you have a lot of lead in your body or mercury, do a blood test. If the lead level is not high, you don't have a lead problem. But if you look a little deeper into the real research, it will show that's not true.

[00:21:30] You could have normal levels of lead in the blood, but the tissue could be full of lead. The same thing with thyroid hormone and the TSH level coming from the pituitary. It may look normal in the blood, but that doesn't mean that within the tissues themselves—within the thyroid, within the pituitary,

[00:22:00] within the tissues of the body—that the thyroid hormones are up to par. A test that's always been around that I kind of resurrected was called the TRH stimulation test.

Lo and behold, since I've resurrected it in 1997, in 2007, there were a number of peer-reviewed studies that came to the same conclusion. Frequently, you cannot rely on routine thyroid blood testing, including TSH, in certain populations. Many of these researchers say that we should bring this test back into clinical practice.

[00:22:30] By doing this test, I have seen that so many untold number of patients—I'm talking about over 50,000 patients that I have seen on my own, maybe more in this period of time, probably a lot more—that would never have been diagnosed with an underactive thyroid if not for the types of testing that I'm doing like the TRH stimulation test. That being said, what's important here is its profound effect on the

[00:23:00] brain. So many people are being diagnosed with dementia, various brain diseases, and a broken brain, and the thyroid is being missed.

If you're missing a thyroid problem, how are you going to be able to correct the brain problem? The thyroid hormone is so critical for brain function. It's the gasoline for the neurons. It's the gasoline for

[00:23:30] every cell in our body. How is the brain going to work if it doesn't have gasoline? If you're going to rely on the routine testing—even if you change the reference range like some doctors are doing who are realizing we can't rely on this anymore—even then, you're going to miss it.

There an S-Y-M, a big advocate of the TRH stimulation test, to improve the brain. In fact, there was a

[00:24:00] study in patients with dementia, with Alzheimer's on autopsy. They found that in the blood, the thyroid levels were completely normal, but in the brain tissue itself, the levels of T3 were extraordinarily low.

The studies have also found this in autopsy on children with autism. Normal blood, thyroid blood test, low T3 in the brain. How could we miss this? If we miss it, we're not going to sufficiently be able to help

[00:24:30] our patients with all kinds of brain diseases and disorders. If we find it and understand that it's a high, high chance, that will set the stage for all the treatments to work that much better to be able to heal various types of brain disorders.

You know, I'll tell you something. The problem with the TRH stimulation test, I'll be very honest, is that

[00:25:00] it's been forgotten. This was the main test that was used to diagnose thyroid disease until 1996. It's a challenge test. It's like, you could do an EKG on somebody. Looks fine. The next day, they die of a heart attack. How is it possible? Well, resting their cardiogram is normal. Put them on a treadmill, which is a stress test, and you're going to see how well the heart is functioning.

That's the premise of Functional Medicine. How is are the organs, the system, the body functioning? Okay, it doesn't have a disease, but is it healthy? Are you healthy? You don't have X, Y, and Z, but are

[00:25:30] you healthy? That's the incredible value of understanding health from a totally different paradigm.

[00:26:00] Erroneously, they stopped using the TRH stimulation test in 1996, because they thought they were using the test only because the assays to pick up TSH were very crude. Unless the numbers were very high, they couldn't detect it. So they figured, well, let's do this stimulation. We can get this TSH up very high in someone who's healthy and someone who has a low thyroid.

[00:26:30] TSH comes from the pituitary. When you inject TRH, it stimulates the pituitary to release TSH. If there's a brisk stimulation, the pituitary is telling us it thinks the thyroid is low. But the doctors or scientist, medical community was thinking, "Well, that's the only reason why we're doing it, but now that the assays are better, we don't need it anymore."

[00:27:00] Anyone who comes from a different way of thinking like we do in Functional Medicine, in holistic medicine, or even if you don't use that title to describe how you practice, but you're a doctor who is broad-minded, you'll come to the conclusion that, of course, we should use this type of a test to be able to look deeper. To see more about functionality, to improve the whole way of understanding how thyroid works and how this whole system works.

[00:27:30] It was forgotten. I started using it at that point, because when I first started practicing, and the people that were coming to me ... Because I was practicing holistic medicine in 1996, they didn't even know what holistic medicine was. They just went to me because every other doctor threw them out of their office. They were being bounced around. It's like, "We'll go to Dr. Kellman, we never went to him." They didn't know what holistic medicine was all about. I would see one after another after another, and they all had typical symptoms of a low thyroid.

[00:28:00] Many of these people had various brain diseases: depression, cognitive issues, brain fog. Many of these people—some were in their 40s and 50s and 60s—really believed they were developing early Alzheimer's. They were petrified. They couldn't remember what they did 30 seconds before. The depression came out of the blue. There was nothing that changed in their lives, and they were depressed. They would go complain to the doctor of all their symptoms, and the doctor would say, [00:28:30] "Well, you're depressed. Let me give you an antidepressant." "But doctor, I wasn't depressed two years ago. My life is better. Why would I be depressed?"

Some of them would take it and then they would go downhill. Some of them would take it and they would feel nothing, because that wasn't the root cause. Many would just live in despair. Many other people had issues like weight gain and gastrointestinal problems. And then with the gastrointestinal [00:29:00] problems, anxiety, and then more anxiety. And then panic attacks, and then more gut problems—and they went to this gastroenterologist and to this neurologist and that psychiatrist, and on and on and on. They all had typical symptoms of low thyroid, but the routine tests were all normal.

[00:29:30] That led me to look deeper, and I remembered this TRH stimulation test while everyone forgot about it. I learned it from an old timer how to use the test, and because I was interested in Functional Medicine back then, it was a test that became my cornerstone. It was what everyone tossed out that actually became the cornerstone of many of the tests and the treatments I offer.

[00:30:00] The problem now is, how are other doctors going to learn to do this test? It's not that difficult. First, there has to be the desire, the will, and the understanding that this is important, that we can't rely on the routine testing. Then, with that, people will find a way to learn about this test. I've offered so many times to teach doctors and scientists, even patients, so that they try to convince their doctors. But in such a medical environment that we are in today, people don't want to start something new, especially if it's another blood test and you have to inject the hormone, even though it's totally safe. So, people [00:30:30] kind of shy away from it, but it's a must that we bring it back into the clinical setting.

[00:31:00] The whole brain protocol is a protocol that heals all kinds of brain issues. It sets the stage for all kinds of treatments, but it really has to be the foundation. The whole brain protocol is based on the idea that, of course, the microbiome and the brain are part of one whole. We have to restore the integrity, the power, and the healing capacity of the microbiome.

[00:31:30] If you think of the coral reef, think of it with the way it used to be with beautiful colors of the rainbow, and what it looks like now. That's what's happening to our microbiome. We have to restore the color and the abundance back to our microbiome. When that happens, the brain will also be full of color. But until we restore the microbiome, like restoring the coral reef, we can't expect the brain to become healthy again.

The program is premised on this in order to heal the brain. First of all, we have to start introducing the foods that our bacteria like to eat. The foods for the bacteria are called prebiotics. Prebiotic foods.

[00:32:00]
[00:32:30] Prebiotic foods are basically different types of fiber—one is inulin, another one is called arabinogalactan—and these compounds are found in various foods. For example, Jerusalem artichoke is a prebiotic food, jicama, radishes, you name it. There are so many different vegetables. Even fruits, like kiwi, for example, is another very good prebiotic food. But just vegetables and salads in general, I consider prebiotic foods. Like polyphenols—a very important compound found in fruits and vegetables that absolutely heal the microbiome and heal the gut.

[00:33:00]
[00:33:30] These foods are all part of the whole brain protocol, so now we're really nourishing the microbiome. If we nourish and heal the microbiome, the microbiome will heal us. The best portal into healing the brain is by healing the microbiome. It's, first and foremost, introducing these types of foods, introducing fermented foods. You don't even have to focus on telling people what to remove, because by starting to eat these foods, they're not going to want to eat those unhealthy foods. It's going to happen within a week, that now, they're just more oriented. They're eating in more of a primordial way that they're only seeking the healthy foods our bodies are really craving.

The symptoms of poor brain function, to a great degree, depends on the person. For example, if someone had an incredible memory two years ago, and now their memory is just average, that's a brain dysfunction. If someone now is feeling anxiety that they've never felt before and there's a change, but there's a change in the brain.

[00:34:00]
[00:34:30] All of these factors have to be taken into account in a very individualized, personalized way. But in general, you know if your brain is functioning well, if you have a sense of vitality and optimism and your cognition is clear. You don't have to be the most brilliant person in the world. You don't have to have a memory that's just amazing. You just have to feel that everything is falling into groove, that all parts of the brain are focused in the same direction. There's just a right amount of resistance, right amount of stress, and the brain is nourished by it. Everything falls into place, and there's an ability to overcome a certain degree of stress in a healthy way. That's the way the brain really should work.

[00:35:00]
[00:35:30] With a proper balance between emotions and intellect and sensory experiences, there's a flow, but the flow frequently is so discombobulated in many people. The reason and rationality becomes like the highest point of the totem pole. If someone is oriented and too deeply rooted to that part of who we are, then I know there's already some dysfunction. The rational part of us—the reasoning ability, so to speak—really grows from the emotional and psychological. If the emotional and psychological have been just swept under the rug—and you see there's a hypertrophy of just the rational part of who we are—then you know the brain is not functioning as well as it should.

[00:36:00] I'm adding this part because this is not what's usually asked or looked for. It's a subtler way of detecting brain disorganization. It's so important to realize there's a flow. The brain is organized by a sense of a desire. I want something.

[00:36:30] Like a baby, a newborn baby. The baby is an expression of a will. The baby, what are the baby's needs? The needs are to survive, to live. It needs the mother's milk. It needs comfort. It needs the nurturing. It needs to be cleaned. From those needs develop emotions. When the baby is fed, the baby is comforted, then the parts of the brain begins to develop of the emotions. Ah, that's a good feeling. Unfortunately, if there's deprivation, the bad feelings start developing.

[00:37:00] From these primary experiences, emotions and our psychological state develop. From that, our rational part develops. That's the healthy flow. But it's also important to know what has happened to us at the earliest times of our life because that will set the stage in setting the needs and the will in the first place.

[00:37:30] So many people who've been traumatized early in life have closed down. Their will has been shattered. Then, you see that it left its footprints in all parts of the brain. There are ways of picking up on this. We can pick up on this even by looking at the microbiome, because the microbiome develops its fingerprint early on in those first few months after birth—in year one, year two. God forbid if there's

[00:38:00] early trauma, or lack of nurturing. It leaves its marks in the microbiome, and we can detect these problems by asking the right questions to our patients.

[00:38:30] I always ask my patients to give me one word that describes their earliest experiences in your life. Unfortunately, I hear negative words. I hear gray. I hear being alone. I hear sadness. I hear scared. Sure enough, they're here to see me because they have autoimmune diseases. Because they have depression, because they have anxiety. Even, unfortunately, autoimmune diseases of the brain like MS.

[00:39:00] We have to go all the way back and understand what it means to have a healthy brain and where does it start from, and how to detect subtle problems in the way the brain needs to be organized.

One thing about learning about the microbiome is that we're all part of a whole. It's just incredible that the bacteria on Earth in mass are greater than all the fish in the sea and animals on Earth, and we can't

[00:39:30] see any of the bacteria. All the bacteria on Earth are really acting like one organism. They're acting with a concerted will. They're all doing the same job, and they're all responsible for life on Earth, and they're not fighting with each other. They're working together as one whole, one organism to set the stage for life to develop on Earth.

[00:40:00] Without bacteria, we would have no carbon or nitrogen. The only thing we would have on Earth are rocks. We would have no plants, trees, cattle, fish, or humans. Without bacteria acting as one organism, all of which we can see, we would not have rain. We would have 50% less oxygen on Earth,

[00:40:30] so they're working as a whole. It's one whole. We're part of a whole.

We're part of nature, too. We now know, it's quite obvious, that nature works as a whole. Everything works in fellowship. That's the way life works, and if we want to be healthy, we have to follow the template of life. If that's the case out in nature, and we're part of nature, the same rules should apply

[00:41:00] to us. We're also part of a whole. We work best, we function best, we feel best, we heal best when we're part of our natural environment—when we're part of a whole where we're really being the beings that we're supposed to be, which is part of a whole.

The real question is, how could we even function when we're alone and independent, thinking that we're independent. That's not our natural state. Of course, the studies are showing this. We shouldn't

[00:41:30] be so surprised. "A new study has come out that elderly people who live in a community do much better. They live longer." Well, of course. It's self-evident. What's amazing is that's how the microbiome works too. That's what we're learning from the microbiome: the understanding of

[00:42:00] interconnectedness, to work with one team, to work as one whole in the desire and the will to support life for all.

People have frequently asked me, "Well, how do you speak to the microbiome? Can I just visualize or think certain thoughts that will get my microbiome to feel better?" I said, "I don't think so. I doubt it." You could wish that your microbiome gets better, but it's probably not going to listen to you. It has its own language. We now have the ability to really eavesdrop on the conversations of the microbiome,

[00:42:30] the conversations to the brain. As we eavesdrop, we're going to hear, we will hear, and we are hearing, an incredible conversation.

[00:43:00] Remember what I said before, that the earliest moments of our lives—whether they were nurturing and healing and loving or God forbid, if they were not so—those recordings are right there in the bacteria, in the microbiome, and becomes disorganized. It's not the same as a healthy, healing, healed microbiome.

[00:43:30] What is the language of the microbiome? It's not a rational language. It's not a computer language. It relates to something below the radar. It's not reason. It's not intellect. It's not even emotions. It's something so primordial that really touches upon the essence of who we are, and I call it the will.

[00:44:00] It's a word that's been used in philosophy for thousands of years, but it hasn't really been formulated and described clearly to understand what is the will in a human being. But I could say this, once we begin to know what the will is—and it's parts of two arms of the will and how to integrate them—we'll never be able to speak to the microbiome because the microbiome remembers the shattered will. That's what it remembers. It also was listening for a healed will. And that will, that inner point of who we are, is instantaneously transmitted to the brain. When that wakes up, the brain wakes up and it heals.

[00:44:30]
[00:45:00] I'll give you an example of what I mean. If you look at the CNN Hero Awards, all of these incredible, powerful individuals who've turned around their lives and created great organizations to help so many people, they have one common feature. They all came from a broken will. They came from a horrible childhood of deprivation, of emotional pain, physical pain, and with a crushed will, and their lives were going downhill in every which way.

[00:45:30]
[00:46:00] But somehow, they decided to turn it around and to take the will that was shattered that was only focused on themselves, and understandably so. And their lives were really falling apart, and they said, "I'm going to put an end to it, and I'm going to turn it around, and now I'm going to awaken this will, and I'm going to focus it on the same kids that was so similar to me and to what my life was like. I'm going to help them." That's the hero of CNN's Heroes because they took that shattered will, and the remaining parts of that shattered will that was only this way to try to survive, and they said, "Enough. I'm going to focus on the others who need my help from my experience." Then, they healed themselves, and look how many people they're healing.

That's the example, that's what speaks to the microbiome. We all can't do that, but we don't have to. We can apply the similar ideas, similar concepts every moment of our lives.

[00:46:30]
[00:47:00] To optimize our brain to improve brain health, we have to go about it from a few different ways. One is to understand the relationship between the microbiome and the brain, that they're really part of one. We have to think of the microbiome and the brain—meaning whatever it is from the neck up—as one whole. We've said that they're similar. They communicate in a similar way. They have the same point of origin. They know each other. They're constantly producing the same molecules. Let's think of them as one. And if you want to heal this, don't only focus on the problems, what's missing here ... Focus on what's depleted down here in the microbiome, number one.

[00:47:30] Number two is think about what are the right foods for our microbiome? What's the primordial diet? The microbiome diet is really the primordial diet because it's really what the bedrock of life needs to eat. Since the bedrock of life is within us, if we heal and feed them with the right types of foods and nutrients, it's healing us as well.

[00:48:00] The next thing, is the seamless integration of what seems to be a disparate concept of something that people relegate to. Something spiritual, and they use metaphysical terms, which you don't have to use. You could talk about the inner point of the human being as the will, and to think about where is your will today, and to extricate the will from self-imposed shackles and the prisons we impart on them.

[00:48:30] And like those heroes, extricate them, and see its power unfold.

[00:49:00] It's going to transform your microbiome. Your microbiome will be so happy. They'll praise you and thank you forever. And then they'll heal you, and you'll help to heal others, and then a community will be healed, and mental illness would be healed. And it would be healed through the power of the origins of life: the microbiome, and even deeper, the human will.

RICK HANSON, PhD | Author: *Buddha's Brain*

Dr. Rick Hanson:	Stressors do not equal stress. In other words, we can face all kinds of challenges and not be triggered in our body along with negative emotion. That's really the functional definition of stress. For example, I've done a lot of rock climbing. I've been in really hazardous situations, lots of stressors, storms are coming in, I'm standing on little ledges half the width of a pencil and my body is activated. It's alert. It's energized. There is some anxiety floating around the edges, but deep inside, I'm having the time of my life. There's a sense of strong calm and capability as I meet the challenge.
[00:00:30]	
[00:01:00]	People often assume that, because there's some sort of stressor, they necessarily need to feel stressed or driven or pressured by it. Not so. We can actually grow resources in the mind and body that function as shock absorbers between us and stressors, which is extremely useful to have for a full life. Of course, in a full life, we do want to deal with challenges of various kinds, including ambition and raising a family or whatever we're interested in, including helping the world become a better place, while doing so with a resilient happiness hardwired into our own nervous system. That's the possibility.
[00:01:30]	There's a natural range or distribution, kind of like a bell curve roughly, of response to stressors of different kinds. Probably about a third of what creates that range is hardwired, if you will, into our own DNA. It's baked in. The other half to two-thirds of what creates that range of resilience or lack of resilience is based on the experiences that people have and what they do with them. On the one hand, having experiences that sensitize people to painful, stressful experiences, such as trauma; on the other hand, people having experiences of gratitude or meaning or worth or relatedness to other people or positive emotions in general—experiences like that are internalized and push people toward the resilient end of the spectrum.
[00:02:00]	
[00:02:30]	Wherever you are on that spectrum, there's tons of hope. This is all about where you go from here from now on. Three of the most helpful words in the language: "From now on." As a psychologist, it's deeply interesting to consider how to turn these experiences we're having into lasting changes inside so we actually become more resilient and happy along the way.
[00:03:00]	There's been a lot of research on what stress does to the brain. Now, small amounts of stress that are managed successfully tend to grow coping resources embedded in our own nervous system. That's good. That's pain with gain. Most pain has no gain. Most stressful experiences, in part because of the brain's evolved negativity bias, which means that it tends to overlearn from stressful emotionally negative, emotionally painful experience, and it tends to under-learn from beneficial, usually enjoyable experiences. Maybe we'll talk about that later.
[00:03:30]	To really focus here, in terms of the effects of stress on the brain that are outside of mild experiences of stress that actually make us stronger, when stress is harming the brain, it does so through multiple pathways. One of the primary pathways involves the stress hormone, cortisol. The same neuro hormonal machinery that evolved to help our ancestors run away from sabre-toothed tigers and threats prior to that, that machinery is active today when we're stuck in traffic or having an irritating interaction with our partner or kid or our bosses, coming at us too fast and too hard. We are experiencing releases of cortisol then, just as our ancestors did, running for their lives.
[00:04:00]	Then up in the brain, cortisol has kind of a one-two punch. First, it overstimulates and sensitizes the alarm bell of the brain, the amygdala. Technically, there are two amygdali, one on either side of the brain. People speak of them in the singular. Now we have an alarm bell that reacts easier and louder. Cortisol also overstimulates and gradually kills neurons in a nearby part of the brain, the hippocampus, which does three important things in terms of managing upsetting experiences. The hippocampus puts
[00:04:30]	

things in context. "My boss is not my mother. She looks like my mother. She's authoritative like my mother. She's not my mother." It puts things in context. This is now.

[00:05:00]

The second thing the hippocampus does, is it literally inhibits, it puts the brakes on the alarm bell of the brain, the amygdala. It calms down the amygdala so it's not so intensely sounding the alarm. Then third, the hippocampus tells the hypothalamus—a very important part of the brain that's at the center of the stress hormone cascade, "Enough stress hormones already. No more." That creates a vicious cycle. Stress today overstimulates the amygdala, weakens and damages the hippocampus, which makes us a little more irritable, anxious, prickly or blue tomorrow, a little more vulnerable to stress tomorrow, which then releases more cortisol, sensitizing the amygdala, damaging the hippocampus, which in turn makes us even more vulnerable to stress the day after that.

[00:05:30]

[00:06:00]

Another negative or damaging effect of stress on the brain travels through inflammation. Stress and broadly-defined negative emotions, being irritated or anxious or hurt or sad, particularly with moderate to severe negative emotion, is inflammatory. It creates inflammation, and among other things that occur when there's inflammation, these chemical messengers called cytokines are released by the immune system. Many of them travel up into the brain and then lodge in the brain, including in the hypothalamus, making a person increasingly depressed. This is called the Cytokine Theory of Depression.

[00:06:30]

You can see different pathways of negative impact, stress, in this case, traveling through inflammation, releasing cytokines that go up and actually change the brain for the worse, lowering mood. A key takeaway from that, for me at least, is to disengage from stressful experiences as fast as one can and, in particular, grow resources inside so that when challenges and other stressors land, we're not so stressed by them.

[00:07:00]

Then the amygdala and hippocampus, what do they do? Inside the head are about 1.1 trillion cells out of roughly a hundred trillion in the body altogether, so 1.1 or so trillion cells, about 10% of which, a hundred billion or so, are neurons. There are roughly as many neurons between our ears as there are stars in the Milky Way Galaxy. A typical neuron makes about 5,000 connections with other neurons, called synapses. These little junctions give us our own internal world wide web with several hundred trillion little microprocessors, all sparkling away, all interacting, firing or not firing, doing all kinds of things, representing and communicating and changing information coursing through the nervous system, including that fraction of the information coursing through the nervous system that's the basis for our experiences, moment to moment to moment.

[00:07:30]

The brain altogether has been actually called the enchanted loom, continually weaving moment to moment, the fabric of our own mind. In that larger context, the brain evolved over six hundred million years and it did so, roughly, in three stages, kind of like building the floors of a house from the bottom up. We have the more-or-less reptilian brain stem first floor, the more-or-less mammalian subcortex, the second floor, and the more-or-less primate human third floor, the cortex, the neocortex of the brain.

[00:08:00]

In the different floors of the brain, different parts do different things. In the second floor of the house of the brain, the subcortex, there are a couple of really important regions or parts that we all have that do useful things, but they can take us into trouble. One of them, in particular, is called the amygdala. There are two of them, one on either side of the brain. They are an ancient, roughly 200 million-year-old part of the brain in terms of the origins of the amygdala that are continually tracking whether things are relevant-salient. They're called salience detectors.

[00:08:30]

[00:09:00]

Since so much of what's relevant to early humans that are Hominid and then Primate, Mammalian, etc. ancestors, so much of what's relevant is a threat, the amygdala for most people are biased toward threat detection, toward being alarmed at anything that might be harmful, including signals coming up from inside the body. If a person has a physical illness, a dysfunction of some kind, chronic pain of

---

[00:09:30] some kind, this bias says something's wrong, something's not quite right. That triggers alarm systems inside the tissues and organs of the body, which then travel up in the nervous system, eventually, which is to say within seconds or less, to arrive at the amygdala, which then sounds the alarm, which then initiates the stress response cascade, ending up in the release of hormones such as adrenalin and cortisol.

[00:10:00] The good news is that the amygdala can also track opportunities. It can track friends, not just foes, and it can see carrots, not just sticks. Over time, it's very likely that we can train this alarm bell of the brain to become increasingly joyful. The title of one of my favorite research papers I've read is *The Joyful Amygdala*. For example, the amygdala has receptors for oxytocin, a neurotransmitter and hormone that's associated with feeling cared about or feeling caring, feeling connected. As people repeatedly have and internalize healthy, authentic, usually mild but still completely genuine experiences of feeling

[00:10:30] cared about or caring, that tends to sensitize oxytocin receptors in the amygdala, and probably grow additional receptors as well, which then has the effect of calming, soothing, easing and relaxing the amygdala so it's not so reactive to stressors.

[00:11:00] To put it simply: love is love, flowing in or flowing out. In other words, we're so profoundly social as human beings, arguably the most social species on the planet. I think there are probably five major ways to feel cared about to create opportunities for people to feel included, seen, appreciated, liked or loved—any one of those counts. Even without total soulmate love, we still have opportunities to feel cared about.

[00:11:30] Similarly, when we are caring, when we have compassion for others, we wish they didn't suffer. When we feel moved empathically, when we have kindness for others, we wish they were happy. When we delight in their good fortune, when we're happy they are happy, when we stand in solidarity with others in terms of social justice, social change, etc., when we're just hanging out with a friend and we feel fond of them and friendly toward them, we like them. We love them maybe. When we're having those experiences, wonderfully protective hormones and other neurotransmitter activity occur that

[00:12:00] exert a reparative, repairing influence over the nervous system, slows and protects the heart rate through processes that involve different branches of the nervous system that both go into the face and are very engaged with relationships, as well as go down and calm down the lungs and the heart and regulate the visceral altogether, so that's really good.

[00:12:30] Also, the positive emotions that come with feeling caring, not simply feeling cared about, we reduce the production of stress hormones, increase our sense of oxytocin-based relatedness, and I would say also have an opportunity to learn that we are cared about and we are caring. Which then, if that's learned in some general sense, can become a resource we can draw upon to meet the next challenge. When we're caught in the moment and, in a sense, things are flashing red inside our head, what can

[00:13:00] we do in the moment, right? Then, maybe we can also talk about what we can do when we're not upset or not stressed out that can grow, embody my resources inside of us, so that the next time that thing happens, that parent that gives you unwanted advice, that co-worker is snarky, your bus is late, the next time those things happen, we're not so triggered by them.

[00:13:30] Okay, so in the moment, there are three great little quickies that Mother Nature has evolved to help her little critters, her little babies, including us, move out of spikes of red zone stress and recover rapidly back to the by-design resting state. I call it the "green zone," an ongoing equilibrium condition of basic safety, satisfaction, and connection. How do we get out of that spike of red zone stress,

[00:14:00] because a little bit of that goes a long way? One is to experience some form of safety, that you are protected. In the moment, maybe you're anxious about something. Maybe you've got a real challenge to deal with but register in this moment, "I'm not dying." For example, I've had a lot of situations in the wilderness where I wasn't physically comfortable. I was uncomfortable and it was a tough situation, but I knew I was going to live through it. Just that alone, establishing to the maximum that's authentically available, a sense of safety.

[00:14:30] If you think of the evolution of the brain, the reptilian brain stem is associated most fundamentally with safety needs, because first and foremost, in the wild, eat lunch today; don't be lunch today. Safety comes first. First and foremost, establish a basic sense of safety. Okay, it's this bad but it's not this bad. All right? The yuckiness is going to last my whole evening, but tomorrow is going to be

[00:15:00] another day or yeah, they really got me on this one, but there are these other parts of my life that are still fine, or I don't like it; it's uncomfortable, but I've lived through this kind of thing previously. I know I can do it. I'm going to draw on that knowing, and I'm going to keep going, establish a basic sense of safety. Notice protections around you. One is an environment that is physically safe. Whatever you can do for five, ten, 20, 30 seconds, it doesn't take forever to do it, register safety.

[00:15:30] Second, in terms of the mammalian subcortex, look for a healthy reward. Eat something sweet. Have that cookie. Make sure it's gluten-free, but something pleasurable. Look out and see something beautiful. Brush your hair. Wash your hands. Basic wholesome pleasure of one kind or another. Watch a kitten video on YouTube. Watch somebody doing something goofy and funny, just something that is

[00:16:00] momentarily rewarding, activating the satisfaction need system in the brain. That, too, tends to bring us right out of something that's a spike in stress.

Then third, in terms of the most recent layer of the brain, look for some sense of connection. Who do you love? Who has loved you? Who are your friends? What groups are you part of? Can you mobilize in that moment a sense of compassion for the person who has wronged you? You're not necessarily

[00:16:30] forgiving them. You're not necessarily letting them off the hook. You may still want to pursue justice, but it's interesting that having compassion for people who have wronged us, if it's authentic, alongside having compassion for ourselves and sticking up for ourselves, but having compassion for them, which is a very social emotion, actually helps people feel less upset. It seems paradoxical like compassion, a sense of the suffering of the person who has been a jerk, would make me feel better. But in addition to whatever is moral about it, it's enlightened self-interest to do that, for example. Those are the big three: safety, pleasure, and connection are real quick fixes to reset the brain, to pull it out of the red

[00:17:00] zone and back home to its resting state, its home base, which is the green zone of calm, contentment, and confidence, rather than fear, frustration, and heartache.

People often ask, "My life is hard. My life's tough. This thing and that thing. Are you saying look on the bright side and smell all the roses?" I'm saying no. Sure, smell the roses if they smell good but the

[00:17:30] more a person's life sucks, the more important it is to look for authentic opportunities, to experience something beneficial, a moment of relief, a moment of drinking water when you're thirsty, a moment of finally getting on the bus and being able to take off your shoes, a moment of connection with your friend, a moment of relaxation when you finally get into bed. The worse your life, and the less that outside sources are taking care of you, the more important it is to take care of oneself and to look for

[00:18:00] those opportunities to have beneficial, usually enjoyable, experiences in the flow of your day and then really, really, really take them into yourself.

That's true for people in general, not just people whose lives are really hard and really challenging. It means that we have opportunities in the flow of everyday life based on experience-dependent neuroplasticity, this idea that the experiences we're having are leaving lasting changes behind them

[00:18:30] for better or worse. That means you can use your mind to change your brain to change your mind for the better. That means that you can work backwards. If a person understands a little bit of, "Wow, what would help my life be better? What, if I had more of it inside myself, would help me deal with this challenge, this relationship breakup issue, this really tough job, this long commute, this child with special needs, this aging parent with a health condition? Inside myself, what if there were more inside

[00:19:00] me, would this improve my treatment outcome?"

Half the disease burden in the developed world is caused by mental factors. 50% of the problem and yet routinely, when people focus on a physical health condition, which is what I'm talking about here, 50% of the medical conditions worldwide are the result of mental factors of one kind or another, a lot of which have to do with lifestyle choices. Physical factors matter, of course. We should pay attention

[00:19:30] to them, but mental factors matter, too, like being able to be compassionate for one's self or to calm down one's reactivity to pain in the body or to develop more resilience in other ways, to become more grateful, to become more skillful in interacting with care providers. When people have medical conditions, that often drops them into a foreign country, the healthcare system. They have no background with it. They don't know what to do about it. They are flooded already. They are

[00:20:00] bombarded with unwanted advice or wanted advice from all kinds of quarters. What to do? There are skills that will help people be better patients, basically, and make use of the system in more effective ways. That, too, is a mental factor that can be learned.

[00:20:30] My larger point here is that once we start to identify what, if we had more of it inside ourselves, would help us to cope more effectively and also help us experience more well-being, more peace of mind, more fulfillment, more quality of life, when we start to zero in on what those things are, including happiness altogether. If the pharmaceutical companies could patent happiness, based on the research already established for how happiness is a major beneficial factor when grappling with illness, disease, dysfunction, and so forth, including neurodegeneration, if the pharmaceutical companies could patent happiness, we'd see the ads for it every night on television.

[00:21:00] Once you identify that which you want to grow inside yourself, as a mental factor, as a psychological attribute, much as once you identify certain kinds of proteins you'd want to develop inside yourself or certain kinds of hormonal activity you'd want to improve or certain kinds of protective factors you'd want to have inside your own brain to slow the progression of dementia once you identify the good that you want to grow, then in terms of growing mental factors, it's usually much easier and much

[00:21:30] more straightforward than growing positive beneficial physical factors. The fundamental process of growing mental factors has two simple steps to it: experience what you want to grow or the factors related to it and then really internalize that experience. Help that experience, which is just passing and impermanent, transfer into long-term storage in the brain so you move from state to trait and over time grow, for example, trait resilience, trait gratitude, trait understanding of how to be a more

[00:22:00] skillful, more effective patient.

That fundamental process, to finish on that point, to identify what you want to grow, look for ways to experience it that are real, and then when you get that song playing on your inner iPod, turn on your recorder, take the extra dozen or two dozen or three dozen seconds with it, a few breaths with it, to really keep those neurons firing together so they wire that beneficial experience into your nervous system.

[00:22:30] Let's suppose that someone is dealing with a chronic health condition, maybe an autoimmune condition, maybe a neurodegenerative illness, maybe they're recovering from an injury, a traumatic brain injury or some other form of injury. Let's suppose also that that person is being advised by their healthcare providers, or they know it themselves, or they remember what their grandmother told

[00:23:00] them, that fountain of wisdom. They realize, "Oh, it would be better if I could find more calm that will help me think better about all this craziness that's happening in my life. It will feel like a shock absorber between me and the pain in my body and the fear that's understandably coming up in me." Fear can come up in a person without it invading and hijacking them. If they can establish an authentic kind of calm, not a numbing, not a suppressing, but a certain fundamental equanimity or stability of

[00:23:30] one's self so that we're not overwhelmed by what's happening.

Let's say a person goes, "Oh, it would be good if I could acquire more of an inner peace or calm or steadiness, a sense of calm strength in my own core." For example, someone could think, "Oh, it would be really helpful for me to acquire more gratitude for the things that are still good in my life or

[00:24:00] were good, and therefore will always have been good." Gratitude would be good to develop, more of an attitude of gratitude, whatever it might be, and one can think of other sorts of things, commitment to treatment, commitment to exercise, commitment to dietary changes that are initially boring. Rice flour, boring, right? That, too, is a mental factor much like a physical factor that would be very beneficial for a person, motivation and commitment.

[00:24:30]

[00:25:00]

Now you know what it is, so in the flow of everyday life, you'd look for opportunities to experience it. Maybe opportunities to experience calming. Most of these opportunities will come in a flow of a day, not in some kind of formal meditation session, or formal gratitude practice, or formal psychotherapy appointment, or formal listening to some kind of audio program. That's great. That's great stuff, but what about the rest of the person's day or week or life? That's where most of the opportunities really are. This is, in effect, self-directed neuroplasticity. You know what you want to grow in the garden of your mind, the flowers you want to grow, in part, to crowd out the weeds there, so you look for opportunities to experience that resource.

[00:25:30]

Calm, you look for opportunities to find calm's strength, often in other areas, unrelated to your illness, which is great because it creates more opportunities. When you are exhaling and naturally relaxing a little bit as you exhale, that's an opportunity to experience some calming. When you have that experience, for a single exhalation or three in a row or ten in a row, really register that experience, taking the good of it so it sinks in.

[00:26:00]

[00:26:30]

Maybe you're in a situation where you just have to wait. You just have to be patient. You're in line at a store. The bus isn't there yet. You have to keep listening to your Uncle Bob rattling on after a few beers. You've got to be patient. Okay, right there. You're calm. You're centered. It's not an enjoyable moment, but you're still calm. You're still centered. Right there—an opportunity for learning. Similarly, gratitude. Walking down the street, things you could feel grateful for. Thank you, people who made sidewalks. Thank you, streetlights. Thank you, people walking past me who don't whack me with your shoulder like kids in junior high school might. Thank you, buses that show up on time. Thank you, cell phones. Thank you, ESPN. Thank you, ibuprofen. Thank you, refrigerators. Right? Gratitude. A person might have opportunities for gratitude as well.

[00:27:00]

I'm a big believer in formal practice, but as someone who has done a lot of formal practice and takes people through formal practices, whether it's psychotherapy, say, or meditation, or meditation retreats. As someone who does that, boy, oh boy, oh boy, I've really come to appreciate the value of taking in the good on the fly, in the flow of everyday life. In a way, it really boils down to three things, if you think about it. It's amazingly simple but, of course, we have to do it. See the good facts. Don't miss them. Notice them. Eyes wide open. Notice the good facts.

[00:27:30]

Second, a lot of people notice good facts, but they don't feel anything. They notice people are smiling. They notice they got something done at work. They completed that email. They finished that weird interaction with somebody. They notice it but they don't feel anything as a result. The second step, after seeing the good fact, is feeling the good fact. Slow it down. Take the extra breath or two or three to really feel it. Stay with it. Then once you're feeling it, once you're actually having some kind of appropriate experience, take it in. Turn on the inner recorder. Slow down the experience five, ten, 20, 30 seconds in a row to really help that pattern of mental neural activation that is the basis for that beneficial, useful experience to help that pattern of activation leave lasting traces behind as durable changes of neural structure or function.

[00:28:00]

Those three things can make an enormous difference for people if they just deliberately do them half a dozen times a day, less than half a minute at a time. That's less than five minutes a day and yet research on my own work shows, and also research in other disciplines and domains, also shows those kinds of little deliberate changes taking less than five or ten minutes a day can lead to major accumulating benefits for people, including reduction of the course of a disease.

[00:28:30]

One of the most interesting findings from neuroscience that's relevant to people, is what scientists call the brain's evolved negativity bias. What that means is something I think we've all experienced. Ten things happen in a day in a relationship, let's say, with our partner or with somebody at work. Ten things happen in the day. Nine are positive. Nine went fine. One was negative. One was irritating. One was worrying. All right. Ten things have happened. Do we put 90% of our attention on the nine that were good and do we put only 10% of our attention on the one that was bad? No. The one that went

[00:29:00]   wrong, that's the one we tend to think about. That's an ordinary example of the negativity of bias.

[00:29:30]   It's the idea that the brain basically over-learns from negative, painful, stressful, harmful experiences and under-learns from positive ones because that really helped our ancestors survive and pass on genes and then helped their babies pass on even more genes. If you think about it, in the wild, early humans and our ancestors needed to both get carrots and avoid sticks, carrots like food, etc., sticks like predators. Both are important but if you fail to get a carrot today, you'll have a chance at one tomorrow. If you fail to avoid that stick in the wild, no more carrots forever. We have a brain that,

[00:30:00]   today, routinely does five things. Scans for bad news, over-focuses on it, overreacts to it, fast tracks that whole package into memory, especially what's called implicit or emotional memory, somatic memory and then fifth, gradually sensitizes the brain through cortisol to become even more reactive

[00:30:30]   to stress the day after. That's our nature. The way I describe it is we have a brain that's like Velcro for the bad but Teflon for the good. It's the result of having a brain today that's optimized for peak performance in Stone Age conditions.

This negativity bias creates a lot of excess suffering. It's useful if you're in combat or if you grow up in what's like a combat zone, but most of the time, this negativity bias makes us over-preoccupied with painful experiences, even though we might be having relatively frequent mild or mildly positive

[00:31:00]   experiences over the flow of our day. They just wash though the brain like water through a sieve while those negative ones get caught every time. One of the major takeaways from that is if you're having a negative experience, be with it. Step back from it, hold it in spacious awareness, observe it. Right there you're stopping a process of reinforcing that experience because you've stepped back from it and you're starting to associate that anger or that fear or that shame or the sadness, with spacious mindfulness, which helps to counter-condition it. That said, as soon as you can, start moving on to

[00:31:30]   something else, because neurons that fire together wire together and the longer that negative preoccupation is active, ruminating about it, looping about our worries or the case we're making against other people, our resentments or self-criticism, the more that we tend to marinate or ruminate about that, the more we are wiring that negativity into our own nervous system.

[00:32:00]   That's one takeaway, to really appreciate how vulnerable the brain is to absorb painful, upsetting, stressful experiences, including mild chronic ones in the flow of everyday life. The second takeaway is to tilt toward the positive deliberately, not based on looking at the world through rose-colored glasses, actually based on a very tough-minded, hard-headed understanding that we've got this negativity bias

[00:32:30]   and that Mother Nature is tilted toward survival but therefore against, in many ways, quality of life.

When we tilt toward looking for good facts, helping ourselves have a good experience as a result, which we take into ourselves, if we tilt into that direction, we're just leveling the playing field.

[00:33:00]   One of the great things about the science that's emerging about experience-dependent neuroplasticity is how we, ourselves, from the inside out can turbocharge the learning process. In other words, we can steepen our own growth curve, our own development or healing or learning curve as we go through an hour, a day, a year, a life. There are things we can do from the inside out that really help beneficial experiences land and not just wash through the brain like water through a sieve. One of the major ways we can do that is to tune into what's fresh or alive or new in the experience because the brain is a big novelty detector and what's new, right? That's what we're always looking for.

[00:33:30]   We can become kind of jaded, "Oh, yeah, gratitude, shrug, oh, yeah, feeling connected, whatever, move on, oh yeah, dodged that bullet, fine. The boss liked my stuff, good, so what?" No. If we bring more of what might be called beginner's mind, Zen mind, or if we bring more of a sense of looking at the world or inner experience through the eyes of a child, we're exploring new aspects of a familiar,

[00:34:00]   although beneficial, experience like gratitude or compassion or connection with other people. If we bring that quality of novelty to bear, we're going to increase the conversion rate of that passing experience into being some kind of lasting beneficial trait, hardwired into ourselves.

[00:34:30]

[00:35:00]

The question of how to use our mind to enhance our brain is a fundamental and deep one. Really briefly, in neuroscience, essentially by mind, people mean something really down to earth as a natural phenomenon, not something supernatural or transcendental, simply mind being all the information represented by the nervous system. That may sound kind of strange, but routinely, we're having experiences in which immaterial information is being represented by some kind of material substrate or basis. For example, right now, if we're talking, the information, the meaning of the words I'm expressing here is being represented by changes in frequencies of sound, which are embedded in the air in this room.

[00:35:30]

In the same way, the information, the mind, altogether is represented by the nervous system. The question then becomes, "How do you use the mind to change the brain in a simple kind of way?" The trick or the way, the method, which is wonderfully useful, is that any kind of experience, a sound we're hearing, a thought we're having, a memory that's emerging, a lovingness toward another person, a feeling of our own worth and healthy entitlement, healthy, deserving of care and concern from others, whatever experience we're having is presumably based upon some kind of pattern or underlying neural activity. Otherwise, we're left with supernatural explanations.

[00:36:00]

[00:36:30]

[00:37:00]

Inside the natural frame of science, any sort of experience, as well as unconscious information processing, requires underlying. It entails some underlying pattern of neural activity. Here's the thing. Repeated patterns of neural activity, based on repeated patterns of mental activity that enlist them, so the two going along together; repeated patterns of neural activity leave lasting traces behind in changes of neural structure or function. By deliberately looking for beneficial experiences of various kinds, most of them mild and in the flow of everyday life, we're already having them, by looking for those opportunities of a beneficial pattern, beneficial eddy in the stream of consciousness, if you will, a beneficial pattern of activation, then we can help our brains learn and change for the better by truly taking in the good and maximizing the conversion of that passing pattern of mental neural activation into the lasting residues left behind. That's how we can use the mind to change the brain to change the mind for the better.

[00:37:30]

[00:38:00]

That's the essence of what Jeffrey Schwartz at UCLA described a couple of decades ago as self-directed neuroplasticity. Neuroplasticity is a fancy word, a lot of syllables, right? The root of it is plasticity, which just means the changeability of something, so the plasticity of a substance is how wiggly and bendable and so forth it is. Neuroplasticity simply means the capacity, the property of the nervous system to be changed by the information moving through it, particularly that fraction of the information moving through the nervous system that's involved with the conscious experience. In other words, neurons that fire together wire together, for sure, throughout the entire body, but that process of firing becoming wiring is on steroids for what we pay attention to. Attention is kind of a combination spotlight and vacuum cleaner. It illuminates what it rests up, and then sucks it into the brain.

[00:38:30]

The mechanisms of neuroplasticity, the experience-dependent neuroplasticity, are multiple, and it's really quite striking to appreciate how continuously and dynamically the nervous system is changing. Neuroplasticity is often talked about as if it's breaking news, or even, gosh forbid, being invented by somebody. No, it's been understood for a long time that if there's any sort of learning, children learning to walk instead of crawl, adults learning how to navigate tricky conversations with their partners, if there's any sort of learning, there must be some kind of underlying change. If the mind changes, the body must change as well. Otherwise, we're left with magic, so the body's got to be changed.

[00:39:00]

What is news, though, about neuroplasticity, is our understanding of its profundity and pervasiveness. It's happening continuously. It tends to be biased negatively, so watch out for that. Also, we can make use of the opportunities in it. There are many mechanisms of neuroplasticity, if I were to just list a few really quickly here. One is in the famous saying that neurons that fire together wire together. Existing synapses get sensitized. New synapses form. New neurons are actually born in the hippocampus and

[00:39:30] maybe other regions of the brain, but primarily in the human brain in the hippocampus, through neurogenesis. Regions that are active and busy, if we're repeatedly engaging some mental function, we're going to activate repeatedly the part of the brain that does that thing, which will increase blood flow to that part of the brain.

[00:40:00] Different parts of the brain connect with each other in new ways. There are changes. That's another mechanism of neuroplasticity. Changes in the expression in genes, little strips of atoms in the twisted-up molecules of DNA, deep in the nuclei of individual neurons so that certain genes that do good things become more expressed. Certain genes that are involved in problematic things become more inhibited. That's another mechanism of neuroplasticity. Just to finish, as well, there can be changes in the flows of neuro chemicals, greater serotonin activity in terms of building up a kind of underfloor to protect mood, so that we don't fall through the floor into depression, changes in the activity of, let's say, dopamine or norepinephrine or natural opioids or oxytocin, other neurotransmitter systems.

[00:40:30] That's another mechanism of neuroplasticity.

[00:41:00] Now to finish, the amazing thing isn't so much that the brain changes. The amazing thing is that there are parts of the brain that don't change at all, and they are few and far between. I grew up in a loving home in a relatively ordinary middle/low class environment and along the way, for various reasons having to do with my parents not being very empathic while also being loving and also being very young and dorky going through school, I skipped a grade and have a late birthday, so I was very young and kind of shy and so forth, so I didn't get a lot of the social supplies, they're called, that people normally need, even relatively introverted stubborn and independent people temperamentally, like me. It was a little bit like trying to breathe through a straw. You can get enough air but it's just not enough. The supplies were more like a thin soup.

[00:41:30] I ended up, then, when I went off to college and my early adulthood, in my late teens, with what felt like a huge hole in my heart. Also, I should add that in school, I wasn't particularly bullied but I was left out a lot, and I ended up feeling, as my dad who grew up on a ranch in North Dakota put it, like the runt of the litter. That left me with this kind of hole inside, the absence of the good is often as painfully problematic as the presence of the bad. Then the question is, "What can you do about it?"

[00:42:00] In my own story, I learned, amazingly kind of early in college, that if I just looked for those good facts of being included, seen in value, typically small but real in the flow of everyday life, and then if I let myself feel included or seen or liked or wanted. Some girl would smile at me and, "Oh, I'm not such a loser after all." Something would happen inside me and then, in particular, I just started doing this thing of feeling like it was sinking in, like water into a sponge, or it was shifting inside me. Something was happening. That gradually, slowly but surely, filled the hole in my heart. One of the takeaways

[00:42:30] from that in terms of how to deal with situations with others who are confronting us, is that through internalizing those supplies, it's really simple and basic, which I love about this. It's simple and usually enjoyable, but we have to do the work. We have to do it. We earn our gains but we have to do the work to get them.

[00:43:00] If a person repeatedly internalizes those beneficial experiences, including, for example, a sense of confidence that I am also loved, that I am also liked, that I'm not a complete loser, I'm not damaged goods. As we build that up inside, then, when other people are challenging, we have more of that shock absorber. We have more layers of resilience and depth that that challenge is landing upon or triggering and even if we do get rattled, it's a little bit like with repetition, one synapse at a time, one

[00:43:30] neuron at a time, one moment at a time. It's as if we are deepening as we internalize and grow resources inside. It's as if we are deepening the keel of our personal sailboat, deep, deep, deep in the water so that even if someone is confrontational or challenging or dismissive or devaluing and knocks us off balance with that deeper keel, we right ourselves more rapidly, and we're then more able to mount a response that's appropriate, that's neither too weak nor too combative.

[00:44:00] That, to me, is one of the great double benefits of this kind of work. We can use it to both heal old wounds and fill old holes in the heart, and also grow resources for dealing with real world challenges here and now and moving forward into the rest of our life. If there is one takeaway for me from all this material, it's to appreciate the power of little things with a brain in which neurons are typically firing 5

[00:44:30] to 50 times a second, in which coalitions of millions, if not more, of synapses are firing synchronously at the same time, many times a second, thus producing brain waves that are detectable in EEGs and so forth. It's all happening extremely quickly. That means that an experience that lasts half a breath or a breath or two or three in its duration can make a big difference.

[00:45:00] It's lots of little things added up over time that usually take us to a bad place, and it's going to be lots of little things adding up over time that take us to a better one. I like that because it's very hopeful. Even in the midst of a life that's really challenging and difficult, there are always these authentic little moments of beneficial experience, reassurance, relief, completion, gratitude, some kind of pleasure, some kind of ending of pain, some kind of connection with another person, that right there are our

[00:45:30] opportunities, multiple times a day, to take in the good, let it land, and then have it with us wherever we go.

ROBERT MELILLO, DC | Author: *Disconnected Kids*, Co-Founder Brain Balance Achievement Centers, drrobertmelillo.com, brainbalancecenters.com

Dr. Robert Melillo:

[00:00:30]

My background is I started out as a chiropractor. I went into chiropractic because I was an athlete and played college football, something I grew up with. When I was in chiropractic school, I fell in love with neurology. It was one of the first courses I had. When I graduated, I got to do a subspecialty in neurology and then rehabilitation. Neurology and rehabilitation has always been my focus as well as diet and nutrition, something I've always been interested in, even personally most of my life.

[00:01:00]

When I was in practice, teaching clinical neurology, and doing rehab, I had a friend and neighbor that actually approached me about her son who had severe ADHD. She had started a large organization of parents and teachers that were all focused on learning challenges, in ADHD in particular. She asked me if I could look into some of the alternative approaches that were being presented to her. She had people coming up to her talking about nutrition, and diet, and eye exercises in chiropractic, osteopathy, and craniopathy.

[00:01:30]

[00:02:00]

She didn't know if any of it was valid or not. She knew I had a pretty varied background. She asked me if I would look into it. I didn't know a whole lot about ADHD or childhood developmental issues at the time, but I felt like I should. I was a father of three young kids. When I became aware of how much it was expanding, it really concerned me both professionally and personally. Statistics came out in 1995 that actually showed that the use of Ritalin had increased in the United States 250% between 1990 and 1995.

[00:02:30]

Nobody really knew why. That was something a lot of people paid attention to. Here was this medication for significant behavioral issues that was increasing dramatically. No one really could explain that. I started looking into it. At the same time, I went to a parent-teacher meeting. The teacher told my wife and I that she thought my son had some issues, whether learning issues or attention issues, really couldn't pinpoint, but he was pretty impulsive and hyperactive. Now, it became something that was personal for me. From that point of time on, I really focused on looking at what the problem was.

[00:03:00]

I think the challenge with the conventional approach to neurological disorders is it doesn't really take into account the brain. I think very few people out there really understand what I refer to as functional neurology, meaning the way the brain works, and the way it develops. I think that's another really major issue, is looking at developmental neurology.

[00:03:30]

I think a lot of the things we're looking at now that are adult issues, we realized that they really start in development either in the womb or early in the first few years of life; things like schizophrenia that may not show up until into the 20s. Actually, we know that if you have two identical twins, and at six months of age, you basically go back and look at their videos, and one of them ends up with schizophrenia and one of them doesn't, you can already identify differences in the way they're moving and their motor developmental milestones. I think that's a critical piece.

[00:04:00]

Many people are really focused on the biochemistry of the brain, but they're not really understanding how the brain actually works and the way networks develop, the way networks integrate, or when they don't integrate with one another. What I look at is different developmental imbalances in the brain and understanding that the brain controls everything so that not only can problems in the body with the digestive system, metabolic issues, toxins, not only can that affect the brain in the way it functions, but it also, I think more commonly, goes the other way around that when the brain doesn't develop appropriately, when there are imbalances in different areas of the brain, especially between the two

[00:04:30]

hemispheres of the brain, that actually alters the biochemistry.

[00:05:00] It creates imbalances in the immune system, the digestive system, and the autonomic system. It can affect the way the body metabolizes blood sugar and the way we detoxify. Understanding that there is this two-way street, but also understanding that the brain in many cases takes the lead. I don't think that is considered typically when people are looking at the brain issues. They're looking purely at more obvious things, like attention problems, psychological, psychiatric, learning, or memory, but they're not

[00:05:30] realizing that even things like autoimmunity, food sensitivities, chronic bowel issues, and all of these issues could actually be caused by problems in the brain and in development of the brain.

Functional disconnection, what it is, is that as the brain is developing, there are a number of different things that happen. Obviously, the brain is growing, but what's also happening, and more importantly,

[00:06:00] is that the brain is actually developing connections. It's also developing specific networks. It's becoming localized so that areas of the brain and the brainstem are carrying specific types of information or controlling different types of functions and movements. What's really critical is as the brain is developing, those networks have to become more coordinated and synchronized with one another.

[00:06:30] They have to really be able to communicate and integrate. What makes your brain really unique is the fact that we have this really large brain, but what we have is areas of the brain that are really perfectly integrated. One of the things that the human brain does better than anything else is that we can activate multiple areas of our brain at the exact same moment of time, simultaneously. If there is some disruption in that timing, even we think on the nanosecond time level, it can disrupt the way the brain

[00:07:00] actually works and the way we're able to remember things, the way we're able to learn, the way we're able to recall different memories and the way the brain will then control the body.

Functional disconnection is basically saying there's something that's disrupting the way that integration and communication develops that there's not anything specifically wrong with any one area of the brain. Most of the issues we look at like autism, when we look at their brains, they look pretty normal.

[00:07:30] That's one of the things why most people I don't think really understand what autism is, or what ADHD is, or what many of the learning challenges like dyslexia are, because when we look at an MRI, or an image of the brain, it looks pretty normal.

There isn't anything that stands out unless you really start looking at the dynamics of the brain and the way that communication is or isn't taking place. Essentially, functional disconnection is that there isn't

[00:08:00] any damage in the brain, but there's a problem with communication between areas of the brain that they're not sharing information appropriately. Therefore, the person can't really use all areas of their brain in a learning process or a memory process or in just day-to-day thinking skills.

[00:08:30] What we often see are certain types of imbalances that develop in their functions like as in autism, we see that for the most part, in the main type of autism which is what we call an essential autism, there's this unevenness of skills and really in all of these issues. This is something that stood out in the literature for many years that no one really was able to completely explain, that when you look at dyslexia or autism or ADHD or OCD or threats, all of these individuals have certain areas of their brain

[00:09:00] and certain functions that are delayed, or behind, or immature, whereas they have other areas of their brain that are very advanced or maybe even genius level or even savant level.

This imbalance in their skills is often confusing when people look at it, but what it really represents is this imbalance in networks of the brain where we have certain networks that are stronger, over-

[00:09:30] connected, and even process information faster than what most humans do. Then, in the same individual, we see other networks where they're underdeveloped and they're really more immature. That represents the cause, I believe, of a functional disconnection.

When we look at the idea that people automatically think that something, especially autism, is genetic, most people don't really understand what that means. I think they get it wrong in the media a lot.

[00:10:00] When somebody says that it's genetic, when a researcher or when a paper comes out, the implication is that there's some genetic mutation, that there's something wrong with the DNA—that it's actually been physically altered in some way.

[00:10:30] For many years, people believed that the only way you could pass a trait on through different generations was if you literally had a physical alteration of DNA. In autism, going back to the 70s, I believe, the first study was done looking at twin studies. They looked at identical twins and fraternal twins. What they found in that study was there was a very high rate, 80%, 90% of identical twins that had autism as a diagnosis. There was a much, much lower rate for fraternal twins.

[00:11:00] This was a very small study. I think there were only 10 or 12 people in the study. At that point, the idea was, "Oh, autism must be genetic because if there's such a difference between identical and fraternal twins." There's been about 25 different studies throughout the years looking at that. All of them correlated that, until a study in 2001 out of Stanford where they really looked at the largest study, which was about 162 different pairs of twins with autism.

[00:11:30] What they found was very different from previous studies. They found that there was actually a higher rate with fraternal twins than there was with identical twins. What they stated in that study was that 60% or more of the factors that contributed to autism were environmental and only about 40% or 38% were actually genetic. This really speaks to the concept of epigenetics, which is what we really know [00:12:00] now that governs most of what happens, is that there isn't actually physical damage to genes, but rather segments of genes are turned off and inhibited, usually by different chemicals and molecules in our body—methyl molecules in particular—that basically cover up and prevent that from being read.

[00:12:30] In the old days before the 1990s, when epigenetics started to become out and really in 2000 when a landmark study came out, we used to believe that during the period of conception, these epigenetic marks that basically cover up our genes and prevent them from being read, and can cause many different types of disorders or issues. We believe that during conception, all of the marks were wiped clean. Then, a baby would start with a clean genetic slate.

[00:13:00] We now know that's not the case, that many of those marks, let's say, the sins, if you will, of the adults, of the parents, can actually be passed on to the children. We know now that different studies have shown that can go for at least up to 11 generations that we know. In practical terms, what does that mean? It means that if someone smokes, and they have children, it's possible that some of those chemicals may actually block some genes that may not affect the adult who is smoking, but actually [00:13:30] may affect the genes of their children and their children's children. The genes, 85% of our genes are actually there to build our brain. The genes that are most commonly affected are the ones that actually have to do with brain development.

[00:14:00] With regards to epigenetics, and what can turn genes on and off—almost anything. In my book, *Autism: The Scientific Truth*, I identified around 50 different really well-documented, well-researched environmental risk factors that may elevate the risk of somebody or a couple having a child with autism or some other developmental issue. We know things like age are a factor. We know things like diabetes, hypertension, and obesity are significant factors.

[00:14:30] We know stress and how someone metabolizes or how the stress affects their body is something. We know if they have different vitamin or mineral deficiencies, things like they don't have enough folic acid, iron, or things like that. We know if they have activation of their immune system, or if they have things like a gluten sensitivity, or they have autoimmunity, or if someone, in particular if the mother gets a flu virus, we know that that elevates the risk significantly.

[00:15:00] The fact is though, all of these risk factors really do primarily one thing to the body. They really contribute to causing inflammation, increasing production of stress hormones and all of those chemicals that are released during that or activation of the immune system and inflammatory immune regulators. They are the ones that really primarily interact with genes and can alter it. All of the different factors really do, for the most part, the same thing.

[00:15:30]   In my experience, and from my perspective, one of the biggest risk factors that nobody really talked about is if the adults have imbalances or functional disconnections in their own brain. If they have imbalances or if there are areas of their brain that haven't really been as active, that haven't developed

[00:16:00]   as well as they should, those imbalances create imbalances in their body. Those imbalances in their body are more likely to lead to an activation of their fight-or-flight system and cause inflammation, production of cortisol, all of those different chemicals in their body that may then block the expression of genes in their own children, so any of those factors.

              There are many of them. We're really learning them every day, different things like pollution. It's

[00:16:30]   confusing because there's one study—a really good study—out of California that shows people, and mothers in particular, who live near highways and were exposed to pollution, exhaust fumes, mercury, and heavy metals, that the risk of having a child with autism went up significantly. But then, there was another study that showed if you live on a farm and you're exposed to pesticides and fungicides, and things like that, your risk of having a child with autism goes up dramatically.

[00:17:00]   That's why probably the most important thing is not only looking at your environment, but being able to really understand what's going in your body and measure those things. The good news is that almost all of these risk factors are modifiable or avoidable and can be eliminated. What we need to start thinking more is really what I think preconception more than what we've been doing. Obviously, giving

[00:17:30]   prenatal vitamins and trying to make somebody healthy, but really being more specific and looking at all of these distant different factors in trying to get them into a good functional range before you get pregnant because if the genes are already turned off in the parents, then when you get pregnant, it's already there.

[00:18:00]   The good news is because there are environmental factors in the womb, and even after the child is born, and even into adulthood, we can modify gene expression or at least we're pretty sure we can so that it's never over. It's never too late, but it's also never too early. The way we know it that somebody has a functional disconnection or a brain imbalance, there are a number of different clues throughout our life. Like I said, most of these start in development, really start in the womb or maybe even preconception.

[00:18:30]   One of the earliest signs is really looking at developmental milestones, in particular motor milestones, the way the brain develops. One of the most important things for brain development in children is movement. In my first textbook, *Neurobehavioral Disorders of Childhood and Evolutionary Perspective*, I was trying to really go back to the beginning. We're looking at learning problems.

[00:19:00]   We're looking at behavioral issues. We're looking at brain issues. The question I had was where do brains come from? Why do brains develop, to begin with? What we know, it's been very well-documented in the research, that brains develop because some living thing decided to move, and that brains are only necessary for moving creatures. Movement is what really initiated brains to begin with on this planet. Movement is what initiates development of brains in children.

[00:19:30]   Looking at that and looking at how we move, if a child doesn't roll over at three to five months on both sides, if they don't crawl in a normal way, if they don't really crawl in what we call a cross-crawl pattern, if they don't do that in a specific timeframe, and really, they should then stand up and walk

[00:20:00]   almost exactly at 12 months. What I hear all the time is parents come to our centers or come to my office and will tell me how their child had some delay in crawling or walking. Then, maybe in speaking or in their nonverbal communication, their social skills, their eye contact, something like that.

              When it starts somewhere in development, it then progresses. It doesn't usually go away on its own. It usually gets worse. What we see is that they're often told that it doesn't matter. One mother actually

[00:20:30] said to me, "Why do we get this list from the pediatrician of all these developmental milestones? Then, when you go back to them and you tell them that your child didn't meet it, they say, 'Well, it doesn't matter.'"

[00:21:00] We know it does matter. I know that pediatricians are mostly just trying to not be alarmist, and they're trying not to make the parents worried, but it's important because also they do it because they don't know what else to do about it, meaning they're delayed. What are we really going to do? We know, and a lot of what I do, is really look to work even with small children on, if they're not crawling properly, then try to change that and intervene at that point. We know the earlier you can intervene, the better the outcome. Getting them to move better and getting them to walk on time, all those things are really important.

[00:21:30]
[00:22:00] I think the problem with autism research is that most of it has been really geared towards looking for genetic mutations. I think, obviously, pharmaceutical companies and people looking for that answer. Yes. I've seen estimates that 95% of the research dollars over the past 25 years have been spent looking for that genetic mutation. We haven't found it. I would like to look more at the actual functional neurology of the brain. We have actually published a lot of research in that area. Whenever I go on and I lecture, and I lecture to all different types of audiences all of whom either work with or have kids with different types of problems and especially in professionals, the first question I ask them is, "Who can tell me what's actually happening in the brain in someone with autism or ADHD or OCD?"

[00:22:30]
[00:23:00] When I ask that to an audience and I say, " Raise your hand if you think you could answer that." Almost in every audience for the past 10 years I've been doing this, nobody raises their hand. Even in MDS and PhDs and really sophisticated audiences, I think the majority of people out there working with these issues don't really know what the problem is. Therefore, I think really understanding the way the brain works, understanding where there is a problem with the functional neurology, the functional connectivity in the brain itself, understanding the epigenetics, and being able to try to identify and really show that there is an epimutation or where something is blocking a gene, and then being able to show that we can do different things that might be able to wipe off those methyl marks and change gene expression.

[00:23:30]
[00:24:00] I think that's really important. I think looking more at nutrition and diet and how that plays a role and looking at physical activity and exercise. There's one researcher, John Constance, out of the University of Washington St. Louis, who has published some really good research looking at, again, identical twins of kids with autism. And following them out and really identifying that the difference between an identical twin who gets autism, and it doesn't get autism, is really looking at their motor development, and that is probably one of the main features we're looking at.

[00:24:30] I think looking at real practical functions of the brain, really mapping out networks and looking at how they don't connect with each other, and looking at different interventions that really focus on creating connectivity in the brain itself, rather than looking and spending a lot of time for genetic mutations that don't exist. If we're going to really look at factors like that, let's look at environmental factors that affect the epigenome and gene expression more than looking for gene mutations, I think, because what are you going to do if there are gene mutations anyway? There's not much you're going to do.

[00:25:00]
[00:25:30] If there are epigenetic factors, those are things that we can fact for pre-conception, during conception and after conception, and really make a huge difference. I think we're just finding out a lot about the nutrients, and all of the different factors that come into play when we look at pregnancy, and during that period of that antenatal period. Folic acid, we believe, is important because it has to do with what we call a methylation pathway. Methylation is really important, as I said for gene expression, but it's also important for a number of different pathways and the way we metabolize certain substances and even as it affects our detoxification process.

[00:26:00] The way we break down different toxins in our body, those are really important factors. Again, we know that a lot of environmental factors and a lot of what that's related to is the way that our digestive system is working. Why does somebody not have enough folic acid? Really, that comes down to that we need to have proper levels of acid in our stomach to be able to do that. We need to have the right digestive enzymes to be able to do that. We have to have proper blood flow to our digestive system to absorb these different nutrients. B12 is associated with that as well.

[00:26:30] Then, the way I think is we see people that have issues where they're deficient in folic acid or deficient in a vitamin or mineral or they have food sensitivities. I look at it. I go, "Why? Why does this person have it and these people don't?" A lot of that again goes back to how the brain may be regulating those things. If our brain isn't developed and isn't working properly and isn't balanced, we get an imbalance between our fight-or-flight and our rest-and-digest systems—our sympathetic and our parasympathetic system.

[00:27:00]
[00:27:30] Generally, we get under-activation of what's called our vagal system. Our vagal system really slows our heart rate, increases blood flow through our digestive system and our organs and allows us to rest and relax and feel safe and repair. The fight-or-flight system we're born with is on in the womb that's already very active. What that does is it takes blood from our digestive system and our organs and moves it out to our muscles so we can fight or run away. If we're in a chronic state like that, if our brain doesn't develop in that first year appropriately in our brain stem, we don't inhibit those things.

[00:28:00] Therefore, what happens is that we don't produce the proper level of acid in our stomach to digest food and digestive enzymes. We can't break down proteins as well as we should. We don't have proper blood flow. We end up with malabsorption of vitamins and minerals and nutrients and amino acids. We end up where our stomach lining becomes more porous. It's not as healthy as it should. The cells start to separate a little bit. We get what is called a leaky gut or intestinal permeability.

[00:28:30] Now, foods that aren't fully digested, especially proteins that normally wouldn't get through the stomach lining, can get through the stomach lining. When they do, they may come in contact with an immune system that's overactive because if our brain is out of balance, our immune system can be out of balance. I think this is what may set up the situation as to why we have vitamin and mineral deficiencies or why we have food sensitivities or why we have chronic immunity issues and inflammation.

[00:29:00]
[00:29:30] All of those factors and environmental factors and chemicals we're exposed to, all of us are exposed to these things. We can go back and see that heavy metals have been around for probably millions of years in our environment. It's really more the way our body is interacting with our environment. A lot of that has to do with our own lifestyle. Most of the factors that influence gene expression and most of the factors that are driving an epidemic rise in things like autism and ADHD and even adult issues are the same factors that are actually causing an epidemic of obesity and diabetes and heart disease in adults. It's mostly lifestyle factors, and especially things like not moving and not eating properly and exposure to different chemicals.

[00:30:00]
[00:30:30] But a lot of it has to do with the fact that our brain isn't developing as appropriately as it should. It's affecting our body's ability to interact with the environment. Obviously, when we look at what nutrients are important for the brain, it really depends on what that individual needs. To a certain extent, that's the whole point of Functional Medicine and Functional Neurology, is that it's really directed towards the individual. It's based on measuring what their individual needs are, but certainly, there are some basic things that I tell just about everybody. Omega-3s and, in particular, DHA, are very important for the brain, for the membrane of the brain itself, so that it remains fluid, so that it doesn't start to break down, and so that we can get a proper exchange of nutrients and ions. That's really important.

[00:31:00]   Vitamin D, I think, is hugely important because it helps to balance out the immune system. It helps to really support a lot of our digestive functions and maybe limits what foods we become sensitive to. I think it's probably the most important immune factor. If we have an imbalance in the immune system, like I said, that really can cause a lot of problems, cause a breakdown of our blood-brain barrier or breakdown of our gut and really lead to some big issues.

[00:31:30]   As we've discussed, folic acid and B12 I think a lot of the B vitamins are very important for brain itself. I think that CoQ10 and looking at things that help support mitochondrial function are really important. We know that a lot of the issues that we see are when the mitochondria, which is really the energy source of the brain cells, when that starts to break down and become dysfunctional, that's when all hell breaks loose in our brain. That probably ends up leading to many chronic neurodegenerative issues, a process what we call excitotoxicity.

[00:32:00]

[00:32:30]   Magnesium can be helpful to diminish that. It helps to lower that fight-or-flight response in our body and helps to improve blood flow. I think probiotics obviously, because the gut health is really important, and especially for the brain that the brain and the gut interact with one another. Therefore, if the brain isn't working properly, we get a breakdown of that gut biome, but being able to try to reestablish that and restore that is very important as well.

[00:33:00]   I think at the most basic level, I look at the omega-3s, vitamin D, probiotics. Then, in addition to vitamin D, we usually recommend vitamin A and vitamin K to go along with that. Then, I like to look at the individual person and see what they need. I do recommend that if you can try to eat foods that are rich in those particular nutrients, because if the person has this high fight-or-flight system on, you can give them a lot of vitamins and you can have them eat food, but they're not going to digest it properly.

[00:33:30]   If their brain isn't working properly and their digestive system isn't working properly, they can eat a lot of food. They may have a great diet. I see this all the time. The parents are really aware and feed their children great foods and great diet, but the child isn't digesting any of it. They're not breaking it down because they're not producing digestive enzymes. They're not producing acid. They don't have the blood flow in their gut. They can't absorb these nutrients.

[00:34:00]   In that case, then trying to supplement them and give them more, I think is really important. Sometimes, we have to use things that are more sublingual or might be absorbed through the mouth or the mucosa because they're not going to be able to break it down or absorb it in their gut properly. I think that a combination of both. I prefer food, whole foods. In most cases, if their digestive system isn't working properly and if their brain isn't working properly, then they're not going to get it from foods, even if they're eating a really healthy diet in there.

[00:34:30]

[00:35:00]   Therefore, we need to supplement them. When you have kids, they're in this fight-or-flight, which again anybody that has a developmental issue. We're born with our sympathetic fight-or-flight system more active. We've actually shown that kids with autism and ADHD have a persistence of that through their life, meaning they're always more in this fight-or-flight. The most effective thing you can do is actually to create balance in their brain and stimulate brain growth and development so that we look at where in the development did something go awry.

[00:35:30]   What we see is that as the brain is building from the bottom up, meaning that it starts in the brainstem, when we're first born, we really only have about 25% of our brain there. In the first three years, we'll develop 90% of the adult brain. There's this massive growth phase that occurs after we're born. It can't happen before we're born because the head wouldn't get out. It's important.

[00:36:00]   All of these environmental stimuli like light, sound, heat, temperature, and especially movement and gravity, actually stimulate and turn on genes that help to build our brain from the bottom up, basically like layers. What we find is that the two sides of the brain develop in series rather than in parallel, meaning that the right side of the brain really develops in the womb for the first two to three years.

Then, we get the left brain, then the right brain, then the left brain.

[00:36:30]

This being exposed to different environmental stimuli and experiences at different stages of development—what we find is that is what creates the difference or what we call lateralization or asymmetry of our brain, so that the right brain ends up being better at certain things and the left brain ends up being better at other things. This is really something that is advantageous to us as humans. That makes a huge difference in our ability to think and learn, and why we're smarter than other animals.

[00:37:00]

What we know is that if something interferes with that development, we get almost like an arrested development of certain networks at different stages, so being able to identify where that is. A lot of that is looking at the movement and looking at something that we call primitive reflexes, which are reflexes we're born with. We said that we have to move to build a brain. But we don't have a brain yet, so how do we move to build our brain when we don't have a brain yet that's going to move us? We're born with these reflexes in the brainstem.

[00:37:30]

In that same area is where many of the basic nuclei for the fight-or-flight system and the vagal system really come from. The maturity of these brainstem areas have to develop first. Then, ultimately, they go, and create the brain. Then, the prefrontal cortex, which is really where all of our thinking skills, our personality, and what makes us human literally grows out of the motor cortex. Then, that all comes down and ultimately ends up controlling things.

[00:38:00]

[00:38:30]

The best way to modify that fight-or-flight and to stimulate the vagal centers, or the rest-and-digest—is really to stimulate those brain networks on the way out with brain activity, and making sure they're moving the way they should. There are simple exercises we can do that will inhibit these primitive reflexes and will cause brain stem development. Then, there are things we can do to the brain itself. There's what we call bottom-up types of approaches. Then, there's top-down approaches, but there's nothing more important than really getting the brain to inhibit these mechanisms themselves.

[00:39:00]

You can do other things like eliminating foods or eliminating triggers. If the digestive problems, inflammation, or the things that are also triggering some of this fight-or-flight, are from the brain, then all you're doing is really just putting out fires. You ultimately need to really deal with the brain issues by identifying foods, or identifying different environmental triggers that might lead to inflammation, or activation of the immune system or toxins in our body.

[00:39:30]

Those are also very, very important to help reduce that fight-or-flight system. Basically, using a bottom-up or a top-down approach, or both, is what we do with every child we work with. We have centers all across the country. We'll work with thousands of kids this year. We've worked with tens of thousands of kids and families. In all of those, what I developed was a way of assessing their development and looking at their bottom-up processes—did the maturity and development of their brain happen the way it was supposed to, or did they get stuck somewhere along the way?

[00:40:00]

Then, also looking at if it did get stuck, did it affect more right-brain development or left-brain development? Then, what do we have to do to try to stimulate growth at that level? It's very important to really identify where in the development the problem came about. Then, we need to go back to that and build that bridge again. Looking at primitive reflexes is really important. We do that with pretty much every kid, but what you see with primitive reflexes, it's pretty fascinating.

[00:40:30]

I'm actually presenting a paper in Oxford this summer at a conference called *Movement and Cognition,* that right now, one of the big things that the psychology and psychiatry community is realizing, is the importance of movement and development of the brain, and development of cognitive and emotional abilities, cognitive abilities, social skills, learning, and attention. All of those are built on top of movement and sensory stimulation.

[00:41:00]

[00:41:30] Those are things we're getting less and less of in our society. I just did a lecture in Sweden to a group of doctors. What I often do is ask someone to come up and/or a bunch of people to come up. We demonstrate that many of these doctors, who are really well trained and obviously bright, still have some of these primitive reflexes. Many of them still have a history of a developmental issue, but because they're so gifted in certain areas, they've been able to compensate.

[00:42:00] I've seen people that have gone through med school, or chiropractic school, or physical therapy, who are severely dyslexic and you think, "How can they get through school if they can't read very well?" But they compensate because they have other areas of their brain that are so gifted that they find ways around it, but they're still struggling. Once we identify these primitive reflexes, we can actually get rid of them pretty quickly through different exercises and through creating balance in their brain.

[00:42:30] Then, everything changes. All of a sudden, people are able to read who couldn't their whole life, or anxiety that they've had forever suddenly goes away. Finding that, not everybody has these primitive reflexes and not everybody has these bottom-up problems. Not all problems are developmental. Other problems may be acquired. People can get brain injuries, or have traumatic emotional experiences, or get sick, or get into a car accident. There are all different types of things that can happen. That's the important thing is when I look at somebody, whether it's a child, a teenager, or an adult, the first thing I look at is to see if there's a developmental issue here.

[00:43:00] One of the best ways to see that is, do they still have some primitive reflexes and do they have a developmental history? Did they miss some of their milestones? Did they skip over them? Did they walk late? Did they talk late or did they struggle? A lot of people don't know that. Their parents never knew or said, "You didn't walk on time." But they know that they struggled in school as a kid. They know they couldn't pay attention. They know they were hyperactive or they know they couldn't read.

[00:43:30] Looking at that tells us, is this something that's been there their whole life and what we're looking at is the end result of that, or is this something that was acquired later on because of some other factor? That makes a big difference, whether we're going to use a top-down approach or whether we're going to use a bottom-up approach, or both.

[00:44:00] Any parent that is struggling with a child with any of the labels, learning disabilities, ADHD, autism, and quite honestly in our centers, maybe up to 50% of the people who come in don't even have a label, but they know they're struggling. There are two things parents should be aware of. We'll give them a clue if the problem is primarily a brain imbalance. Did they meet all their developmental milestones and, also, does your child have a real unevenness of skills?

[00:44:30] This is something we see parents come in with all the time that they're really good at certain things and really good at playing with Legos, or they're really good at remembering directions, or they have great eye contact, but yet they can't read or they can't remember something. Most parents are aware. That's confusing to them because they see these really great skills their child has, and the teacher may even see that. But then, they struggle so much in other areas.

[00:45:00]
[00:45:30] The important thing to understand is what you're looking at is this developmental imbalance. The good news is that those things are changeable at any point. Many parents are out there. It really kills me that they believe their child is broken or their family is broken, and over 80% of families end up in divorce if they have children with developmental issues like autism. It's so important for parents to understand that the child is never broken, that you can change these things at almost any stage, and not only change them, but most of the kids I work with are really gifted.

[00:46:00] They're so gifted in certain areas of their brain. Certain areas of the brain are so strong. Certain networks are so good relative to other people, they're more susceptible to an imbalance because if the environment doesn't properly stimulate the growth and development during one stage of development, they're more likely to develop an imbalance because they're so good in certain areas.

Never give up on the child. There's always hope and we see it all the time.

[00:46:30]　　I think people really need to educate themselves and stay away from anybody that tells you, "There's nothing you can do, just accept it, just be happy with the small stuff." Anybody that's saying that to you, just run away from them as fast you can and really educate yourself. I think my books are a really good source of where to start, because it gives them a different perspective on what actually is out

[00:47:00]　　there, but also exercises, diet, nutrition. There are so many great people doing so many great innovative things that I think they can really see things that will change their life, and really get their children to be who they always knew they would be.

[00:47:30]　　That's the greatest thing when parents come up to me and say, "You really gave us the child we always knew was there that couldn't get out. Now, here he is (or here she is)." Usually, of course, they're crying. I'm crying at that point. But to me, there's nothing more important. There's nothing more important than being able to help a child that's struggling, to be able to help a family, and to be able to restore their hopes and dreams. My main message is never give up, and always keep hoping, and you'll find the answers.

ROBIN BERZIN, MD | Founder/CEO Parsley Health

Dr. Robin Berzin: The challenge in the conventional medical way we approach chronic disease is that medicine has been designed for an era where acute illness was our main concern. Today, that's just no longer the case; 86% of our disease burden today is chronic and lifestyle-driven or lifestyle-modifiable. We have a system where we really should be managing a lot more of our medical needs on the primary care level. We should be integrating nutrition, wellness, and prevention into primary care. We should be

[00:00:30]   having amazing longitudinal relationships with our patients, and spending a lot more time with them than we do.

Instead, what we have, because of the way we pay for primary care, and the way our healthcare system has evolved, is we have a system where we don't really pay very much for primary care. People either bounce in and out of emergency rooms or urgent care, or they go to specialists who are highly expensive. Yet, we know that most people don't need medication, most people need to change their lifestyle. They need to change the way they're eating, moving, managing stress, and their overall toxin

[00:01:00]   burden. We see that when we change these things or help people change these things, they're able to restore vitality. They're able to resolve a lot of the common chronic cardiometabolic, immune, inflammatory, gastrointestinal, what have you. All sorts of diseases can be resolved or at least modified in these ways, and we're not doing enough of that. As a result, our costs are skyrocketing.

At Parsley Health, we integrate nutrition, wellness, and prevention into cutting-edge medicine. We

[00:01:30]   believe you need to take a whole-person approach to primary care. We need to look at all aspects of your life from when you were born, your family history, your genomics, your environment, maybe even your microbiome, all the way through to now, the medications you're taking, the foods you're eating, and even the diagnoses that you have. We need to take a global view of you, which we do, get to know you over time, and help you manage and resolve chronic diseases. Put nutrition and wellness first, but also using cutting-edge diagnostic testing and medicine along the way. Really, Parsley Health is a hybrid

[00:02:00]   of the best of both worlds. It's bringing together cutting-edge medicine as well as a nutrition, wellness, and prevention-first approach.

We have physical offices at Parsley Health, but you can also work with us via tele-medicine. After your first doctor's visit at Parsley, any visit can be virtual or via video. We believe that medicine should come to you. We send mobile phlebotomists to your house to do a blood draw. We really believe that medicine should be embedded in your life and come to you where you are, as opposed to constantly asking you to come in to the doctor's office.

[00:02:30]   I definitely think Parsley Health is the future of medicine. Both because we're incredibly tech-forward—we've built our own platform that allows you to interact with your doctor and your health coach completely seamlessly. Because we're not fee-for-service—we operate entirely through a membership model—we're not incentivized to see you more and have you come back over and over again like regular doctors are. We're incentivized to have you be our member and help you get healthy over time, and not necessarily just to use more care.

[00:03:00]   We're absolutely the future of medicine in terms of our clinical approach, which is unique to any conventional doctor out there. All of our doctors are board-certified and trained in conventional medicine. They've all additionally been trained to use a functional, whole-person, health approach. That's been game-changing for our patients. We actually show that we have 72 times the engagement of a regular primary care doctor. You spend 225 minutes with your doctor each year instead of 15 minutes with the average primary care doctor and we're reducing prescription drugs 70%. The average primary care doctor results in a prescription drug at 80% of encounters. At Parsley Health, that's 10%.

[00:03:30]   What we're able to do is help people live their way healthy, in addition to managing their illnesses along the way.

[00:04:00]   The idea of functional lab testing is just that we look at more than what a conventional doctor might to understand the root cause or the underlying issue that could be driving a problem. Instead of saying, "You're depressed. Let's give you an anti-depressant." We'll say, "You're depressed. Let's look into why." For some people, depression can be driven by a hormone imbalance like hypothyroidism or an imbalance in the female hormones or even low testosterone. For other people, depression could be driven by inflammation and we can look at that in the body. We now know that the microbes, the bugs in your gut actually are linked to your mood, and we can test those and look at them. We can look at nutrient deficiencies. We can look at toxin levels.

[00:04:30]   A Functional Medicine approach to testing is simply saying, "Let's look at more than just the surface." Then, instead of waiting until you're incredibly sick and only testing those markers to prove to us what we already know—that you're sick—we look at more than that. We look at underneath the surface, and we get a lot more data. Thousands of data points as compared to 10s or 100s in conventional medicine. That helps us put together a complete picture of you, so we can understand the root of why you might be feeling depressed or dealing with any other chronic illness.

[00:05:00]   Thyroid dysfunction is really common. One in eight women in the United States will be diagnosed with a thyroid problem in her lifetime. It goes under-diagnosed a lot, so to start off, we look at testing that reveals changes in hormones before things have gone too far. We look at more thyroid hormones than usual. Then we also look at things like inflammation levels, food sensitivities, and nutrient deficiencies. There are a lot of things that can be corrected that can help the thyroid thrive without replacing thyroid hormone through a medication. That said, sometimes people need thyroid hormone, and it completely helps them. They might have an autoimmune condition driving their thyroid, and that can be something we address with medication. We can also sometimes address it with food and lifestyle change. It really depends.

[00:05:30]   At Parsley, we believe that everyone should have a health coach. We include unlimited health coaching in everyone's care. When you sign up as a member at Parsley, you get a doctor/health coach team. The reason we believe health coaching is so important is that your health is defined by the 99% of your life you're not in a doctor's office. If your doctor gives you a fancy plan and tells you to take this drug or eat this food, and you don't go do it, you're not going to get better. You need to take action on these things out in your regular life.

[00:06:00]   Our health coaches are there for support, for accountability, for motivation. They're there to troubleshoot any challenges you hit along the way, explain to you how to get testing done, follow up with you, and make sure you even got that test. We talk a lot in conventional medicine about how people aren't taking their medications, and they're not getting their tests done, and they're not implementing lifestyle changes. It's because they don't have a guide in how to do that in their regular life. Our health coaches are working side-by-side with our doctors at Parsley; they're all trained.

[00:06:30]   They're experts in their own right, but they're helping our members actually implement the changes we're recommending on a regular basis, so the outcomes are better.

            Meditation is incredibly powerful, and there are reams and reams of research on it showing that it can do everything from help increase gray matter in the brain, to improving plasticity, to lowering hormones like cortisol that can lead to inflammation and can also lead to brain damage over time. We know that meditation is a powerful tool, and it's being studied more and more. At Parsley Health, we

[00:07:00]   actually prescribe meditation, and we prescribe it infinitely more than we prescribe medication. We certainly prescribe both, but meditation and also practices like yoga, which lower cortisol in the body, can actually lower the chronic stress response, can infinitely improve focus, concentration, sleep, all of the things that then ultimately improve brain health over time.

[00:07:30] Cortisol imbalance is something that gets thrown around a lot, and not a lot of people understand it. Cortisol is one of our main stress hormones and it's produced by the adrenals, which are two little glands that sit on top of your kidneys in the body. When you make cortisol in response to stress, that's your body working. We developed a fight or flight response, so we could run away from a lion or survive, right? Today, in our worlds that we're living in now, what I see is patients living in emergency all day long. They're feeling like they're in emergency from the moment they wake up until the moment they go to sleep. They're running, running, running, from work to maybe exercise, to taking **[00:08:00]** care of family. They're eating too much sugar, they're living on caffeine, so both of those things are stimulants. They're constantly hyper-stimulated.

As a result, their body stays in fight-or-flight mode and never gets to go into the opposite of fight-or-flight mode, which is rest, digest, relax, and heal. That side of your nervous system needs to take over so that your body can rest, digest, relax, and heal. What I see is that a lot of people are never actually getting to heal. They're living in a state where their fight or flight hormones like cortisol are always **[00:08:30]** elevated or constantly spiking. High cortisol leads to blood sugar spikes, which leads to insulin spikes, that leads to insulin-resistance and metabolic syndrome and ultimately diabetes. That can also imbalance some of your sex hormones, testosterone, and the like, so we see hormone imbalances as a result of those chronic high-cortisol states.

[00:09:00] We see imbalances in sleep. When you don't sleep, your brain doesn't get to take out the metabolic trash that it creates during the day through regular metabolism. It's literally like your brain doesn't get to clean up its house overnight, which is one of the reasons sleep is so important. What we see is that people are chronically sleep-deprived, exhausted, they're gaining weight. Their blood sugar is imbalanced, and that is the beginning of disease, of dysfunction, and many of the huge chronic diseases we see that are crippling our healthcare system.

[00:09:30] Pregnant women aren't necessarily susceptible to high cortisol levels. That's really dependent on the person. Women who are pregnant are susceptible to pre-diabetes because your blood sugar balance naturally changes. When you're pregnant, so many of your hormones are in flux, and that's a key thing to remember. They're not static throughout your pregnancy. They're changing all the time. You also make more liquid volume in your bloodstream, so your blood pressure can go up. You also have higher blood sugar so you can make that sugar accessible to the baby. All of these things are adaptive mechanisms for pregnancy that are meant to happen.

[00:10:00] In a world where we are living on refined flours and sugars—refined carbohydrates—where these things create the basis of our diets, we're constantly pressing on that sugar balance system in ways that our bodies were not designed to handle. Then you add to that the changes that happen in blood glucose in pregnancy, and it's often too much for the body to handle. What you see are people developing diabetes in pregnancy because there's so much pressure on the system, because of the way we're eating, because of our stress levels, because of lack of activity. When you add pregnancy on top of that, sometimes that normal shift in your blood sugar balance is the straw that breaks the camel's back in that case.

[00:10:30] We teach a lot at Parsley Health on how to have a healthy pregnancy, how to get healthy before you're pregnant, so true prenatal care. How to stay healthy while you're pregnant, and how to get healthy or get healthier postpartum and heal from delivery. Some of the most important things you can do for your brain and for your baby's developing brain when you're pregnant, first of all, avoid the toxins. We are swimming in a sea of neurotoxins. Things like mercury in fish, particularly tuna and swordfish, but other fish, too. We are swimming in a sea of toxins from everything from dry-cleaning, to pollutants in **[00:11:00]** the air from gasoline and from car exhaust, to some of the products even in our furniture. Even your couch might be filled with flame-retardants that are neurotoxins.

What we and top researchers at Harvard and Mount Sinai Hospital have discovered is that there are numerous of these neuro-toxic chemicals that are building in our systems, and they're affecting our

[00:11:30] children. They're building up in babies, and we're detecting them in babies' bloodstreams after they're born. Some of the things you can do to protect yourself: certainly avoid sources of mercury in particular high-mercury fish. Avoid non-organic dry cleaning. Avoid sources of arsenic—that can be certain types of rice. Really "green the cleaning," as I call it. Get a lot of these toxins out of your personal care products and your cleaning products.

[00:12:00] Aside from that, fill your body with the good stuff. We know that in America we have too much ingestion of omega-6 oils and too few of omega-3s, and those omega-3s are what are building your baby's brain. Also, you want to stock up on those omega-3s, so that if you're breastfeeding after you have your baby, you have good stores to feed your baby. That baby's brain is still growing after it's born. Get lots of low-mercury fish, and good sources of healthy omega-3s, including flax oils, walnuts, and wild salmon, which are great sources of omega-3 fatty acids. Make sure you're not eating foods with too many toxins. Really watch your sugar intake.

[00:12:30] We got schooled as women that when you're pregnant, you should sit on the couch, and eat that extra pint of ice cream. What I see is women who are becoming even more de-conditioned and out of shape, and developing metabolic syndrome in pregnancy. I'm a new mom, I can tell you, after you have that baby, you're even more busy. You have even less time for yourself and to work out and to cook for yourself even. So, if you're already in a state that's not optimal when you're pregnant or before you get pregnant, that just gets perpetuated.

[00:13:00] We try to help a lot of our pregnant patients see that they don't necessarily need extra calories. You only need about 100-200 extra calories a day in the second and third trimester. That's like a handful of nuts. Yet people are eating too much. They're not exercising. Their mood becomes imbalanced because they're not exercising, because they're overeating, or they're eating sugary, high-carb foods that are not great for the brain. Everything compounds, so I always say to our pregnant women, stay active, eat [00:13:30] clean. You really don't need to eat extra. Generally, especially in the United States, people aren't eating too little, they're eating too much of the wrong stuff.

We hear a lot about burnout, and people always ask us or ask me is it a real thing. It absolutely is, and what it means is that you have physiological biochemical dysfunction as a result of chronic stress. You could have thyroid dysfunction. You can have imbalances in your cortisol levels. You can have imbalances in your digestion, and we know that stress is one of the major triggers for autoimmune [00:14:00] disease. While there's a genetic component to autoimmune diseases of all kinds, genetics plus environment are always a thing that add up to displaying the disease, and stress is often the trigger.

What I see are people who have hormone imbalances, weight gain, insomnia, anxiety, and now increasingly autoimmune conditions, which are skyrocketing, particularly amongst women. That constellation is what we refer to as burnout. It's from living in a way where you're literally living in emergency from the moment you wake up until the moment you go to sleep. I see people all the time [00:14:30] who tell me, "Well I got up, and I ran all day. I went to work, then went to dinner, and then I went to that spin class. Then I looked at social media until the moment I went to sleep, and I'm fine. I'm not stressed at all." What we see is that they really are deeply stressed, and biochemically they're stressed chronically.

[00:15:00] Our bodies are meant to have stress turn on and then turn off, but not to be chronically stressed. So, when you are chronically stressed, and you're not sleeping on top of it, that leads to this global dysfunction. It becomes a level of dysfunction that people can't actually recover from, right? We all just think, "Oh I'll just get that one good night's sleep, and I'll be fine." That might have been the case five years ago or 10 years ago or at some point, but if you're living in chronic stress, sometimes that one good night's sleep or even a weekend off isn't enough to recover.

By helping people understand that while they want to be incredibly successful and productive in their lives, they're actually undoing that productivity and undoing that success by destroying their bodies

[00:15:30] and ignoring themselves from the neck down, is a huge component today of what we need to help people understand in order to achieve health. We are fighting an uphill battle, right? Everything is conspiring against us. We look at computer screens all day. The average worker looks at the screen eight hours a day. The average American consumes 11 hours of media between desktop, television, and mobile every single day.

[00:16:00] We are sitting, eating, and stressing our way to really, really poor health. It doesn't mean that you quit your job and move to a tropical island, although that sounds great sometimes. But it does mean that you have to make changes in the way you move, eat, and conduct your daily life. Otherwise, your body's going to give out on you, and you're not going to have it there to enable you to do everything that you want to do.

[00:16:30] One example I have of a patient who has really benefited from this approach to medicine is a new mom. Her daughter was about one years old. The mother was exhausted. She'd developed hypothyroidism and adrenal fatigue, her digestion was off, she developed insomnia, and she wasn't sleeping. She was in her 30s, and wasn't particularly overweight, but had developed high blood pressure. We literally went step-by-step to address her nutrition, the way that she was sleeping, giving her some time-outs every day, so that she wasn't always working or taking care of her child. She had

[00:17:00] some help two hours a day, so that she could relax and do some yoga and meditate. She also had some food sensitivities, so we helped her recognize those and cut some of those foods out of her diet. And literally within six months, all of her dysfunction had resolved, including things like high blood pressure and hypothyroidism. We spared her what have would have otherwise been a lifetime of chronic medications.

I absolutely believe that your community is one of the most important determinants of your health. We know that the social determinants of health are more important than the genetic determinants of

[00:17:30] health. We know that the health status of your Facebook friends can actually be a really good indicator of how healthy you are. So, I try to remind people that they need to deliberately cultivate people in their lives who make them healthier. Of course, we can't control every person we come across day to day, but we can choose to work with people. We can choose to be friends with people. We can choose to have social lives that include people who make us healthier, who encourage us to move, who encourage us to eat better.

[00:18:00] We all have those friends, who we get together with, and we end up having too many beers, or eating pizza, or skipping the workout. Those are the friends who can be amazing for us, but we need to counteract those friends with some of the friends who help us live a little bit differently. I've literally done that in my life. For instance, I practice yoga, and in my yoga community, having people in my life who also like to practice yoga really contributes to making sure that I practice yoga and am active more than I would be if I just had to remind myself all the time.

[00:18:30] Top neuroscientists around the world have now codified that mobile phone addiction, or mobile device addiction is real. These devices we're using day to day are actually addictive. They give us a dopamine rush every time we look at them. Dopamine is the same chemical in the brain that's activated when you eat sugar or when you take cocaine. We know that these phones that are now literally attached to us, are addictive, and that it's really hard for people to put them down. When dopamine, that important neurochemical that you get this rush from, goes away, how do you feel? You feel dropped.

[00:19:00] You feel down. You feel anxious. The same way you feel when you crash from having too much sugar, right?

People are caught in this cycle of wanting that dopamine rush, feeling that crash when it's not there, and then getting it again. That's creating anxiety. We know mobile phones contribute to insomnia through affecting the way our hippocampus controls our circadian rhythms. We know that the effects of these devices are real and I believe we're literally conducting the largest uncontrolled experiment on humankind that's ever been done with our use of mobile devices and screens. We don't know how this

[00:19:30] is going to affect us long term because it's so early. It's 2017 right now. The iPhone came out in 2007. In 10 years, we have radically changed the way we work, shop, communicate with everyone in our lives, and the number of people with whom we're communicating on a regular basis. That is radical, and that is a very fast and quick period of time to change all of these fundamental ways in which we live our lives.

[00:20:00] I think it's important we recognize that. It's not that we have to throw the baby out with the bathwater and reject all technology, but I do think we need to understand that technology needs to serve us and what I see is people who are in a race against tech. They're in a race to keep up with technology in their workplace, at home. It's always more and more and more, and they can't turn it off. I think there

[00:20:30] is going to be reckoning where we understand that these devices are awesome, but they're really affecting our health, and we have to change the way we interact with them, and make sure they're serving us. Otherwise, we're going to be a slave to technology, and that's not why we created it.

I always recommend people avoid social media at key points in their day, where they're getting habituated to looking at it just reflexively, right? Typically, that can be in the morning or at night. Make a choice, make a decision, not to start your day with social media and not to end it with social media. It

[00:21:00] doesn't mean you can't check it all day, but I always recommend having some sort of routine in the morning that's screen-free. We know that most people are going to spend eight-plus hours a day looking at a screen. Don't make that the first 30 minutes you wake up. Get up. Take a shower. Get dressed. Make your breakfast. In my case, walk the dogs or take care of the baby. Do something that doesn't involve your screen, and resist that temptation to look at it. Just sort of time-box it, right? Set that limit, and say I'm not going to look at screens for this period of time.

[00:21:30] Do the same thing in the evening when you get home. People are going to bed too late. They're staying up for an extra 30 minutes, an hour even, looking at media before they go to bed. Keep your phone out of your bedroom. Again, remind yourself you have plenty of time to look at your phone all day, but create these special hiatus times at the bookends of your day, where you can get used to not always having it. I think that's really important.

[00:22:00] My top tips for addressing stress in the moment are number one, develop a breathing practice. Develop something that is your go-to. We know that if you inhale for say a count of three, and you exhale for a count of five, so your exhale is longer than your inhale, that activates your vagus nerve, which is your parasympathetic nervous system. That's your rest, digest, relax, and heal side of your nervous system. That will immediately lower your heart rate, relax your digestive system, even lower your blood pressure. This is an active basic cue. You can do it in public because no one needs to know you're doing it. You can immediately relax your nervous system. If you find yourself in a meeting, on a

[00:22:30] call, in a conversation, or wherever you are, and getting anxious, getting stressed, immediately turn to this simple breath of breathing in for three and out for five. It could be a different count as long as the exhale's longer than the inhale. That can relax your parasympathetic nervous system.

It's also really important to have a period of time every day where you put your body in a relaxed state. That can be yoga, walking, cooking, meditation, breathing practice, listening to music and not doing

[00:23:00] anything else—some period of time where your body gets to redevelop that muscle memory, that visceral intuitive memory of what it's like to feel relaxed. So many people are anxious and stressed all day long, their body doesn't even remember what it's like not to be coursing with some of those stress hormones.

Another tip I have, and I think this is where technology can be really empowering, there are some really interesting new technologies that can actually sense your cortisol levels, sense your heart rate variability, sense when you're stressed and give you some of that biofeedback to notice, hey I might

[00:23:30] not have noticed that I was so stressed. I might not have felt it. Especially when I talk to men, they often have suppressed their sensation of stress. They don't even feel it, and they think they're not stressed, but their body says otherwise. Some of the wearable technology is actually showing us that.

That's where I think some of this tech is getting really exciting.

[00:24:00] I do think we are over-prescribing antidepressants for mental health issues. I see over and over again patients coming to me who have been prescribed antidepressants often for a variety of off-label uses that aren't mood disorders, where all sorts of specialists are using them in ways they haven't been researched at all. In addition, I often see really well-meaning primary care doctors and psychiatrists who aren't sure what else to do or aren't sure how to help somebody, and so they just start an antidepressant. That's problematic because we know, in many cases, exercise actually goes head-to-head in the literature with antidepressants, and it's just as effective. We know that some of these antidepressants aren't much more effective than a placebo. We know that some of these

[00:24:30] antidepressants actually have really concerning side effects and can lead to higher rates of suicidality.

There are certainly cases where antidepressants and medications of the like are absolutely appropriate and can be really helpful, but they shouldn't be a first-line treatment. They should not be our go-to, and they are. We have millions of people who are prescribed antidepressants, and now more and more I see stimulants for conditions that aren't pathologies, aren't a disease, aren't even a mental health

[00:25:00] imbalance, but are just the result of their lifestyle. It's the result of not sleeping, having too much caffeine, eating too much sugar, being inflamed, having poor digestion. We know there's a big gut-brain connection, even having infections going on that haven't been detected. Why aren't we looking for these things before we prescribe a drug that then ends up being a lifelong drug because people are afraid to get off a drug they didn't even need in the first place?

[00:25:30] We're actually really effective at Parsley Health in some cases in helping people safely get off of these medications they didn't need. We use genetic testing often, to help us do that because there are genomics that teach us which drug is more appropriate for a certain person, whether or not that person would have responded just as well to exercise, and we can use this information that's truly cutting edge to help people get off of unnecessary medications. I also think we need to sound an alarm about the number of stimulants that are being prescribed. These stimulants are speed, effectively, and

[00:26:00] they are drugs of abuse, and they are addictive. What I'm seeing is that patients are able to get off of some of the antidepressants. They are not able to get off of some of the stimulants.

Telling someone who's just tired and having trouble focusing because they're looking at their mobile phones too much, and they're not sleeping well, and they're eating poorly, that they need a stimulant, that they're then going to be addicted to for life, is really problematic. I think we've sounded the alarm

[00:26:30] amongst physicians for the opioid epidemic that physicians in part created, and we're really addressing that, as a field, today. I think that's incredibly powerful. We need to sound the same alarm for stimulant medications that are being over prescribed.

There are numerous neurotoxins we're being exposed to on a regular basis. While any one of them in a minute amount on its own might not make you sick, the cumulative burden of a lot of them, which are stored in fat tissue, we all have may. Our brains are actually made of fat, and a lot of these neurotoxins

[00:27:00] get stored in our brains. The cumulative burden of these neurotoxins is bad. It's bad for our hormones. It's bad for our brains. It's bad for our metabolisms. I think we're only beginning to see the cumulative effect of them. Some of the common neuro-toxins we're exposed to are things like pesticides, flame-retardants in furniture, chemicals used in non-organic dry cleaning, heavy metals like arsenic and mercury, lead in the past, although luckily to a lesser extent because that's been highly regulated.

[00:27:30] One of the number one things you can do to avoid these toxins is just eat organic foods. A lot of these toxins are in non-organic food, and while it is more expensive, the investment in your body, the only vehicle that you have for your entire life, is so much more important than the little bit of extra money you're going to pay for just buying organic. That's a number one way you can avoid neurotoxins. Also, the NRDC and others have great resources on high-metal levels in fish and which fish to avoid. At

[00:28:00] Parsley Health, we educate all of our patients on which fish are high in mercury and which ones to avoid.

[00:28:30] Then getting organic dry cleaning, avoiding furniture that is treated with chemicals. There are a lot of furniture makers these days who are making non-toxic furniture. All of these things, these are little choices that you make day to day, but they add up to a life that's toxic or not toxic, and the research is bearing out from top researchers at Harvard and Mount Sinai Hospital for instance, that these neurotoxins are not only affecting us, they're affecting IQ points of our children.

My top tips for optimizing your brain every single day are pretty easy. The first one is get sleep and prioritize sleep. Try to go to bed by 10-10:30pm, 11pm at the latest. And get seven and a half to eight hours of sleep a night. You can take magnesium at bedtime and that can really help you have a higher quality sleep without any addictive side-effects, so that's a great one.

[00:29:00] The second one is green your life a little bit. Avoid some of the common neuro-toxins, whether it's in non-organic dry cleaning or high mercury fish or pesticides. Choose organic wherever you can. Get some of these common chemicals out of your cleaning products and your personal care products and avoid the heavy metals that are in our food. These are some of the simple ways that I know that I'm protecting my brain for the long-haul. We're living longer and longer, so we want our brains to be there for us.

[00:29:30] The third way is to find some sort of relaxation practice every day. It could be a two-minute breathing practice. It could be yoga. It could be meditation. But the effects of chronic high cortisol and stress hormones on our brains is really depleting our brainpower. One of the things you can do is recognize how stressed you are, then find some way even for two minutes, to breath your way or meditate your way out of stress. There are great apps out there and videos that tons of people are making that make it really easy online for free to learn a simple practice that reduces your stress response.

RUDY E. TANZI, PhD | Harvard Professor of Neurology and Author of *Super Brain*

Dr. Mark Hyman:	Dr. Tanzi, you've been a pioneer in studying Alzheimer's and you were on a team that discovered the genes that lead to one of the factors that causes Alzheimer's, or the pathology of Alzheimer's, which is amyloid. How did you discover these genes, what is amyloid, how does it play a role, and what can we do?
Dr. Rudy Tanzi: [00:00:30]	Back when I started working on Alzheimer's disease and wanted to find an Alzheimer's gene, there were none known yet. There was one person out in California named George Glenner who was picking apart the senile plaques and found out what it was made of. It was a little protein, a peptide, that he named "Amyloid Beta Protein." Most people didn't believe it mattered. In fact, even at Harvard in my department, when I said I was going to go after the gene that makes this little thing, they said, "You know, the senile plaque is just a big junkyard, and you're pulling out ... He pulled out one little tin can, and now you're going to chase the tin can down the street."
[00:01:00]	When I was a kid, I was pretty stubborn and a little bit rebellious, and I said, "No, I'm going to do it." And they said, "Well, you're going to waste your time." The prediction was there'd be a gene that made that little amyloid protein and that gene was going to be an Alzheimer's gene on chromosome number 21, because Down syndrome folks have an extra copy of that chromosome and get Alzheimer's pathology almost inevitably by middle age.
[00:01:30] Dr. Mark Hyman:	Yeah.
Dr. Rudy Tanzi:	So that was the prediction. A lot of ifs, and a lot of speculation. And it all turned out to be true. It turned out to be an Alzheimer's gene, it turned out to be on chromosome 21, it explained Down syndrome, and why they get the pathology, and they never turned back.
Dr. Mark Hyman:	Amazing. So, how does amyloid get involved with Alzheimer's? How does it lead to Alzheimer's?
Dr. Rudy Tanzi: [00:02:00]	When we first found the amyloid gene in 1987, and then we found two more genes called presenilins in 1995. What they all had in common was they led to much more amyloid deposition, plaque deposition in the brain. That led to the idea that the plaques caused the disease.
Dr. Mark Hyman:	Yeah.
Dr. Rudy Tanzi:	So, there was then about two decades of debate, fiery debate, because when you put those Alzheimer's genes into mice, they got the plaques.
Dr. Mark Hyman:	But they didn't get Alzheimer's.
[00:02:30] Dr. Rudy Tanzi:	Well, eventually the mice got sick, because there was enough amyloid in the brain that there's some inflammation, but they didn't get the tangles. So, the other pathological hallmark is the neurofibrillary tangle, and it's made up of another protein called tau. In the field, there were the "Tauists," who said, "It's the tangles." And there were the beta-amyloid protein Baptists who said, "It's the amyloid." And they would fight at these meetings. Mostly they would fight because the mouse didn't make tangles, which really are what kill the nerve cells, and respond to the amyloid they were making in their brain.
[00:03:00]	
Dr. Mark Hyman:	Yeah.
Dr. Rudy Tanzi:	This went on for two decades, and then only a few years ago, we said, "Maybe it's because it's mice. Maybe humans are not big mice." Who would've thought? And so, we decided to create a mini

Yeah.

— end —

human brain organoid in a Petri dish, using stem cells.

Dr. Mark Hyman: You made a brain in a Petri dish?

[00:03:30]
Dr. Rudy Tanzi: Yes. People were taking stem cells, making nerve cells, and then throwing them in a Petri dish in liquid, which was kind of silly because the brain's not made of liquid. So, we said, "Let's do it in gel," like the same gelatinous substance that the brain is made of. So, this is called Three Dimensional Cell Culture, or 3D Cell Culture. And when we did that, these nerve cells, these neurons, came alive. And they started making connections, and then we looked at whether they were signaling and talking to each other. We don't know what they're talking about, but they're having a blast in there firing and

[00:04:00] signaling with each other, wiring together just like they do in a brain.

And then, when we forced them to make amyloid, with the Alzheimer's genes, we saw plaques in the dish in six weeks, and the fellow doing the work in my lab came and said, "We have plaques, we have plaques!" And I said, "Well how about the tangles?" And he's like, "Okay, I'll be back." Literally after eight weeks they came in, and there were the tangles. And then, the proof of concept was: if

[00:04:30] we added drugs to stop the plaques in the dish, we didn't get the tangles. So that was the first proof of the amyloid hypothesis, that the amyloid is sufficient to cause the tangles, as long as you don't do it in mice.

Dr. Mark Hyman: Yes.

Dr. Rudy Tanzi: And I don't even know why it doesn't work in mice.

Dr. Mark Hyman: Because they're not humans?

Dr. Rudy Tanzi: Well, they're not humans, and because they're not humans, the tau protein they have is the wrong
[00:05:00] type. The tangles they made are this protein called tau, and the mice have a different version and combination of that protein than we do. We were able to figure that out as well.

Dr. Mark Hyman: There are people challenging that amyloid is the big deal that we all think it is, because there may be other mechanisms going on.

Dr. Rudy Tanzi: People challenge the amyloid for good reason, because all of the trials have failed. Every trial that started in amyloid, and either cleared it out of the brain or stopped its production, has not helped Alzheimer's patients.

Dr. Mark Hyman: So, there were like what, over 400 studies ...

Dr. Rudy Tanzi: Oh, plenty of them.

Dr. Mark Hyman: Billions of dollars, and 99.6% don't work.

[00:05:30]
Dr. Rudy Tanzi: Right. As usual, the devil is in the details, and while Wall Street might treat that as a binary event and say, "Okay, the amyloids there, then any company working on it, sell their stock." Well, what we've looked at were imaging of the brain for amyloid over time. There were studies in Australia and the US looking at how amyloid accumulates in the brain in people who don't have Alzheimer's onto
[00:06:00] people who have Alzheimer's. And what those studies figured out is that the amyloid plaques accumulate in the brain 15 to 20 years before symptoms.

Dr. Mark Hyman: Wow.

Dr. Rudy Tanzi: By the time someone has symptoms, has actual dementia, the plaques have already built up in the brain, and now they've peaked and they've plateaued. You have somebody where the plaques aren't even growing any more ...

Dr. Mark Hyman: The horse has left the barn.

Dr. Rudy Tanzi: [00:06:30]	Yes. And you're giving them a drug that hits the plaque. From what we figured out, the plaque lights the match, and the match is the trigger. The tangles are the brush fires that then spread to the brain killing nerve cells. And what we were doing was trying to blow out the match where there was already a forest fire. That means we have to back everything up. First of all, we have to diagnose Alzheimer's disease when there's pathology, not when there are symptoms.
[00:07:00]	Think about if we diagnosed cancer when there were symptoms. Imagine if we did the same thing for cancer, heart disease, and diabetes, that we foolishly do for Alzheimer's, which is, "You don't have Alzheimer's until you have symptoms."
Dr. Mark Hyman:	Yes, wait until you have a heart attack, and then treat it.
Dr. Rudy Tanzi:	Wait until you have a heart attack, or wait until you have a two-inch tumor, organ failure, an immense pain, and say, "Okay, now he has cancer." Now he's given that tumor suppressor.
Dr. Mark Hyman:	Yes.
Dr. Rudy Tanzi:	And that's what's happening. Somebody does not want to have the stigma of saying, "I have Alzheimer's disease," 20 years before symptoms because you have plaques.
Dr. Mark Hyman:	And there's nothing you can do.
Dr. Rudy Tanzi: [00:07:30]	Right. But you can look at it like AIDS versus HIV positive. We're coming up with terms like HAVS, meaning you have amyloid beta in your brain at a level that's concerning, just like you could have some plaque around your heart without congestive heart failure, and that's when you start treating, someone will bring their cholesterol down. We're saying, "At that point, let's bring your amyloid down." At least our group says, "Don't wipe it up. You still need a towel."
Dr. Mark Hyman: [00:08:00]	So, here's the interesting question. With Functional Medicine, we look upstream. What's the cause? What's the cause of the amyloid? It's not just the genes, because genes can be turned on and off, and genes can be expressed in different ways depending on the inputs of the environment, diet, lifestyle, toxins. With the amyloid, what is driving the production of all this amyloid in these patients?
Dr. Rudy Tanzi: [00:08:30] [00:09:00]	In the rare cases of early-onset familial Alzheimer's, where we found those first three genes, that's maybe one or two percent of all cases, we know that the gene mutations cause the production of a longer version of the amyloid beta protein. It's more likely to drive amyloid plaque formation. It's almost like, picture those old chemistry experiments you did when you get a crystal. You have liquid and you add something to the liquid, and you get a crystallization. That's called a nucleating event, or a seeding event. You seed the crystal. In the brain, amyloid has to get seeded. In those rare cases of early onset Alzheimer's, those mutations cause a longer version of that amyloid protein that seeds the amyloid more rapidly.
Dr. Mark Hyman:	So that's like a genetic cause.
Dr. Rudy Tanzi:	That's a genetic cause, and it's one or two percent of cases.
Dr. Mark Hyman:	Yes.
Dr. Rudy Tanzi: [00:09:30]	But that's not happening in 98, 99% of cases. We have to ask, I'd say based on that you then have to ask logically, what's seeding, like a crystallization event, what's seeding amyloid when you don't have more of that longer form of amyloid protein like they have in the rare, early-onset genetic cases? What we figured out over the last ten years, is that pathogenic microbes, bacteria, yeast, viruses, may be doing the seeding of the plaques, where the plaques are actually forming to protect the brain against those microbes.
Dr. Mark Hyman:	So, what you're saying is, really, heresy, right?
Dr. Rudy Tanzi:	It's pure heresy, yes.

Dr. Mark Hyman:	Heresy, which is ... one: that we know that there's a blood-brain barrier that stuff can't get through.
Dr. Rudy Tanzi:	Yes.
[00:10:00] Dr. Mark Hyman:	Two: we know that the brain is sterile.
Dr. Rudy Tanzi:	Oh, of course. Tell the brain that.
Dr. Mark Hyman:	And three: you're discovering something radical, which is this idea of a microbiome of the brain and there's really a trigger, which is this infection in the brain that is subtle, but actually is driving this chronic, long-term process of inflammation, that's really the thing that causes the symptoms of Alzheimer's.
[00:10:30] Dr. Rudy Tanzi:	Well, yes, I mean in essence, what we figured out is, first of all, the brain is not sterile. If you try to look for bacteria, yeast, and viruses, you do find them in the brain. When it comes to certain viruses, we see more of them in an Alzheimer's brain, and we think that might be a major culprit. We used to believe that the brain didn't have a lymphatic system, right? Now it does. Everything we believed about the brain, no lymphatic system, wrong. Completely sterile, wrong. Right?
[00:11:00]	And, the way the brain accumulates microbes is, yeah, you could have the blood-brain barrier integrity go down, so they come in from the blood, and that can happen with age, the blood-brain barrier integrity starts to go downhill. But the gut microbiome is what helps to keep that blood-brain barrier integrity ...
Dr. Mark Hyman:	Well there's more heresy, right? How the gut floor is affecting the brain.
Dr. Rudy Tanzi:	The gut floor is protecting the brain through the blood-brain barrier. And it helps stop inflammation. So, more heresy.
Dr. Mark Hyman:	If it's the right gut micro ...
[00:11:30] Dr. Rudy Tanzi:	If it's the gut, right. In fact, in our Alzheimer's mice, where they're getting inflammation downstream of the amyloid, it's a two-way street. You start to see that the gut actually loses the bacteria, like bifido and Lactobacillus that you get in yogurt and probiotics, they actually start losing it. So, you get this vicious cycle.
[00:12:00]	Getting back to the microbial story, the viruses don't have to come from the outside. The viruses can be dormant, integrated in the genome of neurons, and other cells in the brain. That's what we've seen, is that from infancy, viruses are affecting you, and you develop your immune system against them, and the antibodies, but then they lie dormant in your genome.
Dr. Mark Hyman:	Just like a herpes infection on your lip, it may be there forever and never come out.
Dr. Rudy Tanzi:	It's dormant, it has to get activated.
[00:12:30] Dr. Mark Hyman:	Have stress, or infection, or a cold ...
Dr. Rudy Tanzi:	UV, ultraviolet, yeah.
Dr. Mark Hyman:	Sunlight ... It can get activated, right?
Dr. Rudy Tanzi: **[00:13:00]**	Yes. What we're seeing is that there are a slew of viruses that are dormant in the brain, and they seem to get more activated in Alzheimer's patients. When they do, you get an instant formation of amyloid plaques. More heresy, right? The field has always said, "It takes years for an amyloid plaque to form. It takes months in a mouse," right? We showed proof of concept that you can get amyloid plaques to form in 15 minutes, an hour. Overnight you can get a whole region of the brain to fill with

---

amyloid in a dish or in a mouse by just having a microbe there where the amyloid is actually being seeded to envelop the microbes and protect the resident cells from the microbial infection.

Dr. Mark Hyman:	Everybody is listening, and wondering, "Oh my God, do I have viruses in my brain, and what do I do about it?"
Dr. Rudy Tanzi:	We all do.

[00:13:30]

Dr. Mark Hyman:	Are there takeaways, or things to think about how to keep the viruses quiet, or prevent the activation of the viruses?
Dr. Rudy Tanzi:	Everyone has these viruses, just about everyone has these dormant viruses in their brain.
Dr. Mark Hyman:	There are things you might get as a kid, an infection, right?
Dr. Rudy Tanzi: [00:14:00]	Yes. Like roseola is a type of herpes virus. When infants get the red rash roseola on their face, arms, and that virus then inserts itself into various genomes, including in the brain. The question is, why does it get activated? How does it get activated? The amyloid doesn't form until the virus is actually activated, and you're making viral particles in the brain.
[00:14:30]	We don't know, but we know that it happens more in Alzheimer's. And, we can look at where the virus is integrated in the genome, what parts of the genome is integrated in Alzheimer's patients versus those of the same age who don't have Alzheimer's. You can start to see there are common integration spots in the genome where you get the human DNA, and the virus has inserted itself and integrated, and it looks like, for some reason, we could have never predicted that they may get integrated in areas of the genome involved with inflammation.
Dr. Mark Hyman:	Yes.
Dr. Rudy Tanzi: [00:15:00]	So now you have to think: maybe inflammation, which we usually think of at the end of the disease as the forest fire that's taking you out, maybe small bouts of inflammation early on could be triggering the activation of a virus that causes the plaque. Now you get this fresh cause of disease, plaque, tangles, more inflammation until it's finally dementia.
Dr. Mark Hyman:	Wow.
Dr. Rudy Tanzi:	And this is all totally new stuff. We're still learning as we go.
Dr. Mark Hyman:	And we do know, at a higher level, that what you do in your life has an impact on your immune system.
Dr. Rudy Tanzi:	Yes.
Dr. Mark Hyman:	Your thoughts, your feelings, your diet, exercise, how you deal with stress.
Dr. Rudy Tanzi: [00:15:30]	Deepak and I just wrote a whole new book on that actually, yeah. Our book is exactly on that topic.
Dr. Mark Hyman:	What's the new one?
Dr. Rudy Tanzi:	It's called *The Healing Self*. It's about the power of the mind, and lifestyle over your immune system.
Dr. Mark Hyman: [00:16:00]	The news is, you actually can modify your risk by doing something before you get Alzheimer's. You make a big point of that, we're often dealing with things after the fact, like you said, like having a heart attack and then treating it, as opposed to going into prevention. You've said that it takes like 20 years before you get Alzheimer's symptoms, your brain is already starting to deteriorate.
Dr. Rudy Tanzi:	We have to back everything up. So, we used to call treating plaques prevention. Because we didn't say you had the disease until you get symptoms. Now, we want to back that up and say that treating

[00:16:30]	plaques is treating the disease. If we have too many plaques early on, and you're perfectly fine, you start treating those plaques just like you treat plaques on the heart so you don't have congestive heart failure later on. If you have HIV, you don't wait for AIDS to get rid of HIV. It's a similar idea, and so now, treatment of Alzheimer's is backed up to pre-symptomatic treatment when you see plaques. That's going to be the future, and the FDA needs to play along with us on this.
Dr. Mark Hyman:	Because of testing, or because ...
Dr. Rudy Tanzi:	Well, the FDA wants you to use an amyloid drug and make people cognitively better who already have the disease. And that's like having someone with congestive heart failure ...
Dr. Mark Hyman:	His heart's already failed.
Dr. Rudy Tanzi:	And say, "Make them better with Lipitor."
[00:17:00] Dr. Mark Hyman:	Right.
Dr. Rudy Tanzi:	All right, we had to use that before.
Dr. Mark Hyman:	Yes.
Dr. Rudy Tanzi:	Or it's like, someone has a two-inch tumor and organ failure, and you say, "Make them live longer with a tumor suppressor."
Dr. Mark Hyman:	Right.
Dr. Rudy Tanzi: [00:17:30]	The FDA has to get that. It's an ongoing dialog we have to have with them. If they make us show that amyloid drugs used 20 years before preventing you from getting to the symptoms, how are we going to do 20, 10, even 5-year trials? Who's going to do that? They would cost tens of millions of dollars, and by the time they're done, you say to the pharmaceutical company, "Thanks very much, but now your drug's off patent too. But thanks for spending 20 million dollars on this new drug." And it's smart to go generic, because it took this long. So, who's going to do it?
[00:18:00]	The FDA has to look at genetics, look at the new Alzheimer's in a dish, look at all of the data and say, "If we have a safe therapy that lowers amyloid, let people take it." On top of that, now primary prevention becomes, how do we stop the accumulation of amyloid in the first place? Then we have to think about ...
Dr. Mark Hyman:	Because that's still a little downstream. If you have someone who has plaque, even if they don't have symptoms and you're treating that, it's still not addressing why the plaque happened in first place.
Dr. Rudy Tanzi: [00:18:30]	Right. So now we're talking about 20-year-olds. Now we're talking about teens and 20s and 30s, what can they do to know whether they're getting more viral activation, if that turns out to be the way it happens. How to bring the viral load down, what can you do with lifestyle to turn down neuroinflammation regarding diet, gut microbiomes, sleep, stress reduction, exercise, all of the things we may talk about. Primary prevention for this disease is going to begin in the 20s.
	And you're going to actively look for issues in your 30s. By the time you're in your 40s or 50s, you're seeing how much amyloid you have, and you're coming up with a plan to dial it back down.
Dr. Mark Hyman: [00:19:00]	You said that 40% of people over 85 have symptoms of dementia.
Dr. Rudy Tanzi:	Yes.

Dr. Mark Hyman:	And that's the biggest, fastest growing segment of our population, and the costs are 200 and change billion dollars, and it's only getting worse. It's affecting 50 million people around the world. This is an epidemic.
Dr. Rudy Tanzi:	One in five dollars already of Medicare or Medicaid goes to Alzheimer's.
Dr. Mark Hyman:	Yes, it's more expensive than heart disease and cancer treatment.
[00:19:30] Dr. Rudy Tanzi:	Yes. 71 million baby boomers, within five years, you're looking at three out of five dollars of Medicare and Medicaid going to Alzheimer's.
Dr. Mark Hyman: [00:20:00]	So, what you're suggesting, and this is a huge issue, but you're suggesting kind of something pretty radical, is that given what we already know about how the brain works and is influenced by our lifestyle, diet, and all of these activities from sleep, stress, exercise, and diet, these are low-cost, simple interventions that can have a profound effect on this epidemic. And even the microbiome, like you said, learning about how the gut affects the brain ... This is a very empowering message for everybody. It's not like, "Oh, shoot, we all have to wait around to get Alzheimer's." We can actually do something about it. This is an important message. For someone who is a Harvard professor, who's been a leader in research, who's discovered genes that could win the Nobel Prize, I mean, you are really saying something pretty radical, because conventional medicine doesn't have that approach.
Dr. Rudy Tanzi: [00:20:30]	No, but the fact is you have to think about Alzheimer's disease as a challenge of management your whole life.
Dr. Mark Hyman:	Yes. How do you know if you're at risk? Not everybody is, right? How do you know if you're the 20-year-old or 30-year-old that's supposed to actually start now?
Dr. Rudy Tanzi: [00:21:00]	Family history is number one. If you have first-degree relatives with the disease, you're at greater risk. The earlier age of onset, the stronger the role of genetics versus lifestyle. But that doesn't mean that even if you have one of these mutations and early-onset familial genes like we discovered that guarantees the disease, those mutations guarantee plaques and tangles. We know, from resilient brains, people who die in the their 80s are cognitively fine, but then you look at their brain and you say, "Whoa, this is ..."
Dr. Mark Hyman:	A mess.
Dr. Rudy Tanzi:	"Alzheimer's levels of plaques and tangles, how did they not get the disease?"
Dr. Mark Hyman:	Yeah.
[00:21:30] Dr. Rudy Tanzi:	The answer, in each case, is no inflammation. There's no neural inflammation in the brain. Those people were lucky, either with lifestyle or with other genes, that despite all those plaques and tangles, their brain did not react to it with inflammation, so they didn't get the disease. Bottom line is, you can live with plaques and tangles in your brain and not get dementia.
Dr. Mark Hyman:	If the inflammation doesn't turn up.
Dr. Rudy Tanzi: [00:22:00]	Right. So even these people who have this death sentence of Alzheimer's gene mutation that causes onset at 40 or 50 years old, if they did things to keep neuroinflammation down, they can live with a lot of plaques and tangles in their brain. Resilient brains have taught us that. Even in these dire cases where it seems hopeless, lifestyle would most likely still be able to make some difference in delaying that age of ...
Dr. Mark Hyman:	Yeah, I recall.
Dr. Rudy Tanzi:	The onset of symptoms.

Dr. Mark Hyman: [00:22:30]	A patient I had who had an APoE 4/4—75% of people will get Alzheimer's with that gene. She was a health nut. She was like 90 years old, she was a dentist and was still working. She ate perfectly, she exercised every day, she handled her stress, and she was like 90 years old and was sharp as a tack.
Dr. Rudy Tanzi:	I know people like that, too.
Dr. Mark Hyman: [00:23:00]	It's a testament to the power we have to actually influence our gene expression, and to influence neuro inflammation. Most of us live a pretty inflammatory lifestyle, with very high processed food diets, high levels of sugar and starch, and not enough fruits and vegetables. We don't eat enough fiber to help our gut microbiome, we don't exercise enough, we're too stressed, we don't sleep. The average American sleeps two hours less than he did 60 years ago. So, all of those things are things we are actually empowered to do ourselves, which is a great message for people.
Dr. Rudy Tanzi:	Right. And that's the best thing you can do, no matter what your family history is. But if you have a family history, you need to take it even more serious.
Dr. Mark Hyman:	Yeah.
Dr. Rudy Tanzi: [00:23:30]	And if you're ... Let's say, some day at 40 or 50 years old, everyone gets tested. Right now, it's imaging, but there might be a blood test someday to see what your amyloid load is in your brain. Just like cholesterol, you might need a drug to help you bring it down, or you might choose not to, you might say, "I can do without the drug," and you choose lifestyle changes to bring it down. But it's going to be very similar to managing heart disease and cholesterol.
Dr. Mark Hyman:	How far away from tracking and testing ... We now have PET scans that are $10,000, and not really practical for ...
Dr. Rudy Tanzi:	Like a dog is $5000.
Dr. Mark Hyman: [00:24:00]	$5000, well that's a big discount. But you extrapolate that to millions of people, it's a lot of money. How far away are we from having a test, whether it's a blood test or a cheaper scan, or some other indicator.
Dr. Rudy Tanzi:	Yes, the blood tests are coming along. Amyloid and tangles can be found in these vessels called exosomes, and you can even find them in urine. In fact, to some extent, urine is a better indicator of what's in the fluid of the brain, or what's in spinal fluid, than blood is.
Dr. Mark Hyman:	The brain-bladder connection.
[00:24:30] Dr. Rudy Tanzi:	Yeah, exactly, the brain-bladder connection. There are people working on everything from urine tests, to blood tests. Right now, let's say worst-case scenario, you only have the scan, and let's say the companies got less greedy and you can do this, the scan only costs $1000, because the price also has to do with demand.
Dr. Mark Hyman:	Sure.
Dr. Rudy Tanzi: [00:25:00]	Let's say that happens. Well, right now when you turn a certain age, you get a breast exam. When you turn a certain age, you get a colonoscopy, which is not cheap. So, I'm sure at some point, people, when they were first saying, "Everyone will have a colonoscopy after 50 years old," they were like, "Oh yeah, like that's gonna happen." But you know what? Now they do.
[00:25:30]	And so even in the worst-case scenario, it might be that by 50 you have your brain scan. Let's say we don't have any other test, and I would say that if you have a family history, you look at the first of your relatives, earliest age of onset, of symptoms, subtract 20 years, and that's when you buy the first check for your amyloid. If someone has someone in their family who had Alzheimer's at 60 years old with symptoms, you would do the test at 40 rather than 50. If nothing else turns up and we have to do imaging, I can still see how that could happen.

Dr. Mark Hyman: [00:26:00]	The future of Alzheimer's could be like the future of colon cancer, which is we control a lot of it through screening. Even more than that, we develop a protocol to actually optimize your brain function, reduce neuro inflammation, reduce your risk factors, and that combined maybe with drugs that are targeted that can help if you're high risk to actually modify it, we're looking at maybe a future of really treating Alzheimer's, or really preventing it.
Dr. Rudy Tanzi:	Right. So, we like to use the mantra, early prediction, meaning look at your family history to know when you need to start getting concerned. Then early detection, meaning you look for the pathology that's beginning 15, 20 years before symptoms, and then early intervention. So early prediction, early detection, early intervention.
Dr. Mark Hyman: [00:26:30]	Amazing.
Dr. Rudy Tanzi: [00:27:00]	We had a meeting with GE, who has computer programs to predict when different parts of jets are going to fail, or large machinery, right? And they do a very similar thing, to have algorithms to learn everything they can about a blade in an engine or something, and they look for the early warning signs and predictions of failure, and then optimization, early intervention to make sure the blade doesn't break while there's someone flying in a plane. We can talk about applying those algorithms as a learning machine, mechanism, machine learning mechanism, to look at all of our data and tell us what we have to do in that same mantra: early prediction, early detection, early intervention.
Dr. Mark Hyman:	It's amazing. Speaking of early intervention, you collaborated with Dr. Deepak Chopra in doing some extraordinary research around different interventions that affect the brain. And one of them was using meditation.
Dr. Rudy Tanzi: [00:27:30]	Right.
Dr. Mark Hyman:	And you found all kinds of extraordinary things that help to optimize, heal, and renew the brain, and also prevent problems down the road. Can you tell us a little bit about that research?
Dr. Rudy Tanzi:	Yes, we did a clinical trial where you had 30 people learning to meditate, 30 expert meditators who were teaching them, and then another 30 people who were just staying at the same resort having fun, but eating the same food. We had control for the diet, right?
Dr. Mark Hyman: [00:28:00]	Yeah.
Dr. Rudy Tanzi:	And what we found was that the folks who were learning to meditate had changes in the right direction for genes involving inflammation. We looked at the expression of all the genes in the genome and built maps. And they were very different for the meditation group versus the resort group. In both cases, resort was good for you, you saw nice changes in genes involving inflammation.
Dr. Mark Hyman:	So, having a vacation is good.
Dr. Rudy Tanzi: [00:28:30] [00:29:00]	Yeah, so a vacation is good, but meditation was much better. With meditation, you saw changes in the anti-aging enzyme telomerase that grows the ends of your chromosomes, that keeps your cells dividing longer. There was a 40% increase in telomerase activity in the expert meditators who were meditating intensively all week. There were changes in the genes involving Alzheimer's, and how amyloid protein is cleared from the brain, they were also in the right direction. I mean, when I looked at all the data, if I was writing a science fiction novel where you lied about the future and the effects of meditation, I would not have gone as far as the results I saw.
Dr. Mark Hyman:	It's pretty amazing. I mean you think about it, you said even in the novice meditators, it's not like you have to be in a cave in Tibet for 20 years to see these changes, they happen within days or weeks.

Dr. Rudy Tanzi:	This is one week.
Dr. Mark Hyman:	One week.
Dr. Rudy Tanzi:	This was all in one week.
Dr. Mark Hyman: [00:29:30]	Yes, that's extraordinary. I think, I found personally that applying it in my practice and in myself has just been extraordinary, and how it works in the brain, and reduces anxiety, helps with sleep, improves mood ...
Dr. Rudy Tanzi:	And stress plays such a huge ... Stress affects your gut microbiome, which then affects your brain, which then affects your gut microbiome ... And stress ties into sleep. You're stressed out, so you can't sleep, and because you can't sleep you get stressed, and then because you're stressed you eat junk food and comfort foods ...
Dr. Mark Hyman:	Sounds like a prescription for Alzheimer's.
[00:30:00] Dr. Rudy Tanzi:	Yes. And the whole time you're forgetting to exercise. So, we just kind of described America.
Dr. Mark Hyman:	Yeah.
Dr. Rudy Tanzi:	And that's what has to change, because that's how you're really going to hit Alzheimer's in a life management scheme.
Dr. Mark Hyman:	Let's talk about exercise, because people really struggle with that. One of the things that's sort of changed dramatically in the landscape of the brain is the idea that we can create new brain cells, and new connections in age, even up to death.
Dr. Rudy Tanzi:	Yes.
Dr. Mark Hyman: [00:30:30]	And that is a radical change from the idea that the brain is fixed, you have a certain number of neurons. If you lost a few in college from too much partying, well that's too bad, nothing you can do. Well now we know that's just a false premise, and there are some very simple things like meditating or exercise. So, how does exercise affect the brain, and neurogenesis...
Dr. Rudy Tanzi: [00:31:00]	Specifically where we see neurogenesis is in pockets of the brain, right? So, the hippocampus, which is the short-term memory area of the brain, if we use Dan Siegel's idea of the handy brain, right? Where you have the 300-million-year-old brain stem, which is instincts, base instincts for survival, right? Then you have the midbrain, which is fears, desires, short-term memory, emotion, and that's 100 million years old. And then, all this stuff here, frontal cortex, which is four million years old, that's the new stuff.
Dr. Mark Hyman:	Yeah.
Dr. Rudy Tanzi: [00:31:30]	Right. So, then you say intellectual brain, emotional brain, and instinctive brain, right? Well, where we see neurogenesis, the birth of new stem cells, is here, and where Alzheimer's hits. Alzheimer's first hits the short-term memory area of the brain. And so how do you induce neurogenesis in that area to have more nerve cells? Number one is exercise. And what exercise does is it turns on proteins like BDNF, which is a growth factor for nerve cells.
Dr. Mark Hyman:	It's like Miracle Gro for your brain.
Dr. Rudy Tanzi: [00:32:00]	It's like Miracle Gro for the brain, yes, very good. But what we also found was that BDNF not only helps the nerve cells to grow, but it cleans up the area so that they can grow in a safe neighborhood. We did an experiment where we used a chemical, a drug, that causes nerve cells to grow, causes nerve cells to divide, neurogenesis. We said, "Let's see if that helps a mouse that's suffering with plaques and inflammation and Alzheimer's," right? A mouse model, but at least we could see what it would do to the inflammation.

Dr. Mark Hyman:	Yes.

[00:32:30]

Dr. Rudy Tanzi:	And when we used the drug that caused tons of new nerve cells to grow in the mouse, nothing happened. The mouse did not get better at all, because what we saw was that the new nerve cells are being born in a battleground. That's like babies being born in the middle of a battle, in a war. They didn't survive, they died on the battleground. If you induced neurogenesis with exercise, you get two for one. You get the birth of new nerve cells, and it cleans up the area of inflammation so the nerve cells can thrive.

[00:33:00]

Dr. Mark Hyman:	That's amazing.

Dr. Rudy Tanzi:	And then, we figured out, because people always want drugs, we figured out that what exercise was doing was causing this BDNF to be turned on. So, then what we did was, we added the drug that causes neurogenesis, plus a drug that causes BDNF to be turned on, and that mimicked exercise.

[00:33:30]

Dr. Mark Hyman:	Yes. That's powerful. And going back to the stress thing, I've seen data that show that people who have high levels of stress, their hippocampus, which is the memory center, shrinks.

Dr. Rudy Tanzi:	Yes.

Dr. Mark Hyman:	And when you have somebody with Cushing's disease, which is a production of cortisol, sort of like high stress, but they get a very shrunken hippocampus because you cut out the tumor that's causing the cortisol, their brains grow back.

Dr. Rudy Tanzi:	Cortisol kills neurons. It's a killer.

Dr. Mark Hyman:	So next time you're worried or stressed about something, think about your brain.

[00:34:00]

Dr. Rudy Tanzi:	Yeah. That's why I worry about some genetic testing now that's direct to consumer. Like you can get an APoE test done.

Dr. Mark Hyman:	And then you freak out.

Dr. Rudy Tanzi:	And let's say, they told you that you have an E4, risk of E4 you have two E4 risk factors, the nocebo effect alone could take you out.

Dr. Mark Hyman:	Yes. Just the stress of having the gene.

Dr. Rudy Tanzi: [00:34:30]	But it depends on the person. Some people might say, "Well if I knew I had two APoE4s, I'll definitely get eight hours of sleep, and I'll definitely exercise more, and I'm going to change my diet, prebiotic, probiotic, etc." It can have a positive effect, but it can also have a negative effect. It's going to be very interesting to see how this all plays out.

Dr. Mark Hyman:	Yes, because some of my patients don't want to know, and others are excited to know so they can ...

Dr. Rudy Tanzi:	I wouldn't want to know, because I think I'm highly prone to the nocebo effect. I would worry about it.

Dr. Mark Hyman:	I'd want to know, because I know what to do to like ...

Dr. Rudy Tanzi:	I'll just assume I have it and kick my old butt to ...

Dr. Mark Hyman: [00:35:00]	Yeah, I mean that's true. The thing is, people think, "Well, there's one treatment for Alzheimer's and one for heart disease and one for cancer and one for diabetes." The truth is that it's not like you need different diets for each of these things and different approaches, the same thing works for

everything, right? So, the diet that's going to prevent Alzheimer's is also going to prevent diabetes and cancer.

Dr. Rudy Tanzi: That's right. What's good for the heart is good for the brain.

Dr. Mark Hyman: Yeah.

Dr. Rudy Tanzi: And throw in the pancreas as well.

Dr. Mark Hyman:
[00:35:30] Yes, exactly. In this documentary, we've talked to scientists who are looking at how to increase brain cell growth, neurogenesis, and increase connections in our plasticity, and they're using the nervous system as inputs to the brain to help it sort of rebuild and rewire. Like music, for example. You've looked at that. Tell us what you've shown about music.

Dr. Rudy Tanzi:

[00:36:00] An amazing thing is, as this pathology spreads through the brain in Alzheimer's disease, the music memory area that's tucked inside does not get affected. You'll see in nursing homes someone with pretty moderate to late stage Alzheimer's who can still remember how to play every song on the piano, or even sing. Even remembering words of a song is a different type of memory, of remembering ...

Dr. Mark Hyman: So, they can't necessarily talk coherently, but they can sing a song ...

Dr. Rudy Tanzi:

[00:36:30] But they can sing or play the piano. Then this brings us to what happens with Alzheimer's, right? Sensory information is coming in from your world, and the thing is, you can't integrate it into your life. So, in other words, you can't make sense of a smell or a sound, because that association you make that comes with learning has now been devastated by the loss of neurons, the loss of synapses. So, at any moment, even listening to me speak, sensory information is going from just behind the nose, your intermodal cortex, that whole cortex there, into the hippocampus here.

[00:37:00]

[00:37:30] And then in the hippocampus, you have to make sense of it, and that's how you're keeping track of your day, keeping track of every moment of your day. So, it used to be thought that the sensory information just couldn't be stored, that the record button didn't work. And now, newer studies have shown at MIT, just a couple of years ago, that the record button does work, and these mice that are impaired because they have lots of plaque and inflammation, it turns out they can't learn the task. And it's not because you can't record the information about how to learn a certain task, you do record it and you can't play it back. So, it's access. That's good news, because it says that that information is still getting stored, what's going around them during the day ...

Dr. Mark Hyman: So, your hard drive is still working.

Dr. Rudy Tanzi: Yeah, but you can't access the neurons and synapses that are storing that short-term memory that allows you to keep track of what's going on, or keep track of a conversation, or cooking, and answering the phone. One question has become, how can we stimulate those neurons to push the play button again?

Dr. Mark Hyman: Yeah.

Dr. Rudy Tanzi:
[00:38:00] And in experiments they did in mice, they used light, and they used something called optogenetics, something we couldn't do in humans. It was just to provide proof of concept. But if you look at how music memory is wired to the hippocampus and the midbrain, there's a chance that music might stimulate those neurons where you need to push the play button.

[00:38:30] So, we came up with an app called Spark Memories Radio—because you're going to spark it up, right? So basically, what happens is, you play music that the patient loved between 13 and 25 years old, because that's what emotionally stimulates you, and see if we can awaken that part of the brain, see if we can awaken those neurons.

Dr. Mark Hyman: Is it working?

Dr. Rudy Tanzi: [00:39:00]	Right now, we have to wait for people to use the app, and they write emails and tell us their experiences, but we're getting incredible emails. People who were in the early stages of the disease, who are depressed and agitated and angry, calm down. Those who are in the later stages of the disease who don't speak much, who are vegetative, not conscious, they tend to not want to hear music with words in it, with lyrics. They like the music that they recognize, but they'd rather hear just instrumentals. They get confused by the lyrics.
[00:39:30]	And that tends to make them wake up. We got an email from someone who said their dad, who hadn't spoken in five or six months lying in bed, after hearing a bunch of songs from when he was a teenager, on in particular, a song "Fever" by Peggy Lee, "You Give Me Fever ..." All of a sudden, he just, for the first time in five months, started speaking and started talking about this red pickup truck that he really loved, and this girl he took out in the pickup truck, and everything he did with the girl in the pickup truck on one of his dates.
Dr. Mark Hyman:	Well that's ...
[00:40:00] Dr. Rudy Tanzi:	So, it was very embarrassing, but they loved it, because he was finally speaking.
Dr. Mark Hyman:	Yeah. So, what you're saying is, the music is a doorway to open access to memories and to cells that were sort of asleep in a sense.
Dr. Rudy Tanzi: [00:40:30]	Right. And in some programs, they're going to nursing homes and playing music very loud from the time, an average time of when they were teens, and then they have a doc there who's analyzing the folks, and what they're seeing is that 15 minutes into that, you start having a conversation with a patient who normally couldn't follow a conversation at all, who is actually following a conversation again. And music is actually allowing them, it looks like, ability to access the incoming words they hear in the conversation, and follow it longer. Like, maybe you push the play button on those access ...
Dr. Mark Hyman:	Amazing.
Dr. Rudy Tanzi:	I mean we don't know for sure.
Dr. Mark Hyman:	So, Spotify is a treatment for Alzheimer's.
[00:41:00] Dr. Rudy Tanzi:	Well ...
Dr. Mark Hyman:	The right song ...
Dr. Rudy Tanzi:	No, you have to use Spark Memories Radio.
Dr. Mark Hyman:	Use Spark Memories Radio, yes.
Dr. Rudy Tanzi:	That one is a very sophisticated algorithm. What music was hits between 13 and 25? And they either push if he or she liked it or didn't like it, and it keeps learning ... But it works.
Dr. Mark Hyman:	That's amazing. Wow, thank you. Are there any final thoughts or words you want to share?
[00:41:30] Dr. Rudy Tanzi:	I think what you do is amazing. I think Functional Medicine is the future, and rock on.
Dr. Mark Hyman:	Thank you, thank you.

Dr. Rupy Aujla:

[00:00:30]

Food is literally the most important health intervention anyone can make. It's a collection of phytochemicals. Those are the chemicals you find in plants. Fiber has a massive impact on things like gut microbes, that have effects on neurotransmitters and information. It is also the process of eating as well, the act of community. It kind of subsides lots of different barriers. It crosses the way we communicate with different people and our cultures. Our ability to nourish ourselves is just one of the parts of how food has medicinal properties.

[00:01:00]

Food is probably the first question I ask after taking a full history. I want to know what they're eating for breakfast, what they're eating for lunch, what a general, typical day looks like or what a seven day plan looks like. I want to be really getting an understanding of how they're using food in their daily lives. If it's something that's rushed, if it's something they don't really pay that much attention to, if they're on a particular diet plan, all that kind of stuff. I work as an emergency medicine doctor as well. So that's probably not going to be the first thing I lead with, but certainly in the clinic environment, when we're dealing with patients with chronic medical problems, that's one of the first things I start with.

[00:01:30]

The process of eating has been lost in our millennial generation, for sure. But certainly, in our modern societies, the process of eating is rushed. When you think about food and the process of eating, it's everything from the smell, the visual element, the sounds and the environment that you're in at that time, and how that has an impact on neural networks. The perception of everything in our environment has massive impacts on our neural networks.

Food and the process of eating is part of that environmental setting. It's part of that sensory stimulation that leads to so many different mechanisms in our body. It's certainly something that is much wider than just the energy and the macromolecules that we have in a plate of food.

[00:02:00]

The process of chewing—I talk to my patients quite a bit about the process of mindfully eating. Making sure you chew your food properly means that you're actually digesting it properly. If you're not chewing your food, then you're not increasing the surface area, you're not getting access to the internal molecules and you're going to be passing a lot of undigested food through your digestive tract.

[00:02:30]

The biggest misconceptions I think are that healthy eating is expensive, it's inaccessible, it's bland, and it's boring. I want to smash those preconceptions because I believe healthy eating doesn't have a price tag. It's not a privilege. It's something that we can all enjoy as a massive community, and really what I'm trying to do with *The Doctor's Kitchen* is to inspire people that the most nutrient-dense ingredients are usually the cheapest on the shelf. It's just about being explorative with them. It's about being inspired by different cultures and different ways of eating. And the different sorts of food pairings, the use of spices, that kind of stuff.

[00:03:00]

Those are probably the biggest misconceptions, and when you actually inspire patients that healthy eating can be fun, enjoyable, tasty, delicious, and culturally relevant, that's when you get people on board, and then you can have a different conversation about how it fits in with their lifestyle, meditation, sleep, and all the other things that we talk about in functional medicine.

[00:03:30]

Fooditis is this concept that's quite unfamiliar for us in the UK, but I've heard a lot about it, and it's quite worrying. This is where the use of technology and food really comes into play because we can have access to lots of different ingredients using lots of different delivery mechanisms. Getting spices, certain types of powders like raw cacao and other things like that can actually increase the nutrient

[00:04:00] density of food we have access to. Also, look at simple foods. They don't have to be particularly exotic. They could be things like Brussels sprouts, any types of brassicas, you can even grow your own as well on a window sill with little plant pots. Just get some soil that you can put in yourself. You can add things like nutrient-dense herbs and spices; coriander, bay, basil. These are all wonderful simple plants we all have access to that heighten the nutrient density of even the most bland of food.

[00:04:30] I say keep it really simple and if you stick to just three or four recipes you master, then you can start with the inspiration, little nuggets of information that people actually enjoy the process. When you break it down like, "I don't like cooking." What don't you like about cooking? Is it buying ingredients? Is it the effort of going to the grocery store? Is it the process of chopping and then burning something? Or the worry that you're not doing it right or it doesn't come out right? Or maybe there's a particular memory of you trying a recipe and it failed and you just haven't gone back to it. You have to figure out what it is that's preventing you from eating or cooking in the first place. Then you can narrow it down where you're going to work on with them and when it comes to inspiring them to cook. And honestly, if you master two, three, four dishes, then you're inspired. "Maybe I'll add a different herb or maybe

[00:05:00] I'll add a different spice or maybe I'll use a seasonal ingredient," and that's where you'll get people on board.

It's a really interesting concept that we as humans have evolved almost intertwined with our environment. We've evolved alongside the seasons and the seasons changing. Our biological mechanisms are matched. We've simultaneously grown alongside the changing of the seasons and

[00:05:30] everything else. Eating seasonally reminds us to add variety into our food and there's lots of different research that shows that variety in our food is actually very good for our microbiome population. For example, eating late summer fruits has a little more fructose in it and evolutionarily that would have encouraged more fat storage around our organs and that would have been protecting us against the winter cold, for example. There are lots of different ways in which seasonal eating is actually relevant but perhaps in modern life, maybe less so. It's just a good reminder to vary up your food because we

[00:06:00] know a variety of food has immense impacts on the gut microbiome and that's actually something we need to probably nurture a bit more.

My top tips for making food a lot more exciting and engaging is to: buddy up. If you have someone at home—kids, spouse, parents—everyone gets involved in having a different role. Doing something called *mise en place,* which is where you have everything prepared, everything chopped up already, and then it's just a case of putting different things in pans or boiling or whatever. Having everything prepared is really good, and then have a buddy to cook along with.

[00:06:30] Music. One of the best things I've found after getting back from the clinic is putting on my tunes, doing my *mise en place*, and then just enjoying the whole process of being on my own. It's actually kind of like a medicinal thing I get into.

The use of spice. There are so many different spice blends that people just don't know about and they're very easy to make yourself if you want. Things like togarashi, harissa, or berbere from northern Africa. These are different spice blends that not only make food more interesting, they add phytochemicals to your food, nutrient density, reduce inflammation, they have wonderful different

[00:07:00] biological effects on our body, and they make food a lot engaging and excitable for people.

You can also make your own pastes. Make a different lemongrass paste that you can just quickly put in coconut oil and coconut milk and then add some vegetables. That whole process is pretty inspiring for a lot of people as well.

Another thing I talk to my patients about is adding a new ingredient to your shopping list every week. Try something new, whether it's sunchokes or a different type of sweet potato like this purple sweet

[00:07:30] potato that we get from South America that has a wonderful purple flesh and a gorgeous texture to it and you can make it in different desserts even, you can have it for breakfast, you can put almond butter on it, those sorts of things. When you do that just once a week rather than putting loads of different exotic vegetables and fruits into your basket then it weaves itself into your normal cooking regime.

[00:08:00] Breakfast is something I get asked about a lot because it's a really hard topic. I think it really depends on your dieting strategy and how convenient it is for you. For me personally, I have breakfast a little bit later in the day usually around 7:30am when I get up at 6am. That's because I like to work out before. When you exercise will determine when you're going to be having breakfast if breakfast is even achievable at all. Sometimes, people prefer to fast up until midday and then have an eight-hour defined eating period. In that case, if it's good for them and they've done it for a few weeks and

[00:08:30] they're not having side effects, then perhaps skipping breakfast for that individual might be the best thing as well. It really depends on convenience, your work-life balance, when you're exercising, and the type of food you have accessible.

As a general rule-of-thumb, I think breakfast is exceptionally important particularly for someone like me who works in the NHS. I know if I don't have breakfast before I go to work I'm going to be snacking on different things, like cookies and chocolate. We're human so we're going to be attracted to those sorts of things. We're going to have sugar lows and if that's going to be the only sorts of food available

[00:09:00] then we're going to crack in most places. In a lot of cases, I think breakfast is pretty important. My general rule-of-thumb for people eating breakfast is have something with fiber and have something with good quality fat as well as protein. That's going to stop you from those sugar highs and lows and keep you away from cookies.

[00:09:30] Smoothies can be a good way to go if people really are lacking on time. I prefer to get food in its most whole form as possible. Something with high fiber like precooked sweet potatoes with almond butter for example. Or some dark leafy greens with added walnuts and spice nuts with some boiled egg. That has protein, fat, and fiber as well. You can actually gnaw through that pretty quick. I actually do Facebook Lives before I go to the clinic just to show people that you can do it in about ten minutes before you go to work. There are lots of different examples you can knock up in about ten minutes and still have nutrient density and not reach for cookies mid-morning.

[00:10:00] Being *The Doctor's Kitchen,* I get asked a lot about what food is good for "X" condition or what food is good for psoriasis or what food is good for eczema or diabetes or whatever. It's really important to get the concept across that food can't be treated like a pill. Food is an adjunct; food is a tool in a clinician's toolbox when it comes to treating a patient for whatever condition they might have. When people ask me about brain food, I have general principles of eating, but I have specific foods. Certainly high-fat

[00:10:30] foods, but high-quality high-fat foods are something I try to encourage as much as possible. Things like walnuts, chia, avocado, and extra virgin olive oil are fantastic wholesome sources of fats. Traditionally, the conventional medical profession has veered against because of our fears of cholesterol, but now we're learning that's completely false and actually these foods have lots of benefits, particularly for brain health and things like long-chain omega-3 fatty acids as well. And yes, oily fish definitely goes into that category.

[00:11:00] When you're having high fiber foods, not only is that great for nurturing your microbiome that has positive effects on brain inflammation, on reducing your instance of chronic disease like heart disease or diabetes that have brain effects. It also means that you're going to be more efficient at removing things like environmental pollutants that Joe Pizzorno is scaring us all about and it's quite interesting

[00:11:30] to see how high fiber foods are actually facilitating that process. They're making our bodies more adaptable to our new environments. The other things with regard to brain health are foods like colorful plant-based foods. The different sorts of food that have high nutrient density are tomatoes and the yellows and the greens and the dark-greenish vegetables and the brassica vegetables. Not only are they good for cardiovascular and diabetes reasons, but those particular chemicals you find in those pieces of food are actually reducing inflammation, neuroinflammation, and generalized

[00:12:00] inflammation that has holistic effects on the body while improving brain health at the same time.

[00:12:30] High fiber foods? Yes, tons. Beans, legumes, things like lentils, pulses. Things like chicory and asparagus stems, broccoli, sunchokes—we call them Jerusalem artichokes—sweet potato, cold potatoes as well (they have lots of prebiotic fiber), garlic, tons of different types of prebiotics as well. There's a ton. I tend to have a list and go through it with patience and just say, "Look, these are different ways in which you can get them into your food and these are the kinds of recipes you can use as well." And then launching as a segway into that you can talk about foods in general that improve microbiomes. Things like probiotic foods—kefirs and kombuchas—as well as things like probiotic yogurts. These are all great, nurturing this microbiome has inflammation-reducing effects on the brain as well.

[00:13:00] Foods that are toxic for our brains are going to be things like refined carbohydrates and sugars. I know it's something that people should be more aware of now but they sneak in a lot of places. We have a lot of added sugar, unfortunately, to our processed foods and convenience foods. Really, the whole act of getting people cooking and using ingredients from scratch is going to have wonderful effects on brain health for that reason. Those are the things that are going to zap our energy. They're going to be

[00:13:30] giving us the highs and lows, spiking our insulins, spiking our cortisol levels, and increasing inflammation.

The other thing is the timing of food. If you're going to be eating too late or over a 12, 14, 16-hour period that we tend to do because of our Western lifestyles, that's going to be causing lots of different effects on things like sleep and causing hormone dysregulation and disruption to our circadian rhythm. That's going to lead to reducing lots of alertness and increasing things like fatigue as well. It's

[00:14:00] really how food fits into a greater picture of how we're able to function and how our brains are functioning as well.

I'm pretty food-centric. I like to start the conversation around food and inspire people with delicious recipes that are simple and quick to make, etc., and show them how it doesn't have to be expensive. The most nutrient-dense foods are usually the cheapest on the shelf like red cabbage, asparagus, and all the different types of brassica vegetables. Once you have had that conversation with patients and they actually see some effects, they sleep better, they're less moody, they have less anxiety, and then

[00:14:30] you can have a wider conversation about how that segways into sleep and how sleep hygiene has effects and when you map out the different hormonal changes over a 24-hour period and they get excited about that, they'll actually start putting away their laptops and electric stimulation (things like phones and TVs and stuff like that that heighten the stimulation). That should reduce different hormones that have effects on our brain activity. Then you can start talking to them about the effects of exercise and how that increases BDNF and how that improves neurogenesis. And then you can start talking to them about things like meditation. Meditation is one of the most well-known forms of

[00:15:00] medicine, essentially, that societies like the ancient Chinese and Indian and Ayurvedic principles have always used for years and years. Now we're actually finding the science behind it. You can start talking to them about how they can instigate mindfulness. Food is a great conversation starter to lifestyle medicines in which you're talking about food, then you can go to mindfulness, sleep, and exercise.

[00:15:30] Counting calories and macros is important if you're an athlete and if it actually has a motivating factor to you. In the vast majority of patients I see, I think it adds a lot of confusion and adds a layer of technicality that doesn't really need to be there. Sometimes when you start counting calories and counting macros, you're reaching for a Snickers bar and putting down the banana. Or you're reaching for processed foods and you're negating things like fruits and things that might have a high fructose

[00:16:00] level or high caloric content. That is not the way to go. Food is a lot more complex than a measure of glucose level. The more wholesome and colorful foods you find on your plate, the better that's going be for your brain health. Once you're reaching for those whole sorts of foods and you're counting colors rather than calories that's when you're going to have the best effect. That's the easiest principle and the easiest way I try to inspire patients when it comes to eating better for the brain health or whatever chronic disease they're suffering from.

[00:16:30]   Dr. Minich is a massive inspiration to me and her subject matter of phytochemicals and the different types of plant chemicals that we have and how they have vast effects and everything beyond brain health is a concept that is really easy to introduce to patients. When you actually talk about it from a scientific point of view (you point them towards the studies and give them some evidence base behind it), that's when you can inspire them to count colors rather than counting calories. When you count in colors you don't need to worry about the calories ... Obviously, you have to make sure you're getting

[00:17:00]   enough fiber and protein, but the majority of people are nutrient deficient and we want to increase nutrient load. The best way to do that is with colorful plants, fruits, and vegetables.

SIDNEY BAKER, MD | Author: *Detoxification and Healing*

Dr. Sidney Baker: My background and how I got involved in integrative medicine starts with my mother, who is an artist, and my dad, who was a Unitarian minister who became Dean of Students at MIT after 10 years in the pulpit. It was kind of a quick rise, you might say, and he was killed in a plane crash when I was 13. And

[00:00:30] that, I'm pretty sure, set me on a path that was more independent. He didn't have my back, so-to-speak, and it influenced the way I sought teachers and father figures as I went through my career, even until now.

I went to Yale and I took a year off between my junior and senior years and traveled in the Far East, studying history of art of architecture. And then, I went to Nepal and I apprenticed with a doctor for three months there, Dr. Miller. He turned to me after each patient and said, Sidney, we've done everything we can for this patient.

[00:01:00] When I was in medical school later, it was: Have we done everything we can for this disease? That's a major fork in the road, whether we're talking about treatment for this disease or treatment for this patient. I stayed on the fork about this is treating the patient from then on, although in medical school it was a little awkward because the paradigm is different. But I then came back, went to medical

[00:01:30] school, and became a pediatrician. I took two years off through my training in pediatrics, between my second and third years, and went to Africa as a Peace Corps volunteer. I was a doctor but I was a volunteer.

In Africa, I got a chance as I did when I was traveling around the world, to live with people who are very different from me. And I realized that they're really cool, and they know things I didn't know and I

[00:02:00] couldn't have learned except seeing it in action. It has tremendous relevance to my understanding of the microbiome, about which I have some things to say in a few minutes.

In Africa, they don't have autoimmune diseases or allergies. The thousands of beautiful people I saw were healthy as could be, except for a few who had some kind of sickness I needed to deal with. They

[00:02:30] don't have what we call chronic illness of our kind, like autoimmune problems, multiple sclerosis, lupus, ulcerative colitis, Crohn's disease, and so on. That made a profound effect on me and I kept it with me until today because it enters into my daily life as a doctor now, and we'll talk later about what might be drawn from that experience.

[00:03:00] I came back from Africa. I was Chief Resident of Pediatrics at Yale and took a faculty position as an assistant professor of medical computer sciences and was very interested in data. And then, I figured, well, the data comes from people, and I like taking care of people so why don't I go be a real doctor? So, I kept my faculty appointment part-time and then I walked into a prepaid health plan where I took care of families. They didn't have family doctors in New Haven that were from Yale, but I had some

[00:03:30] training in obstetrics as well, so I sort of volunteered as the family doctor. I got to listen to patients who told me really remarkable stories.

For example, one was a man who I was doing an intake interview, and I said, "Well, are you allergic to anything?" You know, going down the thing, surgeries, allergies, injuries, and so on. He says yeah. I

[00:04:00] said, "Well, what are you allergic to?" He said, "Eggs." In that part of my career in the CHCP, it was called, we had plenty of time at the beginning, and I said, "Well, what happens if you eat eggs?" And he told me this story. It was just stunning what happened when he ate eggs. If he had told the cook in the kitchen, if he was a guest in somebody's house, "I can't have anything that was touched by eggs at all," but say she took a fork and took it from this pan and put it in that pan and there were a few

[00:04:30] molecules of egg, he would end up on the floor with horrendous gastrointestinal problems. I won't describe them, but you know what I mean.

[00:05:00] And I thought, wow, if that could happen to somebody like his story, but maybe not as severe, how would they figure it out? That became part of the paradigm I now go by, which is if there's something wrong with a person chronically ... See, he had these acute episodes but I'm talking about chronic illness now. You take that idea, and transfer it to chronic illness. If that could happen to him from just the tiniest amount of egg, there are people out there who are having some kind of symptom. Not necessarily on the floor with their GI tract, but other kinds of symptoms and we'd have to figure out what it might be.

[00:05:30] That became part of what I call the avoid-side of my paradigm, which is if there's something chronically wrong with you, maybe if you avoided it, that would hasten nature's strong impulse toward healing. Obviously, nature does the healing but you have to do the thing that would help that along. And so, I thought, well, I probably won't see many people like that but I should keep my eye on the ball, just in case.

[00:06:00] There's another woman, a lovely woman from Cape Verde island with two children. She was a working mom and had horrible, horrible menstrual cramps. They were completely disabling, along with migraine headaches. Terrible, terrible migraine headaches. And I thought I was being clever to say, well, these are migraines and go see the neurologist, and they'll sort it out. All the medicines he [00:06:30] prescribed were not good. They didn't work. And so, she went to see a chiropractor, and I thought, well now ... Mind you, I'm a Yale doctor, right? Chiropractor. And so, she came back from the chiropractor after a while, and she said "I'm all better now." And I said, "Whoa, I better talk to this chiropractor." And what he did was give her magnesium and vitamin B6—that was it. He tested her [00:07:00] with kinesiology and that was it, and she was cured with magnesium.

I would tell my colleagues from Yale, I would say, "You know, I had this patient and blah, blah, blah. This is the story." And they'd say, "You're trying to tell me that a migraine is caused by magnesium and B6 deficiency?" I'd say, "No, no, no, I'm talking about this one patient, not a migraine headache. I'm talking about this patient, isn't that amazing?" I didn't get very far with that talk around Yale, but I got [00:07:30] far with it in my own development, and so, it became part of my, what you call, background. And that background has this get-and-avoid name on it. I just said the avoid part. This was the get part: maybe if there's something wrong with you, you are failing to get something for which you have a special unmet need. I'm not talking about deficiency necessarily but I call it a special unmet need. Special for you, everybody's different, and it's not being met, and it's a need. If you get it, you hasten nature's [00:08:00] buoyant impulse toward healing because nature only wants to heal, so that was a big part of my development.

I'd spent seven years at this prepaid health plan, and I matured as a doctor. There were a lot of specialists there, and I was the generalist. I was on call at night and somebody comes in the emergency [00:08:30] room with a foreign body in their eye, and the ophthalmologist has to come in and take it out, and that ophthalmologist shows me how to do it. I learned how to do a lot of stuff that belonged to the specialties because we were all one family. It wasn't like a complicated referral thing. It was to their benefit that they taught me how to do things.

[00:09:00] I became more and more confident in my sense as a doctor or handling different kinds of things. Then, after seven years, I was asked to be director at the Gesell Institute that had to do with child development. Naturally, my patients belong to CHCP, had to stay there but, some of them would come and ask me questions. One of them said, my neighbor's kid developed this horrible eczema, and she's really suffering from it, and the doctors are not sure. I said, "What was the story?" The patient knew what the story was because she knew me and what my belief system was. She said she took antibiotics [00:09:30] for strep throat and a couple of weeks later she broke out in eczema. She knew the connection between taking antibiotics and the eczema was something Sid would know about. And so, she asked me if I could just talk to her friend and sort of give her a curbside sort of free consultation. I said, of course, it's simple.

[00:10:00]	So, I talked to the mom, and I saw the child for just a few minutes to say, "What you need is a prescription for nystatin," which is a medicine that kills yeasts or funguses and it's the growth of the funguses after the penicillin that cause the mischief. She took it and then a few weeks later, I asked my patient, or my patient called me I guess and said she's all better, and her autism went away. I didn't even know the child was autistic. It wasn't on the menu but her autism went away just like that.
[00:10:30] [00:11:00]	In my development as a physician, that made a big impression on me because, to me at that time, autism was something kind of way out there in terms of different diseases. It was way off campus, so-to-speak, and it had this strange history of having been blamed on mothers. For years, it was your mother's fault. You're a cold mother, that's why you have autism, and that was being debunked. During my education at Yale, that was the belief system. Then along came genetics, which is still taking over, trying to take over the territory, which is relevant in some ways, but it is not a genetic problem in the usual sense of the word.
[00:11:30]	I had known at that time that when people take antibiotics, and they get something after that, it's because the disturbance of the germs that live in the digestive tract, called the microbiome. If you go and reverse that by killing the fungi that had grown up because the fungi don't mind the penicillin, it's the other germs that do. I already knew this had a broad application but I didn't know it reached all the way to autism so autism suddenly became in the center of my campus instead of way out there in the suburbs of my mentality.
[00:12:00] [00:12:30]	I was an attending physician as a part-time job along the way that really awakened me to autism, before this event. I was a consultant for a residential treatment center. Not much treatment, a lot of residents, where I was supposed to do annual physical exams and sort of routine weekly sick calls. And the nurse asked me to do an annual physical on a little 14-year-old boy. She said he's autistic. He's nonverbal.
[00:13:00] [00:13:30]	I had never met an autistic child before, and he's 14. He's a handsome boy sitting on the end of the exam table, and I think I was a little nervous because this verbal thing ... I'm a very verbal person, and I usually like to talk to my patients. And even though I know now that people who can't talk are still listening, I simply said I'm going to examine you, and this is what I'm going to do, and I'm going to look in your eye with my ophthalmoscope, which I usually would remove my glasses when I do that, but I didn't. And so, I went to look in his eye, like this, and he hauled off and socked me right in the middle of the bridge of my nose. My glasses, which were the horn-rimmed type at that time, went in two pieces on the floor, and I was struck by what I had experienced.
[00:14:00]	The accuracy, the precision of what he communicated to me was remarkable. On reflection, what he was saying to me is you're looking into me but you're not seeing me, and I thought, "Whoa, that is something. This is a person with unusual skills buried in a nonverbal 14-year-old boy." And so, that's why I became interested in autism, but only later, did I then come into a setting at the Gesell Institute where I began to see more and more kids with those problems. That was a big part of my background that brought me to my current occupation as a teacher and a doctor of my patients, and they continue to be my teachers too.
[00:14:30] [00:15:00]	Children are often treated, I would say poorly, by doctors even pediatricians. Maybe things have changed some, but I think there's a general misunderstanding of children's ability to listen and understand. Newborn babies listen, and they understand the language of the family they were born into. Well, alright, at the beginning they do. This is standard science but people see babies and because they're nonverbal, they say, well, he's not listening, but they are and understanding most of it.
	So, the baby who is attending the whole process, needs to be given the opportunity to hear the story and have it explained and to be in the room. Not be sent over there, while the parents and the doctor talk about him behind his back. It can be talked about in a perfectly reasonable way, so the child can

[00:15:30]   participate, if you consider the child to be an expert, therefore the expert has to be in the room and be in on the conversation. The expert also gets a chance to say how they feel and this can be done in all kinds of ways, as my story of the communication with the knuckles told me something about what was going on in this boy's mind.

[00:16:00]   Children are the source of all knowledge about them, and they communicate it with their behavior, with all of their symptoms. The symptoms are their means of expression and has a huge vocabulary. As I'll talk about as we move forward here, the idea is that the details of the symptoms provide a rich

[00:16:30]   resource for understanding what the child's body is communicating to us about what's wrong. And this has to get us into, not only in a sense of I'll hear the story, but the mother tells me of all these different symptoms but in a more systematic way, like a 500-item questionnaire. You get to check off all the things the child must have and this includes many things that are not required to make a

[00:17:00]   diagnosis. It's a portrait of the person as an individual. If a painter were to draw a picture of you and only did your fingers and your toes, you would be left out of the picture.

[00:17:30]   The reality is with the total picture of everybody's symptoms and symptoms are the means of communication. The expertise of the baby or the child is to say what's going wrong? This is also important at a collective level. If you have those data from the questionnaire, 500 things you checked off, and you might have checked off 50 or 60 of those things are wrong in a child with autism, say. Those details are a rich source of what's going on, not only in the child, but now collectively in all those children. They're all different, but they express things in ways that I'll talk about in a few minutes.

[00:18:00]   Autism is just a label and a rather weak label. If you trusted things at the grocery store with just that name on it, without the fine print, you wouldn't want it. Nowadays, people are sophisticated. They say, well, let's see what's in here, if they're shopping for something. And so, just a label doesn't say it.

[00:18:30]   A few years ago, the word spectrum came along, and it means that the person belongs to a collection of people who represent a broad set of different colors, as in the color spectrum. It goes on really in both directions, forever. This was very helpful for doctors because they could feel more comfortable with the label, where there was a lot of give and take in there, and a lot of flexibility. It was not as

[00:19:00]   good for patients, in a sense that when the doctor says you have myasthenia gravis, well, it's bad news, but they know what I've got, right? And so, you must know what to do about it. But if they say you're in the spectrum, you feel kind of lost, like what do you mean I'm in a spectrum?

[00:19:30]   While it's been a blessing, because it's an accurate description of reality that there's a wide range of different manifestations of this problem called autism, it is a little bit troublesome to parents who feel, well, now how do we navigate in here? And of course, coming back to the question of the child being the expert, the navigation is done by paying attention to the details, which I'd like to talk about more as I go along here.

[00:20:00]   I feel that because of a certain set of rules, call it tacks rules, it's not about taxation, like getting your money to the government. If you're sitting on a tack, it takes a lot of aspirin to make it feel better. The treatment for tack-sitting is tack removal. Say if you have a headache, where is the tack? You take the

[00:20:30]   aspirin, well sure you can. That's for an acute illness. I'm not going to quibble about that. But for chronic illness, it's a different landscape, and there is something chronically wrong with you. Tack removal is better than taking the aspirin.

[00:21:00]   I'm not saying that drugs don't work. I'm going to leave here and go see a boy, who has been taking a medicine for Alzheimer's disease called galantamine for some years. He's an autistic boy. It has to do with the disappearance of a certain brain chemical. I tried all kinds of things for him years ago, and it was the one thing that made a big difference, even though he's taking like three times the adult dose, but it didn't hurt him at all. It's called galantamine and now I'm interested because he's gotten so

[00:21:30]   much better, maybe he doesn't need it anymore. So, we can take it away. But in general, we're trying to find something that is part of a person's experience, inside, and in the environment that needs to be adjusted as in removing a tack.

[00:22:00] Now, the second tacks rule is: if you're sitting on two tacks, removing just one doesn't give you a 50% improvement, and that's helpful for people to understand that chronic illness is complex. The idea that one drug is going to do it, and the idea that just one intervention is going to do it, works sometimes very well. But sometimes it means that you're caught in an environment, a system as I want to talk

[00:22:30] about soon, a system in which everything is connected. And the good thing about a system is sometimes if you hit a part of the system, which has a good influence, that influence spreads through the system and healing takes place. On the other hand, sometimes a system is difficult because if you have something bad happen, that also can spread through the system and then make for mischief. The

[00:23:00] drugs are important sometimes for acute illness and for killing bugs, but they create a lot of mischief and that's something that we, in Integrative and Functional Medicine, are especially aware of.

The first way the data of children talks to us is by having an embrace of the details of the data, which

[00:23:30] means that the child and the parent must have a mechanism for recording all the little details. Sometimes a tiny detail, and I'll give an example in a minute, can make a big difference in the whole game.

Let's say you're filling out a questionnaire and here's a question, are your child's stools of a pale color? A sort of gray or light brown or beige instead of brown poop. That means something, and it speaks to

[00:24:00] us in a trial of a dose of a support called taurine. People call it amino acid. It's not really an amino acid, but it's like them. It doesn't play the game with making proteins. It's just a free agent, and it works in about five or six different ways in the body, all very different, very crucial ways. One of which has to do with dealing with chlorine of all things, and which is used by the body. Your body makes its own kind

[00:24:30] of Clorox to kill germs and then taurine is used to protect the body cell from being injured by its own chlorine. Chlorine is used for making bile and if the bile is deficient in the taurine, then it makes you have light-colored poops, but the light-colored poops are a clue that if you don't know about it, you're going to miss the boat and that's a good example of how the data talks.

[00:25:00] There's another way and that is the collective data. If you have all the data on a lot of children, for example, 20,000 symptoms that are composed of samples of 60 or so symptoms from different

[00:25:30] children out of this questionnaire of 500 possible symptoms different people have, and you have this on your computer, you can really make sense of it. And so, this is something I've been doing during my career, trying to make sense of it. This data then talks vividly about what's really going on, and I should say that the simplicity that turns up from analyzing the data is just astonishing. It really surprised me.

[00:26:00] I've been treating children with autism for many years now, and so in my head, there's sort of a cloud of stuff that's going on in there about this. But when you sit down and analyze the data about the meaning of the different symptoms ... Let me explain. An itchy hand, itching, it itches here, that means there's an itch, which is a kind of function like pain and a lot of other ones, and where is it? It's on your

[00:26:30] hand and what organ in the body is it involved in? It's the skin. And so, that's the meaning of itchy skin and there are certain symptoms with funny names, but you have to say what does it really mean just in those terms, but it also may have an implication.

[00:27:00] Out of the 500 symptoms, about two-thirds or 360 of them in this huge collection of data have implications, which is more than I thought until I started looking at my data that way. If you boil them down to how many implications that come from them, and you look at them the right way, there are only about six different implications that come from the symptoms that drive decisions about what to

[00:27:30] do, and they have to do with some very simple notions. There's one collection of symptoms that have to do with what you'd call neuromuscular irritability. That's the fancy term for it, neuromuscular irritability.

[00:28:00]   It means that the muscles and the brain are all sort of dancing to the same drummer, and there's something that's making people uptight, is the expression in English. I've asked people speaking all different languages, "Is there an expression for 'uptight' in French, Spanish, whatever, Urdu?" and "No, we just say such and such but not like uptight, which has a sort of feeling of tight muscle and

[00:28:30]   nervous thing." But if you cluster these, based on their literal meaning I was just talking about, and take the implication of things that have to do with nervousness, tension, muscle cramps, menstrual cramps, cold hands and feet because the blood can't get through because the little blood vessels are uptight, difficulty swallowing, or difficulty pooping. Constipation is right up there. And you go on TV at night, you see how many ads there are for all sorts of strange and dangerous medicines for constipation.

[00:29:00]   All of those people, they just need magnesium. Magnesium is a mineral that is globally deficient in our population and if everybody got enough magnesium, then a whole bunch of things would go away. The data talks about that because you find if you look at the records of hundreds of people and see how it filters out, like, wow, there's a lot of neuromuscular irritability. And my experience with them, with many patients, is if they have things like that, leg cramps or any kind of stuff like that, and sometimes people have just one symptom. Constipation is enough to get you there but sometimes

[00:29:30]   they have a number of little symptoms. And so, that drives the decision for the patient individually, but it drives a general decision that applies to the understanding of illnesses that exists in our culture today.

[00:30:00]   Another example is the loss of immune tolerance, LIT, like the initials, L-I-T, loss of immune tolerance. It has to do with sensitivity. Now, the word sensitive, it's a good word to think about. Does it have to do with your senses? Of course it does because it says sensitivity. Does it have to do with other aspects of how they say that guy is a very sensitive guy? It's a compliment, right? But if somebody

[00:30:30]   says, "I'm really sensitive to strawberries. If I get strawberries I break out in hives." We have to think about the customs and immigration at JFK.

You're coming into the country and they're going to be seeing if you're safe to come in and they examine 10,000 people every day. They look at your passport, and then you're gone, like this. And

[00:31:00]   every now and then, they find somebody who has a name that's on a list but there's a little bit of irritability there because they have to stop and check things. There's a little inflammation that happens, and then rarely, they catch a bad guy, right? But if the customs and immigration people got drunk one day, it would be a real mess. There would be inflammation everywhere because they'd start arresting all kinds of people that didn't need to be arrested.

[00:31:30]   The customs and immigration has lost tolerance. Now, tolerance, there are two attributes of a complex system, which could be the digestive system, or chemistry in people, or it could be a mechanical system, or political system, or social system. There are two features of it when it's healthy you can count on, and when it gets out of whack, you have to look at what's missing. One is tolerance and the other is diversity.

[00:32:00]   Diversity and tolerance is what you find in a well-working and smooth, healthy, complex system, such as me or you. When you lose tolerance, then you become sensitive and it is expressed in the sensory

[00:32:30]   system. Bright lights bother me. Sounds bother me. I can't stand the taste of this. Those kinds of things. I can't stand to be touched. These are features we see in our children. If you look hard, you can see them in the general population, and it's all about the same thing. It's the loss of tolerance. Also, I can't eat strawberries because they make me break out in hives and all kinds of things, where my body has lost its tolerance in the immune system.

[00:33:00]   There is a lot of that going on in our world, right? Allergy is a word only invented in the 1920s. There was no such word in English before then. Now, you turn on the TV and it's everything for your allergies. And so, the whole population is allergic.

[00:33:30]	When I was in Chad, Africa, for a couple of years, I never saw anybody with an allergy, except the missionaries and their diplomats. Africans living the old-fashioned way didn't have allergies and they didn't have autoimmune problems so that struck me as an important finding. And then, the question is now another word comes into our vocabulary. A very reassuring word, which is restoration.
[00:34:00]	If somebody says, well, you need to do this and it sounds a little weird, then you kind of feel, well, I don't know. But if they say you need to restore something to your body that was missing, well, okay. "I lost my wallet. What was it?" Okay. But if you lost your wallet, you want your wallet back. If you lost your tolerance, you want your tolerance back. And if you know something that will restore tolerance for people, it's a big deal.
[00:34:30]	It turns out that restoring diversity is one way to restore tolerance, so it all kind of goes together. It's what you call a holistic idea, which is sort of a word that's been tossed around in medicine, like Functional Medicine and Integrative Medicine, and so on. It's all a way of thinking along the lines that I'm talking about, which is if there's something wrong with you, maybe it's something you need to get or avoid that will hasten nature's strong impulse toward healing. And if it's on the get side, you want something that will restore tolerance.
[00:35:00] [00:35:30] [00:36:00]	When someone comes to see me with a child with autism, there really isn't a protocol because it bespeaks a sort of cookie-cutter approach. A group of us got together in 1995: parents, doctors, and scholars, all in one room for three days, about 30 of us, to talk about what's the deal with autism. Dr. Bernard Rimland who was the pioneer who got us to this point and he and I helped put on this meeting along with Jon Pangborn, a biochemist. Out of that came a report I wrote with Jon Pangborn about what would be the approach? What are the answers to the question? What do you do when a person with autism comes in? Naturally, a big part of the meeting, especially because of the scholars, biochemists, and all of us were there, was what lab data should you get to try to find out what's going on? Then Jon and I wrote a little booklet called *The DAN Protocol*. DAN stands for Defeat Autism Now! Bernie Rimland made up the name. I hated the name because it made autism sound like a thing, but anyway.
[00:36:30]	We wrote this thing, we called it a protocol. It was a terrible mistake. For lab data, yeah, you could do that. You could say these are tests that would help show us the path. When it comes to treatment, the idea of a protocol is a terrible idea because it isn't the same for everybody. Individuality is one of the key features of the focus that those of us in Integrative Medicine have, which is we're treating the individual, not the disease, going back to what Dr. Miller said to me in Nepal, back in 1959. Treating the individual, not the disease so that individuality comes out with all the symptoms I've been talking about.
[00:37:00] [00:37:30]	We've learned from what we amassed from experience that there are certain things that work pretty well. And now, I tend to not do any lab tests up front. I do thumbs tests. The thumbs test is, you try something for a little while and you see what happens to the thumbs. The mom's thumbs. She says, "Oh, this was great," or "This was great, but he had a lot of this too at the same time," or "Nothing really happened," or "Whoa, it made a bad reaction." You learn so much from thumbs.
[00:38:00]	One of the things we do are sort of generic because they are now so well-known to be related to these kinds of developmental problems is change the diet. On the one hand, that's one of the hardest things for human beings to do. It's amazingly difficult for parents who just haven't really even thought about that.
	My stepdaughter is a teacher for young children, dance and stuff like that. She has four-year-olds and they're allowed to come and bring a snack because otherwise they get cranky. And the mothers send in these cupcakes and candy for their snack. I mean it's really shocking to see through her eyes what's going on outside of that practice. Getting rid of sugar.

[00:38:30]	Sugar is poorly understood in our culture but it's really bad for people. It's bad for everybody. So, you don't have to worry about do you have this symptom or that symptom, don't eat sugar.
[00:39:00] [00:39:30]	Don't eat gluten. Gluten is bad for everybody. Now, this comes not from me, not my voice. This comes from way up there, at the top of the totem pole. Alessio Fasano is a professor at Harvard, and when he came from Italy to be a professor at the University of Maryland Medical School with $2 million of funding, because he's a brilliant guy, and he learned from the gastroenterologist this thing about gluten is very funny. A lot of people think gluten is bad for you but the gastroenterologists, we don't buy this, except for people with the particular disease that has to do with having gluten not agree with you and you have to do a biopsy for that and special tests. And then, okay, now you shouldn't eat gluten. But for the rest of us, it's not a problem.
[00:40:00] [00:40:30]	So, he looked into it with his scholarly eyes and it turns out that gluten is bad for everybody. It opens up what we call the tight junctions, which is like the mortar between the flagstones on your sidewalk. If the mortar gets loose, the rain can go right through, which is not bad. If it's the sidewalk of your digestive tract, then things that are supposed to stay in your intestine, get through into your blood without going through customs, so-to-speak. You don't want to have poopy stuff going straight into your blood or even undigested tomato juice, and if it does, then it's bad. And these same junctions are what keeps the dirtiness of the blood, because the blood is still not that clean. It's pretty good but it's transporting a lot of molecules that came from your food that got through customs, but they're still not what you'd want to have in your brain. So, the same tight junctions stay closed when the blood circulates through your brain so that you don't get stuff in your brain. That's called a blood-brain barrier and then the one for your bowel is the bowel-blood barrier. They don't use that expression much but those are the same thing.
[00:41:00] [00:41:30]	Gluten opens the tight junctions in the gut. It's going to open up the tight junctions in the brain to some extent. That's not really so much the point but it's the gut thing that's happened. So, say I'm giving a lecture and Dr. Fasano was lecturing, I'm putting on a thing and I'm the moderator, and Dr. Fasano is lecturing and I'm looking at the audience. And he says to the doctors, all my colleagues in my tribe, he says tight junctions are opened by gluten in everybody, and the audience has some pretty stunned faces in it. Not me, no, not me.
[00:42:00] [00:42:30]	When the time for questioning comes up at the end, they're passing in the slips of paper with questions on it and I'm waiting for that. I'm the moderator, so I get to ask the first question. I say, "Alessio, you said tight junctions are opened by gluten in everybody and everybody in the audience was kind of shocked. Could you explain and elaborate on that?" He said, "Yes, they're opened in everybody." I said, "What's the difference between the person who has some awful thing happening from gluten and the person who seems to be fine, eating a loaf of bread every day?" He said, "Well, it's just how long the tight junctions stay open." Then I say, "Well, suppose somebody has a tendency towards some problem, some disease, would it be prudent for them to avoid gluten altogether?" I said, "For example, me. I have this disease called aging, which participates in many of the different things that are wrong with you if you have some particular disease. But aging has certain features of those things so, for someone like that but just to sort of hedge your bet, stay off gluten." He says, "Yeah. Okay."
[00:43:00]	He's not saying nobody should ever eat gluten because he's a professor at Harvard and they can't say things like that because their funding would go away. But the idea from the practitioner's side why people shouldn't eat gluten, sugar, and maybe soy. Those are things I would expect people to latch onto. Many people have come to me. They've already gotten there.
[00:43:30]	The thing I would do now is thumbs testing, and I would say you should take a trial of a medicine to cure fungi, and there happens to be one that's not a medicine. It's very effective and it's completely safe. It has a long name but it's okay. It's called saccharomyces. Saccharo means sugar, myces means fungus. It's the sugar fungus and that's the same fungus that we use for making bread, wine, and beer.

[00:44:00] This saccharomyces has a second name because germs have two names and it's called boulardii. And then, the one that we use for making bread and beer is called cerevisiae, which is like beer. And so, these yeasts for saccharomyces boulardii, know how to kill the other yeasts.

[00:44:30] It's really quite stunning because they're cousins but that's a little bit like the way things work in a large family of criminals. If they have one in their tribe, one in their group, in their gang that needs to be taken care of, the thing to do is to get his cousin, Tony, to do the hit because Tony knows how to get in the door. So, the saccharomyces boulardii, being a fungus that knows how to kill other fungi, is pretty brutal but it's completely safe for people to eat, even in huge amounts.

[00:45:00] One thing I would do up front is do a thumbs test and say, well, just try some saccharomyces boulardii. It comes in a little capsule. You can open it and then you can take one every day and then 1 and 2, work up to 5, or 6, or 7, or 8, or 10, or 20 a day, but it can't hurt you. But it can cause quite a reaction because when the hit is made, it can cause a little bit of an explosion of the yeasts that are dying and their toxins are released that they're making all the time. But now, they get released all of a sudden [00:45:30] because the little yeast blows open and now you have a situation where you need to take some activated charcoal that will cool off the situation, usually like that, and now you have proof of concept. And who does it come from? It comes from the child, who is the expert here.

[00:46:00] You get the expert who says I took that saccharomyces boulardii. It made me feel terrible for a week but the charcoal worked, so we're on board with it, and then get a response which is sometimes miraculous and that's what you're going for. The other thing I would do early in the game, is an injection, a little bit of vitamin B12. It's a naturally red substance that is a part of food we eat. It's only made by germs. It gets into our food supply and comes from meat, not so much from vegetables, just from meat.

[00:46:30] There's a glitch in the chemistry of many people, and the autistic children, and the ones where we learned this about, but that's not exclusive to autistic children, where the vitamin B12 is needed because of a problem in detoxification chemistry. The chemistry where the body takes the garbage to [00:47:00] the dump, and when this gets stuck in a certain way because the chemistry is injured, sometimes injured by poisons, it's kind of a funny deal because the poisons are the thing you were trying to get rid of but they jam up the detoxification system. Then, you give a shot of B12 and now, again, it's a thumbs test. Within a week or two, you frequently, half the time, some people ... Jim Neubrander, a [00:47:30] doctor colleague of mine got into this, and he would estimate a high percentage, and I would estimate a pretty high percentage but how high a percentage does it have to be?

So, a shot of B12 and sometimes you see a miraculous response. Really, even just on the way home, kind of, especially if they came all the way from Detroit or something. And now, you know you've learned something really important that no laboratory ... You can't test for B12 and say, "Oh, he's B12-deficient." It doesn't have to do with deficiency. It has to do with a phrase I used before, which is [00:48:00] unmet special needs. Unmet special needs are common in our kids, so I would do that.

[00:48:30] And then, the other thing I would do is a trial of these HDCs, that one of my patients I think has mentioned in this series. They are little creatures that restore immune tolerance. The word restoration again is what we're talking about. Here's B12, an unmet need for something you're lacking, that you have a special need for.

[00:49:00] Killing the yeast is to get rid of something that isn't good for you and getting the HDCs is a restoration of something that belongs in the microbiome and is the kind of thing that my patients in Africa had and made themselves healthy but we lack. And so, if you have this little creature called HDC, which stands for, are you ready? Hymenolepis diminuta cysticercoids. I call them little dudes. If you have these, it restores immune tolerance and the evidence on this is overwhelming. This is the work of my mentor William Parker, a professor of surgery at Duke. This approach is something I usually do early in [00:49:30] the game so I'm on board. There are other important nutrients that need to be considered and some

---

of them should be studied in a lab to see just how bad things are, such as measuring vitamin D is an important thing, and there are others like that. But those are some of the first steps I would take.

[00:50:00] When we started talking, I said that there's the fork in the road I learned about early in the game from Dr. Miller, like treat the patient, treat the disease. This is something I think many people in my profession really are not consciously aware of and maybe they think it's quibbling a bit, but it isn't. It's really a major choice about where you are with this. If it's acute illness, I have no qualms about that. You just do what ... Put a cast on the leg and let the bone heal. But when it comes to chronic illness,

[00:50:30] there's a different way of thinking that is more than just you're treating the individual or you're treating the disease. There's other baggage that comes with it that helps people understand more deeply what it entails.

First of all, the way doctors learn about diseases is that they live so-to-speak in a big tree. There's

[00:51:00] something called the International Classification of Disease, where the experts have gotten together at the United Nations and other places to decide how many diseases are there in the world, and how do we organize them. They have put them in a big tree so they are classes of things and then subclasses, and then, underneath that, other ones so they go in different categories, and have numbers attached to them, and you put that on the insurance form.

[00:51:30] Now, this model of reality that diseases can live in this tree is a completely false understanding of reality, but it came from one of the most perfect understandings of reality that ever was, which was a scientist named von Linné, or Linnaeus, way back in the 1700s. He started to put together a way of organizing the relationships between living things, like rats, cats, cows, pine trees, spruce trees, apple

[00:52:00] trees, this kind of bug, and that kind of bug. It turns out they live in a big tree, a big classification tree in which there are phyla and then it goes all down to classes and species and subspecies, and so on. When you learn about this in biology, this is an absolutely valid work of a genius, that this was established and it still maintains order in our concept of all of the living things in the world.

[00:52:30]

Toward the end, Linnaeus put together two little booklets on the classification of disease, which was a terrible idea because diseases are not things. They are ideas that we form about things and that's an important thing to keep in mind. The diseases are not things and when doctors talk about entities,

[00:53:00] disease entities, and that the diseases cause your symptoms, that is nonsense. The symptoms are the disease and the label is just the label, but we constantly hear people talking about disease entities and autism causes not being able to talk, which people shouldn't talk that way.

Now, the way these are arranged in conventional medicine is in this big tree, which we'd say is

[00:53:30] hierarchical. There are levels that are bigger, and smaller, and smaller, and smaller. In Functional Medicine, our diagram of the way things are arranged is a big system and the system is something where everything is interconnected. It's like a big circle, like a big basketball but hollow. I mean, hollow like a basketball but with lines that connect everything on the outside and everything on the inside. It's all a very complicated interconnection of all the different pieces. And when you're dealing with a system, it's a very different approach than if you're dealing with a hierarchy. The system, the right

[00:54:00] word is dispositive but it means it's all interconnected this way.

The good thing about a system, if you hit it in a place where the bad influence gets loose and it spreads, that can go and infect the whole system. And if you hit it in a good way, the good thing can spread. Sometimes, you don't have to get it all right. You don't have to find every vitamin deficiency and every food allergy or every single thing wrong. Sometimes you just get one thing right and bingo!

[00:54:30] everything starts working better. This is what happens sometimes with some of these interventions that begin with something like the antifungal medicine or the HDCs.

Now, medical thinking is what I call "name it, blame it, tame it, prescription pad medicine." The

[00:55:00] patient comes in, he says, "I have had this for a couple of years now." "Oh, you have such and such. That disease is the cause of your problem right away." That's stupid because the diseases don't cause

[00:55:30] the problem. The problem simply needs a name but the problem is the details. You blame the name for the problem like you come in and you say you're depressed. You feel sad. They say, well, you have depression. Depression is the cause. Now, we have a pill for your depression. So you tame it with a prescription. So, we call it "name it, blame it, tame it, prescription pad medicine." That's my snide way of describing the medicine I was trained to do back at Yale in the 1960s.

[00:56:00] Whereas the Functional Medicine I practice now is principle-based medicine. It's based on a few fundamental principles, really quite simple, and they are that everybody's an individual. That's so important. Every living thing on the planet is an individual. I mean that's the way it was created. If it's God who created, that was God's design. If evolution created it, it's the way evolution did it to make everything unique. If that's the case, then your approach has to be toward the individual.

[00:56:30] The second principle is balance. Balance is what health is all about and that balance has to deal with get or avoid in terms of therapy. Either you need to get this because you have an unmet special need or you need to avoid it because you have an unmet special need to avoid it because it's allergenic or it's poisonous.

[00:57:00] And then, another basic principle is that all living things are rhythmic, that it all exists with rhythms. Rhythms upon rhythms upon rhythms, pulse and respiration, and all those things. Now, this is not being looked at very closely in medicine these days but it's going to come along. There are certain ways in which we pay attention to it, like brainwaves and EKGs and all that. But it's more like music, and if people understood the body more as music then we would get ways of listening to it that would help us tune it into health and there are certain kinds of devices and things coming along in medicine that are along those lines.

[00:57:30] And then, there's a fourth one that is a fundamental principle, which is the agency of consciousness. The agency means something can make something else happen. So, wheelbarrow is the agency for getting the dirt to the dirt pile.

[00:58:00]
[00:58:30]
[00:59:00] A professor at Princeton, a few years ago, was engaged in talks with the new freshman people coming into the School of Engineering. He said, "If you get to be a senior and you have gotten straight As in everything in engineering school, you can pick your own project for your thesis." A young woman came to him at the end of one year and said, "I want to study the effects of consciousness on people on things. People's consciousness on things, put it that way." He said, "Get out of here. This is engineering school. You ought to go over to the psychology department. You can't graduate from engineering school if you're going to think like that." And she said, "But you said", and he said, "Look, we don't do this kind of work. That's crazy talk you're doing." She said, "But you said. I have straight As in everything and I want to study the agency of consciousness. I want to study the effect of the consciousness of a person on a machine." He said, "Okay, but you're risking your diploma. If you're going to do that, I'll support you."

[00:59:30] They set up a little machine that makes numbers and you push the button and it makes numbers between 1 and 200. It makes 60,000 numbers in a minute because it's like a computer and you make 60,000 numbers between 1 and 200, you're going to come out with 100 as the average or a little bit up or down from 100. The distance between the up and down of close to 100 is expressed by what we call a bell-shaped curve. There's a lot at 100 and then it goes off in each direction. It slows down so it looks like a bell in profile.

[01:00:00] They ran this experiment in the laboratory and sure enough, just regular people off the street were sitting there, making this thing go left or right. And they showed that within a few weeks that it was working; it changed the career of the professor. He became deeply involved in that and there's simply no doubt that his work proved the point that consciousness has agency. That is, we can make things happen. The influence may be small but if you're flying a jet plane at 600 miles an hour and a little bit of consciousness puts you in the wrong way, it does make a difference.

[01:00:30]   This is a feature of science that is now published and true but is generally not even known about or avoided by people because the implications are very strong. We'd have to change a lot of things if we included this factor of reality in our doing. I include that because I think it's a terribly important thing for people to know about. They can roll their eyeballs all they want but this was done at a school of engineering, and of course, there are many people who know this anyway, because they come from a tradition where this is common sense.

[01:01:00]   Finally, the principle we're talking about is that the target of treatment is the individual. It's not the disease. That's really the take-home for what we're talking about.

SUZANNE GOH, MD | Cortica, Founder and Chief Medical Officer

Dr. Mark Hyman:	Dr. Goh, you've been looking at the world through a different lens since you saw this patient, Jake. Tell us how he changed your thinking about autism and how the body responds to various insults.
Dr. Suzanne Goh: [00:00:30]	Sure. This young boy was eight years old when I met him. I met him at the time I was co-director of the Autism Program at Columbia University, and I remember being so moved by him and his mother, because of how much they had done along their journey with autism. He was first diagnosed young — around 18 months—and had received a lot of very important therapy like behavior intervention and speech language therapy. It wasn't until he started to receive mitochondrial therapy at the age of three and a half, that things really started to change.
[00:01:00]	At that time, he wasn't speaking. He had difficulty walking. He wasn't able to run. His mother took him to Johns Hopkins University to have additional testing—mainly metabolic mitochondrial testing, and it was there that a diagnosis of mitochondrial dysfunction with autism was made. He was started on a series of vitamins and supplements, that over the course of weeks and months, radically changed his developmental trajectory. He began to speak, to interact socially, and his gross and fine motor skills improved dramatically.
[00:01:30] [00:02:00]	He continued those therapies up until when I met him, which was at age eight, and at that point he had been doing well. He was mainstream in school, but he was beginning to refuse to take the large quantities of vitamins and supplements. He had been inconsistent with that and he was having a period of regression, so his symptoms were getting worse. He had made dramatic progress and now he was struggling again. He was struggling in social interaction, high levels of anxiety, headaches, daily migraine headaches, and obsessive-compulsive behaviors. They were so severe that he had trouble walking down a sidewalk because he was retracing his steps. It was hard to get out of the house in the morning, and so this was, of course, alarming to his parents. With resuming mitochondrial therapy through L-carnitine, coenzyme Q10, B vitamins, some very basic supplements, he began to improve again.
[00:02:30]	Now, he's a thriving junior high school student, plays competitive travel soccer, is in a mainstream school, and is doing incredibly well.
Dr. Mark Hyman:	Extraordinary story and yet, when you go to the doctor, most of the time they don't know how to diagnose mitochondrial dysfunction, and probably never heard of mitochondrial therapy.
Dr. Suzanne Goh:	That's right.
Dr. Mark Hyman: [00:03:00]	Tell us about your work in mitochondrial discovery of how this is connected to autism because mitochondria is a place where we make energy, and it seems like a lot of his symptoms were an energy deficit.
Dr. Suzanne Goh:	Yes. He had very low tone, fatigue, the leg milestones—all of which are associated with mitochondrial impairment.
Dr. Mark Hyman:	What are mitochondria anyway?
Dr. Suzanne Goh:	If you think about the cells of the body, nearly all cells have, inside of them, mitochondria. Mitochondria are classified as a subcellular organelle, so they're tiny structures inside of cells.
Dr. Mark Hyman:	Like a cell within a cell.
[00:03:30] Dr. Suzanne Goh:	Yes. A cell can have dozens or up to thousands of mitochondria. Mitochondria are sometimes called the

[00:04:00]	powerhouse of the cell because one of their main functions is to generate energy. They do that in the form of ATP, which is thought of as the currency or the fuel, the energy currency for the body. Mitochondria are a powerhouse. They do a lot of other things. It's interesting that they're called the powerhouse because, in fact, they're actually very delicate structures and they're very sensitive to environmental factors, stress, toxins, and oxidative stress.

Dr. Mark Hyman: They're easily damaged.

Dr. Suzanne Goh: They're easily damaged but they're so important for all of the body's functions, and the brain is particularly dependent on the function of mitochondria because it has such a high energy demand. The developing brain is hugely impacted by mitochondrial function.

Dr. Mark Hyman:
[00:04:30]
That's like you run out of gas, right? Your brain doesn't work and so the brain doesn't have a lot of ways of responding to insults. With mitochondria, you have all sorts of problems: Parkinson's, Alzheimer's, autism. As you said, the mitochondria are really sensitive to insult. What have you found are the worst offenders in damaging the mitochondria?

Dr. Suzanne Goh: There's a term that's sometimes used called secondary mitochondrial dysfunction—meaning not due to a genetic cause, but due to other factors like inflammation, physiological stressors, and medications. There are some medications that are known to be toxic to mitochondria.

Dr. Mark Hyman: Like statins.

[00:05:00]
Dr. Suzanne Goh: Yes, very widely-used medications, some antibiotics, some commonly used psychiatric medications that are commonly used in children, in young children with autism.

Dr. Mark Hyman: Like what?

Dr. Suzanne Goh: Like Risperidone.

Dr. Mark Hyman: That's an antipsychotic, right?

Dr. Suzanne Goh: Yes, and it's very, very widely used in the treatment of autism. Mitochondria can be impacted by so many different factors.

Dr. Mark Hyman:
[00:05:30]
You mentioned toxins in your work, that you've discovered a load of environmental toxins. You talk about the work of Phil Landrigan—an amazing scientist—who is really connecting the dots between environmental insults, autism, ADD, and behavioral issues.

Dr. Suzanne Goh: Yes, it's so important: there are many chemicals, industrial chemicals, and pesticides that are widely used that we know clearly have toxicity to the developing brain. Many of those chemicals impact the function of mitochondria. It's very likely that at least one mechanism by which they harm the brain is by impairing the mitochondria.

[00:06:00]
Dr. Mark Hyman: The mitochondria, essentially, are the processing factories for the food, and they respond differently to different foods. One of the big insults, we know, is that sugar is a mitochondrial toxin, and it's ubiquitous. The average kid has thirty-four teaspoons of sugar a day. How does that impact the mitochondria?

Dr. Suzanne Goh:
[00:06:30]
Well, nutrient intake or the lack of certain key nutrients is probably one of the biggest factors that affect the mitochondria. We know a lot about the machinery—the delicate machinery inside mitochondria—a lot of that is impacted by oxidative stress. When there are these molecules in excess, called free radicals, they can do damage to mitochondria.

Dr. Mark Hyman: It's like rusting.

Dr. Suzanne Goh: Yes.

Dr. Mark Hyman:	It's like a car rusting or an apple turning brown, in that process happening inside of us.
[00:07:00]	
Dr. Suzanne Goh:	Yes. The things that we eat day to day impact, even within the course of a day. It's that dynamic. The system is that impacted.
Dr. Mark Hyman:	What other kinds of food actually hurt the mitochondria and what are those that help the mitochondria?
Dr. Suzanne Goh:	We think that the foods that are helpful to the mitochondria are foods that are rich in antioxidants, that are a natural source of, for example, B vitamins. There are foods that are natural sources of coenzyme Q10. Coenzyme Q10 is key in one aspect of the mitochondria, called the respiratory chain, that is directly involved in the generation of ATP.
[00:07:30]	
Dr. Mark Hyman:	What has CoQ10 in it?
Dr. Suzanne Goh:	A lot of foods that we may not want to eat, so liver.
Dr. Mark Hyman:	Liver?
Dr. Suzanne Goh:	Liver has ...
Dr. Mark Hyman:	Liver, yeah, liver's good. Liver has B vitamins and is a mitochondrial food.
Dr. Suzanne Goh:	Carnitine, for example, which is in high concentration in meat products.
Dr. Mark Hyman:	Yeah, particularly lamb.
Dr. Suzanne Goh:	It is a form for shuttling fats into mitochondria where they can then be metabolized into energy.
Dr. Mark Hyman: [00:08:00]	Let's talk about fats. You mentioned fat, so we've seen a lot of literature come out that fats really are an important fuel for the mitochondria. Certain kinds of fats actually help the mitochondria work better, like MCT oil. What do you have to say about that research?
Dr. Suzanne Goh: [00:08:30]	Well, I think we know the importance of lipids in, for example, cell membrane integrity. The mitochondria have their own membrane. The integrity of that membrane is very important for the function of mitochondria. In fact, many of the key processes happen along the inner mitochondrial membrane, so lipids from fats are important for those types of things. We understand that mitochondria are very sensitive to inflammation, and that healthy lipids can help regulate the body's inflammation.
Dr. Mark Hyman: [00:09:00]	What about the actual burning of fuel, because it seems like there are these metabolic therapies that are emerging around ketogenic diets, and it's been very effective in these kids. I had a patient with autism recently who was having a lot of violent behavior and aggressiveness. He was eating a lot of starch foods and sugar, and we put him on a ketogenic diet. All of that went away, almost overnight.
Dr. Suzanne Goh: [00:09:30] [00:10:00]	Ketogenic diet is a type of diet that helps provide the body with a different source of, a fuel to burn, so it allows the body to generate high levels of ketones for fuel. It's sort of a way to shift the body into a different biochemical metabolic state. The ketogenic diet and a related diet—the low glycemic index diet—are known to be effective treatments for epilepsy. They reduce seizures. They stabilize the patterns of electrical firing in the brain. We know that in those with autism, somewhere probably around 20 to 30% have seizures at some time in their life. They have epilepsy, and somewhere between 60 to 80% of those with autism have abnormal EEGs. Whether or not they have seizures, they have an EEG, so they have a brain. The EEG is a way of collecting electrical data about the brain that shows that parts of the brain are firing in abnormal ways, and show excessive firing. Diets like the ketogenic diet and low glycemic index diet can help to stabilize and improve those patterns.

Dr. Mark Hyman: [00:10:30]	What you're saying is pretty radical because we, for decades, thought first that it was bad mothering that caused autism. And then, second, that it was a fixed static brain disorder that could never change. What you're talking about is actually being able to change the brain in ways that help these kids recover, which is kind of heresy.
Dr. Suzanne Goh: [00:11:00]	Autism has been misunderstood from the time it was first described in the 1940s until now. It's really been misunderstood. It was thought to be primarily psychological, and in some parts of the world, still thought to be psychological, not neurological. We've really come a long way. We know that it's not due to bad parenting or refrigerated mothers. We know that's not the case. We know that it's not static. We know that it has a lot to do with the body's biochemistry, which is impacted by the environment. We know that it has to do with the brain's metabolism, and that a lot of that can be influenced and changed.
Dr. Mark Hyman:	It's amazing. It's really helpful. It's a very helpful message. Tell us about this groundbreaking research you've been involved with at UC Davis.
Dr. Suzanne Goh: [00:11:30]	Sure. I had the good fortune, during my postdoctoral research fellowship and then as a faculty member at Columbia University, to be mentored by Dr. Salvatore Di Maio, who's thought of as one of the founders of the field of mitochondria medicine. He and I worked together, along with Dr. Bradley Peterson, who is the Chief of Child Psychiatry at Columbia at the time, to do a brain imaging study to look at whether we could identify markers of mitochondrial dysfunction in the brain in children and adults with autism. That had not been done before.
[00:12:00]	There had been studies showing the peripheral markers like blood or muscle, or other tissues, showing markers of mitochondrial problems, but had never been shown in the brain in living individuals. We used brain MRI, in particular brain magnetic resonance spectroscopy, to look for lactate—elevated levels of lactate—which is a bio marker mitochondria l...
Dr. Mark Hyman:	That's what you accumulate in your muscles when you exercise too hard, right?
Dr. Suzanne Goh: [00:12:30]	Yes. It accumulates in the brain when the brain's mitochondria aren't functioning right. It accumulates during sleep deprivation, in the brain. We were able to show is elevated lactate in the brain of a proportion of individuals with autism, and we were able to show the parts of the brain that can be affected. The part of the brain that seemed to show elevated lactate the most is a part called the cingulate gyrus, which we know is so important for the integration of higher level thought, emotion, behavior, and has been implicated in autism in many other neuropsychiatric conditions.
[00:13:00]	There have been many other important research studies of mitochondrial dysfunction. In autism, one out of UC Davis where they showed increased markers of mitochondrial dysfunction in children with autism, that was in 2010.
Dr. Mark Hyman:	Based on blood or based on brain?
Dr. Suzanne Goh:	Based on blood and lymphocytes.
Dr. Mark Hyman:	How do I know if I have mitochondrial dysfunction?
[00:13:30] Dr. Suzanne Goh:	There are a lot of different tests that can give us insight. In the clinic, they primarily test the blood and urine, but there are routine tests that can be done, really at any lab. It's the interpretation of those test results that's important.
Dr. Mark Hyman:	What kind of tests?
Dr. Suzanne Goh: [00:14:00]	Things like plasma amino acid profiles or urine organic acids. These are all ways of giving us insight into the body's metabolism, how we're processing the things that we take in from the outside world. Even things like liver function tests, total and free carnitine levels, coenzyme Q10 level, vitamin E level—those are all important signs. You don't need to necessarily have abnormal lab test results. There are

signs from a child's medical history and physical exam. Even if the lab tests aren't perfect, we rely a lot on those.

Dr. Mark Hyman: What kind of things would you find in a history or exam?

Dr. Suzanne Goh:
[00:14:30] Probably the most important is a history of a child having lost skills at some time in their life. A history of developmental regression, especially between the ages of 18 months to three years, and especially in the setting of a physiological stressor. For example, a very common history I hear is that a child was ill or a child received an immunization, or the family took a trip to India or to China or Europe, or the child entered daycare, or they moved home. There's something ...

Dr. Mark Hyman: Some insult.

[00:15:00]
Dr. Suzanne Goh: Some insult, but it can come in so many different forms. Or, the child had needed to be under anesthesia for ear tube placement or correction of an inguinal hernia—some fairly minor procedure but that required sedation—and put the body into a state of stress. After that, the parents noticed the child wasn't saying the things they used to say. They were clumsier. They weren't looking at them the same way. It's a story I hear over and over again. It's very classic for mitochondrial dysfunction.

[00:15:30]

Dr. Mark Hyman: You sort of notice in your work that there's a correlation, and again, like mitochondria, it's not something that doctors learn about. Doctors don't understand how to diagnose and treat mitochondria. They don't understand the load of environmental toxins or how to diagnose it or treat it. How do you apply the emerging science into clinical practice?

[00:16:00]
Dr. Suzanne Goh: A first step is exposure, so try to reduce exposure. There are a lot of ways to do that, but fortunately, there are a lot of great resources. One of the things that I and my team are sensitive to: there are so many things being asked of families of children with autism. There are so many therapies, so many interventions: making changes in diet and environmental exposure is a lot of work. We try to guide and help them take things one step at a time, thinking about the environment in the home, air quality, food quality, whether they used pesticides in the home or not. Simple steps like that to try to reduce exposures where we can get a lot of bang, get a lot of yield, without a lot of effort.

[00:16:30]

Dr. Mark Hyman: Which would be good for everybody.

Dr. Suzanne Goh: Yes.

Dr. Mark Hyman: How about the diagnosis, because how do you tell the body burden of a kid? We all should reduce those exposures, but how do we know what we actually have, whether there are metals or pesticides or other chemicals?

[00:17:00]
Dr. Suzanne Goh: We do basic testing for metals. I think it's an area where there's not a lot of consensus—especially in the pediatric, being a special needs field—what testing do you do? It's taking a long time for me, as I've had to, because the answer's not out there. I've had to evaluate the options, and have decided on what I think are the highest quality tests available. We do tests from some of what I think are the leading laboratories in Functional Medicine, and we use those test results to guide us. Are they pointing towards burden, excess burden of specific toxins, or heavy metals? And if so, what can we do to help the body to eliminate those in a way that's as natural as possible and gentle? If you're too heavy-handed and too aggressive in your approach, the child may worsen. When things worsen, it really puts the family into panic, so a working relationship is really important, and the ongoing working relationship, because a lot of this takes time.

[00:17:30]

[00:18:00]

Dr. Mark Hyman: You can also set expectations.

Dr. Suzanne Goh: Yes.

Dr. Mark Hyman:	Are you doing challenge testing or just blood or urine?
Dr. Suzanne Goh:	I don't do challenge testing, largely because I feel like it's an area of my own education that is still to come. I don't really know how to do it and how to do it well.
Dr. Mark Hyman: [00:18:30]	Yeah. I read a paper once in the New England Journal and they were talking about mercury, saying they measured it in the blood. I'm like, "Well that's interesting," because they say it's easy to measure. I was, like—it's like the guy who lost his keys on the street and he's looking at a lamppost. And his friend says, "Why are you looking at a lamppost? What are you doing?" He said, "I'm looking for my keys." He said, "Where'd you drop them?" "Well, I dropped them down the street but the light's better here." The body burden, you know, these substances are clear, they're stored in muscle, brain, and organs, pesticides and chemicals, and environment and food, are stored in fat tissue, so I think it's really important to ask the right questions and think about this.
[00:19:00] Dr. Suzanne Goh:	Yes. I'm always trying to improve. I think we've come a long way in my medical practice. I think we're not doing enough, and trying to figure out how to do that.
Dr. Mark Hyman: [00:19:30]	So great. This is impressive. In major medical institutions, you're helping these children detoxify. You're doing mitochondrial therapies. Let's talk about mitochondrial therapy because how do you, if you're healthy, keep your mitochondria healthy? And two, if your mitochondria aren't working what are the options available to people to actually enhance their mitochondria? They are throughout your whole body, so it's not that you're just treating the brain, you're treating everything. Energy deficits are a huge driver of so many illnesses—everything from Alzheimer's to Parkinson's, to autism, to cancer, to diabetes, to obesity. They all play a role.
Dr. Suzanne Goh:	Yes. You know, sometimes in Western allopathic medical training, we're taught to distinguish how different disease states are really different, how radically different they are.
Dr. Mark Hyman:	They're the same.
[00:20:00] Dr. Suzanne Goh:	They're the same. That's why I feel that the Functional Medicine approach is simple and elegant in a way. The same is true for when you're thinking about mitochondrial function and autism. Diet and nutrition, lifestyle, exercise, activity. And then, you can think about nutritional supplementation.
Dr. Mark Hyman:	That's why they're called supplements. They're not replacements.
Dr. Suzanne Goh: [00:20:30]	Yes. They really aren't medications. There are some devices that may have a role. Thinking about exercise, how do you—for a child with autism—how do you approach an exercise regime? That's where things like occupational therapy, physical therapy, music therapy ... Music can be very motivating. There are all these other tools we have.
Dr. Mark Hyman:	Get the kids to dance to music?
Dr. Suzanne Goh: [00:21:00]	Yes, or sort of similar to how music can be used in Parkinson's. It primes the motor system and we find there are all these tools that can help us. They're non-medical tools but they help us with this fundamental aspect of ...
Dr. Mark Hyman:	They are medicines. Music is medicine. Light is medicine. Movement is medicine.
Dr. Suzanne Goh:	Yes.
Dr. Mark Hyman:	Yeah, those are drugs. They often work better than the other drugs.
Dr. Suzanne Goh:	That's right. I found that approach to be very effective.
Dr. Mark Hyman:	What about the supplement side of things? What are the kind of drivers of mitochondrial function?

Dr. Suzanne Goh: [00:21:30] [00:22:00]	Yes, a basic backbone of mitochondria supplementation would include L-carnitine, coenzyme Q10, B vitamins, creatine—another good energy source. There are many others, N-acetylcysteine. There are sort of direct things, nutritional supplements that you might think of as direct. For example, supplementing carnitine or CoQ10, we think, can help in a more direct way. But, perhaps, antioxidants or anti-inflammatories, or helping increase glutathione, for example, or supplementing with N-acetylcysteine, are other ways that can support mitochondria.
Dr. Mark Hyman:	What about some of the research on nicotinamide riboside, which is a supplement that's been touted to be helpful with fatigue and brain function?
Dr. Suzanne Goh:	I think there's very compelling research that's also a beneficial approach, which is fairly new, so not one that I use in my clinic as of yet.
Dr. Mark Hyman: [00:22:30]	Yes, Flint Beal from Cornell has done a lot of work in this sort of mitochondria and Alzheimer's, the other end of the spectrum. I'm a family doctor and, you know, had the insight by treating and looking at the biology of Alzheimer's, the patients and autistic patients. They were almost the same—they had often the same methylation SNPs, the glutathione SNPs, variations in their genes. They were the same problems with the same biochemical pathways, and the same results on their organic acids. I just thought, "Wow, this is like this underlying issue that's going on across the spectrum."
[00:23:00] [00:23:30]	I was just remembering a patient I had recently who had a mitochondrial disease. We didn't exactly know what it was; the genetics weren't clear, and he had severe symptoms of inability to exercise. He would get severe muscle damage and his muscle enzymes would go through the roof. His CBKs would go to thousands. It should be less than 200. I didn't know what was really wrong but I said, "Well let's just treat your mitochondria and see what happens." I gave him carnitine, CoQ10, lipoic acid, N-acetylcysteine, and ribose, and he just was completely cured. He could exercise. He could work out. His muscle enzymes weren't elevated, his muscles didn't hurt. We were just working from first principles, which is what you're doing. You're really going back to first principles and sort of revolutionizing your thinking about how we deal with autism.
Dr. Suzanne Goh: [00:24:00] [00:24:30]	One of the exciting lines of research related to mitochondria and autism has come from University of California San Diego and the laboratory of Bob Navio. It's taking it one step further, even to say that mitochondrial dysfunction encompasses a lot of different things. We classically think of it as impairment of the respiratory chain, and a depletion of ATP and energy. But for a subset of those with autism, it may be an upregulation of certain elements of the mitochondria. This state that Dr. Navio has called the cell danger response, he's finding similarities between autism, Alzheimer's, and other nerve ...
Dr. Mark Hyman:	Really, because I just noticed this clinically.
Dr. Suzanne Goh:	Yes, in terms of metabolomic profile. We're still at the beginning of understanding mitochondria and autism. We know it's critically important, but there are going to be, I think, more subtlety and more options for treatments, yeah.
[00:25:00] Dr. Mark Hyman: [00:25:30]	You talked about the role of diet, exercise, mitochondria, and environmental toxins, but there are other factors that are potentially driving autism. Dale Bredesen talks about the 36 holes in your roof and if you just fix one of them, it's still going to be raining. Or, you fix 10 of them, it will still be raining in your house, so it's similar with autism. I think one of the areas we're discovering is the microbiome playing a role in autism, and how we can think about changing the gut, as far as a way of changing the brain. How have you found that in your work?
Dr. Suzanne Goh:	I'll say that was certainly not something that was ever part of my training. That was something I've learned more recently, and I think the research is also more recent. I think just the idea, newer understandings about how connected the brain and the gut are, have helped us understand there's a relationship between gut health and developing brain and autism.

Dr. Mark Hyman: [00:26:00]	95% of autistic kids have gut dysfunction, right?
Dr. Suzanne Goh:	Yes, and maybe more.
Dr. Mark Hyman:	Right, maybe even more.
Dr. Suzanne Goh:	Maybe more.
Dr. Mark Hyman:	Maybe all.
Dr. Suzanne Goh: [00:26:30]	It's hard to imagine they wouldn't, given how abnormal brain development affects the gut, and the bi-directionality of that. A basic way to think about the mechanism by which the gut is impacting the brain in autism is that when there is gut inflammation, it impacts the integrity of the intestinal lining, and so things enter into the system of circulation that stimulate inflammation. Inflammation in the brain as well, and we know that there is microglial activation.
Dr. Mark Hyman:	Oh, the brains of autistic kids are inflamed.
Dr. Suzanne Goh:	Right.
Dr. Mark Hyman:	Yeah.
Dr. Suzanne Goh:	In sort of a chronic, low-grade inflammation—that's one way that gut health impacts autism.
Dr. Mark Hyman:	Yeah, and it can also affect the mitochondria, right? Because any source of inflammation can alter the mitochondria.
Dr. Suzanne Goh:	Yes.
[00:27:00] Dr. Mark Hyman:	Tell us about some of the extraordinary cases. You mentioned Jake, but I'm sure there are other patients you've seen since then, and you've refined your approach. What are you seeing?
Dr. Suzanne Goh: [00:27:30]	I would say the most common, and probably the most rewarding, are when children come early. When they come to my clinic younger than three years of age, and when we identify the pattern of the child having lost skills, in the setting of some type of stressor, especially if the child can come to us quickly. When that occurs, the pediatrician recognizes it and sends them to us early. We can do the appropriate lab testing to identify the mitochondrial markers, and start treatment early. Remove the stressors and the harmful exposures and begin mitochondrial therapy early, the turnaround is just incredible. We have dozens and dozens of children recently, who've come to us, where that's been possible.
[00:28:00] Dr. Mark Hyman:	Wait a minute, you're saying that we can actually now start to reverse autism?
Dr. Suzanne Goh:	Yes. I think there's no question now that for some—not all—but for a proportion of children with autism. It's possible with the right therapies at the right times, that within six months, a year, they would no longer meet the diagnostic criteria for autism.
Dr. Mark Hyman: [00:28:30]	That's extraordinary. I mean, you know, when most patients, or parents bring their kid with autism to the doctor, they say, "This is incurable. This state is going to be for the rest of his life. You can do behavioral therapy to help a few things, but essentially your child is going to be locked in forever."
Dr. Suzanne Goh:	Yeah. I think the message is changing. I also think it's important to say that there are so many different subtypes within autism. Yes.
Dr. Mark Hyman:	Not all have mitochondrial dysfunction.
Dr. Suzanne Goh: [00:29:00]	Not all have mitochondrial disease or dysfunction. For a portion—and we don't know what that percentage is—but for a portion, a reversal of symptoms is possible, probably because what they have

is reversible metabolic syndrome or reversible metabolic encephalopathy. For some children, the cause of their autism is a little bit harder to change. It may be problems in synapse formation or a more severe type of brain injury. Even in those cases, tremendous progress is possible.

[00:29:30]
Dr. Mark Hyman: Yeah, it's true. There's no case where you can't do something. There may be rare genetic cases, but even in those cases, you can still modify the whole metabolic processes and actually see improvements?

Dr. Suzanne Goh: Absolutely. There's a reason why, for example in Down's syndrome ... Children with Down's syndrome have very different levels of intelligence and levels of social interaction, and why? They have the same gene. They have the same underlying genetic chromosome abnormality.

[00:30:00]
Dr. Mark Hyman: They also have mitochondrial issues, and they get Alzheimer's. Interesting. Well, you mentioned that there are other causes, not just mitochondrial dysfunction. In that subset of patients, how do you approach those kids?

Dr. Suzanne Goh: We do a comprehensive evaluation to try to get a better understanding, because there can be many different factors, many different causes. As one example, there are types of ...

Dr. Mark Hyman: There's no such thing as autism. There are autisms.

[00:30:30]
Dr. Suzanne Goh: That's right. It's just an umbrella, sort of label, that we've developed. Within that, there are so many different, unique types. It's important to identify, if you can help identify that early on with the right testing, you can target therapy to be much more successful.

Dr. Mark Hyman: What are the different types?

Dr. Suzanne Goh:
[00:31:00] There's a subset of children for whom epilepsy is one of the main causes of their developmental problems. The cause of their autism symptoms, language delay, and maybe cognitive disability. Identifying the epilepsy and treating it properly can lead to dramatic improvements—that's one example. There are some individuals who have difficulty in the stabilization of information of synapsis. They have gene mutations that affect that specific process. There are supplements and medications
[00:31:30] now that affect and can help with the process of synapse formation and stabilization. If you identified that, you could then target therapies in that way.

Dr. Mark Hyman: This is going where the rest of medicine has gone, which is personalized medicine. There's no such thing as autism; it's a whole series of different insults that can cause the same symptoms.

Dr. Suzanne Goh: That's right.

Dr. Mark Hyman: We've been coming out through the symptoms instead of the causes.

Dr. Suzanne Goh: That's right. Identifying the autism is not the end, it's just the beginning.

Dr. Mark Hyman:
[00:32:00] Right. I always say in medicine, we call what we do naming and blaming. We name the disease and we blame the name. The reason for your symptoms is you have autism. It's actually not the cause, it's just the name for the symptoms. That's what I call thinking and linking. In Functional Medicine, the thinking starts when you make the diagnosis. It doesn't end, and that's a huge shift in our approach in medicine.

Dr. Suzanne Goh: Isn't that amazing?

Dr. Mark Hyman: That's why you call it the medicine of why, not what, not what disease you have, what drug do I give— but why is this happening and how do I deal with that?

Dr. Suzanne Goh: Yes, I see too often that once the label of autism is given ...

Dr. Mark Hyman: [00:32:30]	Incurable disease with no real treatment, yeah.
Dr. Suzanne Goh:	Right.
Dr. Mark Hyman:	It's such a discouraging message, you know.
Dr. Suzanne Goh:	Yes.
Dr. Mark Hyman:	Those of us on the frontline, you have to believe what you see, not see what you believe. A lot of physicians just see what they believe instead of believing what they see, which is, you've seen it. I've seen it, in the case of autism, regressing or reversing. Not all the kids get 100% better but they can be functional, they can live better lives. Some get cured. It's really extraordinary. You're right, the younger you get them, the better it is.
[00:33:00] Dr. Suzanne Goh: [00:33:30]	Yes. There are lots of possibilities for improvement when children are young. We work with a lot of young adults who can also show really meaningful gains and improvement quality of life. We recently worked with a young adult who, when he came to us was 19, and he was living at home but on just the edge of needing to be instituted, and was placed in a residential institution because he was aggressive and destructive. The parents were having a very hard time keeping him at home. And so, the path that typically leads to for a young adult with autism is one of living in an institution and polypharmacy. Multiple psychiatric medications and all of the side effects that let these two, and the medications often aren't that effective.
[00:34:00] [00:34:30]	When we have the opportunity to work with an adolescent or young adult like that, we can provide the types of therapies that can send the child or young adult down a totally different path, where we begin to target the causes. We look at the biochemistry. We look at their nutritional status and exercise and provide therapies—like physical therapy, occupational therapy and music therapy, speech language therapy—because the brain still has the capacity. It's not that at age 18 the brain somehow stops being able to learn. The capacity is still there, and so one of the most gratifying aspects of the work that I do and my team does, is to be able to change that trajectory, even for adults.
Dr. Mark Hyman:	That's extraordinary. It's never too late.
Dr. Suzanne Goh:	That's right.
Dr. Mark Hyman: [00:35:00] [00:35:30]	Yes. I've seen this over and over again and it's pretty extraordinary when you look at the metabolic factors. When you see kids who literally can't talk, won't look you in the eye, won't interact, won't hug, and within days of instituting various therapies, they're connecting, they're talking. I had one physician who had an autistic kid and he read my book, *The UltraMind Solution*, which is about how to address these responses. And he said they changed his diet and got off gluten and dairy, and all of a sudden, the kid started talking. There are all these things that are outside the brain that are affecting the brain. Martha Herbert calls it—instead of a brain disorder—a disorder that affects the brain, so we're talking about dealing with gut flora. We're talking about mitochondria. We're talking about environmental toxins. We're talking about nutritional status. These are systemic therapies. They're not just targeting the brain.
Dr. Suzanne Goh:	Yes, and I think the research clearly supports that. The research has to be interpreted, and I think sometimes there are barriers to allowing us to interpret it properly. The barriers are conventional ways of thinking.
[00:36:00] Dr. Mark Hyman:	Yes. It's an extremely important point because most physicians will say there's no evidence that this is true. I think the evidence is that they haven't read the literature. The literature is there.
Dr. Suzanne Goh:	It is.

Dr. Mark Hyman: If anybody is curious to go down that rabbit hole and you start to see the patterns and connections—and if you just focus on one line of thinking—you'll miss stuff and you'll miss the connections between everything. I think that's really the beauty of Functional Medicine: it connects the dots. It's the medicine that connects the dots.

[00:36:30]

Dr. Suzanne Goh: Yes. For autism in particular, what I found over the course of my training and my early practice was that what allopathic medicine had to offer was really, really limited.

Dr. Mark Hyman: Sort of diagnose and adios?

Dr. Suzanne Goh: Mm-hmm. (affirmative)

Dr. Mark Hyman: Yeah.

Dr. Suzanne Goh: You have to look elsewhere. Then, when you start to look elsewhere, you realize how rich the
[00:37:00]   resources are. Whether it's in different types of therapies, movement-based therapies, sensory motor therapies. Whether it's from Functional Medicine and the grid of medicine world, yeah.

Dr. Mark Hyman: Is there anything else you want to share about your work or the future of where this is all going?

Dr. Suzanne Goh: In the work I do, the parents of the children I work with have been a real inspiration to me because of their dedication, how they educate themselves, and how they are the ones pushing physicians a little bit out of our comfort zone. I think that's great. I think it's so important.

[00:37:30]

Dr. Mark Hyman: Yes, it's so great that you have a mind willing to listen to what presents to you?

Dr. Suzanne Goh: Yeah.

Dr. Mark Hyman: Not seeing what you believe, but believing what you see. We hear these stories over and over again—you can't help but wonder why, and ask new questions. Very few of us, though, have actually done the hard work of asking the hard questions, doing the research, and putting the evidence behind it. And that's what you've done—such an incredible contribution to the community.

Dr. Suzanne Goh: Thank you. Feels like a privilege to be able to do it.

TERRY WAHLS, MD | Author: *The Wahls Protocol - How I Beat Progressive MS using Paleo Principles and Functional Medicine*

Dr. Mark Hyman: Dr. Wahls, you've had an extraordinary story that has revolutionized the way you practice and the way the rest of the world thinks about MS and neurodegenerative disease. Sadly, you had a debilitating disease, but it led you to discover a way of treating these conditions, like MS, with a whole new paradigm.

Dr. Terry Wahls: Yes.

Dr. Mark Hyman: I'd love for you to share your story and tell us a little bit about what happened, how you discovered this and what, as a result, you learned.

[00:00:30]

Dr. Terry Wahls: I'm an academic internal medicine doc. In 2000, I was diagnosed with relapsing remitting multiple sclerosis. And being an academic doc, I thought I should treat my disease aggressively, so I sought out the best MS center I could find, the Cleveland Clinic. I took the newest drugs and still within three years, my disease had converted to secondary progressive MS.

Dr. Mark Hyman: Which is not good.

Dr. Terry Wahls: Which is not good at all because that means you're going to go steadily downhill, that functions once

[00:01:00] lost, are gone forever. And so that is when I took Mitoxantrone in a form of chemotherapy, then I took Tysabri, the new biologic agent.

Dr. Mark Hyman: Suppress your immune system.

Dr. Terry Wahls: To suppress my immune system, and I continued to decline. And that is when I realized, you know,

[00:01:30] conventional medicine is not stopping this decline. I was on track to potentially becoming bedridden by my illness, potentially demented by my illness. MS-related pain was a big part of my illness and that was getting more and more difficult to control, so I was worried that refractory pain was going to be a big factor. That's when I went back to reading the medical literature and would discover the ancestral health movement. I would discover vitamins and supplements. I would discover The Institute for

[00:02:00] Functional Medicine, and I would integrate all of that into a comprehensive diet and lifestyle program that not only stopped my decline, which was pretty incredible, but to my amazement and the amazement of my physicians, was associated with a remarkable return of function.

Dr. Mark Hyman: But you were in a wheelchair.

Dr. Terry Wahls: Yeah.

Dr. Mark Hyman: And it was only a one-way street, worse.

Dr. Terry Wahls: In the wheelchair I couldn't sit up anymore, I was in a zero-gravity chair where I was fully reclined, knees

[00:02:30] higher than my nose. I struggled to walk 10 feet using two walking sticks. I was losing my keys, my phone. I had severe MS pain, was having to go to the pain clinic, take frequent Solu-Medrol to try to control the pain.

Dr. Mark Hyman: Powerful steroids.

Dr. Terry Wahls: Life was very tough, and that's where I was in 2007. I was still doing my little tiny workouts, like a 10

[00:03:00]	minute very simple little stomach curl. If I did 12 minutes, I couldn't function for a day and a half, but I could do 10 minutes and go to work. In 2008, after doing my diet and lifestyle protocol, I was able to do a 20-mile bike ride with my family. That's how much transformation had happened in that 12-month period. So that, of course, changes how I think about disease and health. It changes the way I practice medicine, and it started me on this new path, and, ultimately, it would change the focus of my clinical research.
[00:03:30] Dr. Mark Hyman: [00:04:00]	Extraordinary. One of the things you discovered was that there's a part of our cells that's required for energy, and, by the way, you had terrible energy, that's a classic feature of MS, which is you're fatigued all the time. You discovered that these little parts of the cells called mitochondria, it's like the energy powerhouse of the cell, were critically important, and they were part of the therapy you used to treat the mitochondria through diet and other things. So, tell us, why are the mitochondria so important in your degenerative disease?
Dr. Terry Wahls: [00:04:30]	The mitochondria are the little bacteria that were engulfed by bigger bacteria about a billion and a half years ago, and they were very efficient at converting energy from the food we ate into biochemical energy that our cells use. That would allow cells to become multicellular, to develop organs, tissues, locomotion. It would let us develop brains, hearts, retinas, etc. The cells that need the most energy, which are brain cells, our retina, and our heart cells, have like 10 thousand mitochondria per cell.
Dr. Mark Hyman:	Yeah, and the heart, I think 17 thousand, right?
Dr. Terry Wahls: [00:05:00]	It's just so critical, and if your mitochondria are not working very well then that organ doesn't work very well. In the brain, that means you begin to have problems with fatigue, pain, irritability, and cognitive decline. That's actually one of the first things I discovered when I'd gone back to start reading the science, was that mitochondria were at the heart of neurodegeneration for Alzheimer's, Parkinson's, ALS, and Lou Gehrig's. No one was yet writing about that for MS. But I thought, "You know what? I bet it's the same, so I'm going to learn everything I can about what I can do to tune up my mitochondria." And so those were the initial interventions I did, which was a variety of vitamins and supplements to support my mitochondria.
[00:05:30] [00:06:00] [00:06:30]	When I was first reading about that, Mark, I had this supplement cocktail: creatine, lipoic acid, carnitine, B vitamins, CoQ, and after about six months I thought, "It's not helping, and I'm wasting my money," so I quit and I couldn't get out of bed. I was just completely exhausted. And three days later my spouse comes in says, "You know, honey, I think you have to take these again." And I took them, and I could get up and function again. That was very interesting to me. So, two weeks later, I did the same thing, stopped all my supplements, couldn't function, and three days later I started them and I could function again. So, my conclusion was, "You know what? They may not be recovering me, but they're clearly doing something for my fatigue." And that was very energizing, very exciting, because this also taught me that the mitochondria were important, and my neurologist or my primary care doc were not telling me stuff like this. I was teaching myself by using PubMed, reading the literature, and beginning to do self-experimentation.
Dr. Mark Hyman:	Mm-hmm.
Dr. Terry Wahls:	It was a very big discovery.
Dr. Mark Hyman: [00:07:00]	So, great. How do you take care of your mitochondria? They're responsible for contributing to the symptoms and the disease states of the neurodegenerative state, and even things like autism and many other diseases. We may not have the mitochondria be the cause, but it's a big factor that gets damaged when you have that helps. How do you recover your mitochondria?
Dr. Terry Wahls:	There are three things I think about. The first one is, "What's the nutritional need for that mitochondria?" The mitochondria, if you remember from ninth grade biology, there's the little oval with

[00:07:30]	a lot of squiggles in the middle, and that's the cell membrane. This mitochondria has a lot of cell membrane, which means it has a lot of fat. You need the right fats, a lot of omega-3s, omega-6 fats to make healthy membranes. You need a lot of B vitamins, and that's essentially the whole B vitamin family to support some of those insomatic steps. You need a bunch of minerals like zinc, magnesium, as cofactors for a lot of those B vitamins, some sulfur amino acids as well, antioxidants. This is really
[00:08:00]	important nutrition that you need for those mitochondria.

[00:08:30] The next thing you need to think about is, "Why did the mitochondria begin to not function very well?" The most common reason is that they've been poisoned, and they can be poisoned by things like heavy metals, lead, mercury, arsenic, pesticides will do that, the insecticides will do that, some plastics and solvents. Poisoning is the most common thing. The third category would be some of the stealth infections, where an infectious particle has sort of hijacked the mitochondria and taken it away from manufacturing energy to manufacturing viral particles. So, address those three factors and you'll go far in restoring that mitochondrial health.

Dr. Mark Hyman:
[00:09:00] That's so great. The other thing I think might affect the mitochondria and also the immune system, you know, I had a patient with MS many years ago and I found I learn the most from just listening to my patients more than any textbook. This woman said, "You know, when my gut symptoms get worse my MS gets worse." And I was like, "Oh, that's interesting." So, I began to work on the gut and people would get better. And I'm curious what you think about the role of the gut in MS and also neurodegenerative disease and how it affects the mitochondria even.

Dr. Terry Wahls:
[00:09:30] So, the evidence about the link between the gut and brain just continues to grow and grow and grow. You can go onto pubmed.gov and put in microbiota and MS, and there are more papers coming out. You can put in microbiota and autoimmune conditions, and you'll find that there are more and more papers identifying that you have a different mix of bacteria living in your gut if you have an autoimmune condition than if you're healthy. As they eat our food and each other's byproducts, they're secreting
[00:10:00] compounds that cross over into the blood and then into the blood-brain barrier, and can increase inflammation, they can shift behavior, they can shift our mood, can shift our cognition, so that's clearly having an impact on the brain.

[00:10:30] Now, in terms of mitochondria, one thing they can do is, I believe about 25 percent of our detoxification capabilities are managed by our gut microbiome. If you have a healthy, vigorous microbiome, a health-promoting bacteria, you'll have improved detoxification, and you'll have less poisoning of your mitochondria.

Dr. Mark Hyman: Amazing. You had both an autoimmune and a sort of a neurologic condition, so you kind of got attacked both ways. A lot of therapies we use in autoimmune disease in this country are problematic. You talked a lot about how there's a hidden cost to the therapy. Can you tell us more about why physicians are just stuck on that and not telling the full story you're telling?
[00:11:00]

Dr. Terry Wahls: There's a really interesting lecture by George Ebers, who's an MS researcher out of the United Kingdom and London, and he reviews that when we're looking at the development of drugs for MS, there's a big question conference with the MS researchers, "What measures should we monitor to decide that an MS
[00:11:30] drug is useful?" It's time to the diagnosis of secondary progressive, time to needing a cane, time to needing a walker, time to being bedridden, time to being dead. Because those are the things that really drive cost and suffering.

Dr. Mark Hyman: Yeah.

Dr. Terry Wahls: And in that research meeting, MRI findings, number of relapses, that was like number 18 and number 19
[00:12:00] on the list of 20, so they were not thought to be important.

Dr. Mark Hyman: Because they just assume the disease is going to progress?

Dr. Terry Wahls: [00:12:30] [00:13:00]	When you look at the epidemiological literature, the number of relapses do not predict time to cane, walker, wheelchair, or death, nor do they predict time to secondary progressive MS. And the number of relapses are very slightly protective, so MRI lesions come and go and they don't appear to have a very clear relationship to, "Are you going to become disabled? Are you going to develop secondary progressive? Are you going to need a cane? Are you going to need a wheelchair? Are you going to become bedridden?" You know, and I'm not surprised, because what I think likely is going on is the neurodegeneration, which is probably driven by mitochondria. It's probably driven by nutritional status and nutritional deficiencies. Now, of course, none of that is going to be treated by suppressing the immune cells, because the immune cells are trying their hardest to repair my brain. They are trying their hardest to come in and quiet that inflammation and to begin to remyelinate. So, it's sort of interesting, what we did, and we looked at our studies, we saw that the people who were the least likely to have improvement in gait were the folks taking disease modifying drugs.
Dr. Mark Hyman: [00:13:30]	The drugs that are supposed to help you actually, they didn't help you.
Dr. Terry Wahls:	May not be so helpful. You can turn off these acute lesions, yes, you can do that, and the drugs are very effective at that. But what we don't know is, will they really change the time to wheelchair, the time to bedridden?
Dr. Mark Hyman:	Yeah, and you got from bedridden almost to riding your bike 20 miles.
Dr. Terry Wahls:	To biking 20 miles.
Dr. Mark Hyman: [00:14:00]	So, you've taken your learnings and your personal experience, and you've not just sort of taken your goodies and went home. You really stepped up and created a research program at university, looking at this approach, not just to MS, but to many other kinds of patients.
Dr. Terry Wahls:	Correct, correct.
Dr. Mark Hyman:	With all sorts of conditions. What is going on with your research? How do you do it at this center and what are we learning from your work?
Dr. Terry Wahls: [00:14:30] [00:15:00]	The first thing we did, we had a case series we used, the e-stim, and I did that with a physical therapist, and we were able to show we had improved gait, then mobility. And so, we got that published. And then the next thing we did, we had a little phase one feasibility study where we had other people with progressive MS. Again people who, by chance, recovery is not going to happen. You'd expect them to steadily decline. So, we enrolled people with secondary primary progressive and we had 20 folks. We were able to show that, yes, they could implement this complicated diet and lifestyle program that I utilized. The biggest side effect, Mark, was if you're overweight you lost weight without being hungry.
Dr. Mark Hyman:	Oh my God.
Dr. Terry Wahls: [00:15:30]	That's a serious side effect. We had the largest reduction fatigue severity that's been recorded to date in the most severely disabled group that's been studied to date, so that was very exciting. We got that up and going, and then did a small pod study, and people were randomized and had folks who got the study diet or randomized to not get the study diet for 12 weeks, and then they got the study diet. We were able to show, once again, that fatigue severity was statistically and clinically significantly reduced in the people who had the study diet compared to control. Function in the hands improved, both dominant and nondominant hand, and walking ability improved, and the how-far-you-can-walk-in-six-minutes improved.
[00:16:00]	Then we got some more money, we were able to go back and analyze. I have lots of data from that first group of progressive MS folks, so we're able to analyze the change in mood and cognition. We're able to show that, again, in progressive MS, we don't expect anybody to improve their thinking or their mood

[00:16:30]

[00:17:00]

because they have a progressive disease. We're able to show that anxiety scores diminished, so they were less anxious, depression scores diminished so they were less depressed, and that verbal and nonverbal reasoning scores improved. Again, very surprising in a progressive disease. We have MRI data in this group we are working on analyzing, so I'm hoping to have that available. We have our videos that we have of before and after. And we had videos of their walking every three months, and we have that analyzed. I have that paper in press, and I'm hoping that that press will finally be out in either June or July. What will be very nice about that, Mark, is the videos, because I put it in open-access paper, the public will be able to see those videos now, too.

Dr. Mark Hyman: That's amazing. It's so impressive. What are the other factors, like stress, and how do those impact? And sleep and exercise, can we talk about those and how they're part of your program?

Dr. Terry Wahls: So, in the program, we talk about how important it is to address stress, and I'm going to step back a little
[00:17:30] bit. For years, I ran a therapy lifestyle clinic. In that clinic we took Alzheimer's, MS, neurological disease, mental health disease, medical problems. And I'd see them in a group, then we'd do a timeline. One of the most common things I saw, Mark, was stress was the trigger that made people be symptomatic. I
[00:18:00] learned that we need to teach people how to engage in a stress-reducing practice. I saw that in all disease states. When we went back and analyzed that, as I said we had a little more data so we could look at the mood and cognition data, we looked at the associations between the diet, the foods that we wanted them to eat, the foods we told them to exclude, the stress-reducing practice, the exercise, and electrical stimulation. The strongest associations were between not eating stuff I told you to not eat,
[00:18:30] eating all those vegetables I told you to eat, and then stress reduction, and they had a very strong association. P-values of less than .0001. Stress reduction was slightly associated, but it was still more important than either the exercise or the e-stim

I was actually quite surprised by that. I had fully expected that exercise and e-stim would be most ...
[00:19:00]
Dr. Mark Hyman: What were the stress-reduction tools you gave to the patients in this course?

Dr. Terry Wahls: It was incredibly simple. We taught them how to do a self-massage of their face, hands, and feet.

Dr. Mark Hyman: That was it?

Dr. Terry Wahls: That was one, and the other was a mantra-based meditation, sort of soft-belly. Focusing on the word soft and belly as they inhaled and exhaled, and they were visualizing the flow of air through the nostrils.

Dr. Mark Hyman: Yes.
[00:19:30]
Dr. Terry Wahls: They're probably getting a whopping five to seven minutes of stress-reducing activity every day.

Dr. Mark Hyman: Unbelievable.

Dr. Terry Wahls: So, not a lot.

Dr. Mark Hyman: So, if they did 20 minutes, then who knows what would happen, right?

Dr. Terry Wahls: Correct, but now keep in mind I was asking people to do a lot of stuff. We had taken away the food they loved and had them eat foods they didn't know how to eat. We taught them how to eat vegetables, we were having them to do e-stim, and we're having them exercise, and so they were spending hours a day doing everything we asked them to do.
[00:20:00]
Dr. Mark Hyman: Now let's talk about the diet part of it, because I think it's going to be surprising to most people what you recommend, because it's contrary to the most commonly given advice around diet. Yet, it's profound and seems to be impacting not only MS, but Alzheimer's, Parkinson's disease, all kinds of

neurologic issues. So, tell us about that.

Dr. Terry Wahls: Sure. So, as I was going downhill, my Cleveland Clinic docs told me about Loren Cordain's work and the paleo diet.

Dr. Mark Hyman: They did?
[00:20:30]

Dr. Terry Wahls: In 2002, Lael Stone mentioned that to me. I don't think she quite understood what she said, because I went to the websites, read the book, like okay. So, after 20 years of being a vegetarian, I gave up all grain, all legumes, all dairy, a lot of prayer and meditation. I went back to eating meat, and I continued
[00:21:00] to go downhill. But I stayed with it because I was doing something, and I thought, "Okay, who knows how long this takes to recover and I've been going downhill for a long time, at least I'm doing something. You know I'm adding the vitamins and the supplements." And eventually, after getting a little more comprehensive understanding with Functional Medicine, I had this insight. You know I should take this long list of nutrients that I'm taking in pill form and figure out where they are in the food supply. And instead of focusing on what not to eat from the paleo world, I should focus on what I need to be eating to feed my brain. So, then I was on this mission: what are the micronutrients that my brain needs, and
[00:21:30] ultimately, again more research to get that stored up, so it takes it several more months. And the program is lots of vegetables.

Dr. Mark Hyman: Oh my God.

Dr. Terry Wahls: Lots and lots of vegetables.

Dr. Mark Hyman: Did you research that to make sure it was safe?
[00:22:00]

Dr. Terry Wahls: Well you know, what's funny is when I did my clinical studies, I did have to show the IRB that this crazy diet I was advocating was safe, because it was so different than the USDA My Healthy Plate diet.

Dr. Mark Hyman: Yeah.

Dr. Terry Wahls: And so, I was required to do a safety study to show that nine cups of vegetables were safe.

Dr. Mark Hyman: Unbelievable.

Dr. Terry Wahls: So, yeah. So, we did do that. I had to keep these detailed food records of what I was eating for a week.
[00:22:30] We did these analyses, and the dietician who did those analyses for us, who had been doing dietary research for I think 25 years said, "You know, Terry, this is the most nutrient dense diet I have ever analyzed." And so, we're like two to eight times more nutrient dense than the average American intake for these various vitamins, antioxidants, minerals.

[00:23:00]
Dr. Mark Hyman: You found out there were certain things in food that make a huge difference, like sulfur and iodine. You were able to analyze the food, and figure out what to eat to give you those nutrients.

Dr. Terry Wahls: Correct. designed this as I was constructing the diet, you know, I had to decide, I have to chase these nutrients and figure out what my brain needs. I also had the insight that bio transformation is probably
[00:23:30] really important to help resuscitate my mitochondria and help me get rid of whatever toxins I have, from all my toxic exposures growing up on the farm, etc.

Dr. Mark Hyman: Biotransformation means dealing with toxin.

Dr. Terry Wahls: Processing, right, processing, eliminating of the heavy metals, the lead, mercury, arsenic, the atrazine that I'm sure is in the groundwater from the farm, and all the years of pesticide and formaldehyde, you know, the mercury that had been in my mouth for all those years. As I was researching what my brain

[00:24:00]	needs and my mitochondria need, I also researched what can I do to maximize the efficiency of my detoxification enzymes, strictly phase one, phase two. The Brassica family, the organic sulfur in the cabbage family vegetables, the onion family vegetables were a big part of that protocol.
Dr. Mark Hyman:	Yeah and iodine you mentioned is in fish and seaweed.
Dr. Terry Wahls: [00:24:30] [00:25:00]	Yes, fish and seaweed, so seaweed was big. I was very big on fermented foods, again for the microbiome aspect. And the ancestral health folks had gotten me keen, you know, fairly fired up about organ meats. As I'm understanding the dietary needs of the brain more, one of the things I discovered is vitamin K, which you and I learned was all about blood clotting, but vitamin K2 is all about myelin in the brain. Well if you have a problem with MS, you need a lot more myelin. need vitamin K2, and where do you get K2? You get it from liver, and you get it from eating a lot of greens, and the bacteria in your bowels have to convert that vitamin K from the greens into vitamin K2 and K7 that your small bowel will absorb.
Dr. Mark Hyman: [00:25:30]	And you need the right bacteria to synthesize vitamin K and you can get it from food, but it's really important, yes.
Dr. Terry Wahls:	In the way to sort out if you have the right bacteria, actually I sort of laugh about this, we have pooping class in my lifestyle class because we talk about how important it is to look at your poop. Are you pooping rocks, snakes, pudding, or tea? So, we all sit in our chairs, we poop together, then we stand up, we turn around and we look into our toilet chairs, and take turns talking to each other about our poop, and what to do.
[00:26:00] Dr. Mark Hyman:	Why don't you just take pictures of it?
Dr. Terry Wahls:	Well, you know ...
Dr. Mark Hyman:	Group poop, I don't know.
Dr. Terry Wahls:	Well we do have the Bristol stool charts, so we have that in front of us.
Dr. Mark Hyman:	Good, I don't know group poop as a therapy, I don't know.
Dr. Terry Wahls:	Well, we try to have a lot of laughter and fun, and so these group pooping classes people are laughing pretty hard.
Dr. Mark Hyman: [00:26:30]	Very impressive Doctor Wahls. You must be a compelling salesman for that sort of thing. You mentioned vitamin K, you mentioned sulfur, you mentioned iodine. Vitamin D seems to be a big factor in MS.
Dr. Terry Wahls: [00:27:00] [00:27:30]	Vitamin D is really important. You know vitamin D ... If we look at the north-south gradation, the further you get from the equator the higher the rates of MS, and Alzheimer's by the way. And part of the assumption is that our vitamin D levels are declining the further we get from the equator. Some studies have shown that epidemiologically as your vitamin D level is lower, your rates of MS are higher. Other studies have shown if you treat people with vitamin D, the rates of relapse are lower, so that's certainly a factor. Annual vitamin D also speaks to over 1,000 genes, and your brain is filled with vitamin D receptors, so yeah. We want people to fix their vitamin D.
Dr. Mark Hyman:	How do you do that?
Dr. Terry Wahls:	We give them vitamin D and we monitor their levels, and I tell them, "Please go out and get a tan without a sunburn," because when light hits your skin, yes, you make vitamin D, but it is also an immune modulator independent of your vitamin D level. I still think there's utility in having sun exposure.

Dr. Mark Hyman: [00:28:00]	So, you might not get MS, but you get wrinkles.
Dr. Terry Wahls:	You may get wrinkles, yes, but you'll get far fewer wrinkles if you're having bone broth and lots of vegetables.
Dr. Mark Hyman:	So, bone broth, what is that and why should we be drinking it?
Dr. Terry Wahls: [00:28:30] [00:29:00]	This was a very traditional food. It's bones, a little vinegar, some sea salt, and we like to put in a little seaweed, and we simmer it all day long. The vinegar helps draw the minerals out, so it's going to be a very nice mineral-rich concoction. If you put in things like chicken feet, a great source of collagen and gelatin, which can help heal your gut and help give your cells more of the collagen. And collagen is a very basic stratus compound that is a structure that is ubiquitous in our connective tissue. It's a very basic structure that ...
Dr. Mark Hyman:	It's gut healing too, right?
Dr. Terry Wahls:	Very good for our gut.
Dr. Mark Hyman:	Great. So, you created something called *The Wahls Protocol*. Can you tell us what the steps of that are, and what that is? I think people are interested in learning about how to implement this.
Dr. Terry Wahls: [00:29:30] [00:30:00]	When I devised my diet and lifestyle program, I did all of that to try and slow my decline. I had no hope of recovery. When I had this unexpected side-effect of recovering, it certainly changed how I practice. After a few months, I decided to call our local food co-op and I said, "You know, how about I give a talk," and it was a huge success. As I began teaching the public, I realized the public was hungry for all of this. I ended up deciding to create a book and to teach these concepts. As I was teaching the concepts, I realized I couldn't just have these lists of food stuffed in my mind. I needed to have a teachable method so I could teach my patients at my clinics, and I could teach the public. I codified that into what I call *The Wahls Protocol*. We have the diet, the foods that you need to eat, so lots of vegetables, greens, sulfur, color.
Dr. Mark Hyman:	So, there are three categories, right?
Dr. Terry Wahls:	Three big categories.
Dr. Mark Hyman:	Dark green leafy vegetables ...
Dr. Terry Wahls: [00:30:30]	Green leafy vegetables to get all that vitamin K going and the carotenoids and magnesium, a great source there. The sulfur-rich vegetables, cabbage family, onion family, mushroom family, and that helps with detoxification, it helps with intracellular glutathione, it helps with making neurotransmitters. And then the deeply pigmented, and pigment's a great source of a good market for antioxidants.
Dr. Mark Hyman:	So, eat the rainbow.
Dr. Terry Wahls:	Eat the rainbow.
Dr. Mark Hyman:	Yes. The other aspects of the protocol besides the colorful fruits and vegetables.
Dr. Terry Wahls: [00:31:00]	Remove things that are particularly inflammatory, so the gluten-containing grains, wheat, rye, barley. Remove the dairy protein, you can have clarified butter, but all other forms of dairy we take out. And also take out eggs because eggs are probably the third most common, unrecognized food sensitivity. So that's the food part.

Dr. Mark Hyman: [00:31:30]	So, it's also a very high-fat and low-carb diet.
Dr. Terry Wahls:	Yes, so the average American has about 250 grams of carbs. My diet, depending on which level you're at, may be 100 grams down to 50 grams of carbs. These are pretty non-starchy carbs. We have less carbs, and I want people to have more fat. I want them to have omega-3 fats, flax oil, hemp oil would be fine, avocados would be great. If you're more ketogenic, then I encourage things like coconut oil or medium-chain triglycerides, clarified butter is good.
[00:32:00] Dr. Mark Hyman:	Or ghee, right?
Dr. Terry Wahls: [00:32:30]	Ghee, yeah, that's great. And I'm okay with people eating chicken skin. I'm okay with having fattier cuts of meat because our cells, and the cell membrane wraps around the axons or the nerve wiring to make myelin. 70 percent of that cell membrane is saturated fat and cholesterol. So, cholesterol has got this terrible rap, but we need it to make our hormones, including vitamin D, and we need it to make our cell membranes, so we need it to make myelin.
Dr. Mark Hyman:	I had a neurosurgeon at Cleveland Clinic once tell me, "I don't know why anybody would take statins. If you're a neurosurgeon you know what it does to the myelin and to the nerve cells and sheets."
Dr. Terry Wahls: [00:33:00]	Yeah, you know I'm very comfortable with people having fat. I think that is a very critical part of brain health is to have enough fat.
Dr. Mark Hyman:	What are the other aspects of the protocol besides the three different categories of veggies, the good fats, low sugar, and carbs.
Dr. Terry Wahls: [00:33:30]	You want to be sure there is enough protein. Many people don't have enough protein in their diet, you know, ask a vegetarian, vegan for many years, clearly not enough protein, probably low in B12 as well. I prefer that people have some fish, poultry, or fruit. I do have some strategies for vegetarians and vegans because I recognize there are vegetarians and vegans for spiritual beliefs and religious beliefs. We have some separate programs for them to help them do that more safely. We are very keen on fermented foods to help populate the gut with a diverse set of microbes. If you have fermented foods, you get many more different species of microbes than you're going to get in your probiotic capsule.
Dr. Mark Hyman: [00:34:00]	Like sauerkraut, kimchi.
Dr. Terry Wahls: [00:34:30]	Kombucha, I teach people how to make fermented chia seed pudding—it's quite delicious. And then we get coconut milk and we show people how to make fermented coconut milk cheese, fermented yogurt, fermented kefirs. You know, and fermented beets, fermented carrots, fermented radishes, so lots of ways to have fermented foods, and that can be fun and easy. I encourage them to begin using seaweed. Our ancestors would have traveled great distances to have the seaweed, or would have traded to get seaweed, and they certainly recognized that it was very important for the reproductive health of the clan. The young men and women who they wanted to have kids got the seaweed.
[00:35:00] Dr. Mark Hyman:	Because of iodine and you need it for your thyroid. And if your thyroid is not working you can't get pregnant.
Dr. Terry Wahls:	Exactly, so we have those things. I also talk about the benefits of ketosis and why that is something to consider. We have some strategies to get people in ketosis.
Dr. Mark Hyman:	Which is not eating many carbs and actually ...
Dr. Terry Wahls:	Having more fat.
Dr. Mark Hyman:	More fat and burning the fat instead of the carbs for fuel.

Dr. Terry Wahls: [00:35:30] [00:36:00] [00:36:30]	Correct. Now the ketogenic diet has a long history. It's been used to treat epilepsy. It started I think about 1919 at the Mayo Clinic and Johns Hopkins got it going again in the 1960s, but they have a dairy-based ketogenic diet with only 20 grams of carbs, which wreck people's microbiome. They wreck their hormonal balance, they have to use a lot of supplements because it's so nutritionally unsound. Unfortunately, a lot of people are using the ketogenic diet dairy-based, again with only 20 grams of carbs, and they have a lot of health benefits initially. But now have concerns that over time they'll develop nutritional deficiencies, the hormonal imbalance it gets to be a problem. So, I'd much rather they use a medium-chain triglyceride based, like coconut oil, coconut milk. If you don't like coconut or coconut disagrees with you, you can do it using olive oil, but then you're going to have to restrict your calories. And so, this is a lot tougher. Now you're eating once a day or every other day. Once you're in ketosis, eating every other day is actually pretty comfortable. I'll eat once a day or every other day when I'm in ketosis, and it's very comfortable. I'll sometimes eat every three days for a longer fast, but that is not easy at the beginning. You have to very gradually ease your way into that.
[00:37:00] Dr. Mark Hyman:	Not eating doesn't sound fun.
Dr. Terry Wahls:	No, no, no. I think for most people it's easier to do it with a medium-chain triglyceride on the ketogenic diet.
Dr. Mark Hyman:	Powerful, and so you can be on a ketogenic diet if it's more well designed, you don't necessarily have to become nutritionally deficient, you can do a healthy version of it.
Dr. Terry Wahls: [00:37:30]	When I design my diets, I have level one, two, and three, level three is the ketogenic diet. We went back and did a nutritional analysis of each level to verify it was nutritionally sound: do they have enough fiber, can it maintain a healthy microbiome, and so, yes, you certainly can if you're following our protocol. If you're doing a dairy-based ketogenic diet, I think you're at a definite risk of long-term problems.
Dr. Mark Hyman: [00:38:00]	The other thing I want to cover is what your experience is with the resistance to your ideas, because you did a TED talk and had some challenges around that, as you mentioned. I think that you've been able to work in a major university to implement this, which is a huge breakthrough, but there's still a lot of resistance, and can you talk about why that is?
Dr. Terry Wahls:	Sure.
Dr. Mark Hyman:	What kind of resistance have you encountered with this ground-breaking idea?
Dr. Terry Wahls: [00:38:30]	I've certainly had lots of resistance, and I think some of the reasons I'm successful is I'm a little socially not attuned. I've always been into doing my own thing. I just do what I think is right, and I can let the world roll off my back, so I think that was critical to my success.
Dr. Mark Hyman:	Yes.
Dr. Terry Wahls: [00:39:00] [00:39:30]	Early on when I had this transformation, I was assigned to the traumatic brain injury clinic, which, by the way, I was assigned to that as an attempt to force me to take medical retirement. Because I was assigned to that in 2007, I went home, told my family, and my spouse said, "You know there's no way you can do that job," and I knew there was no way I could do that job, because I was going to be seeing traumatic brain injury patients without residence, and I just physically would not be able to do that. It said I'd start that in the end of January 2008. Well, as it turned out by the end of January 2008, I could do that job. And so, I'm helping in the traumatic brain injury clinic, but, unlike my colleagues who were saying, "Well, there's nothing you can do," I'm like, "Well as a matter of fact there is a lot you can do. We can teach you how to eat a more nutrient dense diet, we're going to teach you how to meditate, and we'll talk with you about exercise, and we're going to have you do Epsom Salt baths, get a pedometer

and start walking." And my chief of staff calls me and says, "Terry, people are really upset. What are you doing?" And so ...

Dr. Mark Hyman: Can you please not help them?

Dr. Terry Wahls: [00:40:00] So, I took down 85 different papers that say, "Okay, this is what I'm doing and why," and he was like, "Well, but it's still not FDA approved." And I'm like, "Well okay, and I'm happy to do only what's FDA approved if you'll send out an email to all of my partners here at the university that that's the only way we can treat our patients is using FDA-approved treatment protocols. They can no longer use the latest science."

Dr. Mark Hyman: Right.

Dr. Terry Wahls:

[00:40:30] And I stopped and smiled, and then he goes, "Okay, I see you have a point." And he actually would become a huge fan of mine. He started telling folks who were criticizing me saying, "Okay, if Terry harms somebody we'll do a peer review and we'll see what's going on, but vegetables are not a problem. Meditation is not a problem. Exercise is not a problem."

Dr. Mark Hyman: Is meditation FDA-approved?

Dr. Terry Wahls:

[00:41:00]

[00:41:30] No, that's the whole point. So, he became a huge fan, and in fact a couple years later he gave me two unfunded days to do my research. My chief of staff became very, very supportive. The chair of medicine at the university saw my recovery and gave me the job of writing a case report, which writing a case report on yourself is not an easy task. I got it done and we got it published, and then he called me back saying, "Okay, we need to do a little clinical trial." That took about a year to get that through and got that going, and I could not get it through the IRB, because there's no safety data other than me. He had become the Dean of the Medical School, and so he'd facilitate behind the scenes to let the IRB know that work with Wahls and the physical therapeutics committee, she needs to be able to do this study. So, then I met with the Head of Affairs of Pharmacy Therapeutics, and we identified what were all the labs they would have to do, who we would have to exclude to be able to safely do this study. We got that study up and going.

[00:42:00] Then, next what they started doing was lecturing the public. Again, I get warned like, "You can't be doing this," "You don't have any studies saying this is really safe," so I got some coaching on how to more carefully talk about it. This is my experience, this is the scientific rationale, and you could talk to your personal physician, and if this makes sense, try it out and see how you respond. I had to learn how to talk about it in a way that was culturally acceptable.

[00:42:30]

Dr. Mark Hyman: What an extraordinary story. You know you've gone from someone who was basically debilitated, almost on disability ...

Dr. Terry Wahls: Oh, yeah.

Dr. Mark Hyman: To someone who's healed herself, to someone who's begun an initiative that educated patients and consumers, to being a research scientist, proving the concepts over and over again.

Dr. Terry Wahls: [00:43:00] We had our little pile of studies going, and it was small, private foundations that funded our work. We're doing little stuff, and the university is giving me PhD students and some grad students to work for free in my lab, and I'm writing grants to the NIH, MS society, and they're giving me scathing reviews like, "Clearly Doctor Wahls has no understanding about the pathophysiology of MS," but you know I keep writing anyway. And, finally, we're having some preliminary data, and I slowly get these scathing

[00:43:30] reviews, but I publish my book, *The Wahls Protocol*, which creates a firestorm in the MS world, and drives a huge consumer interest in diet and lifestyle, which causes the MS society to take notice and rearrange their research priorities.

Dr. Mark Hyman:	Yeah.
Dr. Terry Wahls:	And ...
Dr. Mark Hyman:	And I talked to them a decade ago and it was just like talking to a wall.
Dr. Terry Wahls:	Well, you know I was a banned speaker because I was creating false hope. So ...
Dr. Mark Hyman:	There is no such thing.
Dr. Terry Wahls:	As false hope?
Dr. Mark Hyman:	Hope is a medicine.
Dr. Terry Wahls: [00:44:00]	Hope is a medicine, but you know I was a banned speaker and my book came out in 2014, and then in the fall of 2014 I get an email from the MS society that they want me to come to their Wallace Meeting, and I'm a preliminary speaker at another event that same day. But I'm thinking, "Okay. Well that sounds sort of interesting." So, I call the MS society and say, "Do you know who you're inviting? I'm a banned speaker." They were very apologetic, "Oh, no. Yes, we know about you. We know about your work. We know we banned you. We're very apologetic. We really want you to come." So, I rearranged with that other organization and I spoke on a different day, and I went and helped them see the light.
[00:44:30] Dr. Mark Hyman:	Amazing. Well, thank you for your work and inspiration for so many people, and I'm sure we're going to see a lot more of what you're doing and it's going to change how we think.
Dr. Terry Wahls:	It's very exciting.
Dr. Mark Hyman:	Thank you.
Dr. Terry Wahls:	Thank you.

Dr. Titus Chiu: [00:00:30]	I went to undergrad to study biology. When you're in high school, your place for those tests is kind of to figure out what your specialty is, or your gifts are. I was good at science, I guess. Honestly, I wasn't very passionate about it. But still, it's like, this is what you're good at, I was smart, I was good at that, and it came easy to me. I just went to school, went through the whole program, did what everyone does after they graduate high school and that whole path. As I went through school, I was really good at it, it didn't light my fire. It was, how should we say? It was kind of boring, actually.
[00:01:00] [00:01:30]	I didn't want to really study medicine, because I didn't really agree with the philosophies and the framework of conventional medicine. I didn't want to study in a lab, I studied biology. So, I did what any confused 20-year-old would do, I moved to Japan. As I was in Japan I was teaching English to little kids. One day I was driving home from work, I was on my scooter, and out of nowhere, this lady hit me and it was very traumatic, like I flew 10 feet through the air. I ended up breaking three ribs, dislocating my shoulder, I had a road rash, and suffered a mild concussion. At the time, I actually didn't even know that, because I didn't know what a concussion was.
[00:02:00]	I tried everything. I was in chronic pain. I tried conventional medicine, I tried pain killers, I tried physical therapy, and nothing worked. I was at a point where I was pretty much giving up hope, because I couldn't do any of the things I loved doing anymore. Thankfully, at that time, my brother was already practicing natural medicine. I went home for a vacation and before that point, you hear natural medicine, or Functional Medicine, or chiropractic, well, I was like, "I don't really trust those quacks." It's just what we're taught.
[00:02:30]	I came from a family of medical doctors and nurses, and so, that was a paradigm. I was at this point where ... and it's funny now, because patients come to me all the time and they're just like, "I'll try anything." I was at that point and I went, and after a few treatments with him and some lifestyle recommendations, dietary changes, supplements, my pain was gone. It was like three sessions. Yeah. I was just like, blown away. It's in my nature, I'm a curious person. When something like that happens, I want to figure out why. "How did that happen, number one, and, how can I take this information and share it with others?"
[00:03:00] [00:03:30] [00:04:00]	Without a second thought, I went back to Japan, finished my contract, came back to the States and I dove right into medical school—chiropractic school to be specific. It was from there I had found my calling. All that stuff I studied that I was really good at, that I had no drive or passion really, all of a sudden it had meaning. It's like, I could apply this to my life and I can apply this to my patient's life. From there I was just like, before, I was kind of unmotivated, suffered mild depression, and I was getting sick all the time. I was just kind of weakly to be honest. I wasn't driven to do much of anything. After that, not just the healing process of the techniques and treatments, but also, wow, this is what I was put on this planet to do. I had this huge fire to learn as much as I could.
[00:04:30]	What got me interested in neurology, I was seeing patients, I was practicing Functional Medicine, I got a Master's in nutrition because I love food. I was using all these protocols. About 80% of the patients would get better and would respond phenomenally. Then, about 20%, especially the ones with a little bit more chronic issues, a little more-slippery neurological conditions, like Alzheimer's, or concussion, or just brain fog, wouldn't. Again, it's in my nature, I was born to be curious and want to answer that question, "Why aren't they responding to care? and what can I do about it to take that to the next level?"

BROKEN BRAIN

[00:05:00] I decided to dive deeper into neurology. It was awesome, because neurology for me is a way of understanding myself. It's also a way for me to understand what's going on with my patients and get to the root cause for a lot of these chronic neurological symptoms that are just persistent, and slippery, and subjective.

[00:05:30] Some early warning signs of Alzheimer's and dementia are forgetfulness, like when you're in an interview and you're on the spot and you don't remember the question that you practiced 30 minutes ago. And, when you walk into a room and you're like, "What did I come into this room for?" Or, "Where are my keys?" Or, even things like just a slowing of overall processing speed, like, your thoughts aren't as sharp or clear like they used to be, or even your movements, your reaction time. You might have issues of balance and coordination. These are very significant because they're early warning signs for potential neuro degeneration. Things like Alzheimer's and dementia, but maybe even

[00:06:00] chronic traumatic encephalopathy, you know, a sequel or a sequel, something like that, in result of a concussion that wasn't treated properly.

These are all clues as to what's actually happening. They're windows into your nervous system, because it's our brain. The reason why it's so important, I think, and one of my missions is to share with the world, why the brain is so important and relevant to everyone is that, it allows us to think. It

[00:06:30] allows us to feel, to move, to have dreams, and to create. If that's not working well, you can experience things like forgetfulness, because you experience things like having brain fog, or you're just not feeling sharp.

It's really subjective, and if it gets bad enough, you might go to a doctor, they run all the tests and everything's normal and they're just like, "It's in your head." But they were right, it actually is in your head, but not in the sense they thought, because it's a specific neural network, specific areas of the

[00:07:00] brain, that if they're not as strong as they were maybe five, 10 years prior for you, then you can experience those symptoms.

It really depends on what's going on with you as an individual. The reason for Alzheimer's and dementia, there are these root causes for it. If we can address the root cause for Alzheimer's or for

[00:07:30] dementia, there are so many things we can do. For example, for my patients, I put together customized menu plans or dietary supplements targeted to their imbalances, their physiology, what their body and brains need. There are other lifestyle recommendations we can make. Give them stress management techniques like a simple breath in and a breath out, which can just totally calm a person's nervous system and prevent further degeneration or further inflammation. It can allow

[00:08:00] healing to happen.

We are at the forefront of the evolution of neurology. What is possible with healing in the brain? I'm so excited for that. Everybody should be doing these things. We don't want to wait until someone develops Alzheimer's or dementia, because that's kind of like the end game. We want to make sure we catch those things earlier on. The exciting thing is, even if it is the end game, there are things we can

[00:08:30] do to reverse that. Everyone talks about cardiovascular health. We want to make sure that our heart's healthy and so we exercise, we change our diets, and we do all these wonderful things, but the brain, same thing. The brain can respond to those things as well.

[00:09:00] There's this radical new field. It's been around in the scientific community for a long time called epigenetics. That speaks to our ability to take control of our health and that applies to the brain as well. We can do things like change our diet, we could change the way we think about things—our mindset. We can make changes in lifestyle. We can exercise more. We can connect more with our

[00:09:30] loved ones. All those things have been proven to actually slow, stop, and even reverse any type of neurodegeneration. Things that are good for the heart are also good for the brain. Things such as exercise, diet, lifestyle, specific supplements, and stress management. The brain is unique, not only does it respond and require nutrition to thrive, but it also needs exercise and activation.

[00:10:00]	Exercise and activation, what I mean by that are things like playing chess. Or, mental stimulation like mindfulness practices, meditation, or learning Sudoku, learning how to play a new instrument, rocking out, learning a new language. That's what I call a top-down approach, where you can use your mind to train your brain. There's also another way that I call sensory genomics, where we can use all the senses, like sight, sound, smell, taste, touch, and this other really curious and essential sense known as proprioception or body awareness.
[00:10:30]	Proprioception allows us to get a sense of our own groundedness in being on this planet. If that's off, you can have problems with balance and coordination, but it could be so subtle that it's just in the back of your mind. One of the main functions of the brain is to allow us to move on this planet and not fall over, really.
[00:11:00]	We weren't born reciting poetry, playing music, all those wonderful creative things. You know, filming with the Red cameras. We were born to walk and navigate on this planet. If the systems in our nervous system start to break down that allow us that, then we have to use all of our mental resources to be able to balance. All of a sudden, we can experience brain fog and not really know why, or forgetfulness, or our capacity to deal with stress is just right at this level because those systems aren't working well.
[00:11:30] [00:12:00]	We should always be challenging ourselves to learn new things. Whether it's learning how to play the piano, learning a new instrument, a new language, or spending time with family or meeting new people. All these things grow and strengthen the brain. In addition, like I said, all these different senses, we can use the senses. The next time you're washing the dishes, close your eyes and really bring your attention to how that feels. How the water feels, and the warmth of it, and the soap suds, and the sound of the water. When you do that, when you bring your awareness to your senses, you actually powerfully activate the brain.
[00:12:30]	In Norman Doidge's book, I just have to geek out about that for a bit. He talks about all these neuroplasticians. That's what I do in my practice. I do things like aromatherapy, where a person smells like rosemary or lavender, and it can help with their anxiety. It's not actually impacting our nose, it's activating specific areas within our nervous system that can calm our emotions. That's sensory genomics. Another example is what I call the vestibular rehab, where we spin someone in a chair and it activates these little canals in their inner ear. If they have problems with balance, coordination, or anxiety, a lot of times it's because they have an imbalance in their inner ear and we can retrain that. That's sensory genomics.
[00:13:00]	Go out with me for an enjoyable glass of wine, and then I will teach you the differences between Pinot Noir from Sonoma and from Willamette Valley, that's sensory genomics. You're not expanding your palate, you're expanding this area called your orbitofrontal cortex in your frontal lobe that allows you to differentiate between the different ones. That's sensory genomics.
[00:13:30]	The way I use dye in my practice is very personalized, number one. And number two is therapeutic. We're finding out we can actually use food as medicine, as a therapy that can be more powerful than a medication. It depends on what my patient is coming in for. For example, a patient came to my office with Alzheimer's. I did the whole workup and found that they would best respond to a low sugar diet, plus removing all inflammatory foods, such as gluten, dairy, grains, those are the most common.
[00:14:00] [00:14:30]	My patient with post-concussion syndrome, it was horrible. She was a student of mine actually, and she had suffered a traumatic brain injury. She developed bilateral subdural hematoma, which is bleeding in the brain. And because of that, she was in the midst of medical school and could no longer do what she had set out to do, to become a doctor. She had brain fog, balance problems, headaches, and when she tried to study and read, she'd just get really tired and would crash out. I did the workup and in my experience a lot of those patients with concussions, they respond really well to what's known as a ketogenic diet. That looks at higher fat, but healthy fats. Middle, moderate protein, you

know, meat and things like that and really low carbs.

[00:15:00] Everyone's different in how much they can tolerate. For example, my wife can drink juice upon juice and still be in ketosis—I'm impressed. Whereas, with me, I have to keep it down to about 15 grams of carbs a day. I did that myself and *oh my God* ... this is probably speaking again to that concussion I had suffered. When I did the ketogenic diet, I didn't think I had issues with blood sugar, or brain fog, but all those things went away. I was like the Energizer bunny. I just kept going, and going, like I'd go through

[00:15:30] this entire day at work, I'd see patients back to back to back to back, yeah, like for nine hours straight. Maybe, with a little break. I'd get home, hangout with my family and my wife, and they'd be like, "Who is this guy? He has so much energy, he's not irritable anymore and he's like, really focused and on point."

[00:16:00] Yeah. The ketogenic diet works really great for people suffering from concussion and people with Alzheimer's disease, they do really well with the low sugar diet anti-inflammatory. Again, it's totally personalized based on the root cause for that unique individual. The ketogenic diet, it's so fascinating when you actually look at the history of it. Initially, originally, it was used way back in the day that dude named Hippocrates, right? The father of modern medicine. He was using it way back in the day to address things that he described, what we know now are seizures. In addition, about, I believe the

[00:16:30] 1930s, they had found that children suffering from pediatric epilepsy would do phenomenally with the ketogenic diet because it stabilizes their brain cells. People who have neuronal or neurological disfunction, their brains are no longer communicating in this synchronized fashion, it's just like noise in the system. It's this instability.

[00:17:00] Have you ever not slept for a day and then you woke up and you're just really groggy and you're irritable? You're just like, "I don't want to see anyone, I don't want to do anything." The lights are just like, "Get me outta here." That's because this area of your brain or underneath your brain called the brainstem, is just like that. Any little stimulus like light or sound, you're just like, it's too much. Imagine now a patient with seizures or with a concussion, or Alzheimer's, they're like that all the time. The

[00:17:30] ketogenic diet helps to balance and smooth this out, the neuronal communication. So, we're able to handle a lot more. So then, you go into a bright room, you don't squint, you don't get a headache. When you wake up, even if you don't sleep that well, you don't feel irritable or brain foggy.

[00:18:00] When I work with patients suffering from neurological symptoms of Alzheimer's, or concussion, or just brain fog, I take a very comprehensive and investigative approach, to get to the root cause of why they're having those symptoms in the first place. That can involve the very comprehensive medical history, where I sit down and talk with you one-on-one to really understand your unique situation, because your brain cells don't live in a little Petri dish. Your brain is connected to every single organ in your body. It's connected to the world around you. All those things can influence your brain health.

[00:18:30] From there, when I tease out some root causes, then I move on to an advanced neurological exam. In that exam, I check for things like balance, coordination, I look at how your eyes are moving because those are all windows into how well your brain is working. From there, if necessary, I run some more advanced tests. I might run stool tests, saliva tests, blood tests, urine tests, to actually understand

[00:19:00] what's happening with your biochemistry. Imbalance is biochemistry or neurochemistry and can throw off brain function as well. When I gather all that information, I dive deep into what's going on with you, and understand your unique situation, then I put together that plan, a very personalized plan that looks at diet and a very personalized diet. Targeted supplementation, lifestyle recommendations,

[00:19:30] exercise, and like I talked about before, sensory genomic therapies, where we can actually activate and exercise the brain very specifically.

Some supplements I might recommend: everyone's unique, everyone's different. There's a thing called biochemical individuality. With that being said, there are patterns. I've been doing this for years. One

[00:20:00] of the main things the brain needs is essential fatty acids. Things such as omega-3 essential fatty acids, specifically DHA, docosahexaenoic acid. This essential fat, docosahexaenoic acid, allows your brain cells to smoothly communicate with one another. If you're lacking in that, again, you can experience that noise in your brain. You might not hear anything, but you might experience irritability, brain fog, or mild forgetfulness.

[00:20:30]

[00:21:00]

When it comes to nutrition and supplements, one of the root causes I'm trying to address with those tools, is neuroinflammation. Neuroinflammation is one of the root causes for all neurodegenerative diseases. Whether it's Alzheimer's, Parkinson's, chronic traumatic encephalitis, chronic traumatic encephalopathy, or post-concussion. Neuroinflammation is one of the root causes that needs to be addressed in these conditions. The great news is, that we can address those things naturally. Again, using things like supplements, diet, stress management, taking long deep breaths, even long walks in nature with your loved ones or your dog. It's really calming and it helps calm neuroinflammation.

There are specific brain exercises you can do to calm those things through a top-down approach, that I was talking about before. Your brain is unique, in that it not only requires nutrition, it needs brain activation. If we can target and activate the specific areas of your nervous system that are contributing to neuroinflammation, even without the use of diet and supplements, just through your own mental machinery, which is amazing, you can calm those things down and address the root cause for your symptoms.

[00:21:30]

[00:22:00]

Sensor genomics is a revolutionary way where we can activate specific pathways in your brain to heal the brain. By using all the different senses that we have available, so it's not invasive, it's safe, anyone can do it. There's a simple three-step process that, through many years of research, seen patients with neurological conditions, teaching, educating doctors about these different ways. I've put together this three-step-program. Step one. To prime yourselves for healing. Step two. To activate these specific areas in your nervous system and brain. And then finally, what's so overlooked in modern society these days, is step three. Integration. That's where, after we prime ourselves through proper nutrition, and exercise, and breathing, and then we activate our brain using these specific exercises.

[00:22:30]

[00:23:00]

Step three is where we allow our bodies to integrate all of this and embed it into our neural network. We integrate by unplugging. The world we live in today is just so phonetic and non-stop. There's so much value placed on getting things done, doing this, being successful, achievement, achievement, achievement. That's great, I'm all about that, but so many patients I see, one of the main root causes for their inability to heal, is not integrating. Not unplugging. It could be something as simple as lying on a patch of grass and taking a deep breath in, connecting with mother earth and letting that sun hit your body. Like I said before, that ties in with step two, activation. When you're actually feeling that you bring your awareness, your attention, to that moment. And you just unplug from everything. You turn your cell phone off, you turn your TV off, you don't check your emails. You turn off the mental chatter happening in your own brain.

[00:23:30]

[00:24:00]

[00:24:30]

Integration is one of the most important steps in this three-step process, that I see so many people not doing today. It's one of the main reasons why they're still suffering. What's the correlation between poop and brain function? A lot of the latest research is showing us that there's a strong correlation between gut health and brain health. In fact, the brain, the second brain and the first brain are intimately related embryologically, they come from the same tissue. There's this bidirectional communication pathway we call the vagus nerve, where the brain can talk to this brainstem vagus nerve and then the gut can talk back. If you have imbalance in your gut, whether it's dysbiosis or infections, maybe even what we call leaky gut, that can release chemical signals crossing the blood-brain barrier causing all kinds of problems, like brain fog, memory issues, headaches, and problems with focus and concentration.

[00:25:00]

At the same time, the gut can communicate with the brain by what we call the vagus nerve, where it's an electrical signal that communicates with our brain. By testing the stool, we get this beautiful window into the microbiome, it's the environment of our guts. That can give us clues as to, is there an infectious process, maybe a bacterial infection, a parasite, causing neuroinflammation, by traveling

[00:25:30] and attacking the brain. We can see if a person has leaky gut. Or, big food particles cross and enter, and then the immune system launches a response, again, causing neuroinflammation.

[00:26:00] We can get a window into the health of the actual cells themselves. We can get windows into inflammatory markers. The stool test is a great way of getting a really important window into what's happening in a person's microbiome, which could then impact the health of their brain. The neurotransmitters are the special unique chemical messengers that allow your neurons, your brain cells, to communicate with one another. They can talk to each other. The different neurotransmitters are kinda like different personalities. We have something called dopamine, which is really excitable and motivated. We have things like GABA (gamma-Aminobutyric acid), which is really chill and just the guy you want to just hang out with on the beach.

[00:26:30] We have things like norepinephrine, where it's just like that fight-or-flight response, they just have to get things done, right? When it comes to neurotransmitters, when it comes to brain health, it's all about balance. If we have too much dopamine, what happens? We can develop things like mania, or we can develop things like movement disorders where there's too much movement. Or, have you ever gotten that thought stuck in your head? Or, that song that keeps playing over and over? That's too

[00:27:00] much dopamine. If you don't have enough dopamine, you can have a slowing of your movements or a slowing of your thoughts, like we see in Parkinson's.

The same thing with GABA, it's about balance. If you have too much GABA then you're just like, "I don't want to do anything, this is very comfortable." If you don't have enough GABA, you're always anxious and you always feel like you have to do something, you can't shut that off no matter how many exercises you do, breathing exercises, etc.

[00:27:30] With neurotransmitters, it's all about balance. When it comes to food and its impact, neurotransmitters, artificial sweeteners, like food coloring, things like that, specifically artificial sweeteners, they can mimic one of the neurotransmitters we call glutamate. Now, glutamate is

[00:28:00] extremely important. It's one of the most abundant neurotransmitters in our nervous system. It's like the on switch. When we turn it on, things happen in our brains overall, but if a person takes aspartame found in artificial sweeteners, it mimics glutamate and it's just too much for the brain to handle. It's like the on switch is happening over and over and over again. The brain can't calm down. What ends up happening is what we call excitotoxicity, where the brain cells literally get really unhealthy, to the point they can actually die.

[00:28:30] For example, you've heard of cocaine? You've heard of coca, right? Where it comes from? Coca leaf has been used all throughout history as a healing traditional medicine. What happens when you take that coca leaf and you break it down to that specific compound, we call now cocaine, and someone

[00:29:00] uses that and it exceeds the brain's ability to handle it, it literally destroys brain cells. That's the same thing for things such as MSG. MSG was actually isolated by a Japanese scientist from Kombu. It's this delicious seaweed that naturally flavors soups and things like that. This Japanese scientist is like, "How can I isolate that and get that umami flavor without taking the time to steep and soak that seaweed into that broth." They found a shortcut. With that shortcut, it became this powerful substance, that if

[00:29:30] consumed at too high a level, guess what? Excitotoxicity. The brain can't handle it.

Most people think MSG is found just in Chinese food, but it's found in so many different processed foods. It comes with these hidden names, because everyone's just like, "Oh yeah," most people know, right? We're a lot more conscious. We want to choose the foods we eat and be very conscientious. A lot of people read, and if you don't now, please, start reading what you're eating. A lot of people these days are reading, "Oh, MSG." So, what the food companies have done is they've hidden it. They

[00:30:00] disguised the name, camouflaged it.

TODD LEPINE, MD | The UltraWellness Center

Dr. Todd LePine:

I'm trained in internal medicine—very traditional, straightforward internal medicine. I trained at Dartmouth, and I went through what most physicians go through. I actually have an interesting story because I took over a very traditional practice. It was Dr. Campbell who was the town doctor in Stockbridge for 50 years. He is the doctor who is portrayed in that Norman Rockwell painting—of a little boy who's bending over to get a shot in his buttocks. It was like taking over a piece of history for

[00:00:30]

traditional, family-style medicine, and that's what I wanted to do.

After I had been in practice for a number of years, I started banging my head against the wall because I wasn't really helping patients get healthy. I was just treating symptoms. It took a while for me to start saying, "You know, I need more tools in my black bag." All I had was either a scalpel or a prescription pad, and those things have their use. Using surgery for certain kinds of conditions and using prescription medications—they're definitely strong and valuable tools, but I needed more things to

[00:01:00]

help patients acquire health and get healthy and stop treating symptoms.

I started doing my own research. I started reading, I started attending conferences. I also was introduced through the Functional Medicine organization when I worked at Canyon Ranch, where a lot of us in Functional Medicine in the Berkshires had worked. We also were introduced through Jeff Bland, who was friends with Kathie Swift, who is a nutritionist. That's sort of how I evolved. Then, once I heard Jeff Bland speak for the first time, who is a brilliant, brilliant synthesizer of complex biochemistry, nutrition, and genetics, the light bulb went on in my head and I said, "This is the kind of medicine I need to practice. This is real medicine. This is why I went into medicine."

[00:01:30]

[00:02:00]

Functional Medicine, it's not a sexy term, but I like to tell patients that it's really about creating health as opposed to treating disease. When patients come to doctors, they come in usually with some kind of symptom: "I have pain. I'm tired. I'm overweight. I can't remember." Whatever. Then you say, "Here, take this pill. Try this. See if it works," without asking the question: "What kinds of things are you doing or what kind of things are you not doing that's causing you to go down this path of ill health?" Our

[00:02:30]

bodies are really incredibly designed to have resiliency.

We also have health built into it. Our bodies naturally want to be healthy, so if you give it the right things in terms of sleep, nutrition, exercise, movement, relationships—all those things create health. When we're out of balance, we are dysfunctional and our bodies are dysfunctional, and when we bring that balance back into the body, then our bodies are optimally functional. That's really what Functional

[00:03:00]

Medicine is. People also say, "Well, what do you do?" I say, "I do clinically-applied nutritional biochemistry. That's what I do, and lifestyle medicine. I tell people how to live their lives in a healthy fashion."

I've always been pretty aware of my own health, always exercised, and always tried to eat right. I don't eat right 100% of the time. I sneak potato chips, ice cream, and beer every now and then, but it's a

[00:03:30]

matter of balancing things. Is there a right diet for everyone? No, there is no right diet for everyone. Everyone's different. Some people can tolerate gluten, while for other people it's like arsenic or kryptonite. There's not a one-size-fits-all kind of a diet that you give to everyone. Diet is really important. With a foundation of Functional Medicine, because I can prescribe all the supplements, I can give all the prescription medications, but if a person eats a crappy diet, they're never going to get

[00:04:00]

healthy.

Some of the tests I'll do for patients who come in complaining of brain symptoms are really just observing the patient. I'll see how their language skills are. Are they able to engage in conversation? Do they laugh appropriately? What's their mood like? You can read a lot of what's going on in the patient.

[00:04:30] As far as some of the tests go, we do organic acid testing, amino acid testing, fatty acid testing, and gut health testing. Then, also genomic testing and toxicology testing are some of the key things I look at when a patient comes in complaining of brain symptoms.

[00:05:00] What we do in Functional Medicine is really we dig much deeper. Traditional tests, blood chemistry panel, CBC, liver function tests, cholesterol, and thyroid tests—those are all good tests, but Functional Medicine really gets into the underlying complexity of biochemistry, nutrition, functional metabolomic analysis, and genomic analysis. It's really much more complicated. You have to dig deeper to really uncover what's going on with a person when their brain is not working.

[00:05:30] The gut-brain connection is a big, big part of depression. How do we label depression? What does depression mean? When somebody says, "I'm depressed," it basically means that your brain's not working and your mood is not normal. You're either flat, sad, depressed, or isolated and withdrawn. There are many things that can trigger and tie in with depression. We're told, when you watch television commercials for big pharma, that depression is a serotonin deficiency. All you need to do is take an SSRI, get your serotonin up, and we cure your depression.

[00:06:00] Guess what? That's not true. In the same way, heart disease is not a cholesterol problem. It's much more complex. Heart disease in the same way is really an inflammatory process, the latest data shows us that depression is really an inflammatory process, and it probably originates in the gut. There's a huge connection between the gut and the brain, and when the gut is out of balance, when the bacteria, yeast, and/or parasites get out of balance. Those things can trigger systemic inflammation. That systemic inflammation, in turn, can trigger withdrawal behavior. It can increase molecules in the body

[00:06:30] called cytokines. It's sort of like when you get the flu and you're really sick, you want to just withdraw. That's what you do, and that's what depression is.

Depression from an illusionary standpoint has a role that if you get really sick, you're going to withdraw, you're going to be depressed, you're going to sit in a corner till your body gets over that sickness, you get healthy, and then you're fine. When that process becomes more chronic, we label that depression, but it's really an inflammatory process, and there are other things. The gut is highly

[00:07:00] tied in with depression in the brain, but there are other things that can also trigger depressive symptoms, like not getting enough sunshine.

How do we spend our lives? Actually, let's ask a better question. How did we evolve? If you go back 10,000 years, we were basically outside pretty much 24/7. Occasionally, we'd go into a cave. We were pretty much naked, and we were hunting and foraging for our food, and we were in rhythm with Mother Nature. When the sun got up, we got up. When the sun went down, we went to sleep.

[00:07:30] Light is a huge factor. In fact, there's actually a condition called seasonal affective disorder. Seasonal affective disorder means that during the fall and winter when there's less sunlight, you're going to become more depressed. You're going to withdraw more. You're going to sort of semi-hibernate. That's a natural thing when you think about it in an illusionary standpoint. However, if you are in a building all the time and you never see the sunrise—and at nighttime you're on your iPad, your computer, your

[00:08:00] video games—and the sun never sets, you disrupt that circadian rhythm. And that is a big, big contributor to depressive symptoms.

Anxiety can be triggered by a variety of different things. It can be related to a person's genetic predisposition. There are some people who are more anxious and hardwired. I call them squirrely, the people who are always vigilant and watching out. There's a natural sort of personality that each of us have. From an evolutionary standpoint, it's actually good to have anxiety. You're watching out so you

[00:08:30] don't get eaten by a sabre-toothed tiger. It's okay to watch out, but if we're in an environment that's not hostile to you, you don't want to have anxiety 24/7.

[00:09:00] It's okay to have anxiety when you need to be vigilant, but if you can't turn off that hyper vigilance ... There are some people who also have difficulty in detoxifying stress hormones. I can almost literally predict if a person has a Catechol-O-methyltransferase deficiency (COMT). That's a big mouthful. COMT basically means that when you're under stress, your stress hormones linger in your body longer. That fight-or-flight response you get when you're anxious, is basically like a merry-go-round. It keeps circulating in the person's body and they remain anxious all the time.

[00:09:30] It's natural if you get more adrenaline, you're going to get more anxious. If I shot you with adrenaline, you would get on edge, and that edge should go down as your body detoxifies those stress hormones. But there are some people who can't detoxify those stress hormones. Those are the people for whom mind-body types of behaviors where meditation, deep breathing exercise, visualization, relaxation are really, really key for dialing down their anxiety.

[00:10:00] Also, other things that are highly tied in here are gut bacteria. Some of our gut bacteria when they're out of balance have been shown to increase anxiety because they actually consume a compound in our gut called GABA. GABA is that compound that helps with relaxation. If you have an imbalanced gut, it can trigger anxiety-type symptoms. I've had a lot of patients who come to me, not necessarily with, "My stomach hurts," or whatever, but when I test them, I ask them, and I treat their gut and get their diet back into balance, their anxiety melts away.

[00:10:30] In my training, I was trained to treat anxiety with prescription drugs. Some of the medications would include benzodiazepines, things like Valium and Xanax. Yes, they do treat anxiety, and there are times when I will use those prescription medications under a really ... Let's say somebody is in an accident and their system is so hyped up that they need something to sort of short-term calm them down for a couple of days. That's perfectly appropriate, but long-term use, they actually have more of a disadvantage.

[00:11:00] The things that I'll work with nowadays—besides just giving a prescription medication—is looking at their nutritional biochemistry, looking at a gut analysis, and teaching them deep breathing exercises. Another thing I've learned is that anxiety is also related to the brain pH. If you have an acidic brain, that causes anxiety. Most people say, "Well, how do I know if I have an acidic brain?"

[00:11:30] We've all experienced having an acidic brain. An example of that is when as a kid you go underwater and you hold your breath to see how long you can stay under, the thing you get at the end when you "run out of air"—you get this incredible, "Oh, my God, I have to get up. I have to get oxygen." Well, guess what? That actually does not happen because of low oxygen. It happens because the carbon dioxide builds up in your body and the carbon dioxide causes an acidic brain. That acidic brain is telling your body that we need to ... There's panic that's going to happen.

[00:12:00] Things that you can do to prevent your brain from becoming more acidic—which is a strong trigger for anxiety—is regular exercise. The number one thing you can do for people who have panic attacks and anxiety is regular exercise with interval training. That teaches the body how to clear out those acid buildups—what we call organic acids—in the brain, which then decrease anxiety. I think in today's world, there's lots of information. We get bombarded by information.

[00:12:30]

[00:13:00] Some of it goes along with aging to some degree. In the same way that when I'm 70 years old I can't run as fast as when I was 20 years old, so you may not be able to think as fast. You may not be able to recall people's names or places, but what you really want to do is catch memory problems early. I think one of the great talks that we went to at this year's Functional Medicine Conference was Dale Bredesen's talk about catching Alzheimer's early. You really do that by asking the patient a variety of different questions, doing a mini mental status where you have a patient remember a series of numbers, have them draw a clock. There are a variety of different things you can do to determine early on if this person is showing signs of cognitive impairment way before you develop Alzheimer's.

[00:13:30] We have the same analogy that I don't want to wait till a patient has Frank diabetes and their blood sugar is 230 before I treat them, because guess what? The horse is out of the barn. It's a lot harder to treat a patient who has diabetes when the diabetes presents as uncontrolled, versus, "Can I treat this patient when their blood sugar is normal?" After they have a meal their insulin goes up, their blood sugar goes up. I can treat that very, very easily and early, in the same way you can treat Alzheimer's very easily and early before you have an end-stage process going on.

[00:14:00]
[00:14:30] Aging is "inflammaging." What we call aging is really chronic inflammation affecting the body and in certain cases affecting the brain. We know it affects your joints because it's harder to get up from the chair when you're 85 years old and you haven't taken care of yourself, or if you're overweight. The autoimmune process is really a continuum, so when you have inflammation, and inflammation, in turn, can change the molecular structures of certain proteins in the body where the body now perceives self as non-self and you start attacking your own self. There really is this continuum between aging, inflammation, and autoimmunity, and it's sort of an all-in-one spectrum. It's not like we can put something in this box and say this is just autoimmunity and this is just the aging process. It's really a continuum effect.

Lyme disease is a topic all unto itself. Living in the New England area, especially in the Berkshires, we see a lot of patients with Lyme disease. If you go back in history and you actually understand the history of syphilis, syphilis is a spirochetal disease. It used to be called "the great mimicker," meaning it could present any different way. It could present as a heart problem, as an arthritic problem, or as a memory problem.

[00:15:00]
[00:15:30] Lyme disease is a bacterium, which is a spirochete, and it has a tendency to go towards connective tissue and neuronal tissue. A person who gets a tick-borne Lyme disease bacterium—oftentimes it can sit silent in the body, and then over time, it can cause neural inflammation. I've seen patients come to the office here who had presented with multiple sclerosis as their "diagnosis," memory problems or, "early Alzheimer's," patients who presented with Parkinson's-type symptoms, and their true underlying cause was actually tick-borne Lyme disease.

[00:16:00] A Functional Medicine approach of Lyme disease is really multi-faceted. I think one of the big things you can do with a patient who has Lyme disease is improve their diet. There's some substantial evidence that a ketogenic diet in patients with Lyme disease can be highly effective because the bacteria lives off of sugars. A ketogenic diet where a body goes into ketosis, where you're burning fat as opposed to burning sugars, can be very effective for switching metabolism.

[00:16:30] You think of your metabolism as like a car that you can either drive with gas or you can ride it with electricity, and you can make that switch and you can flip it over. Rather than burning carbs, you're now burning fat. That process of burning fat is much more fuel efficient and a cleaner engine, if you will, and that allows you to help a variety of neurodegenerative conditions like Lyme disease.

[00:17:00] One of the other things I should mention is actually hyperthermia. This is sort of a little pearl I learned, is that most people who have Lyme disease—especially if it's chronic Lyme disease—they usually never develop a fever. I always ask them, "When was the last time you had a fever?" Say, "I can't remember the last time I had a fever." Well, how does your body get rid of a bug when it's sick? You raise the temperature. You cook the bugs, if you will. Hyperthermia, doing sauna therapy ... In some cases, over in Germany, they actually have boxes they put people in and raise the body temperature to revoke heat, shock proteins, and other things that stimulate the immune system to help naturally fight off the bacteria.

[00:17:30] There are a lot of people who are bitten by ticks, get infected, but never manifest with the disease. It's not like everyone who gets a Lyme bacterium is going to have the disease. It's when the immune system is not working properly to identify and get rid of outside infectious agents is when you can then manifest as having "Lyme disease."

[00:18:00] I had one patient, a young girl—I'll never forget her. She was 22 or 23 when I saw her, and she was a vegan. She was hospitalized prior to seeing me. When she came in, she was on three psychiatric drugs. She was on anti-anxiety medications, and she was not functioning well. When I did a full nutritional biochemical genetic analysis on her, she was markedly deficient in amino acids. Amino acids are the building blocks of your neurotransmitters. She was deficient in fatty acids. Fatty acids are basically the fats that build the lipid membranes in the body, especially the brain. Well, your brain is mostly fat, and if you don't eat good fat, you're not going to have a functioning brain.

[00:18:30] She was also deficient in trace minerals, and there were a lot of different nutritional underlying causes. She had B12 deficiency because she was a pure vegan. She had iron deficiency. In her case, her "depression" was really mostly just a nutritional deficiency. She actually had been hospitalized for three weeks and never once did she ever have any kind of nutritional testing done. She was thrown SSRIs and

[00:19:00] the benzodiazepines, and it sort of put the lid on the symptoms. But it didn't really cure her. That was a really good case where this young person was really on the path towards long-term pharmacology, and I was able to get her off of her medications and get her back to feeling whole and happy.

[00:19:30] There are a couple of things people do every day that's really affecting their brain health in a negative way. In today's society, what we do is we are out of rhythm with Mother Nature. I'd probably say one of the biggest things people complain of is fatigue, and I ask them, "Well, what time do you get up and what time do you go to bed?" I think light pollution—especially for young kids on their iPads, on their iPhones, on their computer games, watching TV late at night—that suppresses melatonin, which is the hormone that helps to induce sleep.

[00:20:00] It's also a natural antioxidant. Just having good sleep hygiene is really, really key for affecting one's health in a good way. The other thing is probably just inactivity. People spend lots of time sitting. Most people's activity for the day is moving a mouse. You can just move a mouse and that's actually a computer. That's about all they're moving. That's not a good thing for your body when you do that.

[00:20:30] "I don't have energy." There are multiple reasons for that. Patients come in and say, "You know, I'm tired." There's a whole laundry list of different things that can cause people to have low energy. The thing we get our energy from is our mitochondria, so it makes me think, "Hey, maybe your mitochondria are low." They produce ATP, which runs our body. And if we run out of our ATP, we will die instantaneously. That's why people die of cyanide poisoning. It can kill you in a matter of minutes. I think about low B12. I think about the thyroid.

[00:21:00] I think about their sleep. I ask them, "Do you snore?" If someone is overweight, if they snore, maybe they have sleep apnea. Those are all different things that can do it. Are they pounding down alcohol and caffeine? Those things disrupt the sleep. Disrupted sleep can also cause no energy. Are they not exercising? Some people say, "I'm too tired to exercise." Well, guess what? Exercise will actually give you more energy. Those are all different things that come to mind when someone says, "I'm too tired," or, "I don't have the energy to do things."

[00:21:30] The best thing to keep your brain sharp is to exercise. Exercise is the best medicine, but it's a hard pill to swallow. Exercise actually has multiple effects on the body. What it does, it increases oxygen and increases removal of toxins. This is happening on a very, very small level called the arterioles or where capillaries are. When you exercise, all those blood vessels dilate and they bring in oxygen; they take out the waste products. When you're not exercising, you really are building up toxins in the body.

[00:22:00] Another thing that is highly important for helping with health is to keep mentally sharp—using your brain to think, doing puzzles, engaging in conversation, reading books. The brain is like a muscle. If you don't use it, you lose it. It's really important to keep the mind stimulated, but not overstimulated. Not like multitasking and you're doing a whack-a-mole kind of a thing, which most people are doing every now and then.

[00:22:30]   Community is really important, and community happens on a family level, on a neighborhood level, and it happens in a broader context. There's a wonderful book called *Alone Together* by Sherry Turkle, and she talks about how technology in some way is bringing us together, but it's also making us separated.

[00:23:00]   Real connection is what I call "vitamin O", vitamin oxytocin. Oxytocin is the thing that mammals get when they're in community, they're touching one another, hugging each other, and sitting down and eating together. That sharing, that social bonding that happens, that glue that cements us together is really, really important. Look at the Blue Zones. That's what Blue Zones are really. The striking thing is they have that sense of community, and a sense of purpose and cohesiveness. We're social animals. That "vitamin O" is really, really important.

DR. TOM O'BRYAN | theDr.com

Dr. Mark Hyman: Tom, thanks for joining us.

Dr. Tom O'Bryan: No, thank you. It's a pleasure. It's a real pleasure.

Dr. Mark Hyman: You've become an expert in gluten, which is kind of the latest fad. You think it's quite a lot more than a fad. How did you get into this? What's your background? What made you interested in this whole field?

Dr. Tom O'Bryan: How I got into it?

Dr. Mark Hyman: Mm-hmm

Dr. Tom O'Bryan: [00:00:30] Well, that's interesting. It was 34 years ago when I was an intern. My wife and I couldn't get pregnant. I called the seven most famous doctors I'd ever heard of, holistic doctors at that time, this was 1979. Guys like Jonathan Wright, who had just come out in practice and was writing articles in *Prevention* magazine—I don't know if you read it back then—but it was a godsend to read those kinds of concepts. They all told me what they do and I put a program together. We were pregnant in six weeks.

[00:01:00] My neighbors in married housing heard about this and asked if I'd work with them. We lived on campus. Would I work with them? They'd been through artificial insemination and nothing had worked. I said, "Well I don't know what I'm doing, but I don't think it will hurt you, sure." They were pregnant in three months.

I was treating people out of my dorm room.

Dr. Mark Hyman: You got a lot of women pregnant.

Dr. Tom O'Bryan: That's right, that's exactly right. We came out in practice wanting to help the whole world get pregnant that wanted to get pregnant.

[00:01:30] As we all know, there's not much in medicine that's "all or every," but this was an every. In clinical practice, this was an every. Every person that had hormone imbalances of one type or another were eating things that were causing inflammation in their body and they didn't know it.

The most common food was wheat. That got me interested in starting to study this. Ever since then, it's been going on and on.

Dr. Mark Hyman: That's extraordinary. We think of Celiac disease as sort of an allergy to wheat. It's really a lot more than that. It's an autoimmune disease. Can you tell us about how we really understand Celiac as an autoimmune disease, and what autoimmune disease is anyway?

[00:02:00]
Dr. Tom O'Bryan: You know, there are two questions in there I'd like to address. The first is Celiac disease and we all cut our teeth in studying the pros and cons of wheat by learning about Celiac disease. Unfortunately, so many doctors think if you don't have a problem with Celiac, you do not have a problem with wheat. But, that's not true. Celiac is one manifestation of a problem with wheat sensitivity.

[00:02:30] We know about one percent of the population has Celiac disease in the U.S. and in Europe, about one percent. In my practice I look more deeply and I can find as many as 60 percent of the people that come in have an immune reaction saying, "You have a sensitivity to wheat." They don't have Celiac disease. They have a sensitivity to wheat.

[00:03:00]	That concept bore out the term Non-Celiac gluten sensitivity, which has become known much more in the last 8 to 10 years. Celiac is really important.
	As an autoimmune disease—your immune system is attacking your own tissue—for some reason, when you eat wheat, if you have this genetic vulnerability, you attack the tissue of your gut. We know a lot of the mechanisms of what causes that. That's the autoimmune component of it.
[00:03:30]	There are many other manifestations of a sensitivity to wheat outside of celiac disease. It can be fatigue; it can be a brain fog; it can be numbness and tingling called peripheral neuropathies; it can be hormone imbalances; it can be recurrent miscarriages. The list goes on and on and on, not just celiac, but wheat sensitivity.
Dr. Mark Hyman:	It's fascinating when you're talking about it. As a doctor I learned that you had it or you didn't.
Dr. Tom O'Bryan: [00:04:00]	Right.
Dr. Mark Hyman:	You had Celiac disease that was demonstrated by an abnormal biopsy. If that was negative, it was fine to eat wheat. We know that while Celiac can cause literally dozens of diseases—everything from osteoporosis, to colitis, to schizophrenia, to autism, to depression, on and on—most doctors just dismiss any reaction that's not full-blown Celiac. They don't want people to be restricted in their diets because they think wheat is essential for health, which it's not.
Dr. Tom O'Bryan: [00:04:30]	Right.
Dr. Mark Hyman:	Dr. Fasano, who is one of the world's leading researchers in gluten and Celiac, said to me once that if you have antibodies to gluten, it means that number one: you've been eating it. Number two: you have a leaky gut, meaning the proteins from wheat are getting into your bloodstream. Number three: your immune system doesn't like it and it's pissed off.
Dr. Tom O'Bryan:	Right.
Dr. Mark Hyman: [00:05:00]	Is it true that anybody with any level of antibodies to gluten, whether they're normal or above normal or below normal but still elevated, should be off wheat?
Dr. Tom O'Bryan:	If someone has antibodies to any of the parts of wheat, and there are many different parts of wheat that your immune system might react to, the testing has to be comprehensive enough to look at the different components of wheat, not just one component. If you have what's in the normal reference range of antibodies, that's probably okay.
[00:05:30]	If you have elevated antibodies outside the normal reference range as determined by the laboratory, you have a problem. Your immune system says, "I don't like this." And what happens when you have these elevated antibodies, is that you can have what's called cross reactivity, or molecular mimicry. The antibodies going after the wheat, the signature of the wheat is kind of like saying, immune systems ...
Dr. Mark Hyman:	It's a protein.
Dr. Tom O'Bryan: [00:06:00]	Yeah, it's like saying, "Go after everyone who's wearing a black vest." The protein signature that it's looking for, it's looking for black vests in the bloodstream. If it sees a black vest, it's going to shoot its chemical bullets to attack the black vest.
	That protein signature on wheat looks identical to the Saran Wrap around your nerves called myelin, or to parts of your brain, like the cerebellum ...
Dr. Mark Hyman:	Which affects balance and stability and coordination.

Dr. Tom O'Bryan:
[00:06:30]

Exactly. You may develop antibodies because it looks like a black vest, so the immune system goes after the black vest; it doesn't matter that it's your myelin, the cerebellum, the liver, or your kidneys. There are hundreds of studies that show this.

Dr. Mark Hyman:

That's why gluten sensitivity and Celiac often have neurological manifestations, everything from MS, to like you said peripheral neuropathy, gait issues, ataxia, all sorts of problems that are driven by damage to the nervous system.

[00:07:00]

Let's just back up a little bit and talk about the brain and gluten, and this whole idea that it's somehow affecting our brain. How do we even tell if it is? Are there biomarkers of autoimmunity in the brain we can look at?

Dr. Tom O'Bryan:

There are. In my practice, I took 316 consecutive patients, that meant everyone that came in, two years to 90 years old, all got this one blood test irrespective of what their complaints were. I was looking to see, "Do they have a problem with wheat or dairy or antibodies to their brain?"

[00:07:30]

They all got this blood test, and what we found, and this was just in my practice, but what we found was, if you had elevated antibodies to wheat—any of the components of wheat—26 percent of those people had elevated antibodies to the cerebellum, which is the part of the brain that controls balance, which is why most old people can't dance up and down the stairs. It's not that their muscles can't do it, but their brain doesn't coordinate balance well enough to do it.

[00:08:00]

22 percent of those people with elevated antibodies to wheat had elevated antibodies to the Saran Wrap around the nerves called the myelin. That's what causes MS. 22 percent of everyone that had a sensitivity to wheat had this molecular mimicry where the antibodies were also going after the myelin. That meant they had increased antibodies to myelin.

[00:08:30]

There's a normal reference range for antibodies to all of our tissue. Why is that? It's because, Mrs. Patient, you have a whole new body every seven years, right? Some cells regenerate really quickly, some cells are really slow. Every seven years you get a new body. How do you do that? Well the immune system has to get rid of all the old and damaged cells to make room for new cells to grow. Your immune system makes antibodies to all of your tissue, brain, heart, lungs, and liver. You have a normal reference range. When you have elevated antibodies, you're killing off more cells than you're making.

[00:09:00]

If you have elevated antibodies to cerebellum and you don't know because you can't feel it, and that goes on for years, when you're an elder, it's not likely you'll be dancing with your granddaughter at her wedding. Except, you'll do the two-step: one, two, one, two, because that's all you can do anymore. You can't shake it up. Your cerebellum won't do it. It's been slowly killed off for years and years and years.

Dr. Mark Hyman:

It's fascinating you're talking about looking at these tests. It's important to point out that these are not tests that your normal doctor will check. They'll only check two different proteins. You're checking maybe 20 ...

Dr. Tom O'Bryan:
[00:09:30]

That's exactly right.

Dr. Mark Hyman:

Different proteins that are connected to wheat or gluten, which by the way, is not just wheat. It's barley, rye, spelt, kamut, triticale, and even oats.

Dr. Tom O'Bryan:

That's exactly right. Oats don't have toxic gluten in them when they grow in the ground. When you buy them off the shelf, they have toxic gluten in them. It's contamination. There are companies that have gluten-free oats; they're labeled. The FDA has done some studies on that. They've found that if the

---

foods are labeled, 97.3 percent are gluten-free. If they're not labeled, and it's just oats, then 24.3 percent of them have toxic levels of gluten.

[00:10:00]

Dr. Mark Hyman: Yeah. It's interesting you say that. I've been practicing for 30 years. I've observed, and I wonder if you have ever observed the same thing, patients who do a gluten-free diet but eat gluten-free oats often still don't get better.

Dr. Tom O'Bryan: That's right. That's exactly right.

Dr. Mark Hyman: I don't know why, because if you're saying 97 percent don't have gluten, if they are gluten-free ...

Dr. Tom O'Bryan: If they're listed gluten-free on the label.

[00:10:30]

Dr. Mark Hyman: I'm talking about gluten-free oats. People are still eating gluten-free oats and still reacting. I remember a girl with total body psoriasis. She was still struggling, she got a lot better off the gluten. But then, she was eating oats every day, and they were gluten-free. She still had trouble. I got her off that, and she cleared immediately.

Dr. Tom O'Bryan: I remember a few years ago the conversation you and I had about this. What I was doing in practice - and I still do, is that when people come in, if they need to go gluten-free, I tell them it's probably okay to have oats, as long as they're gluten-free oats. They're labeled gluten-free. But, if in three weeks we aren't noticing that you're feeling better, that things are going right, we're going to get all the grains out of there for a while.

[00:11:00]

Dr. Mark Hyman: We know there are so many different ways that gluten can actually drive health changes, symptoms, diseases, which is like a chameleon. You think you have X, but you have actually gluten problems.

Dr. Tom O'Bryan: That's a really good visual, the chameleon, yes.

Dr. Mark Hyman: Yeah. It's often misdiagnosed or often not diagnosed. Probably 90 percent of people who have it are probably not diagnosed. One of the things you mention in your work is that it actually affects the brain in a unique way. It has to do with your blood flow. Can you talk more about that?

[00:11:30]

Dr. Tom O'Bryan: Yeah, you bet. These studies were done with Celiacs. If they have Celiac disease, 73 percent of those people have a lack of blood flow into the brain. It's called hypoperfusion. It's a good scrabble word, right? It's actually more than seven letters but it's a good scrabble word.

[00:12:00]

Hypoperfusion means lack of blood flow. There's an MRI called a SPECT Scan that looks at blood flow into the brain. You can see these areas of the brain that aren't getting very much blood. It happens to be the areas for people who get seizures, and it was that area of the brain, in the occipital area, where there was hypoperfusion.

[00:12:30]

When you put those people on a gluten-free diet for a year, only seven percent of them still have hypoperfusion. 73 percent goes to seven percent. Now, what does all that mean?

When I'm talking on stage, I'll say, "Docs, could everyone please cross your legs." No one moves. I say, "Cross your legs." They do. "Okay, thank you. Leave them like that for three hours. Now stand up and run." Everyone giggles. You can't because there's no blood in your leg.

[00:13:00]

Give your child toast for breakfast, if they have a sensitivity to wheat, and send them to school to learn. 73 percent of them have a lack of blood flow to the brain. That's why in the Journal of Attention Disorders in 2006, they published a study of 130 kids diagnosed with Attention Deficit Disorder. They put them on a wheat-free diet, gluten-free diet. Within six months, every child, or their parents, reported significant improvement. That's the key term, significant, with researchers. Significant

[00:13:30]	improvement in all 12 DSM-4 markers for attention deficit: fails to pay attention, interrupts frequently, blurts out answers, can't sit still ...
Dr. Mark Hyman:	I do that.
Dr. Tom O'Bryan:	Right. I did too in school all the time. Every child, every symptom improved within six months, just by going wheat-free.
	If that were a drug, it would be all over the front page of every paper in the country. But, there's no profit in going wheat-free.
Dr. Mark Hyman:	Yeah, well for the gluten-free companies there is.
Dr. Tom O'Bryan:	That's true.
Dr. Mark Hyman:	They should be sponsoring this research.
Dr. Tom O'Bryan: [00:14:00]	Oh, but that stuff is ...
Dr. Mark Hyman:	Yeah, I always say gluten-free cake and cookies is still cake and cookies.
Dr. Tom O'Bryan:	It's still cake and cookies. It's white paste. I have no issue with having a gluten-free blueberry muffin once in a while.
Dr. Mark Hyman:	Yeah. I'll also say, "Avocados are gluten-free. Almonds are gluten-free."
Dr. Tom O'Bryan:	That's right. That's true.
Dr. Mark Hyman:	Chicken is gluten-free.
Dr. Tom O'Bryan:	Some people think they can eat the substitute gluten-free pasta stuff to fill you up and get healthy. No, you can't.
Dr. Mark Hyman:	Right.
Dr. Tom O'Bryan:	Once in a while, who cares.
Dr. Mark Hyman:	Right.
Dr. Tom O'Bryan: [00:14:30]	You can't do it every day.
Dr. Mark Hyman:	No. No, right, it's true. What are the common symptoms people can identify that can cause various brain disorders? What are the symptoms of gluten sensitivity? What kind of brain disorders actually are resulting from gluten sensitivity?
Dr. Tom O'Bryan: [00:15:00]	Oh my goodness, it runs the gamut. There are a number of papers of reversing schizophrenia. In the medical literature, reversing schizophrenia with a wheat-free diet... These are not Celiacs; these are gluten-sensitive people. Reversing schizophrenia, a year later they're still checked out of the treatment centers and they're not on any meds. They published a year later, these people are fine now, as long as they're wheat-free.
Dr. Mark Hyman:	Yeah.
Dr. Tom O'Bryan:	It can be schizophrenia, most common is depression or anxiety. Those are called the affective disorders

[00:15:30]   with wheat sensitivity. That's the most common. Anxiety, depression, schizophrenia, migraines, seizures, any function of the body, if the tissue is being compromised by inflammation, and if wheat is the gasoline on the fire, when you calm down the fire, any symptom may improve.

Dr. Mark Hyman: Arthritis ...

Dr. Tom O'Bryan: Arthritis, psoriasis ...

Dr. Mark Hyman: Autoimmune diseases, skin disorders ...

Dr. Tom O'Bryan: In the last number of years, my emphasis has been on the autoimmune manifestations that occur with wheat sensitivity and other triggers.

Dr. Mark Hyman: [00:16:00]   You don't have to have Celiac to have an autoimmune manifestation.

Dr. Tom O'Bryan: Absolutely not. Actually, some studies show there are more patients with gluten sensitivity that have elevated antibodies to their own tissue, than the patients with Celiac.

Dr. Mark Hyman: Mm-hmm.

Dr. Tom O'Bryan: Non-Celiac gluten sensitivity will have more antibodies elevated, ANA antibodies, different types of antibodies, than the Celiacs will.

Dr. Mark Hyman: You know, we keep talking about antibodies, which is the body's intelligent evolved immune system with very specific targets. It's like a laser-guided missile against a specific protein.

Dr. Tom O'Bryan: [00:16:30]   Yes.

Dr. Mark Hyman: That's a newer evolutionary adaptation to deal with immune threats.

Dr. Tom O'Bryan: Yes.

Dr. Mark Hyman: But, there's also an ancient part of our immune system called the innate immune system, which is essentially run by our white blood cells, but it's an all or nothing reaction. It's basically nonspecific. It just creates a lot of aggressive attacks on the immune system, but it's not very specific, so it's a generalized response.

Dr. Tom O'Bryan: [00:17:00]   Right.

Dr. Mark Hyman: It's like it's just pissed off, it's mad, it's not specific. We now know that gluten can also cause problems through that part of the immune system, and yet it's impossible to measure.

Dr. Tom O'Bryan: It's the first trigger. The first trigger is called the innate immune system. They're not shotguns, they are like pistols. These pistol shots in our blood stream are trying to destroy whatever the irritant is.

Dr. Mark Hyman: But it's not specific.

Dr. Tom O'Bryan: It's not specific, it's general.

Dr. Mark Hyman: [00:17:30]   You can't measure it like you can measure antibodies.

Dr. Tom O'Bryan: It's more difficult to measure. All you can measure is the total amount of some of these things, like IL1 Beta and IL6. You can measure those but it's not commonly done. When that ancient immune system, the innate immune system, can't get the job done, then the big guns get called in. That's the adaptive immune system, that's when the antibodies get produced. I refer to them as bazookas.

Dr. Mark Hyman: Yeah.

Dr. Tom O'Bryan: They come in and they just blast away.

Dr. Mark Hyman: The reason I mention is because you might have a reaction to gluten even if it doesn't show up on your blood test.

Dr. Tom O'Bryan: Right.
[00:18:00]

Dr. Mark Hyman: The only way to know is to stop it for a little while and see how you're doing. Then re-introduce it.

Dr. Tom O'Bryan: Well that's a primary way, but not the only way. That suggests if you don't have symptoms, you don't have a problem.

Dr. Mark Hyman: Mm-hmm.

Dr. Tom O'Bryan: When you have the elevated antibodies to myelin, for example, or to cerebellum, or your heart, you don't have symptoms that you notice. When you go off wheat, you can't tell that the myelin antibodies
[00:18:30] have gone down, because you didn't have symptoms with the elevated antibodies. Until the antibodies are elevated long enough, for a number of years, and you've killed off enough myelin, now you start getting the symptoms of MS.

Dr. Mark Hyman: What about what Dr. Fasano says? He's noticed that everybody who eats gluten has some level of reaction? It causes some level of inflammation, some level of leaky gut, and maybe we shouldn't be eating it at all?

Dr. Tom O'Bryan: Right. That's exactly right.

Dr. Mark Hyman: He's Italian, which is saying a lot ...

Dr. Tom O'Bryan: You know, here's the problem with that. We're talking to him at dinner and he's eating a roll.
[00:19:00]

Dr. Mark Hyman: Right.

Dr. Tom O'Bryan: Alessio, "What?" He said, "What? I'm healthy." When he does that, what he's saying and—it's loss of oral tolerance. That's really the big picture. That's what my book, *The Autoimmune Fix* was about, is that everyone has a minor sensitivity to wheat. That's what the science says. Everyone does. But, it's a minor problem, until you cross a line.

[00:19:30] When you've crossed that line, it's called oral tolerance. The immune system starts attacking it. When it the immune system really starts to go after it, now you get all the potential complications down the road, years later from that.

Dr. Mark Hyman: Mm-hmm.

Dr. Tom O'Bryan: Why do we lose oral tolerance? It's all of the toxins we're exposed to in this world today that our immune system is trying to protect us from. Eventually our immune system is so active trying to protect
[00:20:00] us from Bisphenol A, mercury, lead, polysorbate 60, and red dye #3, and all of the things we're exposed to. It's working so hard it becomes trigger happy. It doesn't have the tolerance anymore for the mild irritant that wheat is for most people.

Dr. Mark Hyman: Basically, there are so many irritations to our immune system, it's just generally pissed off.

Dr. Tom O'Bryan: It's generally pissed off and it's going to shoot anybody that it thinks is a problem.

Dr. Mark Hyman: Mm-hmm.

Dr. Tom O'Bryan: That's when you've crossed that line of oral tolerance. Wheat becomes a serious problem. Now you've
[00:20:30] developed Memory B cells to it. Now you have a problem for life with wheat.

Dr. Mark Hyman: You know, one of the emerging concepts in medicine today is this idea of inflammation, that most chronic disease is caused by inflammation: diabetes, obesity, cancer, heart disease, and even dementia.

Dr. Tom O'Bryan: Yeah.

Dr. Mark Hyman: Even depression, autism, and ADD, we find are all linked to inflammation.

Dr. Tom O'Bryan: Yes, yes.

Dr. Mark Hyman: You've been involved with development of certain tests that actually help us look at the immune system response that affects the brain. Can you tell us a little bit more about that?
[00:21:00]

Dr. Tom O'Bryan: You bet. As far as I know, all degenerative diseases are diseases of inflammation. At the cellular level, the cells are inflamed. The basic rule is, first, to identify, is there inflammation going on? Then, why is it there? Stop throwing gasoline on the fire. That's where wheat comes in or other toxins.

[00:21:30] With the brain, we want to look for antibodies to your brain. Once again, there's a normal level of antibodies. That's to be expected, just to keep having a healthy brain make new brain cells. There's a normal reference range. When you have elevated antibodies to different parts of your brain, you have a problem. There's some mechanism going on which may not show symptoms yet, or the symptoms
[00:22:00] are not being associated with the elevated antibodies, like depression, anxiety, brain fog, migraines, or seizures. It doesn't matter what function you talk about in the brain. If it's inflamed, that may be the trigger causing that dysfunction.

We want to look for, are there elevated antibodies to brain tissue? There are a few labs that will look at that for you now. They will look to see: do you have elevated antibodies to myelin? Do you have
[00:22:30] elevated antibodies to cerebellum? Do you have elevated antibodies to gangliosides, which is a component of all nerves?

The value of looking is that you see, "Wow I have inflammation going on in my brain. I feel fine." But, if it's elevated ...

Dr. Mark Hyman: You may not know you don't feel fine.

Dr. Tom O'Bryan: That's right.

Dr. Mark Hyman: Half of people don't know how badly they feel until they start feeling better.

Dr. Tom O'Bryan: They don't know. Right. Because if they go on a diet or something, they say, "Oh, I feel so much better. I'm thinking clearer." They didn't realize they weren't thinking so clearly before.

Dr. Mark Hyman: It's like the frog in boiling water. You drop the frog in boiling water, he'll jump out. If you start with cold
[00:23:00] water and put the frog in, they'll boil to death thinking it's normal as the temperature rises.

Dr. Tom O'Bryan: That's right. That's exactly right. Looking at blood tests to see, do you have elevated antibodies? If you do, you have inflammation in your brain. Those antibodies are killing off that tissue, whatever it is.

[00:23:30]	I did this test on myself. I had three different antibodies to my brain. I had myelin basic protein, which causes MS eventually. I had cerebellum, which causes your loss of ability to move your muscles and keep balance. I had gangliosides, which causes a shrinkage of the brain. I had all three of these.
[00:24:00]	This is when I was 44 and was doing triathlons regularly. I was 44 and I was scoring in the top 10 percent of the guys age 30 to 35. I was walking. "I'm a stud. I'm doing great." I thought I was healthy. I did this blood test to find out, "Wait a minute." I called the lab and I said, "This is a mistake." They said, "No, it's not." I said, "Do it again." "We did. We know it's you. We did it again." That's when I got religion. I realized that ...
Dr. Mark Hyman:	You quit the rolls and pasta?
Dr. Tom O'Bryan:	That's right.
Dr. Mark Hyman:	The carb loading ...
Dr. Tom O'Bryan: [00:24:30]	Exactly. Carb loading, I stopped the carb loading that year. I did stop because I realized there was a mechanism going on that I wasn't having symptoms to that causes MS, or that causes shrinkage of the brain. I was grateful that I found it before it had killed off so much tissue that symptoms were then obvious.
Dr. Mark Hyman:	Those were just a few tests.
Dr. Tom O'Bryan:	Exactly.
Dr. Mark Hyman:	There are many more we haven't discovered. There are ones we know that we should be looking at.
Dr. Tom O'Bryan:	Exactly.
Dr. Mark Hyman:	For example, you were mentioning schizophrenia and autism. About 20 percent of schizophrenics have elevated antibodies to gluten.
Dr. Tom O'Bryan:	Yes.
Dr. Mark Hyman:	17 percent of autistic kids do.
Dr. Tom O'Bryan:	Yes.
Dr. Mark Hyman: [00:25:00]	It's profound and, like you said, when you get these kids off of it, and when you get these adults with schizophrenia off of it, they can recover. It doesn't mean that every case of schizophrenia or autism has this problem.
Dr. Tom O'Bryan:	No.
Dr. Mark Hyman:	That's why our naming issue with disease is so wrong. We think we know what's wrong. We say, "You have autism." Well, not necessarily. It's a spectrum of symptoms that can have many causes.
Dr. Tom O'Bryan:	That's exactly right. It would be really silly to say wheat sensitivity causes autism. It's silly and doesn't make sense. But, it's rational to say wheat sensitivity may cause autism.
Dr. Mark Hyman: [00:25:30]	In a subset of patients ...
Dr. Tom O'Bryan:	In a subset of patients ... Or, it may cause schizophrenia or Alzheimer's in a subset of patients. That's why our friend Dr. Bredesen in his programs to reverse Alzheimer's, and reverse cognitive decline, one

of the first things they look for when talking about food is, get wheat out of there because it's so very common.

Dr. Mark Hyman:	Mm-hmm. And gluten ...

Dr. Tom O'Bryan:	And gluten, Mm-hmm.

Dr. Mark Hyman: [00:26:00]	Fascinating. Let's talk about some patients who had brain disorders that were connected to gluten. I know you and I have been in practice a long time. I've seen this over and over again. It's just astounding what you see when you start to shift the diet. Can you talk about some of the stellar cases you've had?

Dr. Tom O'Bryan: [00:26:30]	A 14-year-old girl: her parents checked her into a psychiatric facility because all of a sudden she had a kidney infection. She had a little kidney infection; she got an antibiotic. After that, within a week or two, she wasn't focusing in school. She didn't do very well and went downhill over the next few weeks until she was hallucinating. She was seeing things and seeing people. They tried different medications, nothing worked. They checked her into a psychiatric facility for three months. She wasn't recovering. She lost weight when she was in there.
	The nutritionist in the psychiatric facility said, "We need to get some weight on you, but let's ..." She just made her gluten-free. The gal got better in two weeks, completely better.

Dr. Mark Hyman:	Mm-hmm.

Dr. Tom O'Bryan: [00:27:00]	They came to see me. We did the blood tests, there it was: high sensitivity to wheat. I confirmed what they had already experienced, and at that point it was education. You don't touch this, ever. She had a couple of relapses and started to hallucinate again within a day or two.
	Seizures: I've had a couple of patients I can think of offhand that their seizures just reduced and were gone within a few months completely and were off their medications, with the support of the doctor who gave them the medication.

[00:27:30]	What I always say to patients, "Go back to your doctor that prescribed this medication and say, "I'm changing my diet. I'm feeling better. I'm having less symptoms. Can you monitor me and see if we can reduce this medication a little bit?" In both cases I'm thinking of right now, they were able to do that over the course of a few months. They were off their seizure medications.

Dr. Mark Hyman:	Yeah, powerful.

Dr. Tom O'Bryan: [00:28:00]	Depression: it's like the lights get turned on when they get the immune system calmed down, when the inflammation goes down.
	Anxiety: same thing. It calms down, they calm down.

Dr. Mark Hyman:	The brain's not so irritated and inflamed.

Dr. Tom O'Bryan: [00:28:30]	That's exactly right. I don't know how many parents have come to me and said, "The teacher said that the new medications are working really well for the child." The parents would say, "We haven't given him any medication. We had him go gluten-free." The teachers have always said, "Oh I've heard about that." The teachers have heard about this, but the parents didn't know. The parents finally tried it and got the results and went back. The teachers validated they had heard this before.

Dr. Mark Hyman:	That's true. I've had parents say to me, "We went on the diet." The kids in school and the teachers go, "Is this is the kid's twin brother because it's not what it was with the other kid ...

Dr. Tom O'Bryan:	Exactly.
Dr. Mark Hyman:	Who was bouncing off the walls.
Dr. Tom O'Bryan:	It's astounding. But see, there's no profit in this.
Dr. Mark Hyman:	No.
Dr. Tom O'Bryan: [00:29:00]	No one's making profit on this. It's not being carried out so our traditionally-trained doctors who don't have time to read all the new studies, who believe what they learned 15 years ago, they just don't know yet about this.
Dr. Mark Hyman:	Yes. People say it's not evidence-based, although they haven't read the evidence, is often the case.
Dr. Tom O'Bryan:	That's exactly right. It's not your library-based evidence ...
Dr. Mark Hyman:	Listen, there are 700,000 new scientific papers every year. It's impossible for any physician to keep up.
Dr. Tom O'Bryan:	Exactly.
Dr. Mark Hyman:	It's unfortunate because a lot of patients aren't being helped.
Dr. Tom O'Bryan:	Yes, that's exactly right.
Dr. Mark Hyman: [00:29:30]	People like you are actually bringing the science to the forefront and helping us understand. Now I just recall a few patients from my practice. One had autism. The parents went on a gluten-free, casein-free diet. The kid wasn't talking one day. A few days into the diet, the kid starts talking in full sentences.
Dr. Tom O'Bryan:	In a few days.
Dr. Mark Hyman:	Yes, very quick.
Dr. Tom O'Bryan:	Wow. Yes.
Dr. Mark Hyman:	Very quick.
Dr. Tom O'Bryan:	That's ... It's startling to see those kinds of results.
Dr. Mark Hyman:	Yes, and you know autoimmune diseases, whether it's psoriasis, MS, rheumatoid arthritis, or colitis ...
Dr. Tom O'Bryan: [00:30:00]	My daughter, when she was a teenager—she's in her 30s now—she always would push limits. Being my daughter, she would revolt against what I want her to do, right, of course. She would eat the way she wanted to eat. She developed vitiligo, which is a loss of color in the skin. These white spots ...
Dr. Mark Hyman:	It's an autoimmune disease.
Dr. Tom O'Bryan:	It's an autoimmune disease. She'd go, "Dad, Dad." I said, "Oh honey, all right, well you know what to do." "What do I do?" "You already know what to do." She would do it. She'd be squeaky clean. It was gone in two months.
Dr. Mark Hyman:	Yeah.
Dr. Tom O'Bryan:	The coloration would come back.

Dr. Mark Hyman: It was just caused by gluten, very often.

Dr. Tom O'Bryan: That's right. Yes.
[00:30:30]

Dr. Mark Hyman: Amazing. Doctors inject steroids and chemicals. It's pretty frightening, the treatments we use for these diseases. They are often very high, in terms of their risk profile, overwhelming infections, cancer. Yet, a simple change in diet can actually reverse those autoimmune diseases.

Dr. Tom O'Bryan: The big kahuna concept here is that diseases are usually inflammatory. Stop throwing gasoline on the
[00:31:00] fire. That's the big concept. The question is, "What's inflammatory? What foods am I eating that are inflammatory?" Let's find out. Then when you do the right tests, when you look with comprehensive testing, you can find the information.

Dr. Mark Hyman: Mm-hmm. Would you recommend that everybody be gluten-free?

Dr. Tom O'Bryan: No. If I did that, I would be fanatical. I recommend everyone who has a health problem gets checked thoroughly to see if they have elevated antibodies to any of the peptides of wheat, including the glutens.

[00:31:30]
Dr. Mark Hyman: It's true. When a patient comes to my office, we check their blood pressure, pulse, temperature, and antibodies to gluten, on every patient if they're ill.

Dr. Tom O'Bryan: Yes, because they're ill. What's throwing gasoline on the fire? That's the way we all need to be looking at this.

Dr. Mark Hyman: On a day-to-day basis, what can people do to avoid autoimmune disease? What should they be eliminating? What are the environmental risks for autoimmune disease?
[00:32:00]
Dr. Tom O'Bryan: Autoimmune disease has a trilogy and its development. There are three things we know are consistently involved. One is, you have the genes. That's the deck of cards you were dealt. You can't do anything about that. The key is turning the genes on or off. The genetics, that's one.

The environmental trigger that sets it off, is the straw that broke the camel's back. The most common straws are the foods we eat, which are most common. But, there are many out there.

[00:32:30] We now know that ... I don't know if you remember back in the 90s, they published studies looking at dogs. Every dog they checked in Mexico City had Alzheimer's, had evidence of beta-amyloid plaque in the brain. That was so startling.

In the late 2000s, they started doing blood tests to check for children. Every child they check in Mexico City has elevated antibodies to their brain—every child.

Dr. Mark Hyman: Why?

Dr. Tom O'Bryan: Because of the air pollution. As we know, Dr. Bredesen talks about inhalation Alzheimer's. It's what
[00:33:00] we're breathing that may be the environmental toxin. Foods are our most common trigger, but there are others. Number two in the autoimmune diseases is environmental triggers—the straw that breaks the camel's back.

Number three is, our friend Dr. Fasano was talking about so often, intestinal permeability.

Dr. Mark Hyman: Leaky gut.

Dr. Tom O'Bryan:	Leaky gut. You can heal the leaky gut and calm down the autoimmune cascade. That's the trilogy in the development ...
Dr. Mark Hyman: [00:33:30]	What foods?
Dr. Tom O'Bryan:	The most common foods are wheat, dairy, and sugar. Those are the most common. After that, there's a whole group of people ...
Dr. Mark Hyman:	Sounds like the diet of the average American.
Dr. Tom O'Bryan:	It does. The SAD diet, the standard American diet, the SAD diet.
Dr. Mark Hyman:	Pizza and a coke.
Dr. Tom O'Bryan:	That's right. That is the problem that you and I grew up with. We're dealing with the health issues as individuals ...
Dr. Mark Hyman:	It's terrible because I love pizza.
Dr. Tom O'Bryan:	I know, me too, man. I'm half Italian. I just had a great gluten-free ...
Dr. Mark Hyman: [00:34:00]	O'Bryan, that's an Italian name.
Dr. Tom O'Bryan:	Well, there was some background stuff going on. I just had a great gluten-free pizza at a detox center in Switzerland.
Dr. Mark Hyman:	There you go.
Dr. Tom O'Bryan:	That was really a treat.
Dr. Mark Hyman:	With dairy-free cheese?
Dr. Tom O'Bryan:	Dairy-free cheese, yeah. That's the trilogy in the development of autoimmune diseases is the genetics, the environmental trigger and intestinal permeability.
[00:34:30]	Now, with the brain specifically, autoimmune brain diseases, what most doctors don't realize is that when you have a leak of the intestinal barrier, the leaky gut, that the identification markers to look to see if you've got that are the same identification markers that affect the blood-brain barrier.
Dr. Mark Hyman:	That's a leaky brain.
Dr. Tom O'Bryan:	It's a leaky brain.
Dr. Mark Hyman:	I had a leaky brain.
Dr. Tom O'Bryan: [00:35:00]	I did, too. I called it a breach of the blood-brain barrier, B4. I believe that in the years to come, we're all going to be talking about, "What's your B4 level? Do you have a breach of the blood-brain barrier?" Without that breach of the blood-brain barrier, you can't get antibodies into the brain.
Dr. Mark Hyman:	Mm-hmm.
Dr. Tom O'Bryan:	Antibodies are too big to get through the blood-brain barrier. There must be a tear in the blood-brain barrier that allows these antibodies to get in and for these antibodies to produce against the cerebellum, as an example, to get out into the bloodstream. There has to be a tear in the blood-brain

[00:35:30] barrier B4, a breach of the blood-brain barrier. I think that's critically important and now there are tests that look at B4 to see, do you have a breach, specifically for the brain.

The tests for the gut, leaky gut, say, "Yup that's the mechanism in the gut and that's also the mechanism of the brain, but now there's exhaust when you tear the blood-brain barrier, and you can look for that in bloodwork.

Dr. Mark Hyman: Stress will do that.

Dr. Tom O'Bryan: Stress will do that, very common.

Dr. Mark Hyman: Toxins will do that.

Dr. Tom O'Bryan: That's right.

Dr. Mark Hyman: Inflammatory foods like gluten and dairy can do that.

Dr. Tom O'Bryan: That's exactly right.
[00:36:00]

Dr. Mark Hyman: We see that all the time. It goes against our prevailing theory about the brain, which has been for decades that there's basically an impermeable barrier. Your brain is protected from what's happening in the rest of your body by this blood-brain barrier. We know now that is not true.

Dr. Tom O'Bryan: That is not true. That's the same that we thought about the gut. We used to think there was a kind of intracellular cement between the cells and the gut. Now we know, thanks to Dr. Fasano, those cells
[00:36:30] open up, and they close. The blood-brain barrier works the same way. The way I explained it to patients, it's like the Panama Canal. The gates open, a little food comes in, the gate closes. New gates open, food goes down a little bit lower between the cells. Gates close, the immune system checks it out. That's happening in the blood-brain barrier also.

Dr. Mark Hyman: If someone has an immune problem and autoimmune disease, and they think it may be affecting their brain, what can they do?
[00:37:00]

Dr. Tom O'Bryan: Identify the markers that show the problem is there, which is critically important. It doesn't matter that you have symptoms and just say, "Okay I have symptoms, let's fix it."

You have to identify, how bad is it so that six months from now, as you're doing the protocols, and you're feeling better you go back can say, "Oh look, it's fixed."

Dr. Mark Hyman: The protocols being ...

Dr. Tom O'Bryan: The protocols being stop throwing gasoline on the fire, take nutrients to help heal brain tissue. Make
[00:37:30] sure you're getting enough fish oils. Make sure you're getting enough N-acetylcysteine. Make sure you have enough glutathione. Look to see if you have heavy metals. What are the triggers that are setting all these things off?

It's the Functional Medicine approach that needs to be taken. There's no package that's going to fit exclusively ...

Dr. Mark Hyman: Take out the bad stuff, replace it with good stuff.

Dr. Tom O'Bryan: Take out the bad stuff, put in some good stuff. That's the bottom line to it. You want to make sure you have your baseline to start. You can then go back and check and confirm. You start feeling better pretty quickly usually, and you say, "I'm feeling better, I guess I can go back and have a little once in a while now." You know?

Dr. Mark Hyman:
[00:38:00]
That's like a patient I had. I put him on a carbohydrate-restricted diet because he had terrible diabetes and obesity. He says, "I know my blood sugar is better, can I go back to eating my carbohydrates?" I'm like, "Sorry, it doesn't work like that."

Dr. Tom O'Bryan:
No, it doesn't. I'm sorry that it doesn't.

Dr. Mark Hyman:
[00:38:30]
You mentioned the importance of an intact gut barrier, and not getting a leaky gut. That often is caused by imbalances in our gut flora. We call it dysbiosis. How do foods contribute to that, like gluten? How can we go about fixing that problem?

Dr. Tom O'Bryan:
Really important question. I know that some of your experts in this series have talked about the gut and the microbiota and how it affects the brain. We know that the bacteria in the gut have a great deal to say about how much neurotransmitters are being produced in the brain, serotonin, melatonin, the catecholamines. The bacteria in the gut have so much say about all that.

[00:39:00]

[00:39:30]
Here's the problem when you go gluten-free: wheat is not really bad for you. There are some components of wheat that are good for you. It's not all bad, but the bad, when you cross the line, is bad enough that you have to stop. The good components of wheat—78 percent of the prebiotics, those are the foods that feed the good bacteria in the gut—78 percent of the prebiotics in the American diet are wheat. When you take wheat out of somebody's diet, you remove 78% of all the food for the good bacteria in their gut that they've grown dependent on.

Dr. Mark Hyman:
Mm-hmm.

Dr. Tom O'Bryan:

[00:40:00]
When you do that, a few months down the road the good bacteria are dying off because they're not being fed. When you eat gluten-free products, it doesn't have the same fibers in it. The good bacteria are dying off and you get worse. You get more dysbiosis problems in your gut when you go gluten-free, unless you understand and replace those prebiotics from wheat with other types of prebiotics.

[00:40:30]
That's why I tell all of my patients, "Mrs. Patient, when you go shopping, preferably at a natural food store or an organic food store whenever possible, buy every root vegetable that's there, turnips, parsnips, rutabagas, Jerusalem artichokes, sweet potatoes, stay away from the white potatoes because of the sugar problem with them. All of the root vegetables, radishes ... Every day, you have two different root vegetables as part of the vegetables you're eating. Those root vegetables are the prebiotics that will feed the good bacteria in your gut. When you vary the root vegetables you're having, you get the diversity, so you're feeding all of the good bacteria."

Dr. Mark Hyman:
Tuesday is turnips.

Dr. Tom O'Bryan:
Tuesdays are turnips, that's a good one.

Dr. Mark Hyman:
[00:41:00]
Tom, we have 80 million people in America with autoimmune diseases; it's more than cancer, heart disease, and diabetes put together.

Dr. Tom O'Bryan:
Yes.

Dr. Mark Hyman:
It can be depressing and scary. What you're saying is that we have a big problem, and that our brains are being affected by it. It's our diet that's causing it. That's kind of a depressing message. What do you see is the future and our possibility of actually addressing this more head-on? What does the future look like for autoimmune disease?

Dr. Tom O'Bryan: [00:41:30]	When you see a Functional Medicine practitioner, or you apply the Functional Medicine principles from your books, from my book, when you apply these principles, you better feel better in three weeks. I don't care what you have. You should notice you're feeling better within three weeks. That gives you hope to know that if you stay with this, dial it down, learn a little bit more, keep learning, you're going to nail this thing. You will get it. Three weeks, that's all it takes. If you're not feeling better, we've missed something. That's been the premise of my practice forever, and in yours.
[00:42:00] Dr. Mark Hyman:	It's true. We had, in our three-week program, a 68 percent reduction in all symptoms from all diseases.
Dr. Tom O'Bryan:	Yes. Yes.
Dr. Mark Hyman:	Which is unheard of ...
Dr. Tom O'Bryan:	Yes.
Dr. Mark Hyman:	It doesn't matter what you have.
Dr. Tom O'Bryan:	Yes.
Dr. Mark Hyman:	It's all inflammatory.
Dr. Tom O'Bryan: [00:42:30]	That's the way it's supposed to be. If we're doctors, and doctors being teachers, and we're teaching people how to be healthier, they should notice they're feeling healthier pretty quickly. Now, depending on how bad you were coming into this, it may take two years. But, as long as you know you're on the right track, and you have validation you're on the right track, it empowers you to stay in the game and stay focused on this.
Dr. Mark Hyman:	That's impressive. There is hope for the future.
Dr. Tom O'Bryan: [00:43:00]	There is hope for all of us, but you cannot follow the traditional approach. I think this is an important visual. When patients have symptoms, it's like they've fallen over a waterfall, down into the pool. The waterfall is coming down at them. The water's all turbulent. They're just swimming to stay alive, trying to get through these symptoms. They want the life jacket that's going to get them through these symptoms. That's where pharmaceuticals are really helpful, to keep people afloat, to keep them going. You have to go upstream to the other side of the waterfall, and look and see what fell into the river before it fell over the waterfall. What fell into the river in my life? What was it I got exposed to? Am I sensitive to foods? Do I have too much mercury? Do I have a toxic environment around me? What is it?
[00:43:30] [00:44:00]	When we can empower people to stay focused, stay afloat, with their pharmaceuticals or whatever they need, but also be asking the questions where is this coming from, then three weeks, that's all it takes. That's all it takes to notice you're on the right track. Once again, it may take you two years. It may take a long time because you've really been at this a while, going downhill or down into the waterfall. You'll know you're feeling better, you're on the right track.
Dr. Mark Hyman:	Basically, a month for every year that you've been sick is what I tell patients.
Dr. Tom O'Bryan:	That's rational.
Dr. Mark Hyman:	If they've been sick for 10 years, it's going to be 10 months.
Dr. Tom O'Bryan:	That's rational, that's really rational. If we can give them that framework, most people can handle that.

Dr. Mark Hyman: Yeah. Very exciting. Well thank you, Tom, great to have you on the show.

Dr. Tom O'Bryan: Thank you.

Dr. Tom Sult:	I was born with dyslexia, which means I don't take tests well. I applied to 42 US medical schools and didn't get a single interview. I went to acupuncture school, and that's where I really was introduced to this idea of holism.
[00:00:30]	In traditional Chinese medicine, an ailment on the skin of your leg, that looks exactly like something on the skin of your arm, they're actually totally different diseases. That introduced me to a bigger idea than standard Western thinking about skin disease.
[00:01:00] [00:01:30]	From there, I learned about foreign schools. I went to Grenada in the West Indies for two years, and while I was there I was able to live with a Grenadian family who was very interested in preserving traditional culture. While living with them, I was introduced to a number of local, what they call, "bush doctors." I didn't understand that term at first. I was thinking like, Australia and the bush, which means the Outback, but really the bush is herbs. They were actually talking about bushes and using herbs. I was able to witness a number of shamanic rituals and herbal concoctions, and it was really fascinating to me and it was such a contrast to the biochemistry, histology, and pathology I was learning in medical school at the time, so that just kept resonating with me.
[00:02:00]	I was able to transfer to the University of California Los Angeles, UCLA, and I met Norman Cousins there. Norman Cousins is a writer. He wrote many books—he's deceased now. He was the current chairman of the Department of Psychoneuroimmunology, which is a fancy way to say holistic medicine. I met him and basically camped in his office for the next two years while I was at UCLA, and we stayed in close contact until his death. He was a major mentor to me in understanding how we're one organism. We're not just a collection of liver, kidneys, heart, and brain. We're one organism. Our mind is a tremendously powerful part of that organism.
[00:02:30] [00:03:00]	From there I went to residency and got most of those ideas drummed out of my head by the workday necessities of taking care of the critically ill. Immediately after residency, my very first patient, oddly enough, was a woman with chronic fatigue syndrome. She asked me if I could help her because her nutritionally-oriented physician was several hours away. My response to that was, "What's a nutritionally-oriented physician?" From there, I rediscovered my roots of being interested in holism; so that's sort of my story.
	I like to say to my patients when they ask, "What is Functional Medicine?" I tell them, and I do what the Lipitor commercial says to do, and that is after a trial of diet and lifestyle, consider Lipitor. Well, if you do the diet and lifestyle right, you rarely need the Lipitor. Functional Medicine is asking a fundamentally different question.
[00:03:30] [00:04:00] [00:04:30]	In conventional medicine we're asking, "What? What's the diagnosis?" Once you have the diagnosis there is sort of a prescribed set of treatments based on algorithms. In Functional Medicine we're asking, "Why?" An individual might have heart disease. Okay, how do you treat heart disease conventionally? Well, you might use some kind of cholesterol lowering medicine, you might send them to the cath lab and they get a stent or whatever. But in Functional Medicine the question is, "Why do you have heart disease and someone else doesn't?" We know that more than half of people with heart disease have normal cholesterol, so clearly, it's not just cholesterol. Asking these "why" questions gets underneath the symptoms and underneath the conventional diagnosis to more personalized medicine. One person with heart disease might have a problem with the way they process folic acid and they have a high homocysteine that causes a problem. Another person might have high inflammatory markers, and so on.

[00:05:00] Interestingly enough, if you have four people with heart disease, all four might have different underlying "whys?", whereas four people with four different diagnoses might have the same underlying "why?" It becomes less about the diagnosis and much more about the individual's relationship with their environment. By environment, I mean their diet, lifestyle, thoughts, beliefs, community, purpose, and sense of belonging. All of those things impact our health.

[00:05:30] In thinking about neurological conditions, whether it's autism, Parkinson's, MS, or dementia of various kinds, there are clearly many different causes. Trying to ferret out the underlying cause and managing that cause is really a much more powerful intervention. Sometimes infectious disease can be an underlying cause. There's evidence that a significant fraction of people with dementia actually have some tick-borne illness like Lyme, Bartonella, or some other tick-borne disease. Treating that can be helpful.

Other people have abnormalities of their intracellular metabolism. We measure their B12 in their blood and it looks fine, but when we measure markers that tell us about how well B12 works inside the cells, it turns out to be abnormal. Looking broader than just the diagnosis is often a much more powerful way to intervene.

[00:06:00] Inflammation is the body's attempt to warn the rest of the system. If almost any bad thing is happening, the cells at the site of the irritation will send out alarm chemicals and these are alarm messenger molecules. These alarm molecules are generally inflammatory. It turns out that if you happen to have a
[00:06:30] ragweed allergy and you inhale ragweed pollen, that will, through a series of biochemical steps, cause your mast cells to release histamine. Histamine causes all the symptoms we know of as an allergy, but it is also telling the rest of the immune system there's something happening that it should be paying attention to. Fundamentally, inflammation is simply the body's attempt to communicate with the rest of the immune system, and the rest of the body, and that there's something going on that should be paid attention to.

[00:07:00] A depressed individual will have inflammation of their brain. Inflammation, just like if you hit your thumb with a hammer, the moment the hammer bounces off of your thumb, the injury is over, but your thumb swells for the next week probably, and it takes another two weeks before your thumb is normal
[00:07:30] again. The same thing happens with your brain. Your brain is inflamed, your thumb isn't going to work particularly well when it's inflamed; neither is your brain. When you have an inflamed brain, something is not going to work right. If you have the flu and you have an inflamed brain, you just feel foggy, and you feel awful, but you also feel depressed. People with acute viral illnesses will say things like, "I feel so awful, I just want to die." Well, that sounds a little bit like somebody in a deep depression, doesn't it? It's the same kind of process.

[00:08:00] How do you reduce inflammation? The first thing you want to do is take away the thing that is causing inflammation. If we go back to our ragweed allergy, you want to try to avoid ragweed, right? You want to get away from the thing that is causing inflammation. Next, there are many nutritional things that reduce inflammation. Eat a diet that has lots of natural color (I don't mean Skittles). The great thing
[00:08:30] about fast food or candy is that every single bite has a full day's supply of food coloring, because we don't need any. Deep, colorful vegetables are anti-inflammatory. You'd think something like peppers, that are just hot as can be, would be inflammatory; but actually peppers are anti-inflammatory. The flavors are not what we're talking about; it's actually the biochemical reactions of these foods.

[00:09:00] The best medicine always starts with food, so a variety of foods. I tell people, you know you've heard about, "Get your five a day," which stands for three vegetables and two fruits. But that comes from, "Get your three to five vegetables and two to three fruits." Nobody talks about get your eight a day, but if you're unwell, you should be getting your eight to ten a day, and then a variety. People eat peas, carrots, corn, and then the next day maybe they have peas, carrots, and corn, and after that they probably have peas, carrots, and corn. But if you really think about it, there are 21 meals in a week,
[00:09:30] right? Three times seven. If you thought about 21 different fruits and vegetables every week, that's variety, and that's going to give you lots of different nutrients.

Expert Interviews – Tom Sult, MD

© 2017 Hyman Digital. All Rights Reserved.

[00:10:00] One of the other things I like to tell my patients, "If you were a carrot, eating carrots would be perfect nutrition." There are some taboos about eating other humans, so let's not go there, but eating a wide variety of different fruits and vegetables is more likely to get you complete nutrition. That's the idea, lots of variety because we need all the different nutrients to function at peak performance.

[00:10:30] Mitochondria are my favorite things. In fact, I purchased an electron microscope at one time in my career to study mitochondrial membrane dynamics. Mitochondria are the power plants of every cell, nearly every cell in the body. It turns out red blood cells don't have them, but every other cell in the body basically has in the vicinity of 200 mitochondria.

[00:11:00] Mitochondria are where you convert your food into energy in the most efficient way. You can turn food into energy in an inefficient way without mitochondria, but you get more than 20 times the energy out of your food if you're utilizing your mitochondria. If you don't have optimally functioning mitochondria, you don't make energy. If you don't make energy ... and by the way, the molecule of energy we're talking about is called ATP. ATP is the common currency for every biochemical reaction in the body. If you're not making adequate amounts of ATP, you can't do anything well. You can't build proteins, make hormones, repair your tissues, repair your DNA, you can't do anything properly. You can't even move your muscles. If you can't move your muscles, that translates into feeling fatigued. If you can't make neurotransmitters, that translates into not thinking clearly, having brain fog, or maybe depression, or

[00:11:30] maybe anxiety, or any other number of psychosomatic or psychological symptoms.

[00:12:00] These mitochondria are critically important for well-being on every level. Mitochondria are optimized in the same way we optimize everything else in our lives; it's diet and lifestyle. So, we go back to that rainbow diet. We go back to that sense of belonging, purpose, meaning, and safety. If you're living in a very unsafe world, or if you're perceiving your world as very unsafe, you get into something called fight-or-flight. When you're in fight-or-flight, you want to shunt blood away from your intestines, so that it goes to your big muscles, so that you can fight-or-flight. Fight or run, right? If you're shunting blood away from your intestines, you're not digesting well, you're not absorbing well, and you're doing something else; you're actually altering your microbiome, which is probably the most important organ

[00:12:30] in our body—the microbiome being this teeming ecology of bacteria that lives in our gut.

[00:13:00] One other thing: 70% of the immune system lines the gut. If you're shunting blood away from your gut, you're shunting blood away from 70% of your immune system. What is all of that doing, and how does that relate to mitochondria? Well, we need that nutrition. If we're not digesting and absorbing our food, if our microbiome is not functioning adequately, they alter our nutritional density. It's not just the nutritional density of the blood, it's the nutritional density inside our cells. As an example, there is 10 times more magnesium in our heart than in our blood. There's 100 times more vitamin C in our adrenal glands than in our blood, and 1,000 times more iodine in our thyroid than in our blood. It's being pumped actively. As we're sicker and sicker, as the ATP is getting lower and lower, as the mitochondria are working less and less, the ability to pump nutrients out of the blood and inside the cells diminishes.

[00:13:30] Somebody with congestive heart failure has 65% less magnesium in their heart than they would normally. When we can't pump this stuff, when we don't have enough ATP to pump nutrients into our cells, nothing works well. If things aren't working well, we go back to the same scenario. You can't make neurotransmitters, you can't repair your tissues, you can't do much of anything optimally and so you

[00:14:00] can't detoxify. So, you make amyloid plaque, and that's one of the features of certain kinds of dementia, and so on.

[00:14:30] Neurofeedback is a kind of biofeedback where we use our own brainwaves. We generally do what's called a quantitative EEG, and that's an EEG where we compare your brain waves to an age- and sex-matched control group. We try to find a normal, right? And then we compare your brain activity to the "normal" and then design a program based on your symptoms, situation, and quantitative EEG, and we try to normalize those areas that seem to be giving you grief.

As an example, perhaps you're a pilot and you're used to flying in bad weather and flying only on instruments without being able to look out the cockpit. You might have a part of your brain that is

[00:15:00] hypervigilant and hyperactive, but that's because of your profession. So, making that normal probably wouldn't be beneficial to that individual. It's not just about taking the stuff that's abnormal and making it normal, it's about understanding the person's symptomatology that is undesirable and normalizing those areas of the brain.

[00:15:30] Fundamentally, in biofeedback, what we're doing is making you aware of something you would not ordinarily be aware of. In EEG biofeedback or neurofeedback, what we're doing is making you aware of those areas of your brain that are not beneficial to you. They're maybe overactive, so you have ADD-like symptoms, or maybe they're underactive and you have depressive symptoms or forgetful symptoms, and we try to bring those closer to the normal parameters that you would find in the control group.

[00:16:00] Who's a good candidate for neurofeedback? Certainly, this is an emerging field, but we use it in our office for depression, for ADD, for dementia. There's a whole other group of people who use it for sort of performance enhancement. We don't do very much of that in our office because we're mostly seeing the unwell, but in the wellness community people who are trying to optimize their brain function, certainly there's a lot of experimentation in that area. We're really focused on treating people non-pharmacologically for their attention deficit, depression, or their dementia types of things.

[00:16:30] Every new patient who comes to our office gets a heart rate variability assessment. Heart rate variability is not variability between 60 and 100. What we're really talking about is variability within 60 beats per minute. So, it's those little microsecond variances of beat to beat variability. That turns out to be governed by the sort of struggle between the sympathetic nervous system, also called fight-or-flight,

[00:17:00] and the parasympathetic nervous system, called rest-and-digest. There's this dynamic play between sympathetic and parasympathetic every single heartbeat. That variability is the result of that interplay. By analyzing that variability, we can actually access the degree of fight-or-flight or rest-and-digest. Every single patient who walks in the office gets this assessment and we determine their balance.

[00:17:30] In my office, virtually everyone is deeply locked in fight-or-flight. My patients have been sick a long time. They've been seen by a lot of doctors, they've been trying to struggle through their illness, they probably have been trying to work through their illness, so they've been driving themselves forward with adrenaline and sheer willpower. They have fried their balance of their autonomic nervous system. This is the first assessment we do: we really try to understand some balance of their autonomic nervous system.

[00:18:00] Once we understand that balance, it goes back to that idea of what happens when you're in fight-or-flight. You're shunting blood away from your intestines, you're reducing blood flow to your immune system, you're altering your microbiome because of the change in peristalsis, food digestion, and so on. As soon as we find somebody who's obviously locked in fight-or-flight, we know we have a lot of work to do in terms of not just getting them back into a balance in their fight-or-flight, but we know they're

[00:18:30] likely to have dysbiosis, leaky gut, and so on and so forth. It's a big big piece of the assessment we do in our office.

Nutritional deficiencies can manifest in a lot of ways. I mentioned earlier there's a big difference between what's in your blood and what's inside your cells. In fact, the idea of deficiency comes from blood levels. You may well have totally normal blood levels of a nutrient, but you may be intracellularly

[00:19:00] deficient. As an example, in dementia you may have normal B12 in your blood, but when we measure methylmalonic acid or homocysteine, those may be abnormal, and that tells us that the utilization of B12 inside your cells is abnormal. The old idea of, "Do you have nutritional deficiency?" is drawing your blood and seeing if you have enough of that vitamin in your blood. As I mentioned earlier, there are hundreds of times more nutrients inside our cells than in our blood. We're really now becoming aware

[00:19:30] that we have to be concerned about intracellular nutrition much more than blood nutrition.

If you don't have a nutrient sufficiency inside your cells, it turns out that you can't do normal machinery. The normal machinery of the cell won't work right, so it's going to have wide-ranging effects. In the most extreme cases, we know that if you have protein deficiency, you can have a disease

[00:20:00] called kwashiorkor, or if you have insufficient vitamin C you get scurvy. Long before you get those

---

[00:20:30] extreme cases of nutritional deficiency, the machinery just doesn't work well. When your machinery doesn't work well, you get these generalized, vague symptoms. You get the symptoms of the walking-well. I just don't feel good, I'm tired. You know I sleep all night, I wake up and I'm still tired, I have brain fog, I just can't think as clearly as I used to. These kinds of general symptoms are usually associated with intracellular nutritional deficiencies.

[00:21:00] The way you determine the intracellular deficiencies is not by looking at the nutrient itself, but looking at metabolites that the nutrient is associated with. I mentioned earlier, homocysteine. Well, homocysteine is in a homocysteine-methionine pathway, which requires folic acid. You need to be able to convert folic acid to 5-Methyltetrahydrofolate, which is just another kind of folic acid. If you can't do that efficiently, then you can't convert homocysteine into methionine, and you start to build up homocysteine. So, by looking at homocysteine levels in the blood, we can infer that there's a problem with folic acid metabolism. There are many of these kinds of biomarkers we can use.

[00:21:30] There's a fancy way you can take a little blood spot and look at it under an electron microscope and look at the x-ray back splatter. That can tell us about the intracellular mineral concentrations. We've talked about magnesium a few times. Magnesium is probably the most commonly deficient mineral and it is extremely common for it to be intracellularly deficient.

[00:22:00] We live in an all-yang, all-the-time society. We are always "go." You know the first question in America is, "What do you do for a living?" It's not, "How are you?" It's not, "What exciting things are you doing?" It's, "What do you do for a living?" We view our entire worth around our output. Every day I talk to patients who can't work anymore and they feel worthless as human beings. We have worth just as being living creatures. Right? That's worthy in and of itself.

[00:22:30] We are always trying to do more. More with less, right? You go to an efficiency seminar and they tell you how to do more stuff. Well, that just makes us more crazy. What we need to learn to do is distinguish the difference between urgent and important. We're all urgency addicts. We're out there running around in circles because it makes us feel like we're busy and important. What we need to do is take a breath, get rid of that urgent stuff, and only do the important stuff. The important stuff boils [00:23:00] down to very simple things. It's eating well. You know people say, "Well I don't like to cook." Okay, so do you like to be healthy? You know? There're some things to weigh out here.

[00:23:30] Part of the ritual of cooking is the ritual of slowing down. It's the ritual of being with family. I tell my patients that our family ritual is, when the kids were little especially, come home from work, hug your spouse. That hug is a separation from the rest of the day. My wife is not going to go slave away in the kitchen, we're going to go into the kitchen, discuss our day, chop vegetables together, we're going to do whatever it is we do to cook together. We're going to probably have a glass of wine. What is wine? Wine is a fermented, whole-fruit, alcoholic extract of grape. Sounds like a health food when you mention it that way, right? I mean, there are a lot of healthy things in wine. Now, hard liquor, it's a little [00:24:00] harder to make an argument for that, but you know, a moderate amount of wine has been shown to have benefits. Have a glass of wine. Wind down from your day, de-stress. Eat a colorful, healthy, freshly prepared diet.

[00:24:30] You do those things and, suddenly it's not cooking. "I hate to cook." Okay, but do you like to spend time with your family? My son's earliest injury was I gave him a gigantic knife to help cutting vegetables, and he tried to add a little extra meat to the dish, and we ended up having a little fiasco in the kitchen. But, guess what he learned? He learned that knives are sharp and you have to be careful. Nonetheless, the whole family is in the kitchen and we're working together. The kids are learning important life skills, they're also learning about how adults behave, how adults interact, and how to do things. It's bigger [00:25:00] than just cooking, it's an entire life skill. I think it's important to incorporate these things in a more holistic manner. It's not, "Oh, I have to go cook." It's, "Oh, we can create a communal event here, and we can find purpose, meaning, and joy."

[00:25:30] In the beginning, we only had each other. We had community, empathy, and sympathy, but we didn't have anything else. There were no medicines when we were tribal. We developed medicines over time,

BROKEN BRAIN

[00:26:00] but it turns out that still, to this day, community is the most powerful medicine. There's famous work from a famous endocrinologist named Hans Selye who really started to understand the stress response. He was able to look at the neuroendocrine effects of stress and isolation, and they're not good. They cause hypertension, heart disease, and even cancers and psychiatric diseases.

[00:26:30] Then, other work has shown something called the relaxation response. The relaxation response really reverses those stress response things. We have this idea that short-term stress, fight-or-flight, is really good. You know if a sabre-toothed tiger jumps out in front of you, it's a really good idea to fight-or-flight, right? You either run, you fight, you climb a tree, or you die. It's pretty straightforward. But when that episode is over, you go back home and you discuss this event. You find purpose and meaning in this event, and you're, perhaps, even hailed as a hero for defeating this object, right? There's all of this ritual and worship surrounding this event.

[00:27:00] But in modern society, we're chased by a sabre-toothed tiger. Somebody comes into your lane when you're driving, lightning bolts come out of your fingers, and you narrowly avert a disaster. Or you get a letter from the IRS and it's like, "Oh my God, what's going to happen next?" Or any number of things happen, and it's a sabre-toothed tiger. We're surrounded by them.

[00:27:30] Instead of being the adaptive phase, which is that single event that goes away, we're in the stress and then the exhaustion phase. When we're in the exhaustion phase of fight-or-flight, nothing is working well. All of those end-stage things of poor circulation to your brain, poor circulation to your gut, poor immune function are happening.

[00:28:00] How do we counter that? We have to do things that help us balance fight-or-flight. The most simple thing I ask my patients to do is go on a walk and just walk. Don't rehash the fight I just had, don't rehash the meeting I just had, don't think about the 47 things I should be doing right now. Just walk. This is the concept of mindfulness.

[00:28:30] Mindfulness, we think of it as somebody sitting in a full lotus position and all of that business, which would just dislocate my hips, so I don't do that. Simply be present. I was driving one time between two clinics and NPR was on and they were talking about mindfulness, and they had a guy on who was making it very complicated. So, I called in. How mindful is this? I'm driving, I'm listening to the radio, and now I'm also talking on the telephone. When the National Public Radio guy came on I said, "You know, being mindful isn't that hard. There are times every day when you can just stop and be mindful." When you're in the bathroom, just pee. Don't balance your checkbook, don't think about everything else going on. Just do what you're doing. Take a moment. Every time you're in your car there's nothing you can do but drive. You can go, "Ugh, the traffic is making me nuts." Or you can take a breath, relax,

[00:29:00] and realize you're only going to get there when you get there. There are many times during the day when we can choose to get uptight and angry, or simply accept what's happening, because there is nothing we can do about it.

[00:29:30] I actually have bracelets I give most of my patients about the Serenity Prayer, which I like to call the Wisdom Prayer. The Serenity Prayer is: "God grant me the serenity to accept the things I cannot change, the courage to change the things I can, and the wisdom to know the difference." If you apply the wisdom, there are many times during the day when we simply have to go with the flow. Being upset about the flow isn't making the flow different.

[00:30:00] I'm an old whitewater guide and I like to tell my patients, "You're jumping in this creek and it's going that way. There's nothing you can do about it; you're going that way. The current is far too strong, but you can go right or left to miss the big rocks." That's really what it's about. It's just moving a little bit to the right or a little bit to the left to miss the rocks and enjoy the ride. Because if you're not, you're just angry, and if you're angry that's putting you in fight-or-flight, and if you're in fight-or-flight, nothing good is happening.

[00:30:30] Learning new skills is the way our brain develops. There's really interesting research that shows language is what develops our brain. There's actually some really interesting research on a group of deaf people in South America who had created their own very rudimentary sign language. It turns out

---

Expert Interviews – Tom Sult, MD

[00:31:00] that their brain development, because of the rudimentary nature of their sign language, brain development is very different than people who have larger language sets. They were able to show in a specific experiment that when this group of people with very different thought patterns were then taught a more robust sign language, within just a few years their cognitive perceptive abilities changed dramatically. It doesn't mean these people were stupid: these people weren't retarded, they were normal, healthy people, but their language inhibited some of their cognitive processes.

[00:31:30] Learning new things creates new connections. The more connected, the more multi-processing. Now notice I didn't say "multi-tasking," I said "multi-processing," so that's a different thing. Multi-processing is the ability to access more data points more rapidly. That really equates to smartness, if you will. If you can analyze a situation from multiple points of view because you can analyze it from multiple data sets, that's going to give you a broader understanding of your situation.

[00:32:00] Multi-tasking is something different, which, frankly, I don't think actually exists. I think that we can rapidly change our attention focus, but we can't actually do multiple things at once. Learning new skills is clearly important. There's an old saying in physical activity, "If you don't use it, you lose it." It's the same with our mind. If you're coming home from work and you're sitting in front of the TV, and you're just doing the mindless activities because you just are too stressed and burned out to do anything else, [00:32:30] you're not exercising your mind. It's the same thing—if you don't exercise your muscles, they atrophy, if you don't exercise your mind, it atrophies.

The idea that it's easier to learn when we're young, I think, is false. There's some truth to it, but it's also true that we're more distracted when we're older. When I was a teenager I had the luxury of being able to spend infinite time doing pretty much whatever I wanted and then complaining about how I didn't have enough time to do my homework, right? I spent an awful lot of time trying to figure out how to [00:33:00] climb up big rock cliffs and I would love to do that now, but I just don't have the time because I've got a lot of other obligations. I think that's really the essence of it. We can learn whatever we put our mind to learning, but we have to put our mind to it.

[00:33:30] When we're young, perhaps we're less experienced and much more curious, so we're able to focus more. When we're older, we think, "Yeah, I know generally what that is so I don't have to focus on it." But, if you dedicate your life to learning, you're continuously making new connections. When you're making new connections, you're building. Unfortunately, we're also losing connections, so hopefully if we're making new connections at a rate as great as we're losing connections, we can maintain some mental acuity and mental health.

[00:34:00] The real question about blood sugar is, "What's driving your blood sugar?" You know, a healthy young person can be given a giant dose of sugar intravenously, and it won't spike their blood sugar. The issues with blood sugar, dementia, mental health, and all of these things, is less about the sugar, although sugar is a problem, but it's really more about what's driving the sugar.

[00:34:30] Why are we getting insulin resistant? We have insulin and sugar. If the sugar starts to rise, the insulin comes up and drives the sugar back down. Then it rises again and the insulin goes up and pretty soon you're making as much insulin as you can, your pancreas is pumping this stuff out as fast as it can, and yet your blood sugar starts to rise because your insulin can't respond, and at some point it turns over a line, crosses a line that we call diabetes.

[00:35:00] What's driving this insulin resistance? In many cases it's cortisol. Cortisol is being driven by our level of stress. So, it really comes back to what we've been talking about all along. It comes back to being in chronic fight-or-flight. If you're in chronic fight-or-flight, you are raising your cortisol. Cortisol by itself isn't good for your brain. But when the sugar starts to rise, maybe you don't have fasting blood sugar problems, but you have after-meal sugar problems, called postprandial. Now you start to glycate protein. All that means is you have so much sugar in your system that, instead of burning it to make [00:35:30] energy, to make ATP, it starts to just glom onto things. It gloms onto a protein and glycates that protein. That alters the structure of that protein and the function and structure are linked. If the structure changes, the function changes.

[00:36:00]	Sugar gloms on to our proteins and makes them not work as well. Now maybe the enzyme that's supposed to detoxify it can't detoxify it as easily. Maybe it's supposed to be doing something important and it can't do it as efficiently. That ends up causing those intracellular machineries to not work as well. If the intracellular machinery isn't working as well, nothing works well.
[00:36:30]	My top tip for brain health is to live in awe and in compassion. If you think about living in awe, what does that mean? That means you're eternally curious. You're always seeking knowledge, you're always interested, you're always engaging.
[00:37:00]	Living in compassion means you're engaged with your community. You're interested in what's going on, what's happening to people around you and how that impacts not only yourself, but them and the larger community. That ends up giving you a sense of purpose, a sense of community, a sense of place in that community. These are powerful, powerful things. Then if you're really engaged, you know every virtue can become a fault, right? It also becomes about balance. Really, the balance here is that fight-or-flight balance. We need to slow down, take a breath, ok, and find and create communal events.
[00:37:30] [00:38:00]	We have been working on creating something I call "social motion." We're trying to bring back community dances in our community, bringing people together with music, movement, community, and fun. Creating this community, it turns out, is hard. We have these capsules we live in. We live in a home, which is a capsule. It's very insulated. Most of us these days don't even know who our neighbor is, let alone anything about them. We get into another capsule called our car and drive to work. We don't even take public transportation where we might accidentally meet somebody. Then we get to our office, go into our cubicle, which is our next capsule. We're living like the immunodeficient Bubble Boy from the Seinfeld series, right? We're isolated all the time. It's not for someone else to create this community. It's up to us to create our community.
[00:38:30]	That's really what we need, is to live in awe, live in compassion, everything that means about community, and about being one as a human family.

VICKI KOBLINER, MS, RDN | www.holcarenutrition.com

Vicki Kobliner:	I feel really blessed that I'm able to spend my life working with functional nutrition. I started out very traditionally trained as a registered dietician and did a lot of the conventional work that most people do. I worked for a doctor who was very ahead of his time. He basically was a GI specialist, and at a time when people believed that celiac disease was one in 1,000, he was diagnosing it much more frequently, because he was simply testing and looking for it. He was one of the first to realize that it was much more prevalent than we thought.
[00:00:30]	

Celiac disease, which is gluten intolerance, has a lot to do with both intestinal health, but also neurologic health, and he was a pioneer in that field. From there, I started exploring more about celiac disease, and learned that there was a link between gluten intolerance and autism, and I began to explore that. Then as I had my own children around that time, I started to incorporate a lot of what I was learning about different ways to look at food, nutrition, and health in my own children's lives, and from there, it just spiraled. Functional nutrition has been something that has both informed me professionally and personally.

[00:01:00]

You know, it's interesting, a lot of people think about when they're going to have a baby, the most important thing to them is, "What is the nursery going to look like?" They worry about, "Is it going to be decorated beautifully?" Are they going to have the right toys to spark their child's neurologic development? But they don't think about the womb, which is actually the child's first home. When it comes to neurological development and prenatal development as a whole, the most important place you really want to start working is in the womb. That's the child's first exposure, and the placenta is not as strong a barrier as we think it is.

[00:01:30]

Many things can cross the placenta. In fact, there was a study done in 2005 which is one I talk about so frequently in almost every lecture I give. It was by the Environmental Working Group, and they took a number of women and checked the cord blood after they gave birth. What they found was over 280 different toxic chemicals in the cord blood of newborn babies. We think that babies are protected from all of the toxins that we may be exposed to, but this clearly showed us that it's just not true. What happens, what we take in is absolutely critical for what our children and our babies are exposed to in utero. That can be toxic chemicals, it can be things like pesticides or BPA and other endocrine disruptors. Children can also be affected by what they don't get and they can be affected by a lack of vitamin D.

[00:02:00]

[00:02:30]

We know that there are studies showing that maternal deficiencies of vitamin D actually increase risk of autism. We know that selenium is linked to depression when there is a deficiency in utero. As I said, vitamin D is another one that's very, very important. Gluten enteropathy, high sugar diets actually are linked to inflammation. Inflammation is one of the things we're going to talk about a lot today, because high levels of inflammation are linked to lots of neurological disorders. When a mom has a high sugar diet that's low in some of the nutrients she needs for development, that's going to impact babies for life.

[00:03:00]

There's a study that looked at famine and its effect on development over time, and what they found was that babies who were born in times of famine who had poor nutrition, actually had a higher incidence of Alzheimer's and cognitive decline later in life. We see that intake at the very earliest stages can impact life for decades. One of the things we struggle with in the United States is what we call the SAD diet, it's the Standard American Diet, and it is really very sad. It's generally really, really high in processed foods, especially foods that are grain-based, so lots of white flour, lots of sugar. These kinds of diets are what we call proinflammatory. Sugar is very proinflammatory, and one of the things we are learning more and more every day is how much sugar and inflammation is linked to

[00:03:30]

[00:04:00] chronic illness, whether it be heart disease or diabetes, but also linked to neurological problems, including depression, anxiety, and autism.

[00:04:30] Inflammation is linked to all of those, and sugar promotes inflammation. The things that help reduce inflammation are vegetables and fruits, high fiber foods, legumes, nuts, seeds. Those are the kinds of things that are not in a typical American diet. The Standard American Diet, that SAD diet, is proinflammatory, and it also doesn't give you the nutrients that you need to counteract some of that inflammation, all those good vitamins, minerals, and other things that help support helping you address inflammation.

[00:05:00] One of the other issues is that high sugar diets actually impair our gut function. Our digestive tract is supposed to be really rich in good bacteria. The good bacteria help our immune system and our brain. Changes in our good bacteria are linked to depression and anxiety, and other mood disorders, including schizophrenia. We know that when we have a good balance of bacteria in our gut, it promotes normal health. When we don't have that good balance, it promotes disease. One of the problems is that sugar actually reduces the level of good bacteria in our guts, and again, things like fruits and vegetables that are high in fiber help grow that good bacteria.

[00:05:30]
[00:06:00] When we eat this typical diet that's low in the good, healthy, nutrient-rich foods, and high in inflammatory sugars and processed products, it promotes inflammation. The other issue we see a lot in a typical American diet is lots of artificial ingredients, whether it be preservatives or sweeteners or colorings, and there are many, many studies that show that those actually have huge impacts on neurological health and how we function and how we handle stress. We know there's a link to hyperactivity, so there are lots of different ways where what we eat impacts our brain for the long term.

[00:06:30] A lot of people are really worried, especially nowadays, we hear a lot about paleo diets and grain-free diets, and I think that those diets do have a place in good health, but I don't believe that everybody needs to be grain-free. There are many people who can tolerate some of the healthier grains, such as quinoa, millet, sorghum, buckwheat, basically gluten-free grains. In fact, I do have clients who can tolerate gluten. I think it is very individualized. The key factor here is really looking at the balance. How much is your diet based on processed grains, and how much of it is whole grains? The predominant part of your diet should really be fruits and vegetables, bright, rich, colorful foods that add lots of nutrients and antioxidants to your diet.

[00:07:00]
[00:07:30] A much smaller part of it should be those grains, if at all. When we think about what we're cooking for dinner, very often the first thing we'll think about, "Well, what's my protein? I'm going to have chicken for dinner, and then I'm going to have rice with it," and the last thing you think about is the vegetable. In truth, a really healthy diet would be, "Well, what's my vegetable tonight?", and then, "What kind of protein am I going to put with that, as a smaller portion?" The vegetable should really be half the plate, and then the protein portion should be about a quarter, and if you're having grains, that should be an additional quarter, but what you really want is the plant produce. You want the fruits, vegetables, nuts, seeds, and legumes to be more of a part of that diet, and the grains are really secondary, and good quality animal protein should also be a part of it.

[00:08:00] When we talk about good quality animal protein, all foods should be good quality. It's not only eating fruits and vegetables, but it's the source. There is research showing that pesticides are also linked to ADHD in areas where pregnant women live near high pesticide spraying—there's a higher incidence of ADHD in their children. We know that pesticides disrupt a lot of different pathways in the body. They're linked to cancer and other chronic illnesses, and we know that neurologically, early exposure can have long term effects. Organic food, food that's free of pesticides and chemicals is really, really important. Another issue we see is heavy metals, and heavy metals in utero can have a really deleterious effect on children's growth and development, and also in the early stages.

[00:08:30]

[00:09:00]

One of the things that's important to remember, is that growing babies and children are so much smaller than we are, that the impact of the same dose of some sort of toxin is going to be much greater on them. They're also developing their brains at that time, so the same amount that we may be exposed to as adults is generally more toxic for them. Most studies aren't done in children of that size, so when we say something may be safe, we really don't know if it's safe in utero, because we really haven't tested it that way. The only thing we haven't tested is combinations of chemicals. We may test a chemical in isolation, but we don't test the synergy of how a combination of chemicals impacts our children, especially in utero. That's an area where we don't know, and we need to err on the side of caution, because we really have no idea.

[00:09:30]

[00:10:00]

When we see what these things can do to adults and growing children, we have to assume the effects in utero are going to be much worse. When we're thinking about having that clean body and that clean womb, the first thing I look at is our food supply. Again, pesticide-free organic food. I also really like to make sure that my meat comes from grass-fed or pasture-fed animals. Animals are growing, and they require their own nutrition, so when they are fed things that are inappropriate to them, they become less nutritionally complete. When we eat those animals, we also don't get the same nourishment. For example, grass-fed beef has higher levels of certain nutrients that are really important for brain growth. When we eat processed, conventionally-fed animals that are fed antibiotics and hormones, and all kinds of pesticides, they are often sick animals, and when we eat sick animals, it has the propensity to make us sick as well.

[00:10:30]

[00:11:00]

We want our animals to be clean, and we want our food to be pesticide-free. There is a high incidence of arsenic in rice, and chicken has been fed arsenic for years. They're actually stopping, that's becoming much less nowadays, that people are aware of it, but we want to make sure that we're not eating heavy metal-laden food. Areas of coal often have higher mercury levels, even in the air. We see a higher incidence of autism and other neurodevelopmental problems in areas where there is a lot of coal in the air. Lead is still around in the ground, so there are a lot of areas where we are exposed to heavy metals. One of the best things we can do is make sure our body's natural detoxification systems work right so we can actually get rid of some of those heavy metals.

[00:11:30]

By doing that, we need, what makes our detoxification systems work? Nutrition. Our body makes something called glutathione, and glutathione is what we need to detoxify ourselves. Glutathione is made from pieces of protein, and it requires a lot of different nutrients for our bodies to make that glutathione, which we need to detoxify. If we don't have the right nutrition because our diet is too high in processed foods and low in fruits, vegetables, nuts, seeds, and other important vitamin and nutrient-rich foods, we can't make that glutathione. If we're not eating enough protein, I see that in a lot of children, they eat a diet that's very high in crackers, cookies, and pasta, etc., and they're not getting enough of the protein they need to make that good glutathione.

[00:12:00]

[00:12:30]

We want our body's own detoxification system to work well. The other thing I see is that we're limited in fat. We're a culture that's been taught that fat is dangerous, and the truth is that's not actually the case, especially for growing children and prenatally. Our brains are predominantly fat. When we don't eat enough fat, when we don't get enough fat, we can't support that good brain growth. There are two components that are really important for brain health that come from fat. One is DHA, which is an omega-3. We've heard about fish oil. Eating good quality fish is a way that we can get that DHA. Now, the problem with that speaks to the problem of heavy metals. A lot of fish is contaminated with mercury, so getting mercury-free, clean fish can be a challenge.

[00:13:00]

It's important to make sure we get our fish oil in a way that's clean, possibly from a supplement. The other thing that's really critical for brain health is something called choline. Choline comes from fats, it's found in high amounts in eggs. Again, we've been taught very often to avoid the egg yolk, but the egg yolk is rich in choline, and it's really important for brain health. There are studies that show that when we supplement with choline and DHA, we grow more neural cells in utero, so that's really, really important and helpful for long term brain development.

[00:13:30]

People look at prenatal diets, and they think about how that should be different from a typical diet, and in most cases, it should be the same. A prenatal diet should be clean, free of artificial ingredients such as sweeteners, colorings, and preservatives. It should be rich in organic produce and good sources of pasture-fed proteins, or vegetarian sources of protein. Some nutrients, though, are especially important for pregnant women, one of which is iron. We also know that iron, or low iron, in utero can lead to cognitive challenges later in life. We see that there are IQ changes in areas where there's chronic iron deficiency. Selenium and lycopene, lycopene is something that we find in tomatoes, those are actually really helpful for promoting normal mood.

[00:14:00]

[00:14:30]

Pregnant women really have to focus on iron. They also need zinc, because zinc is very, very important for cell replication, which is obviously critical in that prenatal time, but things like iron and zinc are not found in very high quantities in processed food, unless they're supplemented. Again, getting the natural form of the food is really important. Another nutrient that's critical in the prenatal period is folate, and we know that deficiencies of folate can lead to things like neural tube defects, so we actually add higher levels of folate to a lot of prenatal supplements, and we also fortify it in the food supply. Unfortunately, we fortify that folate in grains, which is not necessarily the area that we really want to promote lots of high intake.

[00:15:00]

[00:15:30]

The form of folate is also important because folic acid is the form that is supplemented. However, there is some research that shows there are certain genetic mutations that make some women and children less able to move it. Folic acid is synthetic, and it is not the active form. The active form is the one your body uses to do its work, and the active form of folate is something called MTHF. When you can't process that folate and activate it, it's not as beneficial. For some people, it's much more important to get that active form, and make sure that it's the form they're eating or consuming. Supplementation with the active form is actually often more helpful for women who are pregnant than supplementing simply with folic acid.

[00:16:00]

[00:16:30]

One of the things you can do to know if you have this defect is to get tested for something called MTHFR. The MTHFR defect may reduce your metabolism and your ability to activate that folic acid. Knowing that in advance can help you effectively support your own folate status. One of the things I've seen in my career is an epidemic of chronic illnesses in America's children. In fact, I did write a nutrition chapter for a book called *Compromised Generation: The Epidemic of Chronic Illness in America's Children*, and it's such an important topic for me. I'm also actually on the board of an organization called the Neurological Health Foundation. The mission for that, as well as Epidemic Answers, which I'm also on the board of, is to help reduce this epidemic of neurological and other chronic diseases in children.

[00:17:00]

[00:17:30]

I think it's a perfect storm of a variety of issues. We are increasingly living in a toxic society, we have more and more chemicals in our environment. Again, as I mentioned, we don't know the synergy between all the chemicals that are out there—what we breathe, what we ingest, what we drink in our water. We are exposed to more medication, we are exposed to a much more depleted food supply, and one that's filled with more artificial ingredients. When we are exposed to these things, we need to get rid of them. As I said before, the way we get rid of them is through our body's natural detoxification pathways, but when you're not eating the foods and getting those nutrients that help our bodies detoxify, you have no way to counteract this onslaught of toxins. The other key factor here is the gut, and what we call the microbiome. Again, that good bacteria we need in our gut should be like a lawn, it should be like a rich, lush, thick carpet of grass.

[00:18:00]

Instead, what we're seeing is people who consistently have what we call leaky gut, they have brown patches on their lawn, lots of open spaces filled with weeds. Those weeds are other types of bacteria or germs that cause inflammation, and there's a lot of research that actually looks at depression as an inflammatory condition. There are many, many linkages between increased markers of inflammation in the body and increases in mood disorders. When we have this imbalance of good and bad bacteria in our guts, it becomes difficult for us to activate normal enzymes. Those enzymes are necessary for

Expert Interviews – Vicki Kobliner, MS, RDN

[00:18:30]   digesting the food we eat. If we can't digest them right, we can't get access to those nutrients we need.

[00:19:00]   We also know that these probiotics, these good bacteria, modulate inflammation. We also know that probiotics activate B vitamins, and B vitamins are critical for normal brain health. When we can't activate B vitamins, our brains can't function properly. I work a lot with both children and adults who have mood disorders, depression, anxiety, schizophrenia, etc., and autism and ADHD can go with that as well. One of the things I always find interesting is that, we think about medication, medication is often a first line for somebody who's suffering with anxiety or depression, but if you have depression and you get an SSRI ... An SSRI is something that's supposed to help you maintain the serotonin in your brain.

[00:19:30]   Serotonin is a happy neurotransmitter. We make serotonin from protein, a protein building block called tryptophan. We also need a lot of nutrients like magnesium and zinc and many others to make that serotonin. You can take all the Prozac you want, but if you don't have enough zinc, magnesium, and tryptophan to make serotonin, it's going to be hard for you to actually lift that depression. Again,

[00:20:00]   food is one of the primary sources of where we get our mental health, and if we're not eating the right food, it's going to be very hard to maintain normal mood. Again, I think what we're doing is we're feeding a diet that's depleted, so we don't have those building blocks to help support our brains, we don't have enough good fats, we don't have enough good vitamins and minerals, we don't have all those brightly colored fruits and vegetables, we have too much inflammatory foods.

[00:20:30]   When we link that, this deficit in the supportive nutrients, with all the toxins we're being exposed to, there's this huge divide that is becoming harder and harder to overcome when our digestive health is so negatively impacted ... One of the other things that negatively impacts our digestive health is antibiotics. Chronic antibiotic use, those antibiotics will kill germs, but they'll also kill the good bacteria, and if we don't re-establish that, then it's very hard for our immune function and our brain health to be optimal. Another area where our microbiome and our gut is affected is even with things like C-sections. That starts from birth.

[00:21:00]   If Mom has had lots of antibiotics, if she doesn't have good flora, then her birth canal is not going to be populated with flora. Babies get exposed to their own flora from their mom's birth canal. When a baby is born via C-section, they don't get exposed to that good flora, so they can be starting out from birth unable to colonize their own good bacteria properly. When that happens, it can affect their digestion from birth, and when it affects their digestion, it's going to affect all the things we're talking

[00:21:30]   about—their immune health, brain health, gut health, and it's going to have far-reaching consequences.

[00:22:00]   When we see that babies are born via C-section, or even for example, I see a lot in my practice, early on, babies who have colic, who have eczema, who have reflux, these things are not normal in babies, and they shouldn't occur. They often speak to me about a baby who doesn't have good intestinal health, they often are linked to all kinds of inflammation. I love probiotics and there are lots of different ones that can be very very helpful, and it's important to colonize early, but the other thing that you can do is naturally colonize both Mom and baby by using what we call lacto-fermented foods. Lacto-fermented foods naturally contain bacteria, and what's interesting is that every traditional culture in the world except Americans, generally, have some sort of lacto-fermented food in their culture.

[00:22:30]   Yogurt, kimchi, miso, or kavas—they're often bitter, tangy types of foods. Americans don't tend to like bitter, tangy foods, because we've taught ourselves to love sweet, but those foods are naturally found in almost all traditional cultures, and they naturally grow good bacteria in our bodies and are a wonderful way to do that. We're starting to see more of that available in American supermarkets, mostly in health food stores. You can ferment your own foods. Kombucha is a great drink that's naturally fermented, apple cider vinegar often is lacto-fermented and has natural bacteria, natural

[00:23:00] enzymes that are really great for gut health, and that's another really good way to start early with colonizing that good bacteria.

[00:23:30] When we talk about the intestinal bacteria and the lack thereof, or what I call the weeds, another name for that is intestinal permeability or leaky gut, some of the things you can do to help resolve leaky gut issues or help heal them is a multi-faceted approach. Number one, you want to get rid of those things that grow the bad bacteria, like sugar, like processed carbohydrates. You want to eat lots of the things that grow the good stuff, that support its growth, those are called prebiotics. Certain types of fibers are really, really good for that. Again, those fibers are often going to come from fruits and vegetables. You want to add that good bacteria from lacto-fermented foods, so you want to grow

[00:24:00] the good bacteria, and you want to starve out the negative, undesirable germs.

The other thing you can do is there are lots of herbs that are really wonderful as natural antimicrobials, which help normalize that gut. Things like garlic, rosemary, oregano and olive are great at helping reestablish a normal gut. Those are great for managing microbes naturally, and I use a lot of them in my practice. I've seen so many different types of children in my practice, it is not

[00:24:30] necessarily just kids on the spectrum or kids with neurodevelopmental delays. I actually see adults and children. Really, the underlying theme for all of them is chronic illness, and chronic illness, again, often just goes right back to inflammation, and inflammation often goes back to the gut. Those two things are so closely linked.

One of the things people don't realize is that the communication between the brain and the gut is

[00:25:00] two-way, and the gut talks to the brain more often than the brain talks to the gut. A lot of our neurotransmitters are actually produced in our guts, so when our gut is not working right, it's very hard to get that communication back and forth, and to keep our brains healthy. I see lots of people with chronic inflammation, and that can be children with eczema, colic, reflux. It can be children with autism and ADHD, adults with mood disorders, children with mood disorders. I work with people with multiple sclerosis, irritable bowel, any kind of digestive dysfunction, and one of the things I haven't

[00:25:30] really talked a lot about yet is gluten, and gluten's role in inflammation.

Again, celiac disease used to be considered a very rare disease, and we know now that it really averages a little over one in 100. It can have far-reaching consequences, both digestively, but also emotionally and mentally. Gluten intolerance is linked to schizophrenia, there's a lot of research that shows linkages between those two things. It's linked to depression. There's an enzyme called glutamate decarboxylase, and it changes, it breaks down something called glutamate. Glutamate is

[00:26:00] very excitatory, and it makes us hyped up, it can make us more anxious. Normally, we have seesaw in our body, where we go from glutamate to something called GABA, which is calming and relaxing. When you have a lot of glutamate, this glutamate decarboxylase is supposed to break it down and help it move to GABA.

[00:26:30] Gluten can interfere with that glutamate decarboxylase. It actually disrupts that seesaw, so the seesaw remains elevated, and you can't get that calming. Gluten can have that effect. We don't know all the ways gluten may impact mental health, but we know that it can. In fact, there are a number of case studies that profoundly impacted me and impact the way I think, two of which are in the literature and speak to women who suffer from schizophrenia. There are more than two case studies,

[00:27:00] but these two affected me greatly. One of the women, from the time she was seven years old, had schizophrenia, she started having hallucinations, both auditory and visual, she was getting messages to kill herself, she was having hallucinations, and was hospitalized multiple times throughout her life because of the severity of the schizophrenia.

[00:27:30] When she was in her 70s, after decades of severe mental health impairments, she started having digestive problems, and they put her on a gluten-free diet, and her mental health issues decreased exponentially. A gluten-free diet actually provided more help for this woman emotionally than anything else had. There's more in the literature. There's another woman who was 33 years old who

[00:28:00] had schizophrenia, who ultimately started having digestive problems, and when they put her on a gluten-free diet, the schizophrenia abated, so we know that can happen, and we see a lot of impacts of gluten on brain health and neurologic health.

[00:28:30] It's something that has to be considered. I don't think everyone needs to be gluten-free, but I think it's really important for anyone who has any neurological issues, to think about gluten as a factor in their emotional and mental health. A lot of people ask me about testing for gluten intolerance, and that's kind of a little bit of a minefield. If you want to be tested, you need to be consuming gluten when you're tested. If you've been on a gluten-free diet and you test yourself, it's not going to be a valid test. The issue is that you really can't test well for gluten intolerance, and there's a lot of controversy over whether that exists, but we do see more and more research supporting the existence of gluten intolerance that's not from celiac disease.

[00:29:00] You can test for celiac, there are no perfect tests for celiac. A gluten-free diet is truly the only endpoint testing, and if you get better on a gluten-free diet, then you should stay off gluten. If you don't, you may be able to tolerate it, but there are people who test negative for celiac, and still do much better on a gluten-free diet. For those with gluten intolerance, there is no perfect test for that. Very often for me, it's a question of trying it and seeing how you feel both physically and emotionally. One of the other things, when we talk about the toxins that children are exposed to that are really important, one of the other ones in terms of chemicals is BPA and phthalates. Those are plasticizers

[00:29:30] found in things like soft water bottles and some children's toys, but you see them in the plastic containers we may store our food in.

[00:30:00] Those are endocrine disruptors, and clearly, if you're disrupting endocrine, the endocrine system, those are hormones, and those hormones are really important for normal development, especially in utero. Testosterone and estrogen are produced in the growing fetus to help brain growth, to help neurological growth, and also to control for sexual maturation. When we disrupt those things, they can have far-reaching consequences. We can test for things like BPA in the urine, and you see that when there are higher levels of that, they may impact things, what we call externalizing behaviors. Those externalizing behaviors include things like ADHD and aggression, especially in boys.

[00:30:30] We do see that linkage. Avoiding BPA and phthalates is really really important, so again, glass, you know if you're going to drink water, it's better from a glass container than one of those soft plastic water bottles. We want to make sure, again, that our exposure to these toxins is limited so that our bodies can use our detoxification pathways and the nutrients they need to detoxify the things we can't avoid, and avoid the things we can. There are so many areas where we're exposed to toxins, and I don't want this to sound so scary that somebody walks away feeling that it's so overwhelming that

[00:31:00] they can't avoid it. You know, you can. Our bodies have a beautiful detoxification system built in, what we want to do is just limit the exposures that we can, so clean water.

[00:31:30] You know, make sure your water system in your home is clean. You might want to test your water and see if there are heavy metals in it, see if there are different kinds of chemicals that may be coming through in the water, and then put in a system to clean that. Make sure you're avoiding those plasticizers, that's a fairly easy thing to do in your home. I only use glass containers to store my food, because that's a very simple thing to do. I don't use a microwave, but if people microwave their food, they should never microwave it in plastic, because it leaches some of those plasticizers into the food.

[00:32:00] We want to use clean chemicals, so cleaning products in our home and cosmetics can contain a lot of things. Again, our skin is the biggest organ in our body, and it is very absorptive. It's also an excretory organ, so sweat is actually a really amazing way to detoxify. There are studies that show that we can detoxify pretty effectively in saunas, so just another good thing to know, but the skin is a really important organ, both for taking in toxins and for getting rid of them, so you want to make sure that the things you put on your skin are relatively healthful. Then again, getting back to the quality of your food, and making sure your food is clean and free of chemicals and hormones, antibiotics, all those things. That's going to be a great way to support you at the most foundational level.

[00:32:30] For many people, the biggest concern is, especially if they have a child on the spectrum or suffering from ADD, or maybe seeming to be very anxious, or having other mental health issues, it's so scary because this is your baby, and you love your baby so much, and you want them to be as healthy as possible. There are many, many things you can do. My advice to them is, number one, leave no stone unturned. Start exploring everything you can, read and learn, and speak to a professional who understands both the conventional, traditional way of treating these disorders, but also employs

[00:33:00] more of this functional approach, because yes, if somebody is not including food or toxin avoidance in their protocol for your child, then they're missing a really important part of it.

One thing I don't want parents to do is look back 10 years from now, and say, "I wish I had done that 10 years ago," but it's also sometimes hard to walk the line. When you start reading, it's so overwhelming to learn about all the different things that may be affecting your child, so I think,

[00:33:30] number one, work with a professional who understands that can really be helpful, but also being willing to explore all the different things that are available, and looking at lifestyle, diet, and environment, and gut health as key pieces to this puzzle.

In the traditional medical community, when you have a migraine, you go to a neurologist, and when

[00:34:00] you have joint pain, you go to a rheumatologist, and when you have a stomach ache or chronic bowel problems, you go to your gastroenterologist. Although all of them are beautifully, wonderfully trained experts in their field, they're looking at you as if you are discrete parts, but our body is not discrete pieces. Our body is one interconnected web, and there is information that says that artificial ingredients can cause migraines, stomach problems, and joint inflammation. Maybe seek out a

[00:34:30] practitioner who looks at the body as a whole, and finds the root to those seemingly different problems, because maybe they come from poor gut health, toxic exposure, increased inflammation, all of the things that we talk about repeatedly.

[00:35:00] If all of these seemingly disparate symptoms come from one source, you really need to treat the source, and not just the different symptoms, so somebody who's going to look at your child as a whole, and not just a series of parts, is really important. Brain tips: get rid of the things that keep you foggy—things like processed foods, artificial ingredients, making sure you have good fats, because they promote good brain health, making sure you're eating lots of antioxidants and lots of plants, fruits and vegetables, I say the same thing over and over again, but there are also some herbs that are

[00:35:30] really terrific for supporting good brain health. Look at some of those herbs that help you cognitively and can be really, really helpful.

There are some wonderful herbs like ginkgo, and adaptogenic herbs, which can be really, really wonderful for brain health. Adaptogenic herbs don't necessarily help you get higher or lower per se; what they do is help your body adapt. Our body has something called an adrenal system that helps us

[00:36:00] respond to stress, and when we get over-stressed, we get activated. Then, after that stress leaves, we're supposed to calm down again. That's the way the normal body and brain should function. In our society, we tend to have a lot of chronic stress, and we're constantly activated. What the adaptogenic herbs do, is they don't necessarily bring us down or elevate us, but they help our adrenal system to balance and do what it's supposed to do, which is keep us either activated when we need to be, or calm down when we don't.

[00:36:30] That helps our brain, because it keeps our brain from being in overdrive all the time. Some adaptogenic herbs include things like ashwagandha and Rhodiola—they're wonderful. Bacopa is another one, and they have different roles. Some of them are a little bit more for mental health and clarity. Some of them are more for calming and de-stressing, but essentially what they all do is they help bring us back into balance. I would caution families to be careful buying supplements just because I mention one. There's real variety in the quality of supplements out there. They are not

[00:37:00] regulated, so there are certain professional lines of supplements that are phenomenal and highly tested and pure, and there are other ones that are actually contaminated with mercury, lead, and arsenic.

[00:37:30]　　　If you don't know the quality of your supplement, don't buy it unless you work with somebody who does. As we talk about controlling the exposure to toxins, the last thing we want to do is take supplements that may not have any of the actual ingredient in it, but also may have something toxic in it that may be problematic, so we want to be really careful.

WENDY SUZUKI, PhD | Author: *Healthy Brain Happy Life*

Dr. Wendy Suzuki:	I became passionate about exercise and its benefits on the brain when I gained 25 pounds trying to get tenure at New York University, and then I had to lose it. I went to the gym, and I found this amazing class that motivated me to come back to the gym over and over and over again. It's a class called Intensati, and it combines physical movements, from kickboxing and dance and yoga, with positive
[00:00:30]	spoken affirmations. The first thing I noticed was an immediate effect on my mood. I left that class feeling like a million bucks. About a year, year and a half into this regular exercise, I noticed something that really made me sit up and take notice. That was I was writing a grant in my office, like I do as a Professor of Neural Science, and a thought went through my mind that had never gone through my
[00:01:00]	mind before, and my thought was, "Gee, grant writing is going so well today." I've never had that thought before. I realized that it was because I was able to focus my attention deeper and longer, and my memory seemed to be better. That's what made me go back to the neuroscience literature and journal articles to see what exactly do we know about the effects of aerobic exercise on brain function. That was what really got me interested in asking these questions.
[00:01:30]	Exercise does really profound things to the brain, and I think one of the secrets of exercise is that it's affecting so many different systems. It affects heart rate and blood flow. It affects oxygen levels. One of the things we know that is really key, is that it affects the levels of growth factors that are in particular, very important parts of the brain. Two key areas are an area critical for long-term memory, called the hippocampus. We know there's increased growth factors there. The second key brain area
[00:02:00]	important for focusing and shifting your attention is the prefrontal cortex. There are many different effects. I have to say that I don't think we understand the full range of all the different physiological changes that happen in our brain with exercise, but that's just a few of them that happen that cause things like changes in neurotransmitter levels, that improve your mood, and changes in these growth factors that actually improve the function of both long-term memory as well as attention.
[00:02:30]	There are forms of exercise that we know a lot about. The most work has been done on the effects of aerobic exercise. That is, exercise that increases your heart rate. We know that it's particularly useful and effective at improving your brain function. There's less known about resistance training or weight training. There are mixed results there. Some reports say, yes, it is beneficial. Other reports don't find
[00:03:00]	a beneficial effect. It's hard to say whether we just don't have enough studies looking at it, but if you really want to stick to the kind of exercise we know the most about, it is aerobic and cardio exercise that get your heart rate up.
[00:03:30]	Intensati does two different things: it gives you a great cardio workout with kickboxing, dance, and yoga moves, but it also layers on those key positive affirmations, and that does at least two different things to your brain. The aerobic exercise is improving your mood by increasing neurotransmitter levels of transmitters like serotonin and dopamine and noradrenaline. That increases your mood, but also has effects on memory and attention. The affirmations, we know that positive affirmations alone can also improve your mood, so you can think of Intensati as a workout that not only gives you the benefits of aerobic exercise, but gives you a double boost of mood-boosting neurotransmitters in your brain.
[00:04:00]	One of the most exciting findings in recent neuroscience research is, findings showing that if you give rats access to a running wheel, and you can show that they're running significantly more than their brothers and sisters that don't have the running wheel. What happens is you stimulate the birth of brand new brain cells. These are adult rats. In adults, there are brand new brain cells being born in the
[00:04:30]	hippocampus, a key area important for long-term memory. In those rats that have access to the

running wheel, they not only have more hippocampal brain cells, but they actually learn and remember better than those brothers and sisters that are in the cage with no running wheel.

[00:05:00] They are essentially strengthening the function of the hippocampus, which is to allow you to form and retain new long-term memories for facts and events. There is some evidence in humans that this is the case. It's actually been demonstrated much more clearly and much more extensively in rodents. But mice studies looking at the effect of aerobic exercise in healthy, young adults are starting to show the first evidence that recognition memory—memory that allows you to say, "Yes, I've seen you before," or, "I haven't seen you before,"—is actually significantly improved after three months of increased aerobic exercise.

[00:05:30] This was after I realized that exercise seemed to be not only improving my mood, but my memory and attention were better. I wanted to learn more about this topic, and as a professor of neuroscience, I know the best way to learn about a new topic in the field of neuroscience is to teach a new class on it. So, I decided to teach a class called *Can Exercise Change Your Brain?* This class was going to go over all of the animal studies looking at the effects of exercise, as well as clinical studies in people looking at

[00:06:00] the effects of exercise on brain function. I thought "Wouldn't it be fun to actually bring exercise into the classroom?" When I went to the administration to ask could I have some extra money to hire an exercise instructor so we could all exercise together and then I would tell them about the effects of exercise on the brain, they said, "Well, we pay you to teach these classes. There's no extra money for an exercise instructor."

[00:06:30] So, I decided to do the next most obvious thing. I decided to go to the gym myself and get certified as an exercise instructor. Because I was going to all these Intensati classes, of course I decided that I wanted to become an Intensati instructor. That started the first of six months of intensive training to teach a new class. It was the most extensive preparation I've ever done for a class that I've taught at NYU. It really shifted things for me. If I can bring you back to that first day of that first class of *Can Exercise Change Your Brain?*, there were a few things that were really different that day.

[00:07:00] The first thing was I came to class in my best Lululemon, because I had to teach exercise class. I usually don't teach in Lululemon, but that day, I was teaching exercise. The second thing was I was really nervous, and I don't get nervous lecturing in front of students. By that point, I'd done it 15 years, no problem at all, but I'd never taught an exercise class. The third thing that was different was the students themselves. This was the first day of the fall semester. Everybody's a little bit excited and don't know what's going to happen in a new class. These students looked scared. I don't know if it was me in my Lululemon, but I could tell in their eyes, they were not sure they really wanted to be there.

[00:07:30] They were ready, and I knew that the only way to tell whether this was going to work was to actually start class.

[00:08:00] I can tell you that it really shifted the mood in that classroom from one where there is all-knowing professor just talking, a talking head at the front, to much more of an interaction. When you work out and shout silly affirmations and positive affirmations with your class for a whole hour before class, it changes the dynamic. I got so much more interaction, so much more engagement and involvement. It really did change the way that I taught every class since at NYU, but more importantly, did it change their brains? I actually set the class up so that I can test them cognitively at the beginning and the end of the semester, to see if this increased exercise changed their brain. I also tested a control class that

[00:08:30] didn't exercise during the semester. It wasn't very hard to find one of those. I compared the two.

[00:09:00] What I found was significant improvement in reaction times. They answered the memory questions faster if you were in my class compared to the control class. That was really exciting to me. It was a small but significant effect, but that was only once a week. I came away from that class thinking, "If I can get a significant effect after just once a week of increased exercise in these college students, what would happen if I got them to exercise three times a week?" In fact, I've just completed a pilot study with freshmen, in which they did one semester with increased exercise compared to one semester

[00:09:30] with no change in exercise. What we found were significant improvements in attention, significant improvements in mood, significant improvements in short-term memory, as well as significant improvements in that thing I was searching for—long-term memory improvements. We're starting to see these effects, and we're going on to do many more of the thousands of students that I have at NYU to test, but this is one of the big research directions in my lab.

[00:10:00] One of the major goals of my research program is to find out what is the optimum exercise prescription for a student. I'm starting with college students, because that's who I have access to, to improve their ability to learn, retain, and be creative during the learning process. I think it is a huge mistake to take away physical education from everybody from elementary school to high school students. I think it is absolutely clear that exercise can help with attention span, memory, mood, and engagement. One of my goals is to find what is that optimum prescription. When do I have to give you

[00:10:30] exercise to maximally benefit your school day and your learning possibilities? Yes, it's critically important. I'm just trying to develop the data to be able to demonstrate what are those answers.

A key question is how exercise might be able to reverse cognitive decline that you might see in aging. The vast majority of studies looking at the effects of aerobic exercise on brain function and cognition, have been done in older adults where we know that there is a decline in cognitive function. How is it

[00:11:00] doing it? Well, it's doing it because it is enhancing the function of two key brain areas we've already talked about that we know are particularly sensitive to aging. One of them is that key area important for long-term memory, called the hippocampus, and that second one is that key area important for attention and also decision-making, and that is the prefrontal cortex. Through these mechanisms that increase growth factors and help both the hippocampus and the prefrontal cortex work better, you are

[00:11:30] helping these areas work better and work at their maximum function, where in aging they are already starting to decline.

I think it's even more interesting to think about what is exercise doing to young and middle-aged people. Young and middle-aged people are getting even more birth of brand-new brain cells in your hippocampus. You can think of the hippocampus as a muscle. The longer you work it, the bigger, fatter

[00:12:00] and more functional hippocampus you get. Similar for the prefrontal cortex. You don't get new cells there, but you enhance the connectivity and synaptic function of the prefrontal cortex. What's happening, as you're exercising regularly through your young life and middle age, is you're basically strengthening these two key areas. Even if you have Alzheimer's disease or dementia in your genes, it's not going to change that. What it's going to do, it's going to make those diseases work longer and

[00:12:30] harder to show those effects on your behavior, so that you're going to basically last for a longer time with higher levels of cognition. Why? Because your prefrontal cortex and hippocampus are stronger, and they work better because you've been exercising.

There are two reasons why I started to study the effects of exercise on the brain. One of them I've

[00:13:00] already said. I've found this and I've noticed this profound effect of aerobic exercise on my own brain function. I had much more energy. I was in a great mood. I could focus my attention and my memories better. That led to this course that I taught at NYU. That was one of the major reasons why I wanted to study this. This was a critical area of research. I should also say that I wasn't studying this before. I was studying the hippocampus and how it works for memory, but this new area is much more practical.

[00:13:30] How can we use exercise, and what is the exercise prescription to improve your brain function?

In parallel with that observation on myself, my father actually developed a very, very sudden decrease in his memory function. It happened so suddenly and we still don't know why this happened, but what I noticed is from one day to the next, almost several weeks before versus several weeks after, he lost

[00:14:00] some of these key brain functions that were improving in myself. His memory went downhill. He couldn't remember how to drive to the 7-Eleven, which is literally seven blocks from his house. He's been going there for 30 years, and he couldn't remember the way. That's what really tipped us off to something going on. Also, his attention span shifted. He's a very smart man. He remembers, and he could pay attention very, very well. It was clear he still had that knowledge, but those key functions

[00:14:30]   that I study were clearly deteriorating.

[00:15:00]   Now, my father's 86, and I can't just say, "Okay, go out. Go jog around the park a few times, Dad." This kind of became the impetus to think about how can I get more people to have better memory for longer periods of time? For me, the answer was, start young. Start with the college students. Start with the high school students so we can work them through the system and get their brains as strong as possible. Not to say that the work on older adults is not useful and very, very important, but that was my motivation, from my personal experience.

[00:15:30]   So, the title of my book is *Healthy Brain, Happy Life*. It's not to say that you absolutely have to have the most healthy brain in order to have a happy life, but it really was the distilling of my personal experience. For me, it started with losing these 25 pounds I had gained and really getting more fit and noticing how much that changed my brain function. As I said, the first thing I noticed was improved mood. I was just happier when I was going to the gym. You ask whole rooms of people, "Who notices that they feel better when they take a walk?" Everybody's hand goes up. That isn't quite enough for

[00:16:00]   everybody in the room to get on that regular exercise routine. For me, the exercise led me to better mood, and it led me to an area of research that has been just so fulfilling for me right now. How can I bring exercise into the classroom? How can I get more people across the country to improve their exercise regime, because I know what it's doing for their brain?

[00:16:30]   The thing about the brain is that it controls everything. How we see, feel, touch, experience, hear the world. The brain responds to novelty, so a great way to bring new plasticity, new experiences into your life, is to try new things. That could be at lots of different levels. You like food? Go try lots of new

[00:17:00]   flavors. Explore all the different ethnic cuisines or unusual ethnic cuisine. You don't have to eat it all the time, but just exploring that and noticing the differences between what you usually eat and this new cuisine, is going to encourage new pathways to form in your brain. The old suggestion of try to do things with the opposite hand. I'm right-handed. I brush my teeth with my right hand. To encourage new plasticity and new pathways to form in your left hand, try and brush your teeth with your left hand. It may not be as efficient, but with a little practice, you'll be surprised at how good you get at

[00:17:30]   doing these things. Small things like that.

One of my favorites is an exercise that was suggested to me by an artist friend, which is ... This is to enhance your visual system. I love going to a museum, but I like strolling around and looking at art as I stroll past. Maybe I'll stand for a little while. She suggested sit down for a good 15 minutes and really

[00:18:00]   explore all different levels of this painting, each individual sub-section, the overall, gestalt of the painting, and really spend some time and think about what the artist was trying to do. You don't have to be an art critic, but what do you notice? What does your visual system tell you? It's a whole new way to look at art and to stimulate your visual system in a new way, and it's fun. If you're going to a museum, that's one of my best brain hack tips.

[00:18:30]   Creativity is a really hot topic, and I became interested in creativity because this key structure I've studied for the last 20 years of my career, the hippocampus, has recently been linked to a form of creativity. Since the 1950s, the hippocampus has been linked to memory and long-term memory function. Every student of neuroscience will know that the hippocampus is important for memory.

[00:19:00]   More recently, we've realized that the hippocampus is not only important for thinking about and remembering things from your past, but it's also important for imagination and putting things in your knowledge base together in new ways, which is a core aspect of imagination, related to creativity. How do we know that? We know that because people that have damage to their hippocampus have amnesia and memory impairments. That's not a surprise. Recently, it's appreciated that not only can they remember things they've experienced in the past, but if you ask them, "Could you describe a

[00:19:30]   situation that you've never experienced before?"

Let's say you've never been to a tropical beach. You might have been to the beach, but it wasn't tropical. If you have hippocampal damage, you have a very hard time in pulling together that new kind

[00:20:00]   of information. Even though you have the knowledge to be able to understand ... It's not a language deficit. It really does seem to be a specific deficit in pulling together information from your database in new and imaginative ways. That suggests that the same exercise that's enhancing memory function, because you're enhancing new neurons in the hippocampus, may also enhance your ability to imagine new situations. That might be critical if you're a high school student or a college student, and this is one of the questions we're asking in my lab right now.

[00:20:30]   My top memory hacks are based on how we know memory works. How do you form a new memory? You remember things that are very new. A pig walks into your classroom. You remember that, because pigs don't usually walk into the classroom, so novelty. Repetition. Of course, the old adage, "Just

[00:21:00]   repeat, repeat, repeat." The memory system is designed to strengthen upon repetition. Third, association. If you can link a new piece of information you're trying to learn with something that is very well known to you, that will help you remember it. Our memory systems are very good at forming new associations. Fourth, emotional resonance. We remember the happiest and the saddest moments of our lives, because it turns out that another brain structure, the amygdala, can particularly help

[00:21:30]   enhance those emotionally charged kinds of memories, either positive or negative. Those are my best brain hacks.

Exercise is not only enhancing all these great growth factors and helping your hippocampus grow, but

[00:22:00]   it does protect us against stress. It's actually unclear exactly how it's doing that. The surprising thing, the kind of incongruous thing, is stress stimulates the release of a stress hormone, cortisol. Too much cortisol can actually first damage and then kill hippocampal cells. It turns out that exercise is a stressor as well. It will also increase cortisol levels, but the cortisol released with exercise seems to protect the hippocampus from the kind of fire-related, really stressful-related cortisol release that you have.

[00:22:30]   We're still not clear on how it does it, but we know that exercise can protect the hippocampus, in particular, from the deleterious effects of stress induced by negative happenings in your life.

I think my take-home message for everybody is you can start small, but start exercising now. It could

[00:23:00]   be a walk. We know that just walking alone can enhance your mood. It's not going to get you the hippocampal growth of brand new brain cells or the increases in growth factors, but walking is the next step to increasing your aerobic exercise. You don't have to become a triathlete. It can start small, but start it, be regular, and gradually build up. There are so many great apps out there to help you do that in a seamless way, but it's so important to get that regular exercise. My second big tip is, do

[00:23:30]   something that's fun for you. Don't do the most popular thing if you hate it. Find something that you love. If you love working out with your friends, find friends who will work out with you. If you love being outside, find something you can do outside. Everybody can find something to do to make their life more physical and you can start small.

BROKEN BRAIN

PATIENT STORIES

Carolyn:

[00:00:30]

Before I found the UltraWellness Center, I went through kind of a long period of maybe seven or eight years where I was feeling achy. My joints ached. My muscles ached. You know, kind of my whole lower body really was achy and it kind of escalated slowly over time. I remember walking up a hill in the country thinking and saying to my husband, "Don't ever expect me to walk more than two or three miles because I just can't do it. It's too painful." I never thought that I would find something that would help me with that situation.

[00:01:00]

[00:01:30]

There are lots of symptoms that I've had for my whole life that I never really thought were things that could go away. I just thought they were part of me. I've always had anxiety and the anxiety always was located in my stomach. It was like a certain sensation that I would have it my stomach that I associated with different thoughts or feelings. I'm a little bit of an introvert and so if I was going to go to a party or something, I would get this feeling in my gut that was like being nervous about going to the party and that is something that subsequently has gone away since I've been working with the UltraWellness Center, but I wouldn't have necessarily said this was a symptom that I was having.

[00:02:00]

Another thing is a sensation of brain fog. The brain fog would ... come sometimes, when I would get in the car and I would be driving and I would realize that I was a little bit fuzzy. It's a little bit frightening to have that. I mean, it never really caused me a problem. Or if I would sit down at my desk and have a lot of work to do and need to sort it through, I would just be like there was a fog in front of me and I couldn't even see my way through it. So, in retrospect, those were symptoms of things that could go away, but at the time I didn't identify them that way.

[00:02:30]

[00:03:00]

I do remember talking to my doctor about it and I went to a lot of physical therapy for it also, but it turned out that not everything can be cured by physical therapy, as much as I would like it to be. The physical therapist always took it seriously and I'd have exercises that I would work on, but it never really got better that way. I would occasionally talk to my doctor about it but honestly, I didn't really have the expectation that she would be able to help me with it. I mean, what do you do for achiness? You take Advil, and to me that never seemed like a good answer. So, I didn't even have the confidence in my regular doctors to think that they would help me with something like this that was lifelong.

[00:03:30]

[00:04:00]

I had shoulder surgery and I had an amazing physical therapist, and she gave me *UltraWellness* to read. I read it and I was really excited about it. It just sort of opened the door to my thinking that there was some other medical model out there that would be helpful. Then, just coincidentally, my trainer told me one day that a client of hers who had Lyme disease was going to a clinic in Western Mass and just something clicked in me and I realized that those were the same things and I thought, "Oh, I could go there." I did a little research online and I called up and I realized I could go there and it just was exciting and hopeful.

[00:04:30]

[00:05:00]

[00:05:30]

[00:06:00]

I first went to the UltraWellness Center in person about three years ago. That was right after my epiphany that I could come to this place. I had a day-long appointment with Dr. Boham and a nurse and nutritionist and they did some tests, and she really deeply delved into the background of the issues that I brought to her, meaning the achiness and also, I've had an issue with my thyroid for a long time. She was the first doctor that I ever came across who was really willing to sort of deeply delve into the dose of thyroid medication that I took and what the symptoms of thyroid are. I told her all my problems and she made a plan and it was lots of components. One is the gut health component and lots of tests; you know, sort of the mail-back tests where you have to test your stools and lots of blood work and allergy testing. I think the allergy testing came back that I was allergic to a few things including corn and potatoes, and one of her big recommendations was that I go gluten- and dairy-free.

[00:06:30]	The minute I left the UltraWellness Center and I had this new diet, I was on vacation with my husband and I had to eat differently and it was challenging. I remember going out for dinner and thinking there's nothing I can eat here. It was a hard couple weeks of going home and feeling like there was nothing to eat and having to rework my whole diet. I did that and we changed the dose of the thyroid, and at some point, a couple weeks after that I was like, "Oh, my God. That sensation is gone." It was just sort of miraculously I became aware that I wasn't having that anymore. So, I think it happened actually pretty quickly after I made all these changes. I left the UltraWellness Center.
[00:07:00]	
[00:07:30]	I left with this whole new diet. I remember going out for dinner with my husband that night and just feeling like there was nothing for me to eat, and actually for a few days or maybe even a week and a half, I lost a lot of weight because it was hard for me to find food that worked for me. But I worked with Maggie, the nutritionist, and I was able to create a diet that works for me and that was satisfying and I had enough food.
[00:08:00]	I remember one day, maybe two or three weeks later, standing in my kitchen opening the refrigerator and all of a sudden, I realized that that feeling of anxiety that I used to have a couple times a day was gone, and it was miraculous, really! I'd had that feeling for my whole life and honestly, in the three years since then, I haven't had that sensation at all. I've had phone meetings with Dr. Boham over the whole time, the three years, and that was one of the things that I was really excited to tell her, and I've told her over and over again, because it's just so miraculous for me. What my assumption is, is that her work with my gut microbiome is what has helped that situation. It's been teamwork, really between her and I the last couple years to work on my gut. So, I think it's just been implicit in the conversations that we've had that this has been a good thing.
[00:08:30]	
[00:09:00]	
[00:09:30]	Because I'm gluten- and dairy-free, everybody knows, and especially my kids and my husband. Actually, my husband is the cook in our house and he had to start cooking completely differently, so actually it's been a big act of love on his part to restrict his cooking, but I think part of why he does it is because he knows that I'm so much better and I'm less irritable at him. I think that's how I see the benefits of it in the relationship. I talk about the UltraWellness Center and how much better it's made me to anybody who wants to hear about it. My kids know about it, so I'm eager to spread the word, really.
[00:10:00]	My regular internist is a concierge doctor and I have been open with her about my work with Dr. Boham and the UltraWellness Center, and she's been very receptive. I feel very lucky about that. Dr. Boham gives me blood work that I need to get done for my work with her, and my regular doctor is open to doing that. They even talked on the phone at some point and my regular doctor said that she would like to learn from Dr. Boham. I haven't really actualized that but even just doing the tests like the sort of deeper thyroid labs and the blood sugar blood work, I think is educating her that you can look more deeply for the root causes of problems.
[00:10:30]	
[00:11:00]	What has made me feel supported in this process, sort of being a person in the real world, is even just reading Dr. Hyman's book, *UltraWellness*, and believing in it so completely. I'm Facebook friends with Dr. Hyman and he had a little video interviewing women about food cravings and that's actually part of the current phase that I'm working on is dealing with my sugar cravings and the overgrowth of yeast. But the point is, the information I get from the videos and from my work with Dr. Boham and reading, gives me the kind of certainty and the energy to do the things that I need to do. So, when I met with Dr. Boham I said, "Please tell me what you think I need to do because I will believe that and it will help me do them." I think if you are considering going gluten- and dairy-free, reading about it and reading about it from a Functional Medicine perspective, even if that's all you can do, I think can give you some power and energy to defend it from the outside world.
[00:11:30]	
[00:12:00]	
[00:12:30]	We have things wrong with us and there's no reason why you have to think this is something that I'm going to have for the rest of my life. Of course, if you get a dreaded disease or cancer or something, these are lifelong issues, but for something like brain fog or not feeling well during the day for different reasons, there are so many ways of dealing with these issues. I think my experience with brain fog, and

[00:13:00] it being helped, is another illustration of that being true. I just thought brain fog was part of my life. I think I had it since I was a kid. It would come and go. It would come in times of a little bit of stress, so I just thought that that was my way of stress expressing itself in my life. Then also similar to the anxiety,

[00:13:30] I also had an epiphany where I realized that, "Oh my God. I haven't had this brain fog in a couple weeks and time has gone by and it just hasn't come back." So, I think it's worth experimenting with. It's worth reading about, having someone talk through with you and help you to see if there's a nutritional reason or a chemical reason in your body why you're having it.

[00:14:00] When I came to the UltraWellness center, I came with sort of a presenting problem and the problem was that I was feeling achy. When I worked with them, they really worked with me in a whole-body way, so I can't really separate out all these different symptoms and say this helped this and that helped

[00:14:30] that; it was all integrated. Then, there were some wonderful side benefits of my anxiety and my brain fog, but I think from my perspective, working on my thyroid medication was really the key to everything. I believe, and I'm not an expert so I really don't know, but I believe that helped my achiness tremendously. The achiness is gone. I feel like a normal person now and that's part of what just gives

[00:15:00] me so much hope that these people are onto something, because my regular doctors didn't help me with this problem. I think it was the integration of deeply delving into the thyroid issue, and the dose of medication, and what medication, plus the dietary, plus the supplements, and I think it's just the whole package of help has made the whole being of me better.

[00:15:30] Having this help for my whole being, fixing these different problems in an integrated way has just made my life better. I do feel much more physically capable. It helps me enjoy nature more because I don't

[00:16:00] feel like I have to hold back. So, whether I go on longer than two- or three-mile hikes, it doesn't even matter. I just feel capable. I feel like a more at-peace person with everybody and everything, so it's not dramatic but really my whole life and my whole physicality is better because of this.

I did feel overwhelmed with all of the changes and the integrating sort of new knowledge and new

[00:16:30] ways of thinking about my life and my routines. Some of the tests that you have to do at home, you have to get involved with your own bodily functions maybe more than you might want to, and just keeping it all straight and understanding it all. I think over time, what I have realized is that I have a

[00:17:00] tendency to make things feel complicated and if they don't seem like a big deal to me, then it's really not a big deal.

For example, one of the things that is always, in an ongoing way, a little bit overwhelming, is that before I have appointments with Dr. Boham, I have to fill out these forms and keep a log of my food,

[00:17:30] but then I'll meet with her. And she's got my papers in front of her and she works from them and I realize that this is a way that I can efficiently communicate with a doctor who really is going to take this information into account, and it's worth it. So now that I've been doing it all this time, it's really not that big a deal and it's a way of being involved in your own health care rather than watching the doctor input into the computer and then you kind of not knowing what's going to be spewed out. This is much

[00:18:00] more a partnership and it's worth it.

Well, I would say by way of encouraging other people to try this is: you have nothing to lose and you have everything to gain. It's a matter of belief and it's a matter of taking control over your own

[00:18:30] healthcare. You could get so much better, so it's just worth it to try. I would highly recommend Functional Medicine. In a way, to me, it's not even a question of would you recommend it. It seems like the only logical way to have medicine is to understand what causes symptoms and problems. Why

[00:19:00] would you go to someone who's just going to put a Band-Aid on a problem when the problem is still being created in your body and the imbalances and the inputs that are harmful? In a way, I feel like I had Functional Medicine on my mind the whole time and I'm glad I found some place in the world that met that need because how are we ever going to get better just by putting a Band-Aid on a problem?

[00:19:30]   I would recommend Functional Medicine for almost everybody; people who are dealing with dementia at the end of life, people who are dealing with behavioral issues with little children, people who have reflux, people who have headaches, a stomachache. I mean, there are probably some things that you

[00:20:00]   wouldn't go to a Functional Medicine doctor for, but really, I think everybody should go to a Functional Medicine doctor.

COLIN BRUCKER | The UltraWellness Center Patient

Kristin:	Colin suffered from behavioral issues at home as well as some learning difficulties at school. He was very unfocused at school and he also had some digestive issues that were unresolved with conventional medication. We were really looking for a solution for him.
[00:00:30]	I would say from a very early age—maybe around two—we had behavioral issues at home. And then from there, once he entered school, is when we noticed the learning disabilities and the problem with focus. And then around that time also he had stomach issues.
	We sought alternative options by around age five and a half. Towards the end of kindergarten, we went to see Dr. Boham.
Colin:	I used to have stomach problems and rage sometimes. But once I turned my diet, I felt a lot better about myself.
Kristin: [00:01:00]	Colin's behavior was really unpredictable with ADHD. Sometimes he would be okay and then other times he could have an explosive outburst that I would feel difficult to control, especially with my other children around. It was hard.
[00:01:30]	It really impacted all of us because his behavior was so unpredictable. There was one day I remember he had gone to a camp and they fed him a lot of ice cream, candy, drinks that had the artificial colorings in it. He came home and had the biggest meltdown he had ever had. That's where I started to think possibly the diet was related, even though regular doctors had told me no. I just couldn't control him in front of my other kids. I was actually crying I was so upset. And that was kind of my low point. I can't have my other kids seeing me not be able to help Colin.
	I had seen psychological counselors for him, maybe starting at age two, to try to help with the behavior issues. And they gave me some advice, some tactical advice, but nothing that really seemed to make a big difference.
[00:02:00]	Dr. Boham was amazing. She spends so much time with you. She really looked at Colin as a whole person and did some testing that we had never thought to try. And then the diet was just so huge. We worked with a nutritional counselor at The UltraWellness Center and she was really helpful with giving us advice on how to change our diets to something that was better for Colin.
[00:02:30]	It was definitely a little bit hard to change the diet at first. It's a lot of undertaking but we felt that it was necessary to really help Colin. And our whole family adopted the diet as well. So, that kind of made it easier. And also, I think, given Colin's young age, that was helpful, too, that he was more willing to adapt.
[00:03:00]	Our old diet was, I would say, a typical standard American diet. It was what I considered healthy. It was whole grains. We would eat things like whole wheat bread. But now our diet is gluten-free and organic and our meat is pasture-raised and grass-fed. And we also are almost 100% organic. We really cut back on the packaged foods that we used to eat. And if we do eat packaged goods, we really check the labels to make sure they're low in sugar. We certainly don't eat anything with high-fructose corn syrup, things like that. Those were things I didn't know back then that are not good for brain health.
Colin: [00:03:30]	I felt it was a little hard when I was doing it because I was used to eating gluten. And I used to eat whole grain bread. When I changed, it was kind of hard. But now I've gotten the hang of it.

Kristin: [00:04:00]	Dr. Boham was interested in what we were eating. She was very interested to see what our diet looked like. She also was interested in Colin's overall blood work and she did some testing and found out that he was not absorbing B12 properly, which would be a huge thing for brain health. She had him take a sublingual B12 supplement. She really had a lot of supplements to recommend, whereas the regular doctor just had over-the-counter, like for any stomach issues; they just recommended over-the-counter medications.
[00:04:30]	I would say we tried to start them right away but it's a bit of a slow process when you're learning a new way of cooking and a new way of eating. So, it took us some time, but I would say we saw changes in Colin right away. And pretty much within a couple of months we saw dramatic changes.
	We didn't see as many outbursts with Colin, his behavior seemed calmer. He seemed more focused. He really just seemed happier overall.
	Lifestyle-wise, it's really important for Colin to get good sleep. We know that's true. It's also important to limit screen time. We try to do that as best we can. It's kind of hard in this day and age now but that seems to help his focus and calm him down.
[00:05:00]	The biggest things we've found to cut out of Colin's diet that were triggers, I would say would be dairy, gluten, and definitely sugar or anything artificial. Packaged products were probably the number one thing that had to go.
Colin:	Well, I like some of the grass-fed steaks, sometimes, for dinner. I like fruits like oranges, apples, and bananas. I like fruits.
[00:05:30]	I felt good because she would help me, like changing my diet and medicines and I got that. But at the same time, when I heard about I was changing my diet, I didn't like too much about it because I was changing the foods I eat that I sometimes like.
Kristin: [00:06:00]	Colin is such a different kid now. He's more confident, he's doing so well in school, he just finished third grade, he is reading on his reading level. He got into the accelerated math group this year. It's been such a game changer for him. The lifestyle changes were huge.
[00:06:30]	I would suggest other parents look at the diet their children are eating. We've been told for so long that the standard American diet is a healthy option, but really, I think we need to look further and make sure that we're eating more organic. And also, even balancing meals with protein and fat in each meal is really important for Colin to keep his blood sugar stable. I would say that there are other options than just medication.
Colin:	Well I would say they should change the diet. And eat a little bit healthier from a diet they might be eating. So that's one of the things I think they should change.
Kristin: [00:07:00]	I would definitely recommend Dr. Boham and The UltraWellness Center. They have such a personalized medicine approach. They take the time to really listen to you. And they will really get to the root cause of your problems, I think.

Daniel:

[00:00:30]

I think I started to struggle with my health very early in life. I actually asked my mom, "When did I start struggling with my health?" She said, "Really, when you were a toddler," though when I look back and remember it as early as age six or seven, I would regularly get a cold or respiratory problem. I had my tonsils removed when I was seven and adenoids, too. I remember being especially traumatized by that procedure. I had pneumonia at least once or twice, at the age of 10 I had pneumonia. We went on a vacation to Disney World and I got sick and was in bed the whole time with a fever. They put me on steroids and antibiotics, things like that.

[00:01:00]

[00:01:30]

I had chronic sinus infections and missed school periodically. I don't have numbers on it now but I know I was always like, "Oh, I really don't feel well this morning Mom, I don't think I can go to school." I remember starting to be regularly sick as early as age five or six but to me it was just normal at the time, it's just what people went through; they were sick regularly. As far as ADD goes, I think that first came about in third grade; I was eight years old and I started having school anxiety. Of course, I remember this, it was just general nervousness and anxiety about going to school. I would kind of break down when it was time to go to school in the morning or go in the classroom. It wasn't really logical, it was just emotional.

[00:02:00]

[00:02:30]

My parents started taking me to psychologists and psychiatrists. I remember them asking things like, "Well, why don't you want to go to school? What bothers you about it?" I didn't know, it didn't make any sense to me, just like when I got there it was no good. Looking back, especially when I look at pictures, I can see that the anxiety and the illness in my sinuses and things like I got fevers, respiratory infections, it sort of all culminated together and that's also when I started putting some weight on, having asthma symptoms. I remember in gym class we had to do the mile run in elementary school and my chest hurt so much, I was crying afterward; I couldn't finish, I had to walk.

[00:03:00]

I think it was age eight when I was first prescribed ADD medication—Ritalin. I remember I would have to go to the school nurse and take it in the middle of the day, I thought it was special for me. I was on and off those ADD medications throughout school. That was the earliest prescription, age eight in third grade. Then, the last time I took it was in March of 2012, so that's about 15 years. The better part of 15 years I was regularly taking ADD medication and using that to get by.

[00:03:30]

[00:04:00]

The side effects of ADD medication are ... I don't even know how to say. It's like knowing now, having been off of ADD medication for about four or five years, looking back on how I felt every day on ADD medication especially in college and in high school is astounding to recall. It is like, I could just list things. The first thing that I remember ADD medication really messing with is my sleep. In college, I was at the point in my senior year where I would sleep in two-hour blocks because that was how I could manage getting my homework done.

[00:04:30]

[00:05:00]

I would take the Adderall and it would keep me awake. Then eventually I'd start to crash, so I'd try and take a nap. I'd go home and close the blinds and put a blanket over my head and wake up a couple hours later, then take another dose of Adderall and start studying again. Sleep was majorly affected by the Adderall. Another thing I found is that I felt Adderall could enrage me. It actually caused kind of emotional ups and downs. Looking back now, everyone feels angry from time to time but the extremes ... I think Adderall causes more emotional extremes, so if you're frustrated by something, you're more likely to become a little enraged when you're on Adderall.

[00:05:30]

The same thing goes for maybe sadness. If something happens with a friend, you feel more down, like a low afterward and it's really just ups and downs emotionally, I felt on Adderall. I remember pretty distinctly the moment actually that I decided I should not be taking these ADD drugs anymore. It was the

[00:06:00]   day I finished my last final exam of college so I really was ... I have a degree in Physics—I love to tell people that—but I scraped by in college. I was getting Ds, I failed a couple classes and had to retake them. It was the last day of my final exams. I had finished, I was so relieved and so sleep deprived. I had used Adderall to keep myself awake. I'd probably slept six hours in the last 48 or 72 hours.

[00:06:30]   I was doing something around the house and this feeling of sickness, I can still remember, almost in my stomach and my head, a physical sensation of illness from being so sleep deprived as a result of taking the Adderall. I think I went to go close the trunk door on my car and my shoulder did this weird thing and I realized ... I almost had limited control over my body because of how sleep deprived I was physically, I lacked physical control. I said, "Man, something's wrong with me. This feels so terrible, I need to find another way."

[00:07:00]   I ended up Googling something like alternative remedies for ADD treatment and I actually stumbled upon a book *The UltraMind Solution* by Dr. Hyman. It had good Amazon reviews. I had never seen anything like it before, so I ordered it. I think I got through it over the next month or so. Of course, at the time I needed Adderall to even think about reading a book. It's ironic because I was using Adderall at [00:07:30] that time. The only way I knew how to get through a book was on these drugs. I got through the book and I'm reading *The UltraMind Solution* and it was really a little far out to me at the time.

[00:08:00]   I'm thinking, "Food changes the way I feel? I eat bread every day." I remember my regular lunch in college was a baguette and cheese. I actually remember reading *The UltraMind Solution* and feeling a lot of skepticism when I read it. I was thinking, "Is this true? Could this really be true?" It's just coming from this one book but the thing that got me is that there were many references to scientific studies, very established institutions, like universities. I remember looking, the works were all cited in the back of the book and I said, "Okay, this is pretty convincing, maybe I should try some of these things." That was the [00:08:30] beginning. That was my first exposure to it.

        I actually went and reviewed the book now, not having read it in several years. There are so many things in there, so many valuable pieces of advice and ways to improve your health. At the time for me, [00:09:00] because all of these concepts were so new, I was really only able to absorb a few of them into my lifestyle. It was all focused on diet at first. I look back now and realize that he's recommending things like pay attention to your breath to control your stress. In one part of the program, do a breathing practice before lunch to manage your stress. Some of these things weren't even making it all the way into my lifestyle at the time.

[00:09:30]   I remember I started out by, I think I offered to go to the grocery store for my parents. I said, "Hey, let me go to the grocery store. I'm going to get a few extra things that are supposed to be pretty healthy from this book." I came back and the next couple weeks, I found myself having a tablespoon of flaxseed oil in the morning and taking probiotics and not eating bread. It was really quite a big change for me but also for my family who I was living with at the time; my brother and my parents. They were great cooks growing up but we always had at least two cases of Coca Cola in the basement so I drank Coca Cola [00:10:00] every day growing up. No wonder that by the time I was 13, I weighed 230, 240 lbs.

        That was kind of the beginning. Honestly, I think it's important for people to realize that if you're just stumbling upon this information, something like *The UltraMind Solution*, which is extremely robust in all its recommendations for how to improve your health, you don't have to do everything right the first [00:10:30] time. I did not follow the program dogmatically but it was the very beginning for me of realizing that I could really change my brain power and my ability to live the life that I want to by making changes to my diet, eating good foods, eliminating bad foods, and then incorporating these other lifestyle practices like good sleep, exercise habits, things like that.

[00:11:00]   One of the most significant changes I recognize now after reading *The UltraMind Solution* and incorporating some of the diet and lifestyle changes is that for the first time ever in my life, I was voluntarily exercising. This is big. In elementary school, I couldn't do the mile run. In middle school, I

[00:11:30] couldn't even run a lap around the two baseball diamonds, I had to walk half way. In high school, I could get out and go play Ultimate Frisbee or something, but I never had much of an aerobic capacity. Even in elementary school, my parents enrolled me in soccer, t-ball, and I'd be kind of in the middle of the field staring at the grass while everyone else was chasing the ball. I didn't have the physical energy or the mental focus of enjoying those sports.

[00:12:00] A few weeks after making some changes to my diet and lifestyle, I found myself just naturally using the elliptical machine in our basement. Now, I'm starting to move. You look back and it's unfortunate because so many people look at someone who's overweight or unhealthy and they say, "You should be exercising." The truth is, if you are not eating the right foods or if you're poisoning yourself with the wrong foods you have no energy to exercise. You lack the physical energy and you lack the mental interest or energy to get yourself to do those things and to enjoy them.

[00:12:30] That was the beginning. *The UltraMind Solution* lifestyle changes, the first things that I saw were changes in my exercise habits. Within about three years after that, or four years after that, I could say that I had completed three marathons. In 2015, I ran the New York Marathon and the Chicago [00:13:00] Marathon; my wife and I did that together. It's a pretty stark contrast to say I had no interest in running half a lap when I was growing up but now I can call myself an endurance athlete if I want to. I read *The UltraMind Solution* in June 2011 and the last time I took Adderall was March 2012. I don't know ... you can call that a quick turnover or a slow turnover but it was necessary for me.

[00:13:30] I had gotten a job out of college, at the end of 2012. Of course, to even feel comfortable in my first professional environment I was still dependent on Adderall. I wanted to show up to work and have all the focus I could but I started slowly maybe skipping it a day and seeing how that felt. Besides my [00:14:00] hunger changing from not having amphetamines in my system, it was definitely a rough period of change. I remember it was about three weeks of me feeling like I had to be sneaky and get away with things at work. I had to hide the fact that I was not nearly as attentive on Adderall.

It was like a three-week transition period after totally stopping Adderall to feeling normal, like I could actually think. Even with the lifestyle changes that allowed me to wean myself off Adderall, it still took at [00:14:30] least three weeks of pretty heavy withdrawal just to feel comfortable and competent in a professional setting at least. Kids who are growing up now with ADD or who take ADD medication to feel comfortable achieving their goals, I would say that you have to trust me: I was there and there is a better way. If you think that Adderall is the only way you can think clearly right now, you're dead wrong. Once you adopt [00:15:00] the right lifestyle changes you will be miles and miles ahead of where you are right now.

I know in *The UltraMind Solution,* it does really go beyond diet. It also includes supplements and lifestyle changes. Sleep is really an important one, getting enough sleep each night. Diet is kind of the most [00:15:30] important to me because I feel like changing your diet, eliminating sugar, and bad oils is really the critical first step to even give you a chance at focusing on and adopting other lifestyle practices. Growing up, we always had a couple cases of Coca Cola in the fridge. My parents were great chefs and we had great home cooked meals often including many great whole foods as well but the salad had ranch dressing that had sugar and soybean oil added to it. Then there was orange juice on the table that I was [00:16:00] drinking, so a lot of sugar added onto the foods I was eating.

After school in ninth grade, I would walk to 7-Eleven each day and get a Dr. Pepper and a bag of Fritos. I think I was at my heaviest with that daily routine. Generally, I just ate what tasted good. For a while, the [00:16:30] Adderall suppressed my appetite so what I would do is I would go to school and instead of buying a wholesome meal for lunch, I would get chocolate chip cookies because I wasn't really that hungry but I did enjoy eating chocolate chip cookies, just to give you an example of some of the terrible foods I was eating and how much sugar I was consuming.

Now, let's see. I usually will have a cup of Bulletproof coffee for breakfast. I've completely eliminated [00:17:00] sugar from my diet. The last time I had any sugar was July of last year, so it's been 11 months. It's also

[00:17:30] been 11 months since I've eaten any bread or gluten. I have completely eliminated sugar, gluten, and vegetable oils from my diet. I consume organic vegetables now and lots of monounsaturated fats from avocados and olive oil and lots of saturated fat from grass-fed butter, grass-fed meats, pasture-raised eggs, and coconut oil.

[00:18:00]
[00:18:30] Now I'm high fat, low carb, lots and lots of organic green vegetables, even limited fruit, very low fructose. I really just drink water, coffee, tea ... no sweetened beverages at all. Like I said, to compare my mental focus now to what it was like on Adderall there's really no comparison. It's a joke to think that Adderall makes you more focused than a good diet. Another interesting change around nutrition is that once I completely eliminated sugar and breads and things like that from my diet, I found that I'm able to easily go without food for longer periods of time so something I actually practice is intermittent fasting. Today I rode my bike here nine miles and I haven't eaten anything in 22 hours right now.

[00:19:00] What I think that kind of points to is that once you eliminate the sugar and high-carb diet, you realize that your body can energize itself a little more naturally and you're less addicted to sugars. Another thing I noticed after adopting this nutritional lifestyle is that I don't crave alcohol at all anymore. I haven't had a single drink since last summer. I never had a problem with it but I always drank socially in college and even a little bit in high school and after college as well. I'd come home after work and maybe have even just half a beer, something like that, just to relax after work.

[00:19:30]
[00:20:00] I think once you adopt certain dietary changes and stress reducing lifestyle habits, maybe like a regular yoga practice and of course a good, solid sleep each night, you realize that the benefits of alcohol are really not that great. I think that alcohol is used commonly to reduce stress, but if you can manage stress by taking a stressful diet out of your lifestyle and adding good sleep back in, the alcohol becomes kind of unappealing. Then you take a drink once in awhile and realize, "Maybe this doesn't really feel that good."

[00:20:30]
[00:21:00] With these lifestyle changes, I've found that where other people, like colleagues, enjoy alcohol to make them feel more social—maybe an after-work happy hour or something like that—I feel very comfortable without the drink in hand. A good anecdote is that we had our holiday party at work and everyone's drinking sake and soju—it was at a Korean restaurant—and we all went out for karaoke afterward. It's pretty late, like 11pm and I'm only drinking green tea. We all get to the karaoke room and everyone's kind of nervous about singing in front of their colleagues and I'm just like, "Come on, let's do this." I'm the only sober one in the room and I'm grabbing the mic first and kind of showing them how it's done getting people warmed up.

[00:21:30] I feel that adopting these lifestyle habits, which really allow your body to flourish and your brain to flourish, including your mental and emotional state, you can be comfortable all the time. There's actually a great quote. My wife was listening to an interview with Dr. Hyman, I forget where, but the rough quote was something like—not verbatim—Dr. Hyman said, "Every day is an opportunity to show up as your best self and bring a smile and bring happiness and make the people around you feel good." Of course, that's what we all want to do, we want to show up as our best selves. In order to do that you need your best mental state, you need your best brain function.

[00:22:00]
[00:22:30] The big wow moment for me was when I realized that I need bodily health in order to have mental health and bring my best self to every situation. Being regularly sick growing up, I estimate, and my parents estimate, that before I was 18 I had at least 30 courses of antibiotics. I thought it was normal at the time growing up. "Okay, I have a sniffly nose." "We'll figure out how to get you some antibiotics from the doctor." Now, I haven't taken antibiotics in over five years. I also haven't even had a fever in five years. I don't get colds anymore, it just doesn't happen. I feel very confident in my health and my immune system.

Growing up, I questioned that if I was just maybe genetically predisposed to getting sick more. I realize that since adopting these lifestyle changes, you don't need to get sick. That's one of the most beautiful

[00:23:00] outcomes of adopting lifestyle changes like those in *The UltraMind Solution*. If I had the chance to say something to Dr. Hyman now, I would just say thank you. I can see that what he's doing is delivering a really important message that helps people. Dr. Hyman is delivering a message to people that they're not getting in other places; the conventional medical community is not giving patients sustainable wellness. He knows that adopting lifestyle changes through diet, sleep, and exercise provides the best

[00:23:30] outcome so I would say, "Thank you," to Dr. Hyman. Thanks for spreading the message; it's really, really commendable that Dr. Hyman has devoted his life to bringing these tidbits of information about diet and lifestyle to the public. People need to hear it and they're not getting it anywhere else.

DONALD SEGAL | The UltraWellness Center Patient

Donald:

[00:00:30]

My wife and I have been familiar with Functional Medicine, I would say over 20 years. We first encountered Dr. Hyman at Canyon Ranch in the 90s. We both saw him and, matter of fact, it was at that time at Canyon Ranch that he diagnosed me with metabolic syndrome. We used to see him every year when we would go up. We would have a follow-up visit, so we've been very familiar with Functional Medicine since that time. We're firm believers in it.

[00:01:00]

I've been having some memory problems. There was some deterioration of my memory. My daughter was the one who really encouraged me to make an appointment at The UltraWellness Center to see Dr. Boham because, again, we believe in Functional Medicine. We believe in the work that Dr. Hyman and Dr. Boham are doing. It was because of this she felt that it might be appropriate to address my memory problems. I mean I say memory problems. They weren't that bad, but my memory isn't what it used to be.

[00:01:30]

For example, I was having difficulty remembering names. It would take me sometimes an hour or so. I would recognize somebody's face, but I couldn't put a name to it immediately. Then maybe in an hour, it'd come back to me. I mean it's gotten to the point where I feel like my brain is full and so it takes me a little bit longer to pull the information out of it because I've always had a very, very good memory.

I mean, recently, I was just looking at some pictures of some old meetings I attended and I recognize the faces of the people and I couldn't remember their names immediately; It's things like this. There are instances where there were situations that my wife referred to that I didn't remember, but in general, I could notice some deterioration.

[00:02:00]

[00:02:30]

Now, I went to the Columbia Neurological Institute at my son's urging back in 2012 and they tested me. Then I went back for a follow-up visit in 2016, but there, they're not Functional Medicine; they're more traditional medicine. I mean, they did an MRI of my brain and everything and found nothing, which is good. I mean there's a brain there, but no plaque or anything. But they tested me and I remember the doctor telling me in the absolute, she would have said I have no problems. But on the tests they had given me, the memory tests: 2012, I had ranged between above-average and very superior; 2016: I was average to superior. So, she was saying for an average person—hey!—you're doing great, but for me there was some decline. Putting all these things together we decide to go see Dr. Boham and I went right before Thanksgiving last year.

[00:03:00]

Functional Medicine tries to address the causes and treat the underlying causes of a particular condition as opposed to treating the symptoms. When I was there, I underwent a series. They took some blood. They did some blood tests. I believe they did some other genetic tests there, and we had a discussion. She gave me a totally different diet. It's a lifestyle change.

[00:03:30]

[00:04:00]

My diet is now, right now, it is no gluten, no sugar, no sugar substitutes, no dairy and really limited grains as much as I can. I am absolutely amazed at how I have stuck to it. I mean, because I had a sweet tooth. My wife will be the first one to tell you. She would say I was addicted to sugar, but I had a sweet tooth. I loved my desserts: ice cream, cake, things like this. It was a total change. I cannot believe how well I have followed it in terms of ... I mean I can tell you, I've had ice cream exactly twice in the seven months since I've been on it and one was a tiny little profiterole. I've had bites of cake four times and by a bite, I mean literally one fork full. Two of them were gluten-free. For me, this is amazing how I have stuck to it. I have had no dairy other than the couple times I had ice cream. I mean, as I say, stay away from gluten. I am totally away from sugar and sugar substitutes. I examine ingredients much more carefully than I use to. I do my best to stay away from it.

[00:04:30]

I mean they're very, very good there because not only, at the time, did I meet with Dr. Boham, but I met with Lisa Fisher, who's a nutritionist. I've had one follow-up call with Dr. Boham. It's basically six month intervals, but every two months I speak with Lisa Fischer on nutrition, to follow-up and what they do is they ask me how I'm doing. They adjust my diet. They tell me what I should change, how I'm doing. I mean, for example, they say you can cheat a little, but, for example, don't cheat with gluten. I think it's made a difference. I don't think my memory's any worse than it used to be. It's not perfect, but I don't think it's any worse. But it's been an experience working with them and I cannot believe the way I have changed as a result of dealing with them.

[00:05:00]

[00:05:30]

I don't think any other doctor that I know of would have approached my condition this way. I'm eating totally differently. I mean, I start the day with a shake, which is actually the best part of the day. I have a wonderful shake in the morning, protein-based with fruits and seeds and the cacao powder and nibs and everything, but I start the day, and it's delicious. I mean I really enjoy it. For example, when I'm out of town, I don't have my shake, it's not quite the same thing. I'm eating a lot more salads. I have, you know, I'm concentrating on colorful meals, and I didn't concentrate on that as much. I mean this is part of the message that you should have color in your diet because color foods are really good for you and you should have a palatte. I mean ... and I remember this is what they pushed at Canyon Ranch, that you should have a colorful diet so my diet's totally different.

[00:06:00]

[00:06:30]

My energy; I've always been a high energy person, and I don't think my energy is really down. At times, I feel like taking a nap in the afternoon, but that's probably more a condition of my age than anything else. I think it has nothing to do with the style or what I'm eating or anything like that, but I've been surprised how easy the change was even though it was a dramatic change.

[00:07:00]

Functional Medicine is a totally different approach and it's a much better approach than the traditional. It is worth the time and the expense to go up there to visit them. Lifestyle has a lot to do with it. I mean, for example, Dr. Hyman preaches everything starts with the gut and that even includes brain function, and they've changed my diet. I mean, as a result of my change in my diet, I've lost about 20 pounds, which I totally did not expect. That wasn't part of the intent. I didn't think I was grossly overweight. My blood pressure has dropped to the extent that I've been on blood pressure medicine. I'll be seeing my primary care physician in a couple of weeks for my annual physical and who knows, he may take me off the blood pressure medicine. At his suggestion, I dropped to half the dosage I was taking, but there have been these very positive changes as a result of the change.

[00:07:30]

[00:08:00]

I take 31 pills every day, one of which is a prescription pill for my high blood pressure. The other 30 are supplements. Some are what I was taking before and frankly, the ones that was taking before are the ones that were recommended by Dr. Hyman when I saw him at Canyon Ranch. They've added other ones, some of which are specifically intended to improve brain function. There's something called Brain Vitale. There's something called Ceriva. Those I think are specifically for brain function. Oh, I'm on 5-MTHF five, which are 5mg pills, and I think that has to do with a sort of a chromosome type of balance. I'm on a couple of others. I can describe the pill. I remember the name of it, but it is a large range. The protein shake I'm on, it's designed for health; pure paleo protein, unflavored. Very important because all the flavored powders have some sort of sweetener in them so basically, they're keeping me away from sweeteners entirely.

[00:08:30]

[00:09:00]

There are other things. For example, for muscle cramps and everything that they have given me, but those, I would say, are the primary ones they've added. I was probably taking, oh, a dozen pills. At least a dozen a day. Maybe more than that because they've continued those. For example, I take fish oil capsules. I've been taking turmeric and everything so they continue. They probably added maybe eight to 10 of the 31 I'm taking.

[00:09:30]

What have you got to lose? Isn't the whole idea you went to the doctor that you were concerned about your condition, which could be memory loss, and you wanted to do something about it? When the doctor says this is what you can do to help your condition, I mean, you do it. It's as simple as that.

[00:10:00]

Yes, you have to give up certain things. Now the doctor says, yes, you can cheat every now and then and I haven't. I told you, the four bites of cake I had. I mean ... and the one time I had ice cream ... I had an ice cream pop at an actuarial meeting and it was quite deliberate. I knew I was going to have it and I knew I was going off my diet for them, but that's one in seven months. They say it's not so terrible if you break it once in a while and I really haven't, but they're reasonable, but they tell you that this is good for you.

The whole objective is to improve your brain health. If someone else had the same issues I do, the first thing I would recommend is that they see a Functional Medicine doctor, and Dr. Boham is top of the list.

ERIKA HOLLISTER | *Eat Fat, Get Thin* Program Participant

Erika:

[00:00:30]

Over the years, I have always struggled with weight and depression. I'm a seeker of health and trying to figure it out. I've been to many, many doctors for years and years and years, both about the weight and also about the depression and mood issues. They never put the two together. They could never say, "Oh, the depression goes with the weight gain," or "The weight gain goes with depression." Dr. Hyman always says it's not your fault. Doctors always say the opposite, basically. You're not doing it right. You're not taking good care of yourself. It was always a little bit of a blame game.

[00:01:00]

I developed sleep apnea, high blood pressure, tinnitus in my ear, so I could always hear my pulse in my left ear. I felt like I was just falling apart, both emotionally ... I was diagnosed with ADD and depression. It's like, oh my God, it was just everything all at once. I had to reassess and say, "How do I start over again? Learn how to be healthy. Piece my life together." I tried to address my health issues, but honestly, most of the doctors I saw, it's the old thing. They'll take a symptom and they'll give you a pill for the symptom.

[00:01:30]

They didn't know how to say what's the overall picture of this human being. I began to realize I had to sort this out for myself because I never got a clear answer. If I went to see a mental health counselor, they didn't know anything about weight loss. If I went to see a doctor about weight loss, they didn't know anything mental health, and they would just put me on antidepressants—which they did.

[00:02:00]

[00:02:30]

I found Dr. Hyman because I did a lot of research online. There have been a lot of opportunities to watch videos, read books. I read some of his books and he invited people to join the beta group for the *Eat Fat, Get Thin* research. I was already interested in low-carb eating and so I joined that and did that process with him. Man, the sun came up because I stopped eating gluten. I've never heard of gluten before. I didn't know anything about it. But after a few weeks of eating paleo, the depression went away and the arthritis pain went away.

[00:03:00]

[00:03:30]

I started sleeping better. Then I had this couple of crazy experiences of being offered pizza, and hungry, it was lunch time, I thought, "Oh, well, no big deal," and had a slice of pizza, and two hours later I'm in my car weeping feeling as though the whole world has crashed just in a black hole, and I thought, "Wow, okay. This gluten thing may have something to it." I thought, "Okay. That's it. I'll go back to the no gluten for a while and see how that goes," and I felt much better. My mood lifted. My clarity of thought improved. The depression went away and then it happened again with somebody.

[00:04:00]

We were going out shopping and, "Let's have a quick snack before we go," and she put out toast and cheese. I thought, "Well, don't be rude. It can't be that big of deal. No big detour here; let's just have a little snack and then go." Two hours later, this time rather than just a black mood, it was a rage. It's like I blew up. I realized that gluten is like poison for my mind. I didn't have any gastrointestinal symptoms that you associate with celiac.

[00:04:30]

Okay, I said, "Alright, that's it." I can categorically say I can't eat gluten. Finally, I went to my regular family practice doctor and said, "Is there some kind of test we can do about this?" She said, "Well you'll have to eat gluten in order for us to get the antibodies." I said, "No, there's no way I'm going to do that because it's like taking a trip to hell. I just can't do that to myself." She said, "Well that's okay. That's a pretty good sign that this isn't just a sort of fad-ish thing that you've read about somewhere." I said, "No, no. This is scary." It turns out I have four markers for celiac.

[00:05:00]

Through a genetic test, I was diagnosed with celiac. That was at the age of 60. All my life, I've had premenstrual depression, off-the-chart postpartum depression, periodic cyclical depression, been diagnosed with ADD. In between, I try to salvage my good mood, and my joy, and positivity. And I'm a

[00:05:30] teacher, so I have to keep my enthusiasm up. I just feel like I've been given such a gift because I've struggled with it and the therapy didn't help, the pills didn't help. Nobody ever associated my depression with diet—with food—before. They just didn't make that connection.

[00:06:00]
[00:06:30] That was a huge breakthrough. Now, working with the *Eat Fat, Get Thin* program—I did do that beta group—I definitely lost some weight and I felt good on it. I take important parts from various things that I have tried and I ended up crafting my own version. Having done that—and it's been a couple of years now since before that book was written—I still eat more avocados because of that. I used the PGX because of that, and I learned some things about supplements because of that. It helped me to customize what I do. I totally appreciate having a book to read, and to go back to, that has that accumulated wisdom and research in it.

[00:07:00] I appreciate the fact that Dr. Hyman is always sending out new information and writing new books. I definitely do follow it. It's an important piece for me. I appreciate the fact that he's done research both on mental health and on weight loss, and on overall wellness, while most doctors will focus either on weight loss or on mental health, but not so much on mental health through diet. Even though I lost 80 pounds, that's like an outward manifestation of improved health.

[00:07:30]
[00:08:00] To me, by far, the more important part is banishing the anxiety, depression, nightmares, the unbalanced mental health that was far more disruptive to my life, than the weight. Although the two go together, it's very hard to separate them. The fact that Dr. Hyman understands that they go together, has done research on both, and connects them, that to me was very important. It's just so refreshing to read about a doctor who gets it, that what you eat is medicine that cures not just physical things, but also emotional and mental.

[00:08:30]
[00:09:00] It's such a relief to find that, because so many doctors just don't go there. They don't get that. There was a moment in my self-awareness that I understood that depression is a metabolic problem, and that weight gain is a metabolic problem and it's not that you're just weak-willed. Being hungry all the time is a metabolic problem. There are ways to address it and to change that through diet, so that you can change the hormonal balance, so you're not hungry all the time, and so you're satisfied. For me, eating high-fat, low-carb makes it so that I'm not hungry, so that my brain is functioning properly. I can be a balanced and more joyful person.

[00:09:30]
[00:10:00] That is a huge gift. You have no idea. It may seem normal, but in my lifetime, I've been searching for that combination and nobody ever said to me, "Carbohydrates, for some people, cause depression." For 10% of celiacs, the only symptom of celiac disease is psychological. I've been back and forth with, "Should I be diagnosed with bipolar? What's going on? Am I crazy?" Nobody ever had an answer. This is the answer. I am never going to not be a low-carb eater. This is my way of eating that allows me to be healthy and happy. I've gotten rid of fibromyalgia, arthritis, sleep apnea, high blood pressure, and this tinnitus that I had in my ear, and a general inflammation that was causing all repetitive infections and strep throats.

[00:10:30]
[00:11:00] I got rid of chronic yeast infections. I'm just so much healthier, and all those things have psychological repercussions. Just feeling, like Dr. Hyman says, feeling like crap all the time, is no fun. If you can feel like you can control it, wow, big, big, big in my life. When I was at my lowest, I just couldn't understand what could possibly be wrong with me. I knew something was wrong with me. I felt like I was both mentally sick and physically sick. I could not dig myself out of the hole. It was just awful. Coming to a point of discovering that, "Hey, diet has fixed this for me, has alleviated me of that awful, guilty feeling that I'm just an inadequate person, that somehow I was just unhappy, unlovable, unsuccessful, grumpy, irritable, depressed." It's a terrible place to be.

[00:11:30] When I started eating right, the clouds lifted, and I thought, "Wow." I was diagnosed with celiac. I was like, "Wow, okay. This wasn't my fault, and it's getting better, and better, and better." The journey is not over. It's never going to be over, but I just feel like it keeps getting better and better and better. I'm

[00:12:00]   not depressed anymore. I'm often happy, which has eluded me for years. At the darkest, I would just have these deep, black storms of feeling depressed, angry, and frustrated. That just doesn't happen anymore because I know what to do.

[00:12:30]   I feel as though learning to eat a diet that actually supports my brain and my metabolism has been the greatest gift that I have gotten. Literally, for 60 years, I struggled with feeling depressed. It's not fun to be that person who can't get up and go, because the enthusiasm just isn't there. I would say, to people who are suffering from depression, try eating a very strict low-carb, high-fat diet. Don't be afraid of the

[00:13:00]   fats, because it has been an enormous gift in my life, and has completely turned around my struggles. Please, please, please try it, because it's just not to be missed.

            If it helps you, please give it a try. This isn't a sentence that you have celiac; this is a wonderful gift to

[00:13:30]   know that you can control it and change your life. It's new research. There are doctors out there like Dr. Hyman, who are leading the way, and it's actually pretty simple. The food is wonderful. I don't feel deprived at all. When somebody tries to hand me a cupcake, I know that it's going to make me feel terrible, and I'm so glad that I know that, because I used to eat it and then feel terrible for days. The

[00:14:00]   advice is, this may be just the thing that you need to solve big, scary problems that can change your life.

            A lot of people come to a high-fat, low-carb diet because they want to lose weight. Losing weight is like an outer symptom of enormous inner changes that are happening in your metabolism, and overall

[00:14:30]   deep health in my case, and I know for many people, mental health. The weight loss is great, but to me—pardon the connection—but it's like the icing on the cake. Okay, it shows on the outside, but the real benefit is having joy in your life, mental clarity, an ordered way of proceeding forward in your life, and not feeling guilty and inadequate because you can't be on top of things.

[00:15:00]   Being on top of things, not being depressed, solving all kinds of health problems and mental health problems, wow, it's fantastic. Really, really, really, the weight loss is nice. It shows, and it feels good, and it looks good, but the real benefit of it is much more inward and brings peace and joy.

JILL TOMLINSON | The UltraWellness Center Patient

Jill:
In 2015, we had been overseas. We had been in Australia for about ten days and the day after we returned home, I woke up and I couldn't open my jaw. My mouth was pretty much closed because I had so much jaw pain. And I felt very flu-like and thought probably jet lag and maybe I had slept on my jaw wrong.

[00:00:30]
The next day, I woke up with a fever and flu times ten. It was just really horrible and as the days progressed, I felt very unwell, like I had some type of infection. I began to have my migrating joint pain. And it just kind of went downhill from there.

[00:01:00]
Just a lot of different symptoms. This went on for days and weeks. And before long, I knew that I needed some help. I actually went to a naturopathic doctor and he ran some blood work and determined that I did have some sort of bacterial infection, but he couldn't determine what specific kind. So, he put me on some supplements and vitamins and things like that, which probably were useful at the time but it wasn't enough.

[00:01:30]
So, I didn't really have a diagnosis at that time, other than just the vague—you know, the obvious—that my white cells were elevated and something was going on. I followed that treatment for a few months. I followed, I took the supplements and—you know—tried to eat well and take care of myself.

But within a few months, things were just deteriorating. The joint pain became excruciating and it just was to the point that I was not functioning very well. And then September of that year, I'm still kind of rocking along, taking the supplements and things like that, but I became very sick with what I later found out was mono.

[00:02:00]
So, at that point, things really took a turn for the worse. I basically became completely debilitated shortly after that. In September, I also was diagnosed with rheumatoid arthritis. So that explained the joint pain that I was having, but I wasn't satisfied with that diagnosis.

[00:02:30]
I kind of intuitively knew that something else was going on, and I didn't want to live with that diagnosis. I wanted to go the natural route as much as possible and try to reverse rheumatoid arthritis. So, I started searching for answers. I went online, like every good patient does, and I Googled how to reverse rheumatoid arthritis naturally.

[00:03:00]
Everything I was looking up led me to Dr. Hyman's articles. And everything that he said, everything I saw, everything I read really resonated with me and I thought, "This is great." And at that point I discovered the concept of Functional Medicine through his writings and things, and I was really intrigued by that. And I thought, "That's what I really want. I want to get to the root of what's causing all these issues for me." So, that's how I found him.

[00:03:30]
Dr. Hyman listened well. He asked a lot of questions and listened. And he also ran extensive testing just to get to the root of what was going on. So, I would say the extensive testing really differs from a lot of times. You know, you just go in and a Band-Aid gets slapped on things. He didn't just send me home with a pill; he sent me home with the knowledge that we're going to get to the bottom of this; we're going to find out what's triggering these problems.

[00:04:00]
He suspected Lyme from our first visit and that was the turning point for me. Dr. Hyman was very holistic in his approach and his whole team. It wasn't just, what are the symptoms? But me as a whole person. My whole life—what's going on in other aspects of your life that could be—how are you eating? How are you taking care of your body? How is your home life? How is your work life? It's a holistic approach, which was exactly what I was looking for.

[00:04:30]
Looking back, I can see there were a lot of neurological symptoms long before the kind of onslaught of symptoms that started in March of 2015. I actually had experienced all sorts of symptoms. I had vision issues. I actually lost my vision at one point for a period of time. I had ice pick headaches. I had numbness in my face and scalp and just trouble focusing. I'm a writer, an author. I was writing books for not only myself, but for other people as well. And I just, all of a sudden, I couldn't. I couldn't focus anymore. I couldn't focus, I couldn't recall how to spell

[00:05:00]
words. You know, my thoughts just weren't coming together like they always had. Spelling was an issue, which had never been a problem before. And things like that.

[00:05:30] And then, once I emerged, I felt like I had been in the Twilight Zone ... I don't know how else to describe it. Just the brain fog that I had been in. It was like I had zoned out completely. Sometimes you don't realize how bad off you are until you get better. And that was sort of the case for me. So, neurologically it was challenging.

I was experiencing brain fog, severe brain fog. Difficulty concentrating, forgetfulness. I would go to the grocery store and forget what I was there for. I would start driving someplace and couldn't remember where I was going; just difficulty concentrating. I had the numbness in my face and scalp and severe headaches and depression as well.

[00:06:00] At my worst point through this ordeal, I was actually pretty much bedridden. I had to have help getting across the room to my bathroom. I had to have help pulling up covers. I had to have help getting dressed. I couldn't drive. I was pretty much in a mess. It was a dark place and it was a very rough time in my life.

[00:06:30] So, I say that faith, food, and Functional Medicine saved my life, probably my next book. But my faith is really important to me. And then I learned so much about how to eat and care for my body throughout this ordeal and just the importance of, as Dr. Hyman puts it, what's on the end of my fork is so much more powerful than what I can get in a pill bottle.

So, the approach that I've taken to that is, what am I doing to empower my body to heal itself? Because my body was designed to heal itself, so that's been really a powerful thing for me.

[00:07:00] And also, just the concept of Functional Medicine that, hey, let's get to the bottom of this. If I hadn't found Dr. Hyman or the concept of Functional Medicine, I would probably be on drugs for rheumatoid arthritis that I never wanted to take—I would probably be in a really different place. As opposed to I'm back, functioning at life again, I'm back in the world. So, it's good.

[00:07:30] Faith is very important to me. And throughout the darkest of days, throughout this, I held on to the fact that the Lord is my strong tower. And I believe in his promises over my life and so I really clung to that. It got me through. I knew that he was ordering my steps, even in the dark times and just like leading me to Dr. Hyman. He prepared a way for me; he made a way for me. So, yes, very important.

[00:08:00] I really learned throughout this that each of us has a responsibility. I mean, we have this body that we live in on this planet and how we steward it is really important. And how we take care of it. And are we loving ourselves so that we can give away what we were created to give away? I think sometimes we get that sort of out of order, and it was a wakeup call for me.

[00:08:30] One thing I've learned from Dr. Hyman, it wasn't like he just treated me, and treated my symptoms, but he has empowered me to heal myself to walk through the healing journey and make the right decisions. He knows that he's always given me options of different ways we can approach this. There's this way or there's this way. And so, I've always had a voice in how we approached this healing journey, and I really appreciated that because I think
[00:09:00] that's missing in traditional healthcare for the most part.

I highly recommend the Functional Medicine approach to anyone— family and friends. I'm also a certified health coach, so I have people that actually approach me when they find out my story and I always recommend Functional Medicine, because so many times chronic illnesses: MS, autoimmune disorders, and things like that, we
[00:09:30] never get to the root of what's causing them. So many of those things can be reversed and people can walk in health if they just can get to the root of the problem.

If Dr. Hyman was here with me today, I would say, "Thank you. Not only for what you've done for me, but for what you're doing for healthcare in America and just to change the face of healthcare and the way that it works in our country. I think it's amazing."

LEA FRIDMAN | The UltraWellness Center Patient

Lea:	I raised five kids. I now have 18 grandchildren and two more on the way. I'm a professor of English. I did my doctoral studies in comparative literature as my kids were young and growing. It was a wonderful system because I had time to myself and the things I loved. Then after that, I belonged to my kids.
[00:00:30]	Then I had some difficult years. There was a divorce; five children, that was a handful going through that. I had a medical crash—I think it'd been building for a long time. I had thyroid cancer 10 years before, and since then, instead of really feeling stronger, I felt weaker and weaker. I went to all the conventional doctors.
[00:01:00]	My ex was a physician, so I knew how to navigate the system and find very strong doctors. Everyone was telling me—they tested constantly—I was fine. But I was finding myself weaker and weaker. I had an academic job. I was looking after five kids with two abroad and others still in private school.
[00:01:30]	Finally, I just felt so debilitated that I took a leave of absence, a medical leave covered by my union. And at the same time, I also had something that was undiagnosed, but severe pain in the leg—very severe—that debilitated me considerably, and I had trouble walking. So, between not walking and extreme fatigue and weakness that had been building for 11 years, I just thought I saw the handwriting on the wall.
[00:02:00]	It was clear to me: there would be an enormous weight gain and then I would have secondary onset diabetes like my brother and sister. I would have hypertension like my brother and sister. There would be a whole vicious cycle of things that were life-threatening, and I saw it that way. Eventually, I read in a *New York Times* article, which was about a woman who wrote a book called *Crazy Sexy Cancer*.
[00:02:30]	She had a benign tumor throughout her entire body that could turn malignant on a dime and it was clear that she was a celebrity. She had all the time and money to do enormous research, and when I noticed the name of her doctor, I immediately went to my computer to look him up. The name was Dr. Mark Hyman, because at this point, I was ready to jump out of all the boxes and put all of my resources in service of my health.
[00:03:00]	I liked two things on the website. One was, Dr. Hyman talked about looking at root causes because I didn't know the term "Functional Medicine," but the idea of root causes meant that we weren't going to treat specific independent systems of the body. Instead, we were going to look for a cause that manifests across a number of systems, that expresses itself with several systems. So, I liked that.
[00:03:30]	The other thing that I liked was that he used alternative tests. I thought, "Oh, alternative! That means that Dr. Hyman will have additional information that all my other doctors didn't have." I filled out a long questionnaire before that first appointment. On that basis, Dr. Hyman was able to determine what tests I needed, so that when I did go to that first appointment and met with him, he had all this data.
[00:04:00]	On top of that, I brought a loose-leaf, which had about 20 years of all of my blood work chronologically organized, as well as a second loose-leaf with another 20 years of all the reports of other physicians, all organized according to the discipline. So, I had been keeping these records, and I brought it in to Dr. Hyman. He took the loose-leaf with the blood work, and he flipped through every single page.
[00:04:30]	Now, I had brought that to other doctors as well, who kind of flipped it, closed it, and said, "Thank you." This man went through every single page and made notes on some of the pages, and said to me, "Who is this doctor so-in-so who tested you for such-and-such and never told you that you have this-

[00:05:00] and-this?" Anyway, he came up with a list, which was a surprise to me, of about 15 things going on, because I had been undergoing a deterioration of 11 years, and actively visiting various doctors.

And everyone telling me that I'm perfectly fine and suddenly Dr. Hyman finds a number of issues. Now, a number of these had to do with a leaky gut, various food allergies. Turned out that I had a very serious gluten issue. I had something called homocysteinemia; there was something for which I needed antibiotics to be treated.

[00:05:30] He made a diagram to show me, which identified the various symptoms and linked them to their root cause, and showed the connection of them to one another. Really what happened was that I was thrilled to take on his recommendations. His recommendations were, in addition to the opening
[00:06:00] antibiotics, primarily dietary, so it was no gluten, sugar, coffee, dairy, or eggs. Dr. Hyman believed in animal protein. And of course, you know, very balanced meals and all that.

[00:06:30] I was just thrilled to get onto this diet, and my turnaround in energy was so dramatic, and so quick, within weeks I had great energy. What was very interesting was that I remember going through my various kitchen shelves, because I had a variety of deficiencies. So, I had all these deficiencies, and I'm thinking, "I'm going to have to find things to eat that are nutrient-dense," so no longer am I thinking about pounds and losing, I'm thinking about, "Eat, eat, eat! Deficiencies! Oh, this is healthy, take it out."

[00:07:00] This, this, this, my fridge, my cabinets and I'm basically eating quite a bit, and I lose 17 pounds. It was wild. It was like, how did this happen? It's very interesting, this gluten thing. I later on discovered that there are gluten issues in other members of the extended family. I hadn't known about that. But I wasn't eating a lot of gluten. I did like bread, but I really didn't eat any cake.

[00:07:30] I wasn't eating a lot of bread, really quite a little. I was mostly, before seeing Dr. Hyman, a salmon and broccoli person. But being gluten-free means really being gluten-free, and I'm careful about makeup and shampoo—and I'm extremely careful. I keep his diet very, very rigorously, and I keep it and it keeps me.

[00:08:00] From being unable to go to work, I was very conflicted about taking a leave of absence, but it was really the best thing I ever could have done, and I got back a life after 10 years of just doing everything I could, but with no success. So, I think the angels were on my side when I came across that article that
[00:08:30] mentioned Dr. Hyman's name. In terms of brain health, I was feeling as if I had more memory issues.

I had had a life which was one of extreme stress. I have, I think, lifelong high cortisol levels, so there
[00:09:00] had been extreme stress as a young person growing up, all through my marriage, certainly through my divorce, and I had always felt really that the memory was not quite there. Let's say when my friends started finding it a little difficult to remember names, I had started finding that a little before.

[00:09:30] My main symptom that brought me to Dr. Hyman was the extreme, extreme fatigue. But there was a certain amount of memory-loss going on that I felt was probably connected to whatever was happening to me. Not only do I feel that that has reversed, but because there has been some
[00:10:00] Alzheimer's in the family. I signed up with the NYU Langone Center—they have an aging and dementia center, where you join their brain study and I did that so should I have that particular kind of deterioration, I would have resources to advise me.

I thought it was a good precaution, and so I go yearly to be tested and at one point they told me that I
[00:10:30] had actually improved. The change was absolutely in weeks, maybe even within two or three weeks. I was feeling much, much better. I have to say that I have tremendous gratitude, because it wasn't like I
[00:11:00] underwent heart surgery or something like that. But on the other hand, I had no life, and I was in really quite bad shape and Dr. Hyman gave me back that life.

[00:11:30]	I'm 68, I work full-time, I'm not expecting to retire, and I can do that because I have my health. Supplements are costly, and the alternative tests are costly, and I certainly couldn't do that, pay for all that if I retire. On the other hand, I'm paying for a healthy life and a life where I can do other things. I write, I'm a very serious student of the dance, I'm involved in various music and other kinds of projects.
[00:12:00]	So, I'm able to do that because I have my health, and I feel like there was a certain loop I was trying to avoid. My illness, or the weakness bringing about then ... being more in bed and weight gain and diabetes and hypertension—the whole nine yards. On the other hand, Dr. Hyman enabled me to go into a very different loop. You might call it a health loop. Once I got back my health and vitality, when I
[00:12:30]	crashed medically, my goal was to heal, and healing to me meant on all levels.
	So, healing meant the physical, it meant emotional, it meant spiritual. So, it didn't end with seeing Dr. Hyman, and it meant really, you might say, being in tune with my own life, with myself, with my
[00:13:00]	passions, with my goals. Within that, I stumbled into a form of the dance called Gaga. It's developed by Ohad Naharin, an Israeli choreographer.
	It's practiced at various studios here in New York, and I'll just say that when I go to class with a lot of people who are one third of my age, and one young man said to me one day, he said, "I love being in
[00:13:30]	class with you." I said, "Really? Why?" I mean it's really delightful to hear that from a young man, right? He says, "Your energy." I go yearly to Israel because there are many more classes there. Here I can do three classes a week.
	In Israel, I do three classes daily, six days a week, for one month. Sometimes I work with some of the
[00:14:00]	batsheva dancers, Ohad Naharin's company dancers usually teach these classes. Sometimes they work privately, and they tell me, "You inspire me." Just getting back my health meant I could have this really important piece of my life. I'm writing a book called *The Gaga Poems*, interviews of batsheva dancers.
[00:14:30]	It's all a gift based on health. Everything is complex, it's never black and white. There are extraordinary things that conventional medicine can do. And then there are extraordinary holes in conventional medicine. One of the holes is dietary, that conventional medicine doesn't understand nutrition and I can say that because I was married to a nutritionist. The alternative lab test, I'd shown my other doctors alternative lab tests I'd gotten from Dr. Hyman, and they can't read the lab stuff. They don't have the backgrounds to read that.
[00:15:00]	There are gaps in the medical knowledge, and then of course it's the question of you have a whole system that does some great stuff, but it's organized in the silos that don't communicate with one another. Even when there are teams at Mayo and other places, it's different from the Functional
[00:15:30]	Medicine approach, which is always to think of the body as a variety of symptoms that are connected to one another, and looking for those root causes.
	Dr. Hyman certainly looks much more carefully at food and nutrition and their role in health. I don't think I had any other doctor who was seriously talking about it. They might give a little food advice
[00:16:00]	here and there, but nothing too serious. So, it's really completely, completely different. Now the other thing is this is a nice little story, I was going to see Dr. Hyman, I started talking to a woman who was standing right near me, and I asked her, "Where are you going?"
	And she said, "The same place you are." I said, "Dr. Hyman?" She said, "Yeah." Now she had an accent, I said, "Where are you from?" She said, "Yugoslavia." I said, "Really? Why are you coming to see Dr.
[00:16:30]	Hyman?" And she said, "Well, I've read all of his books," and she said, "I'm perfectly healthy, I'm 40 years old, I feel okay." But she said, "But Dr. Hyman says that you should feel vibrant. At any age, you should feel vibrant." She said, "And I don't feel vibrant." She said, "I want to come and see him."

[00:17:00]   So, she had traveled from Yugoslavia and there she was, we got on the same bus together to see Dr. Hyman and I thought that was fascinating because the orientation and the idea of medicine—that's a very radically different idea of medicine. Let's help people be vibrant as opposed to let's fix this issue, let's take care of that issue, and particularly as people age, you know what I mean?

[00:17:30]   The idea of people being vibrant as they age, that's not the same as people in our culture accepting that, "Oh aging means this is going to hurt and that's going to hurt, and I'm going to get up tired, okay, I'm 50, I'm 70, I'm 85, this is how I'm supposed to feel," you know what I mean? That is the thinking that a lot of people have. So, I think that's very different. After I'd gotten better, in the beginning, I saw him every three months, then every six months. Now it might be even longer.

[00:18:00]   But he'd always check my numbers, and then he'd say, "Well, continue such and such a supplement, and then have a test on such and such a date." So, it's always worked out. I do all my tests ahead of time, and whenever I come, he has all the data there. In the meantime, if I have a question, or I need to speak to someone or anything, I just email Doreen, who manages the office, and if I need to ask the nurse something, someone gets back to me.

[00:18:30]   I've never had such a wonderful feeling. It's easy, it makes sense, it's extremely convenient. Unlike the usual, which is you go to the doctor and then they say, "Oh well why don't you have this and this test?" And then you go home, and then you do the test, and then you go back, and then, "What about another two tests?" So, it's a back and forth, etc. So, the fact that it's so nicely organized, and feels
[00:19:00]   very, very welcoming and lovely, I would say really be clear that your symptoms are encroaching upon your life.

[00:19:30]   They're encroaching every minute and every day on your experience, and on who you are with your family, on things you do, the way you spend your time, and resolve to get back your health. I'd say be open and certainly try Functional Medicine, take these things with the utmost seriousness. It's your health and your life that are at stake.

[00:20:00]   Not only did I get back my vitality, at one point I met a guy—the greatest love of my life, really. It didn't work out, but it began with health. Don't let money get in your way. Your health and your daily experience and your life are worth more than anything; they're just priceless.

MARCELA LAWSON | The UltraWellness Center Patient

Marcela:

[00:00:30]

[00:01:00]

Over 16 years ago, I got a stomach infection in the tropics; it's a very common infection there. I was treated with strong antibiotics and after that, I started developing certain intolerances for foods over the years. And then after four years, my digestion issues just aggravated. It was until the point I couldn't function as a normal person. I was searching for help and I moved to the United States. I went to conventional doctors and they didn't seem to have the answer. It was just basically IBS, what I have, and they sent me home and say, "Don't get stressed." But I feel like really, they were not looking for the root of the cause. My symptoms were increasing, so I started losing a lot of weight. My abdominal pain—it was just getting worse and worse since I couldn't even sleep at night.

[00:01:30]

[00:02:00]

[00:02:30]

I knew that it was something else going on and I needed to keep looking, but I just got some general tests—nothing came out. I was desperate at that point, looking for the right help. When I was at that point, I would say the height of my illness, I was desperate. At that point, I couldn't sleep anymore. Looking online, I mean, I tried different things before like changing my diet, going to eating just whole foods and things like that. It didn't seem to work out. Somehow a TED Talk of Dr. Hyman came out in my researching and when I heard his talk and his experience healing himself and a lot of the symptoms were really similar to what I was going through, it caused a lot of different symptoms and also anxiety and all that just resonates so strongly with me. And he was talking about finding the root cause of the illness as well.

[00:03:00]

[00:03:30]

When I heard his talk, I was convinced that he could help me. At the height of my illness, my anxiety was so high that I couldn't walk with my dog two blocks. My body was very weak so I didn't have energy and even riding the bus or going to social events, hiking—I couldn't even do hiking with my husband or dancing—which I love—or basically having a social life. I am a very social person so that made me feel really isolated. But I just didn't feel in control of myself anymore.

[00:04:00]

[00:04:30]

[00:05:00]

When I found the UltraWellness Center, I worked with Dr. Boham. Basically, she knew what I was going through. I needed to fill out a lot of forms about my health history through the years, all the years that I have my chronic illness, because they treat chronic illness. They want to know when that started, all the symptoms over the years, the time, the months, and I did that. When I met with her she had a certain general idea of what was going on with me, she knew what I needed to do. But I feel very confident because also I needed to go through different personalized tests, science-based tests. They do a lot of blood work, but it's based also on your symptoms and what you are going through. After that, she can make any recommendation when she had the results. But she gave me a number of tests also that she would recommend, and I could choose which ones I wanted to do.

[00:05:30]

[00:06:00]

I started feeling better after I changed my diet. The UltraWellness Center also has a nutritionist who will work with you, and she gave me a specific diet and it helped me I would say in the first two weeks. And after that, I was treating with antibiotics and I would say in three months I started gaining weight back progressively. It took some months, because it was a lot of weight that I lost, but you could notice after three months I started gaining weight and feeling so much better.

[00:06:30]

[00:07:00]

I would say that the physical anxiety ... my body in terms of feeling so weak and gaining energy, those kinds of things made me feel uncomfortable, like going outside. I started feeling very ... when I started getting my health back. But psychologically it took at least one year because it was just too many years going through those ... basically being afraid of eating. I had developed a fear of food. What is going to happen after eating this? How will I feel? Also, if I have any reaction, feeling in control of my body and myself and feeling confident again, it took me like one year.

[00:07:30] The root cause of my illness treated at the UltraWellness Center was overgrown bacteria in my small intestine, which was very interesting for me to learn about it because it's not that common—having bacteria there and it's eating your nutrients—it's where you process all of your vitamins. It's the fuel of your body and where you get your energy. But I learned with that, that everything started before when I was treated with the first stomach infection in Costa Rica with the strong antibiotics. They didn't send

[00:08:00] me with probiotics, things that will again help me to build my stomach again, get that healthy bacteria and everything. And that was what caused the whole ... the acid not working appropriately and developed all that bacteria in the small intestine.

[00:08:30] Something I was very happy with the UltraWellness is that they also give you probiotics, they give you supplements that can help you to not just treat with medicine, but also help you to compensate those medicines that can sometimes be hard on you too.

[00:09:00] Some people around me when I started following the program—the UltraWellness program—they were not supportive. I remember in my former job, the boss, it was actually a strong criticism from her ... that she was saying I was not researching the help that I needed and that I was not doing my best.

[00:09:30] And I feel hurt because ... I feel like for some people it's hard to see how it's working and make the connection.

My husband was extremely supportive. He followed the diet at home, he supported every single step of the program. We really have one hope. I just went through a lot of research and I was in a desperate

[00:10:00] state. At least, my close family, and that case my husband, that was the more important for me. But some friends and family were not that supportive ... they didn't understand as much ... the program.

Following the program requires a lot of commitment because you have a specific diet and you need to

[00:10:30] follow rules. Sometimes you need to cook at home. You are restricted to certain foods. Also, going through the test requires sometimes some diet, for a few days, different food, so it required commitment.

[00:11:00] I will highly recommend Functional Medicine if you are really struggling with a chronic illness and you want to know what the root cause is, because sometimes I know a lot of people who struggle for years and years with different symptoms, but they never find out what is the root cause. And you can have

[00:11:30] different symptoms but that can be cause for different reasons as well. And sometimes people also suffer from those medications for years. I would encourage people to try Functional Medicine. I think when there's hope that you can feel better, even if you have questions about maybe something new, and you never changed your diet before, or require certain commitments, I always think you don't lose

[00:12:00] anything. Try it.

[Spanish Language 00:12:05]

[00:12:30] Changing my diet and taking it as my lifestyle reminds me of my roots because I am so ... where I grew up, we grew up with whole foods and I have been changing quickly through the years. But going back

[00:13:30] to that, usually rice and beans, any kind of grain, whole grain ... I try to do it every day. I also try to cook at home as much as I can. But if I go out, I like also to eat organic—a lot of vegetables, grains, and beans—I think food definitely makes a difference. I feel good and never have a problem with that. I think it's like going back home.

[00:14:00] I think self-education ... when you're going through an illness and you've lost hope with your conventional doctors and you feel like you need to find the help for yourself, you start reading a lot of different books and researching for help and I think there are people out there that have been through

[00:14:30] a struggle and they have been helped through diet and through sometimes detoxifying and doing different things, I think you can read those, educate yourself and learn what works for you.

[00:15:00] I know sometimes you need the medicine. In my case, that was the case; I needed the medicine. But I admire people who change their diet and their lifestyle just to be better and they always say it improved their life in so many different ways, and you can start from there. Before, when I was feeling unhealthy, I couldn't eat so many things; that with time I had been able to eat and that had just been a

[00:15:30] great improvement in my life. Physically, I couldn't go for a walk with my dog or even hiking, dancing—that I enjoyed a lot—and didn't have enough energy and now I am able to go and dance as much as I can. I also go to work. Going to work before when I was sick, it was a challenge just the part-time job

[00:16:00] that I had. It was going there and coming home and saving my energy because I didn't have any more. And now going to work, have a full-time job, coming home, cooking or do something else even dancing or going out with friends. It's just amazing. It changed my life completely and sometimes I feel so grateful with this. It feels like a second opportunity. I didn't think about that before.

[00:16:30]

[00:17:00] I would like to tell Dr. Hyman—and also Dr. Boham—that being able to offer Functional Medicine to people and practicing this approach is a wonderful help for a lot of people who are desperate out there with chronic illness. I'm very grateful for Dr. Boham, I think ... the doctor and person that she is, she's very compassionate and I will just encourage them to do what they are doing and I am sure a lot of people with benefit from that too.

MARK KACHERSKY | Patient of Dr. Sidney Baker

Mark: [00:00:30]	Approximately three and a half years ago, I noticed that during certain times, usually later in the day, I would just grow more tired. My eyelids would start to close as if I had lack of sleep, but that wasn't the case. Then, what was very disturbing, I would have double—sometimes triple—vision, which was very difficult to deal with. It happened intermittently and I didn't think that much of it. Then, I had an increasingly difficult time with vision and eye muscles. I found myself in the middle of the day talking to someone and one eyelid would involuntarily start closing, sometimes without me even realizing it until the eye was actually closed.
[00:01:00] [00:01:30]	I just said, "I don't know what's going on here." I thought I had something wrong with my eyes, so I consulted my ophthalmologist, the eye doctor. He checked my eyes and everything like that. He said, "What you have doesn't have anything to do with glasses." He says, "Your eye alignment is off. Instead of focusing in and things being one object, you're seeing two objects." He ran some tests, including blood. He called me back a few days later. He said, "You came back positive for myasthenia gravis." I said, "I don't even know what that is." He explained to me about the muscle disorders and the controlling the eyeballs on the eye movements and the muscles controlling your lids and everything. I said, "What do I need to do now?" He said, "You need to consult a neurologist."
[00:02:00] [00:02:30]	There was a neurologist in my town that I was familiar with. I did that. They were kind of matter-of-fact with me. "Oh yeah. You have ocular myasthenia. Here's a prescription for this, this and this;" Steroid-based prescription medicine. "It really is not going to give you any kind of permanent solution. It's going to put a Band-Aid on it and hopefully lessen your symptoms. Hopefully, you'll be able to function." The way it got, I couldn't function properly. It was very difficult to be out in the world, trying to see things, and you're seeing sometimes two or three of everything.
[00:03:00] [00:03:30] [00:04:00]	I started taking the medication and I found that things really did not improve a lot. A lot of things got worse with the side effects. For example, waking up in the middle of the night with extreme leg cramps and this and that and spasms and everything. I was like, "This is not helping me. This is hurting me." I tried for several weeks and it turned into a couple of months. Where do I go from here? Even driving was almost impossible. I found myself reclining the seat so my eyeballs would be way down like that so they wouldn't move that much to be out of alignment so I could see somewhat. Then I just was really at my end of thinking in terms of where do I go? What do I do? Who has an answer for me that is beyond just taking all these pills that are lined up on the table here?
[00:04:30]	I thought of Dr. Baker. I said, "Wow. It's been over 25 years since I've seen Dr. Baker." He helped my son, who was then four-and-a-half-years-old, with epilepsy. This was on New Year's Eve Day in 1990. I took him to the city in the daytime on the train, because we hadn't been able to come into the city to see Christmas decorations and everything. I took him into Macy's, the main flagship store, on 34th Street. He was singing, having a good time, just a happy kid. I got him on the escalator going up to the second floor, and he collapsed. I was shocked. I was like, "What's going on?"
[00:05:00]	I picked him up and it looked like he couldn't breathe. His face was turning pale white and his lips were purple. I thought his heart had stopped or something. I couldn't figure out what it was. I got on the second floor and laid him on the carpet there. It was a nurse that was doing her shopping that came to help me. They were doing CPR, doing everything. That was one of the worst days of my life at that time.
[00:05:30]	They rushed him to St. Luke's Roosevelt hospital here in Manhattan. You wait in the waiting room for an hour and a half to two hours and you don't know. I wasn't expecting anything good because the last time I saw him, he wasn't showing any signs of life at all. The doctor came out after a period of time

---

[00:06:00] and told me that he had had a seizure. I was confused. I said, "A seizure? He didn't go into any kind of convulsion or anything." He goes, "No, not that kind of seizure. It's a seizure that basically shuts down your body in a sense where you do very slow breathing, almost undetectable breathing. The seizure is like an electrical storm neurologically in your brain that has to pass." Then they told me that he was starting to respond and that I could go in and see him, and he was fine. They said, "This could be a

[00:06:30] one-time event, or it could be something that ... This is epilepsy. You have to keep an eye on him."

[00:07:00] Subsequently, in the following weeks, I was going into the home with him one time, opening the door, and he slumped against the door and lost control of his bladder and he was going into a more classic seizure. I didn't realize the mistake I made was I called 911. After I got my further education from Dr. Baker on the matter, I found that that was the worst thing I can do. The paramedics came. They start sticking him with IVs. He goes into more convulsions. They take him to the ER. They start giving him

[00:07:30] more injections. It made things worse, much worse. I was beside myself, kind of like with my own condition, but when it's your son, it really has a profound effect on you.

[00:08:00] After doing the normal doctor routine and prescription medicine and everything, I called my mom who still lived in Brooklyn, and I said, "Do you have a doctor in that Princeton Bio Center that you go to?" My mother, who was born in Sicily, always went to the best holistic places to get healed. She goes, "Yeah. I know some people down there." She gave me the phone number and I went down there. I walked in and they said, "We have someone who specializes in working with your son, who's here temporarily, Dr. Baker." That's the first time I met Dr. Baker.

[00:08:30] I knew after sitting in his office with my son for ten minutes that this is the right place to be and this is the right person to help me out. Not that I saw any results yet, but you could see the different approach—totally different mindset. He really took his time going over everything in terms of his current diet, nutrition. Then he subsequently did some tests, blood and whatnot. He found out he was

[00:09:00] lacking in things like magnesium and zinc and several other key elements and put him on a program. He said to me, "What are you going to do the next time he has a seizure?" I said, "What should I do?" He goes, "You don't do anything. You keep him calm. You lay him down. Make sure there was nothing in his throat he was eating. He'll get through the storm and he'll be fine. Do not go into this emergency mode." I learned my lesson with that.

[00:09:30] It worked. As he progressed into the program, I'm going to say between three and five months, he became totally seizure-free. I'm proud to say he's 31 years old now. He lives in Seattle, Washington. He has a great life. He's very happy. So am I, needless to say.

[00:10:00] My wife Googled Dr. Baker, and there he was. The last time I had an appointment with him, back in the early 90s, he was practicing at his residence in Connecticut. She said, "He's in Sag Harbor." I said, "Sag Harbor. Is that like the end of Long Island?" She says, "Yeah." "Okay." I took a chance and I gave him a call and I said, "This is what I have. Doctor, I hope you remember me. I was there with my son, Bill, many years ago and you helped him tremendously. Is there anything you can do for me?" Dr.

[00:10:30] Baker said, "I might be able to help you." He says, "I have a lot of associates that are very versed in what you have." He would consult with them and try to come up with a formula. I made an appointment. I went out to see him.

[00:11:00] The approach here is not "Here, take these pills. Let's put a Band-Aid on it." The approach is, "Let's get to the source of what's causing this." In my case it was auto-immune deficiency. He explained to me things that I never knew. Medicine like amoxicillin and different things that the doctors give you for flus and colds actually destroy your gut flora, good germs, whatever you want to call them; defenses

[00:11:30] for your immunity. I just listened, because he never steered me wrong when I went to visit him with my son.

[00:12:00] It was just really an eye-opening experience to see, "All right. Here's the source. The condition that you have does not exist in countries like Africa and India and places where they still live off the land, the soil and everything like that. Only in countries where they have processed food and multitudes of prescription drugs and everything, like the United States, do conditions like this exist." That just made a lot of common sense to me. "Okay, people in this country don't have it." He explained to me even the Iowa farmers don't have much of these conditions because, again, they're living off the soil and the land; it's giving them all they need. We used to think you got your hands all dirty and everything like that. It's actually a good thing.

[00:12:30]
[00:13:00] Then he started me on a program, in terms of what the essentials that I needed for supplements and minerals and different things. Every other week he sends me this extracted larvae, which he gets from grain beetles, which is the natural stuff that you had in your system to begin with, and now has been depleted. It's not a pie in the sky. He says, "You have a 50-50 chance." I was willing to work the program and see where that would end up. I'm going to say in the third to fourth month, it kicked in and I was just virtually normal again. I was just, "Wow. Thank God." It was just a really incredible experience. It's over two years later and I'm still on the program. It's still working for me—I swear by it. There's nothing in the conventional medicine world that could even come close to what I've been given to help my condition.

[00:13:30]

[00:14:00] He recommended less gluten or a gluten-free diet; that would help. Magnesium and certain other supplements that enhance the welcoming of what we call the HDCs, the larvae. Just a good common-sense diet and exercise. Eating the right things. Staying away from the wrong things like sugar and too many carbs. He's given me outstanding guidance. I need someone like Dr. Baker to tell me that potatoes are not really good for you. No more French fries? Things like that. Then all the misconception about the food I love, more than my favorite food, is eggs, believe it or not. He just said to me, "Eggs aren't going to bother you. That's kind of like the little bit out there where they've condemned eggs but they're really okay for you." Just basic natural wholesome things that are just going to help your gut flora and help you have that immune system that are going to give you the proper defenses that you need.

[00:14:30]

[00:15:00]

[00:15:30] We all know that there are tons of viruses and diseases and everything out there that are just lurking in the air, water, wherever, and that could invade any one of our bodies at any given time. The question is, "How good are your defenses?" I think many people in this country don't realize that your defenses, without you realizing it, like mine, may have been broken down due to something that you don't even realize. Like I mentioned, the amoxicillin and different prescription medicines and everything.

[00:16:00]

Unfortunately, in our society here, with processed food and prescription medicine being so dominant and prominent, often people do not even look on the other side of the fence to see what else is available. I'm a very common-sense person. To me, it makes perfect sense that when you ask yourself the questions, "Why doesn't this condition exist in other countries where they're not really developed in terms of food processing, etc.? Why is this condition on the increase in this country, where there are very little signs that it even existed 150 years ago?" What does that tell you? It's the way we're living, the way we're eating, the medicine we're taking, which is intended to do good, often has side effects. Some of them, like in my case, took away my immune system.

[00:16:30]

[00:17:00]

[00:17:30] You really have to think outside the box if you want to get better. The answers are very simple: You just go back to nature versus the conventional world, which is driven by profit and many other factors. Nothing wrong with making profit, but if you're a human being and you have a situation, and all of a sudden your life has been turned upside down, and you're taking conventional prescription medicine ... "Yeah. I feel a little bit better, but I'm not really that much better. I'm still not like I was five years ago before I had this condition, or whatever."

[00:18:00]

[00:18:30]

There are answers. I think if you seek out the answers in the world, there are highly skilled professional people in the medical profession that have answers. They might not be the mainstream, but they are a great stream, as far as I'm concerned. If it's going to get you better and make you feel better, you just have to get back to the basic elements that God gave you for your body and what was put on this earth in terms of what your body needs to function and survive. That, to me, is the answer, versus something that's man-made and just putting a Band-Aid on something instead of really getting to the source of it.

ROOPA TULI | The UltraWellness Center Patient

Roopa:

[00:00:30]

About two years ago, I had just finished a series of fertility treatments. The last treatment wasn't successful and I was upset and decided to go visit my parents in Canada. I lived in India at the time and fully with the intention of going back to India but after about two weeks, I started getting debilitating anxiety. The anxiety was so bad that I couldn't get out of bed. I would have panic attacks. I would sweat profusely and I was scared for my life.

[00:01:00]

[00:01:30]

My parents obviously were concerned with my state and they took me to a doctor, my local family doctor. She asked me a series of questions and she prescribed me an anti-anxiety medicine, which was Effexor, started at a very low dose, started at .25 milligrams and went up to 225 milligrams. Each day for me was excruciating. I used to beg my parents to do something. It was almost like I was suicidal. I used to go to the doctor on a daily basis because she kept increasing the dose but she was only able to increase it every week or every 10 days and I had no relief.

[00:02:00]

I went to a series of doctors in Canada who were naturopaths and they gave me a few remedies, alternative herbs or teas or supplements but it wasn't working. I was lucky one day: I was watching TV and I came across Dr. Mark Hyman's clinic. I went online and did some research and that's it. I don't know what happened. Something just hit me and I said, "This is going to help me."

[00:02:30]

[00:03:00]

My husband was back home in India and he used to visit me frequently, but he wasn't with me in Canada at the time. So, my parents and I, we drove to Massachusetts from Toronto. It was a five-and-a-half-hour drive and there was my savior, Dr. Todd LePine. He saved my life. I can't thank him enough. He's a brilliant doctor. He's thorough, he knows his stuff and he's meticulous in testing, in finding out the root cause.

[00:03:30]

After a series of tests, Dr. LePine told me to remove the gluten, remove the dairy, remove the allergens that were causing leaky gut. Of course, they say that the gut is your second brain so there was obviously a connection between what was happening in my brain and with my gut. Now, it's been almost two years and I'm a different person. I've changed my entire outlook on things.

[00:04:00]

[00:04:30]

When you have anxiety or when someone is watching you, you honestly don't know what to do because you see this person who's in so much agony and it's a very painful experience because it honestly takes over your life. I couldn't interact with anyone in my family. My parents would not leave me alone because it was that bad. It was very difficult for them because they were helpless, my husband and my parents. There was nothing they could do. The medicine wasn't working and my doctor just kept increasing the dose and it just wasn't doing what I needed.

[00:05:00]

[00:05:30]

[00:06:00]

Then, of course, Dr. LePine ran a series of tests. My vitamin levels were all low starting from iron all the way up to vitamin D. My minerals were all low and, hence, that's why a lot of my anxiety was due to the deficit in my vitamin levels. He brought those up to the right level and of course, good food—nutritious, organic food—exercise. It was a host of things that sort of brought me back to normal. They say if you put your mind to anything, you can do it and from day one, when he told me to get off these foods—sugar was another one I used to eat a lot of—I did it and I kept going. Up to today, it's been two years; I've not had any refined, process sugar. It's a journey and it's all about having the courage and the strength to keep going. When you feel like I felt about two years ago, then, you don't want to turn back and you want to fix the problem.

[00:06:30]

I had a host of other symptoms. It wasn't just anxiety. I had hair loss so I'd wake up in the morning with chunks of hair just coming out from the side. I had horrible acne. I had rashes on the back of my body,

---

my face, my neck and that, I think, really affected me because I didn't look how I used to look and I was shy to go out in public because I looked terrible.

[00:07:00] I think I started seeing some improvement after about three or four months. My digestion started improving and my energy levels started getting better and I was moving around and that's when I started doing yoga and lots of walking. I started Reiki and that healed me a lot. In fact, there was

[00:07:30] someone at The UltraWellness Center who was dedicated to healing the body and working through energy blockages and she helped me a lot. I used to do distance healing, distance Reiki with her and, now, I'm a Reiki practitioner so I can do Reiki on myself and I can do it on other people.

I could just think better. I was more in the moment. I was present. It was easier for me to make

[00:08:00] decisions and to be honest, I think I suffered from brain fog for a long time and I didn't know that. My mind continuously would run while I was experiencing the anxiety and now I'm calmer, I'm more centered, and I'm able to make decisions more easily. Of course, I do a lot of meditation so that helps a lot to center yourself and to bring your mind back into your body.

[00:08:30] Conventional doctors do not look at the root cause. The first thing that they do is prescribe you with a medication. They don't look at food intolerances. My family doctor didn't look at any of those. In fact, when I go back to her for my regular checkup, I've taken reports from Dr. LePine to her and she's

[00:09:00] amazed to see that I've made such an amazing recovery. She's never seen these tests before and some of the tests are not your conventional tests that most doctors would use. I think conventional doctors don't have the time to go into what the root problem is and that's where Dr. LePine really saved me and helped me get out of this.

[00:09:30] Aside from the health aspect, I've become a stronger, kinder person. I was very angry before when I went through my anxiety and all the other issues. I was angry. I was frustrated. I was irritable. Now, I'm

[00:10:00] just more centered and I live in the moment and appreciate what I have now. I have faith that everything happens for a reason and I trust the process of life. I think that's very important in healing, to allow yourself to embrace whatever emotional issues you have and to accept them and then, just let them go. I think we live in a society where we suppress our emotions a lot and disease starts from

[00:10:30] blocked or trapped emotions. I was able to look at those as well and overall, I mean it's a tremendous change from what I was about two years ago.

I think there are a lot of young women and young girls who experience the symptoms I had. In fact, I

[00:11:00] have spoken to a lot of girls who've experienced what I had but they're on medicine. I would like to tell them that the medications do not work because they don't address the root cause and they're just a Band-Aid. I think that one can get out of anxiety or depression if you look at your whole body, your mind and your spirit. I think it's a connection and it is possible.

[00:11:30] I highly recommend that you would go see a doctor. I would recommend Dr. LePine, but if you can't, a naturopath or a natural practitioner who looks at the root cause and does all the tests that are required that most conventional doctors don't do. It's not just a six month fix and then you go back to eating the

[00:12:00] way you used to or drinking or doing whatever to, I suppose, suppress what you're feeling or suppress the anxiety or depression. It is a lifestyle. I've chosen it to be a lifestyle and I do not wish to go back to the way I was eating before or my exercise regimen was very different so I definitely would say it is an entire life process.

[00:12:30] To have a better brain, the five things I would recommend are definitely food, which is the energy that you put into your body. Number two: exercise; exercise is very important, any form of movement. The body needs to move. Number three: meditation or mindfulness, taking a pause within the day, whether

[00:13:00] it's for five minutes or even if you can do 10, 15, just to come back to yourself and be with your thoughts, to center yourself and to really get away from the day's stresses. I think it's a super way of de-stressing, especially if you want to de-stress from coming back from work, a busy day at the office.

BROKEN BRAIN

[00:13:30] Number four: connection, connecting with people, with people who you enjoy being with, people who have the same goals or interests. I think we are social beings and so we need people around us whether it's friends, family, your partner but people you can interact with, you can talk to, people that

[00:14:00] you trust. Number five: I think journal writing. Journal writing is a great way to let go of your fears, your stress. In fact, Dr. Hyman, in one of his articles, recommends journal writing at the end of the day just before going to bed. He suggests that one writes down all the things that are stressing one out. Put all those things in a book and close it and have faith that the next day will be brighter and you'll be able to deal with your worries better that way.

[00:14:30] When I first started on this journey, my husband noticed a big difference, obviously, but he would ask me. I'd be doing something or eating a certain way and he would ask me, "What is that that you're doing? Why are you eating like that? Let me try it." He's definitely eating cleaner. He's not entirely

[00:15:00] gluten-free but he is off most gluten products. He exercises and I think he's more mindful. He's happier because they say if one person is happy, that energy is absorbed by the other person so I think that's made a big difference for him, the fact that he's around me and the energy that I emit. I think it's affected him and, of course, my family. They're just, of course, very, very happy that I progressed the

[00:15:30] way I have. They've also started eating clean and looking after their diets and exercising whether it's even just a walk or some sort of movement. I think movement of the body is very important for brain health.

[00:16:00] I was on a flight to Toronto a couple of months ago and there was a girl sitting beside me, a lot younger than I am, and she had an anxiety attack, a panic attack, and it was exactly how I used to face them. For a few minutes, I said, "You know, maybe I shouldn't ask her, let her sort of let the energy pass." I started talking to her and she was in tears and she said, "You know, I've tried everything and it doesn't work." I gave her a few tips and then she took my number and then, she messaged me and she said,

[00:16:30] "You know, just those few tips, I've been able to look at what I'm eating and how my lifestyle is and I've made those changes and it's helped me a lot, so thank you."

[00:17:00] At that time, I knew she was having a very hard time settling her mind so I told her to just deep-breathe and start from her abdomen and to just bring her mind back to the center and as she was breathing, I kept telling her, "You're okay. Everything is fine. You're safe." I said, "I'm just going to guide you but I want you to take deep, long breaths right from your abdomen all the way up to your chest. Fill your chest up and then release and keep doing it until you feel that energy sort of pass."

[00:17:30] She did it and after 10 minutes, she says, "You know, if you weren't here, I don't think I will be able to deal with ... I don't think I would have been able to deal with what I went through." She said, "Each time I feel that wave of anxiety ..." and it's like a wave. It really is and if you don't catch it, you can drown in it and it's a horrible feeling because that's when your thoughts take over and you think that

[00:18:00] something bad is going to happen and that's when you go into the whole fight-or-flight mode. She did that and brought herself back into the moment. She brought her mind back into her body and she was able to release that energy.

[00:18:30] If I can just make a difference and just give some advice: eating is so important. I think we forget that food is energy and whatever you put in is going to reflect on your health. So, I think good food, organic food is really important, sustainable meats which Dr. Hyman and all the doctors at The UltraWellness Center are very particular about. Dr. Hyman calls it pegan (smaller portions of meat, larger portions of

[00:19:00] vegetables and fruits). I still follow up and correspond with Dr. LePine for regular checkups or blood test reviews But if you were to ask him how I'm doing, I think he would have to say that from when he first saw me until now, it's an amazing change and an amazing progress.